Comprehensive Stress Management

THIRTEENTH EDITION

Jerrold S. Greenberg

Professor Emeritus, University of Maryland

Mc Graw Hill

Connect
Learn
Succeed™

The McGraw-Hill Companies

Connect
Learn
Succeed™

COMPREHENSIVE STRESS MANAGEMENT, THIRTEENTH EDITION

Published by McGraw-Hill, a business unit of The McGraw-Hill Companies, Inc., 1221 Avenue of the Americas, New York, NY 10020. Copyright © 2013 by The McGraw-Hill Companies, Inc. All rights reserved. Printed in the United States of America. Previous Editions © 2011, 2009, and 2008. No part of this publication may be reproduced or distributed in any form or by any means, or stored in a database or retrieval system, without the prior written consent of The McGraw-Hill Companies, Inc., including, but not limited to, in any network or other electronic storage or transmission, or broadcast for distance learning.

Some ancillaries, including electronic and print components, may not be available to customers outside the United States.

This book is printed on acid-free paper.

3 4 5 6 7 8 9 0 RMN/RMN 1 0 9 8 7 6 5 4

ISBN 978-0-07-352972-1
MHID 0-07-352972-9

Vice President & Editor-in-Chief: *Michael Ryan*
Managing Director: *Gina Boedeker*
Executive Director of Development: *Lisa Pinto*
Sponsoring Editor: *William Minick*
Marketing Manager: *Caroline McGillen*
Development Editor: *Darlene M. Schueller*
Project Manager: *Jessica Portz*
Cover Designer: *Studio Montage, St. Louis, MO*
Cover Image: *Bear Dancer Studios/Mark Dierker*
Buyer: *Sandy Ludovissy*
Media Project Manager: *Sridevi Palani*
Compositor: *MPS Limited*
Typeface: *10/12 Minion*
Printer: *R. R. Donnelley*

All credits appearing on page or at the end of the book are considered to be an extension of the copyright page.

Library of Congress Cataloging-in-Publication Data

Greenberg, Jerrold S.
 Comprehensive stress management / Jerrold S. Greenberg. — 13th ed.
     p. cm.
  ISBN 978-0-07-352972-1 (alk. paper)
 1. Stress (Psychology) 2. Stress (Physiology) 3. Stress (Psychology)—Prevention. 4. Stress management.
I. Title.
 BF575.S75G66 2013
 155.9'042—dc23
                                                                                    2012019448

www.mhhe.com

brief table of contents

table of contents

part 2

General Applications:
Life-Situation and Perception
Interventions   **109**

CHAPTER 5

CHAPTER 6

part 3

General Applications:
Relaxation Techniques 239

part 4

General Applications:
Physiological Arousal and Behavior Change Interventions 307

part 5

Specific Applications   381

CHAPTER 16

CHAPTER 17

Preface

This book evolved out of two needs. The first pertained to the experiences of my students, colleagues, friends, and relatives who, as I listened to their stories, seemed to be crying out for help in dealing with the stress of life. Upon closer scrutiny, I realized that the only cries I was deaf to were my own. I, too, needed help managing stress.

The second need related to the nature of texts on this subject. I thought they were informative or interesting but seldom both. Furthermore, I didn't think stress management was presented as the complex subject I envision it to be. I thought books on this subject explored parts of stress management but omitted several key components. I wrote *Comprehensive Stress Management* both to address the complexity of the subject and to respond to the very human needs of college students living highly stressful lives.

This book, then, is written in a more personal, informal manner than most, and it is organized around situations in life that, when perceived as distressing, result in the emotional and physiological arousal we know as stress. There is an abundance of scientific and statistical information in this book, but there is also a healthy dose of anecdote, humor, and personal experience to bring the content to life. In addition, numerous means of self-evaluation are provided so that content takes on personal meaning for each student.

Managing Stress in an Increasingly Stressful World

Comprehensive Stress Management empowers students to—

Learn what stress is—emotionally and physiologically—and how it affects their health.

- The science of stress is presented in three chapters covering everything from the role of the brain in stress to the effects of stress on the body.
- New or expanded topics include resiliency, optimism, humor, forgiveness, spirituality, anxiety, budgeting, safety on campus, the relationship between obesity and stress, and many more.

Evaluate their current level of stress and develop a stress profile that identifies their personal triggers and stressors.

- Lab Assessments in each chapter help them identify attitudes, behaviors, and coping skills and target areas for improvement.
- The Personal Stress Profile and Activity Workbook—available on the Online Learning Center for *Comprehensive Stress Management* (www.mhhe.com/greenberg13e)—helps students actively create a personal plan for managing stress in their lives.

Apply what they learn to their own lives by using the tools and activities to become active participants in managing their own stress.

- A chapter on stress and the college student helps students identify and understand stressors unique to their current phase of life.
- Detailed descriptions of stress management and relaxation techniques offer many different approaches to explore and try, including yoga breathing techniques, meditation, progressive relaxation, imagery, behavior and anxiety management techniques, and more.
- "Getting Involved in Your Community" boxes challenge students to participate in projects designed to decrease stress levels on a broader scale.

Content Revisions by Chapter

We all learn from experience, and I am no exception. This edition of *Comprehensive Stress Management* incorporates many changes and updates while still retaining the content and features valued by instructors and students over the previous twelve editions.

All statistics, data, and websites are updated. In addition, the most current research findings are incorporated into the text. New photos and figures have been added throughout the text. The 2020 national health objectives replace the 2010 national health objectives in several chapters.

Chapter 1: A new Lab Assessment is added entitled "What Causes You Stress?" The purpose of this lab is to encourage readers to appreciate the personal nature of the information and skills to follow.

Chapter 3: New boxed material is added entitled "Characteristics of Cardiac Muscle"; the discussion of posttraumatic stress disorder is expanded; and a new Lab Assessment is added entitled "How Are My Health Indices?"

Chapter 4: The chapter entitled "Stress and the College Student" is moved from Chapter 16 in the previous edition of *Comprehensive Stress Management*. The reason for this change is to have readers consider earlier in the text how stress affects college students, and what college students can do to better manage stress.

Two new boxes are added. One is entitled "College Students and Credit Card Statistics" and the other is "The Credit Card Accountability, Responsibility, and Disclosure (CARD) Act of 2009"; recommendations are added to assist college students to better manage credit cards and limit debt; and a section on eating disorders is added that discusses anorexia nervosa and bulimia.

Chapter 6: MyPlate information is included. New boxed material entitled "How to Create a Healthy Diet" has been added. The section entitled "The Heavy Toll of Diet-Related Chronic Diseases" (cardiovascular disease, hypertension, diabetes, cancer, and osteoporosis) has been included.

Chapter 7: Expanded communication coverage has been included. A new section on emotional intelligence is added; a new box entitled "Ways to Improve Emotional Intelligence" provides advice for students who want to become more emotionally intelligent; and a new Lab Assessment is added entitled "How Emotionally Intelligent Are You?"

Chapter 9: A new section entitled "Spirituality and College Students" is added. Updated stress-related national health objectives have been included.

Chapter 12: Body scan relaxation exercises are new to this edition. Repetitive prayer for relaxation information has been expanded.

Chapter 13: 2020 National Health Objectives Related to Physical Fitness has been updated. The presentation of stretching is expanded to include dynamic and ballistic stretching; and exercise guidelines from the American College of Sports Medicine are added. A new table entitled "Adding Physical Activity to Your Life" has been added.

Chapter 14: A new Lab Assessment is added entitled "Can You Use Behavior Change Theory to Change Your Behavior?"

Chapter 15: Two new boxes are added pertaining to mixed race and international college students. One is entitled "How Colleges Can Help Mixed Race Students with Identity Stress," and the other is entitled "Stress and the International Student." The 2020 National Health Objectives relative to gender, race and ethnicity, disability, and sexual orientation have been added, and the discussion of health disparities has been expanded.

Chapter 16: Two new boxes are added. One is entitled "Benefits of Job Stress Management Programs." The other is entitled "Some Facts About Women and Retirement." The chapter has increased coverage of gender and occupational stress.

Chapter 18: "Stress and the Elderly," from previous editions of *Comprehensive Stress Management*, is deleted. Instructor feedback was that the semester did not allow time to consider this material. Therefore, rather than include content that would not be used and thereby increase the cost of the book for the student, this content is deleted. This content can be found on the book's website.

Resources for Instructors

The *Personal Stress Profile and Activity Workbook* is available as an accompaniment to *Comprehensive Stress Management*. The workbook includes numerous other scales to help students learn more about the stressors in their lives and how they can best manage them. How to make the best use of The *Personal Stress Profile and Activity Workbook* is described on page 14.

The Online Learning Center for Comprehensive Stress Management (**www.mhhe.com/greenberg13e**) offers instructors many resources, including a Course Integrator Guide, a Test Bank, and PowerPoint slides.

 McGraw-Hill Create™ Craft your teaching resources to match the way you teach! With McGraw-Hill Create, you can easily rearrange chapters, combine material from other content sources, and quickly upload content you have written like your course syllabus or teaching notes. Find the content you need in Create by searching through thousands of leading McGraw-Hill textbooks. Arrange your book to fit your teaching style. Create even allows you to personalize your book's appearance by selecting the cover and adding your name, school, and course information. Order a Create book and you'll receive a complimentary print review copy in 3–5 business days or a complimentary electronic review copy (eComp) via email in minutes. Go to **www.mcgrawhillcreate.com** today and register to experience how McGraw-Hill Create empowers you to teach *your* students *your* way.

Electronic Textbook Option This text is offered through CourseSmart for both instructors and students. CourseSmart is an online resource where students can purchase the complete text online at almost half the cost of a traditional text. Purchasing the eTextbook allows students to take advantage of CourseSmart's web tools for learning, which include full text search, notes and highlighting, and email tools for sharing notes between classmates. To learn more about CourseSmart options, contact your sales representative or visit **www.CourseSmart.com.**

Acknowledgments

Many people have helped bring this project to completion. They can never be adequately thanked, but perhaps a mention here will let them know that their help has been appreciated.

First were my students, who taught me as much about stress management as I have ever taught them. Not only did I learn from their term papers and other assignments, but the way in which they lived their lives taught me much about managing stress.

Then there were my professional colleagues, who encouraged, stimulated, and provoked me to be as competent and as qualified as I could—if for no other reason than to keep pace with them. In particular, I wish to thank Robert Feldman, who contributed to Chapter 14.

And, there are the academic reviewers, whose comments sometimes exasperated, bewildered, or angered me but who also encouraged me and provided important guidance for revision. Because of them, this book is better than it otherwise would have been. These reviewers include

Jeffrey Anderson
Oklahoma City Community College

Kimberly Ball
Oakland Community College

Muriel B. Gilman
Bemidji State University

Robert Hess
Community College of Baltimore County Catonsville Campus

Keith McCoy
The University of Texas at Tyler

Claudia Rosenberg
Bucks County Community College

Lindsey A. Vacek
Purdue University

Cynthia Welch
Tidewater Community College

Gregory Yon
Tallahassee Community College

I would be remiss not to acknowledge the support of Christopher Johnson and Bill Minick, my editors, and Darlene Schueller, my developmental editor for the thirteenth edition of *Comprehensive Stress Management*, for helping to guide this edition through the sometimes confusing production process. Their support, competence, and encouragement are very much appreciated.

Most important, there is my family. They not only respect my need for quiet time to write but also provide much of the inspiration I need. Karen, Keri, and Todd—I don't tell you often enough how much you contribute to my work and productivity, but you do, and I recognize your support and value it.

This edition is dedicated to Jonah, Zoe, and Garrett—my three grandchildren. When I am with them all stress evaporates away. I wish them that feeling throughout their lives, although I know that to be unrealistic. So, when they experience stress, I hope they are successful employing the numerous stress management techniques learned from reading their grandpa's book and, as a result, achieve lives of satisfaction and fulfillment.

—*Jerrold S. Greenberg*

part 1

Scientific Foundations

1 What Is Stress?

It was a pleasant spring day—about 70 degrees, with the sun shining and a slight breeze. It was the kind of day I would have enjoyed celebrating by playing tennis, jogging, and helping my son learn how to ride his bicycle (an aggravating but necessary task). Instead, I was on the shoulder of a country road in upstate New York with my hands on my knees, vomiting. The story of how I wound up on such a glorious day in such an inglorious position serves as an important lesson.

At the time, I was an assistant professor, imposing my know-it-all attitude upon unsuspecting and innocent college students at the State University of New York at Buffalo. I had become quite successful in each of the three areas the university established as criteria for promotion and tenure: teaching, research and other publications, and university and community service. The student evaluations of my classes were quite flattering. I had published approximately 15 articles in professional journals and was contracted to write my first book. So much for teaching and the proverbial "publish or perish" syndrome. It is on the community-service criteria that I need to elaborate.

To meet the community-service standards of acceptance for promotion and tenure, I made myself available as a guest speaker to community groups. I soon found that I was able to motivate groups of people through speeches and workshops on numerous topics, both directly and tangentially related to my area of expertise—health education. I spoke to the local Kiwanis Club on the topic "Drug Education Techniques" and to the Green Acres Cooperative Nursery School's parents and teachers on "Drug Education for Young Children." I was asked to present the senior class speech at Medaille College on "Sex Education" and wound up conducting workshops for local public school districts on such concerns as "Why Health Education?" "Values and Teaching," "Group Process," and "Peer Training Programs for Cigarette-Smoking Education." Things started to take shape, and I expanded my local presentations to state and national workshops and to presenting papers at various state and national meetings.

My life changed rapidly and repeatedly. I went to Buffalo as an assistant professor and was promoted twice, leaving as a full professor with tenure and administrative responsibility for the graduate program in health education. When I left Buffalo, I had published more than 40 articles in professional journals, and my second book was soon to come off the presses. During my tenure at SUNY/Buffalo, I appeared on radio and television programs and was the subject of numerous newspaper articles. In Buffalo I bought my first house, fathered my two children, and won my first tennis tournament. In short, I became a success.

So why the vomiting? I was experiencing too much change in too short a period of time. I wondered if I was as good as others thought I was or if I was just lucky. I worried about embarrassing myself in front of other people and became extremely anxious when due to speak in front of a large group—so anxious that on a nice spring day, about 70 degrees, with the sun shining and a slight breeze, as I was on my way to address a group of teachers, school administrators, and parents in Wheatfield, New York, I became sick to my stomach. I pulled the car off the road, jumped out, vomited, jumped back in, proceeded to Wheatfield, and presented a one-hour speech that is long since forgotten by everyone who was there.

What I didn't know then, but know now, is that I was experiencing stress—too much stress. I also didn't know what to do. Everything seemed to be going very well; there seemed to be no reason to become anxious or ill. I think I understand it all now and want to explain it to you. I want to help you learn about stress and how to manage it so that your life will be better and you will be healthier.

What Can You Get Out of This Book and This Course?

What if you were told you could buy a drink and feel less stressful when you have an exam in class, or are at a social gathering, or when going to the doctor or dentist? What if this drink also helped you better manage the stress you feel when having to speak in front of a group of people, or when meeting with your professor? How much would you pay for such a drink? Well, unfortunately, there is no such beverage. However, the same benefits can be gained in another way. That is, if you learn, practice, and employ stress management techniques, you can achieve all the benefits above. This book and the stress management course in which you are enrolled will help you become less stressful and, as a result, be healthier and live a more fulfilling, satisfying life. Now how can you beat that? So, let's get started. First we consider how this whole field of stress management developed and how it has achieved credibility.

The Pioneers

I don't know about you, but I found that the history courses I was required to take as an undergraduate were not as interesting as they might have been. On the other hand, the information included in those classes was important to learn—not for the facts per se, but for the general concepts. For example, although I long ago forgot the specific economic factors preceding the World Wars, I have remembered that wars are often the result of economic realities and not just conflicts of ideology. That is an important concept that I would not have appreciated had I not enrolled in History 101.

This wordy introduction to the history of stress management somewhat assuages my conscience but won't help you much unless I make this discussion interesting. Accepting this challenge, and with apologies for my failures to meet it, let's wander through the past and meet some of the pioneers in the field of stress (see Table 1.1).

The first person we meet is Walter Cannon. In the early part of the twentieth century, Cannon was a noted physiologist employed at the Harvard Medical School. It was he who first described the body's reaction to stress.[1] Picture this: You're walking down a dark alley at night, all alone, and you forgot your glasses. Halfway through the alley (at the point of no return) you spot a big, burly figure carrying a club and straddling your path. Other than thinking "Woe is me," what else happens within you? Your heart begins to pound and speed up, you seem unable to catch your breath, you begin to perspire, your muscles tense, and a whole array of changes occur within your body. Cannon was the researcher who first identified this stress reaction as the **fight-or-flight response.** Your body prepares itself, when confronted by a threat, to either stand ground and fight or run away. In the alley, that response is invaluable because you want to be able to mobilize yourself quickly for some kind of action. We'll soon see, though, that in today's society the fight-or-flight response has become a threat itself—a threat to your health.

Curious about the fight-or-flight response, a young endocrinologist studied it in detail. Using rats and exposing them to **stressors**—factors with the potential to cause stress—Hans Selye was able to specify the changes in the body's physiology.

fight-or-flight response
The body's stress reaction that includes an increase in heart rate, respiration, blood pressure, and serum cholesterol.

stressor
Something with the potential to cause a stress reaction.

Table 1.1
**Pioneers in Stress and
Stress Management**

Pioneer	Date	Area of Study/Influence
Oskar Vogt	1900	Hypnosis
Walter Cannon	1932	The fight-or-flight response
Edmund Jacobson	1938	Progressive relaxation
Johannes Schultz	1953	Autogenic training
Stewart Wolf/Harold Wolff	1953	Stress and headaches
George Engel	1955	Stress and ulcerative colitis
Hans Selye	1956	The physiological responses to stress
A. T. W. Simeons	1961	Psychosomatic disease
Stewart Wolf	1965	Stress and the digestive system
Wolfgang Luthe	1965	Autogenic training
Lawrence LeShan	1966	Stress and cancer
Richard Lazarus	1966	Stress and coping/hassles
Thomas Holmes/Richard Rahe	1967	Stress/life change/illness
Robert Keith Wallace	1970	Transcendental meditation
Thomas Budzynski	1970	Stress and headaches
Meyer Friedman/Ray Rosenman	1974	Type A behavior pattern
Carl Simonton	1975	Stress and cancer
Robert Ader	1975	Psychoneuroimmunology
Herbert Benson	1975	The relaxation response/meditation
Daniel Goleman	1976	Meditation
Gary Schwartz	1976	Meditation/biofeedback
Robert Karasek	1979	Job Demand-Control Model
Suzanne Kobasa	1979	Hardiness
Anita DeLongis	1982	Hassles and illness
Dean Ornish	1990	Stress/Nutrition/Coronary Heart Disease
Jon Kabat-Zinn	1992	Meditation and Stress Reduction
Christina Maslach	1993	Burnout
J.K. Kiecolt-Glaser	1999	Psychoneuroimmunology
Shelly Taylor	2000	Tend and Befriend/Women's Coping Style
Patch Adams	2002	Humor and Stress and Health
Johan Denollet	2005	Type D Personality
E. L. Worthington	2005	Forgiveness and Health

Selye concluded that, regardless of the source of the stress, the body reacted in the same manner. His rats developed a "substantial enlargement of the cortex of the adrenal glands; shrinkage or atrophy of the thymus, spleen, lymph nodes, and other lymphatic structures; an almost total disappearance of eosinophil cells (a kind of white blood cell); and bleeding ulcers in the lining of the stomach and duodenum."[2] His research was first published in his classic book *The Stress of Life*.[3] Selye summarized stress reactivity as a three-phase process termed the **general adaptation syndrome** (see Figure 1.1):

general adaptation syndrome
The three stages of stress reaction described by Hans Selye.

Phase 1: Alarm reaction. The body shows the changes characteristic of the first exposure to a stressor. At the same time, its resistance is diminished and, if the stressor is sufficiently strong (severe burns, extremes of temperature), death may result.

Figure 1.1

The General Adaptation Syndrome
in Action

1. Alarm Phase
For example, being
at a party but having
social anxiety.

2. Resistance Phase
For example, when others try to
involve the socially anxious party
guest, he experiences stress
(perspiration, muscle tension,
increased heart rate, etc.).

3. Exhaustion Phase
For example, if the social
anxiety is experienced
often, and over a long
period of time, it can result
in illness and disease such
as coronary heart disease

Phase 2: Stage of resistance. Resistance ensues if continued exposure to the stressor is compatible with adaptation. The bodily signs characteristic of the alarm reaction have virtually disappeared, and resistance rises above normal.

Phase 3: Stage of exhaustion. Following long-continued exposure to the same stressor, to which the body has become adjusted, eventually adaptation energy is exhausted. The signs of the alarm reaction reappear, but now they are irreversible, and the individual dies.

Hans Selye defined stress as "the nonspecific response of the body to any demand made upon it."[4] That means good things (e.g., a job promotion) to which we must adapt (termed **eustress**) and bad things (e.g., the death of a loved one) to which we must adapt (termed **distress**); both are experienced the same physiologically.

Selye was really onto something. His research proved so interesting and important that he drew a large number of followers. One of these was A. T. W. Simeons, who related evolution to psychosomatic disease in his classic work, *Man's Presumptuous Brain.*[5] Simeons argued that the human brain (the diencephalon, in particular) had failed to develop at the pace needed to respond to symbolic stressors of twentieth-century life. For example, when our self-esteem is threatened, Simeons stated, the brain prepares the body with the fight-or-flight response. If the threat to self-esteem stems from fear of embarrassment during public speaking, neither fighting nor running away is an appropriate reaction. Consequently, the body has prepared itself physiologically to do something our psychology prohibits. The unused stress products break down the body, and psychosomatic disease may result.

Other researchers have added to the work of Cannon, Selye, Simeons, and others to shed more light on the relationship of stress to body processes. With this understanding has come a better appreciation of which illnesses and diseases are

eustress
Good things to which one has to adapt
and that can lead to a stress reaction.

distress
Bad things to which one has to adapt
and that can lead to a stress reaction.

associated with stress and how to prevent these conditions from developing. For example, Dr. Harold Wolff became curious why only 1 in 100 prisoners of war held by the Germans during World War II died before their release, while 33 in 100 held in Japanese camps died before their release. Keeping nutrition and length of time held captive constant, Wolff found that emotional stress, much greater in Japanese prisoner-of-war camps than in German ones, was the cause of much of this difference.[6]

Others also helped clarify the effects of stress: Stewart Wolf demonstrated its effects on digestive function;[7] Lawrence LeShan studied its effects on the development of cancer;[8] George Engel studied stress and ulcerative colitis;[9] Meyer Friedman and Ray Rosenman and more recent researchers[10–17] identified the relationship between stress and coronary heart disease; and Wolf and Wolff studied stress and headaches.[18]

Others have found ways of successfully treating people with stress-related illnesses. For example, Carl Simonton, believing personality to be related to cancer, has added a component to the standard cancer therapy: It consists of visualizing the beneficial effects of the therapy upon the malignancy.[19] For some headache sufferers, Thomas Budzynski has successfully employed biofeedback for relief.[20] Herbert Benson, a cardiologist, first became interested in stress when he studied transcendental meditation (TM) with Robert Keith Wallace.[21] Benson then developed a relaxation technique similar to TM and has used it effectively to treat people with high blood pressure.[22–25]

Relaxation techniques have also been studied in some detail. In addition to Benson's **relaxation response** (see p. 243), some of the more noteworthy methods include **autogenic training** (see p. 253) and **progressive relaxation** (see p. 262). Around 1900, a physiologist, Oskar Vogt, noted that people were capable of hypnotizing themselves. A German psychiatrist, Johannes Schultz, combined this knowledge with specific exercises to bring about heaviness and warmth in the limbs—that is, a state of relaxation.[26] This autohypnotic relaxation method became known as autogenic training and was developed and studied further by Schultz's student Wolfgang Luthe.[27]

Another effective and well-studied relaxation technique involves the tensing and relaxing of muscles so as to recognize muscle tension and bring about muscular relaxation when desired. This technique, progressive relaxation, was developed by Dr. Edmund Jacobson when he noticed his bedridden patients were still muscularly tense in spite of their restful appearance.[28] Their muscular tenseness (**bracing**), Jacobson reasoned, was a function of nerve impulses sent to the muscles, and it was interfering with their recovery. Progressive relaxation (see p. 262), sometimes termed **neuromuscular relaxation,** involves a structured set of exercises that trains people to eliminate unnecessary muscular tension.

Although Benson's relaxation response, a form of meditation, became popular in the 1970s, meditation has been around for a long time. In fact, records of meditation date back 2,000 years. Indian yogis and Zen monks were the first meditators to be scientifically studied. The results of these studies demonstrated the slowing-down effect (hypometabolic state) of meditation upon many body processes: heart rate, breathing, and muscle tension, to name but a few. For example, Therese Brosse reported Indian yogis able to control their heart rates;[29] Anand and colleagues showed changes in brain waves during meditation;[30] Kasamatsu and Hirai confirmed and expounded upon Anand's findings;[31] and Goleman and Schwartz found meditators more psychologically stable than nonmeditators.[32]

Later, a whole area of study regarding life changes to which we must adapt and their effect upon health has emerged. Thomas Holmes and Richard Rahe showed that, the more significant the changes in one's life, the greater the chance of the onset of illness.[33] Based on these conclusions, researchers are working toward a

relaxation response

A series of bodily changes that are the opposite of the stress reaction.

autogenic training

A relaxation technique that involves a sensation of heaviness, warmth, and tingling in the limbs.

progressive relaxation

A relaxation technique that involves contracting and relaxing muscle groups throughout the body.

bracing

The contraction of muscles for no obvious purpose.

neuromuscular relaxation

Another term for progressive relaxation.

better understanding of this relationship. For example, Lazarus,[34] DeLongis,[35] and their colleagues have found that everyday hassles (see page 140) are even more detrimental to one's health than major life changes.

More recently, researchers have studied the effects of stress on the immunological system. As a result, a whole new field of research has developed called *psychoneuroimmunology*. Robert Ader,[36] J. K. Kiecolt-Glaser,[37] Candice Pert[38] and others found that stress diminished the effectiveness of the immune system thereby subjecting one to a range of illnesses and diseases. In addition, Shelly Taylor's research[39] identified differences in stress coping techniques used by males and females. Taylor found that females are more likely to use social connections to cope with stressful events than are males. Other current researchers have described a Type D personality (depressed, anxious, irritable). Johan Denollet's research[40] demonstrated that Type D is related to coronary heart disease. In addition, E. L. Worthington[41] showed that forgiveness can be a non-stressful, healthy behavior.

This brief overview, is painted with a broad brush. Subsequent chapters refer to these pioneers and their work, providing you with an even better understanding of the significance of managing stress and tension. When we discuss stress-related illnesses and diseases, for example, you will once again read about Friedman and Rosenman, Simonton, Wolff, and others. When we discuss life-situation stressors, reference will be made to Lazarus and to Holmes and Rahe. When we discuss relaxation techniques, we will elaborate upon the work of Benson, Schultz, Luthe, Jacobson, and others.

For now, I hope you come away from this brief history of the stress field understanding that stress may be not just bothersome but downright unhealthy, and that stress may lead to other negative consequences such as poor relationships with loved ones or low academic achievement. There are, however, means of lessening these unhealthy and negative effects. Stress management is serious business to which some very fine minds have devoted their time and effort. As you'll find out in this book, this study has paid off and is continuing to do so.

Muscle Tension

As you begin to read this, FREEZE. Don't move a bit! Now pay attention to your body sensations and position.

Can you drop your shoulders? If so, your muscles were unnecessarily raising them.

Are your forearm muscles able to relax more? If so, you were unnecessarily tensing them.

Is your body seated in a position in which you appear ready to do something active? If so, your muscles are probably unnecessarily contracted.

Can your forehead relax more? If so, you were tensing those muscles for no useful purpose. Check your stomach, buttocks, thigh, and calf muscles. Are they, too, contracted more than is needed?

Unnecessary muscular contraction is called *bracing*. Many of us are guilty of bracing and suffer tension headaches, neck aches, or bad backs as a result.

Take a moment for yourself now. Place this book aside, and concentrate on just letting as many of your muscles relax as possible. Notice how that feels.

When we discuss deep muscle relaxation, and progressive relaxation in particular, you'll learn skills enabling you to bring about this sensation more readily.

Stress Theory

Now let's get down to business. What causes stress? There are several different theories about what causes stress and its effects on illness and disease.

Life-Events Theory

One theory developed by Holmes and Rahe[42] proposes that stress occurs when a situation requires more resources than are available. For example, if you are taking a test for which you are unprepared, you might experience stress. To measure this type of stress, some researchers have compiled lists of major stressful life events such as the death of a loved one. The rationale is that the more of these events a person experiences, the greater is his or her stress.

DeLongis and her colleagues[43] are supporters of this general approach, but they consider routine stressful life events more significant than major ones that happen infrequently. They argue that daily *hassles,* though appearing less important by themselves, add up and therefore are more stressful than major events. Furthermore, when computing the formula for stress, they consider daily *uplifts,* such as someone saying something nice about you, as counteracting some hassles.

Another theory of how life events affect health is **allostatic load,** first defined by McEwen.[44,45] Allostatic load is based on the hypothesis that there is a cumulative physiological risk associated with exposure to psychosocial stressors over one's life. There is ample evidence for this view.[46–48] Allostatic load proposes that a key mediator of increasing risk for disease is the dysregulation of systems designed to balance the organism's responses to environmental demands. Exposure to stress elicits adaptive physiological responses in regulatory systems, including the sympathetic and parasympathetic nervous systems and the cardiovascular and immune systems. Allostasis (related to homeostasis) is the adaptive maintenance of vitality in these systems in response to changing environmental circumstances. Allostatic load refers to the cumulative biological wear and tear that can result from excessive cycles of response in these systems as they seek to maintain allostasis in the face of environmental challenge. According to the theory, as these systems become taxed and dysregulated, they begin to exhibit imbalances in the primary mediators of the stress response, such as glucocorticoids, catecholamines, and proinflammatory cytokines. Chronic dysregulation is believed to confer cumulative physiological risk for disease and disability by causing damage to tissues and major organ systems.[49]

allostatic load
The cumulative biological wear and tear that results from responses to stress that seek to maintain body equilibrium.

Hardiness Theory

Other researchers conceive of stress somewhat differently. They focus not on how many stressful events you experience but on your attitude toward those events. For example, Kobasa and her colleagues[50] argue that if you perceive potentially stressful events as a *challenge* instead of as a *threat,* less stress will result. This buffering effect—buffering between stress and the development of illness and disease—is termed *hardiness* and is discussed in detail in Chapter 8.

Social Support Theory

Still other stress experts[51] envision stress occurring when there is not enough social support available to respond to the event effectively. Social support may take many forms. For example, it could be emotional support to help you feel better about yourself or about the event as you cope with it, or it could take the form of financial assistance. In any case, social support helps you cope with the event and therefore decreases your level of stress. Social support is discussed in detail in Chapters 7 and 9.

There are many other ways to conceptualize stress and its effects. Each, though, consists of at least two components: a stressor and stress reactivity.

The Stressor

A stressor is a stimulus with the *potential* for triggering the fight-or-flight response. The stressors for which our bodies were evolutionarily trained were threats to our safety. The caveman who saw a lion looking for its next meal needed to react quickly. Cavemen who were not fast enough or strong enough to respond to this threat didn't have to worry about the next threat. They became meals for the lions. The fight-or-flight response was necessary, and its rapidity was vital for survival.

Modern men and women also find comfort and safety in the fight-or-flight response. We periodically read of some superhuman feat of strength in response to a stressor, such as a person lifting a heavy car off another person pinned under it. We attribute this strength to an increase in adrenaline, and it is true that adrenaline secretion does increase as part of the fight-or-flight response. However, there are less dramatic examples of the use the fight-or-flight response has for us. When you step off a curb not noticing an automobile coming down the street, and you hear the auto's horn, you quickly jump back onto the curb. Your heart beats fast, your breathing changes, and you perspire. These are all manifestations of your response to a stressor, the threat of being hit by a car. They indicate that your body has been prepared to do something active and to do it immediately (jump back onto the curb).

So far, these examples of stressors have all required immediate action to prevent physical harm. Other stressors you encounter have the potential for eliciting this same fight-or-flight response, even though it would be inappropriate to respond immediately or with some action. These stressors are symbolic ones—for example, loss of status, threats to self-esteem, work overload, or overcrowding. When the boss overloads you with work, it is dysfunctional to fight with him or her and equally ridiculous to run away and not tackle the work. When you encounter the stressors associated with moving to a new town, either fighting with new people you meet or shying away from meeting new people is an inappropriate means of adjustment.

Stressors come in many forms.

We encounter many different types of stressors. Some are environmental (toxins, heat, cold), some psychological (threats to self-esteem, depression), others sociological (unemployment, death of a loved one), and still others philosophical (use of time, purpose in life). One of the most severe stressors is guilt associated with behaving in ways contrary to one's belief system or moral framework, for example, lying, cheating, or behaving sexually irresponsibly. In any case, as Selye discovered, regardless of the stressor, the body's reaction will be the same. The pituitary, thyroid, parathyroid, and adrenal glands, as well as the hypothalamus and other parts of the brain, are activated by stressors.

The point is, our bodies have evolved to respond to stressors with an immediate action by altering their physiology for greater speed and strength. When we encounter symbolic stressors, our bodies are altered in the same manner, although we do not use the changed physiology by responding with some action. Therefore, we build up stress products, which include elevated blood pressure and increased muscular contractions, serum cholesterol, and secretions of hydrochloric acid in the stomach. We do not use these stress products but rather "grin and bear" the situation. The results are illness and disease when the stress reaction is chronic, is prolonged, or goes unabated.

How Americans Experience Stress

Following are the most common causes of stress in our society along with the effects of stressors. Which ones impact you the most?

What Causes Stress?

Money	75%	Personal health concerns	53%
The economy	67%	Family health problems	53%
Relationships	58%	Housing costs	49%
Family responsibilities	57%	Job stability	49%
		Personal safety	32%

What Are the Effects of Stress?

General Effects:

Lying awake at night	44%
Irritability or anger	42%
Fatigue	37%

Physical Effects:

Headache	32%	Tightness in chest	11%
Upset stomach	24%	Feeling dizzy	10%
Muscular tension	24%	Change in menstrual cycle	5%
Teeth grinding	15%	Erectile dysfunction	3%
Change in sex drive	11%		

Psychological Effects:

Feeling nervous or anxious	39%	Lack of interest/motivation	35%
Feeling depressed or sad	37%	Feeling like crying	30%

This need not be the case. We can learn to take control of ourselves and our bodies to prevent the fight-or-flight response from developing when we encounter symbolic threats.[52] We can also learn how to use stress products once our physiology has changed to prevent them from resulting in illness, disease, or other negative consequences. Remember, stressors are stimuli with the *potential* for triggering the fight-or-flight response; they need not lead to such a response. As our computer programs sometimes need updating, so do our responses to stressors. Reprogramming ourselves in this way means that we learn to perceive events as less stressful, and we choose responses that are healthier and more life-enhancing. With this book and the practice of the skills it describes, you can learn to manage stress better.

Stress Reactivity

The fight-or-flight response is termed *stress reactivity*. This reaction, described in more detail in the next chapter, includes increased muscle tension; increased heart rate, stroke volume, and output; elevated blood pressure; increased neural excitability; less saliva in the mouth; increased sodium retention; increased perspiration; change in respiratory rate; increased serum glucose; increased release of hydrochloric acid in the stomach; changes in brain waves; and increased urination. This reaction prepares us for swift action when such a response is warranted. When we build up stress products that we don't use, this stress reaction becomes unhealthy.

The longer our physiology varies from its baseline measures (duration) and the greater the variance from that baseline (degree), the more likely we are to experience ill effects from this stress reactivity. Of the two, duration and degree, duration is the more important. For example, if you awaken to realize your alarm clock didn't go off and you'll be late for work, you become physiologically aroused from that stressor. If in your haste you accidentally pour too much milk into your cereal, that stressor will result in further physiological arousal. Next, you get into the car, only to learn you're out of gas. Ever have a day like that? Although each of those stressors will probably result in less arousal than having to jump back from a car bearing down on you, it is the length of time that these stressors are with you that makes them more harmful.

People who have learned stress management skills often respond to a greater degree to a stressor but return to their resting rate sooner than those not trained in stress management. An analogy can be made to joggers, whose heart rate may increase tremendously when they exercise but returns to normal sooner than that of out-of-shape exercisers. Try the exercise in Figure 1.2 to demonstrate the effects of a stressor upon your physiology.

Strain

Strains are the outcomes of stress reactivity and may be *physical, psychological,* or *behavioral.* For example, tension headaches and backache are physical strains that result from excess muscle tension. Agoraphobia, the fear of being in crowds, is an example of a psychological strain that stems from stress reactivity occurring when contemplating that experience. And strains such as alcohol abuse and getting into fights are examples of behavioral strains in an attempt to cope with stressors.

Gender Differences in Reactivity

Interestingly, there are some differences between the way males and females cope with stress. Shelly Taylor and her colleagues[53] have found that females tend to exhibit nurturing activities designed to protect themselves and others in coping with stress. These activities are termed "tend-and-befriend." The authors argue that females use social groups more than do males as a response to stress, and that males, in contrast, tend to exhibit more of a flight-or-fight response to stress. This and other gender differences are discussed in detail later in Chapter 16.

strain
The physical, psychological, and behavioral outcomes of stress reactivity.

Figure 1.2

Stress reactivity

While seated in a comfortable position, determine how fast your heart beats at rest using one of the following methods. (Use a watch that has a second hand.)

1. Place the first two fingers (pointer and middle finger) of one hand on the underside of your other wrist, on the thumb side. Feel for your pulse and count the number of pulses for thirty seconds. (See the drawing.)

2. Place the first two fingers of one hand on your lower neck, just above the collarbone; move your fingers toward your shoulder until you find your pulse. Count the pulses for thirty seconds.

3. Place the first two fingers of one hand in front of your ear near your sideburn, moving your fingers until you find your pulse. Count the pulses for thirty seconds. Multiply your thirty-second pulse count by two to determine how many times your heart beats each minute while at rest.

Now close your eyes and think of either someone you really dislike or some situation you experienced that really frightened you. If you are recalling a person, think of how that person looks, smells, and what he or she does to incur your dislike. Really feel the dislike, don't just think about it. If you recall a frightening situation, try to place yourself back in that situation. Sense the fright, be scared, vividly recall the situation in all its detail. Think of the person or situation for one minute, and then count your pulse rate for thirty seconds, as you did earlier. Multiply the rate by two, and compare your first total with the second.

Most people find that their heart rate increases when experiencing the stressful memory. This increase occurs despite a lack of any physical activity; just thoughts increase heart rate. This fact demonstrates two things: the nature of stressors and the nature of stress reactivity. The stressor is a stimulus with the potential of eliciting a stress reaction (physiological arousal).

A Definition of Stress

Now that you know what a stressor is and what stress reactivity is, it is time to define stress itself.

Although Lazarus offered a definition of stress that encompasses a whole spectrum of factors (stimulus, response, cognitive appraisal of threat, coping styles, psychological defenses, and the social milieu),[54] for our purposes that may be too encompassing. Defining stress becomes a problem even for the experts. Mason aptly described this problem by citing several different ways the term *stress* is used:[55]

1. *The stimulus.* This is our definition of stressor.
2. *The response.* This is our definition of stress reactivity and strain.
3. *The whole spectrum of interacting factors.* This is Lazarus's definition.
4. *The stimulus-response interaction.*

Still another view of stress conceptualizes it as the difference between pressure and adaptability—that is, stress = pressure − adaptability.[56]

For our purposes, we will operationally define **stress** as the combination of a stressor, stress reactivity, and strain. That is, a stimulus is presented that has the potential to trigger a fight-or-flight response (the stressor) that elicits physiological changes such as increased muscle tension and blood pressure (stress reactivity) that, in turn, results in physical, psychological, or behavioral consequences such as headache or agoraphobia (strain). Without all of these components, there is no stress. A stressor has only the *potential* for eliciting a stress reaction and strain.

To illustrate this point, imagine two people fired from their jobs. One views being fired as catastrophic: "How will I support my family? How will I pay my rent? What do I do if I get ill without health insurance in force?" The other views being fired as less severe and says, "It's not good that I was fired, but I never really liked that job. This will give me the impetus to find a job I'll enjoy. I've been working too hard, anyhow. I needed a vacation. Now I'll take one." As you can see, the stressor (being fired) had the potential of eliciting physiological arousal, but only the thought processes employed by the first person would result in such a reaction. The first person encountered a stressor, perceived it as stressful, and wound up with physiological arousal and, eventually, strain. By definition, that person experienced stress. The second person encountered the same stressor (being fired) but perceived it in such a way as to *prevent* physiological arousal. That person was not stressed or strained. Table 1.2 demonstrates how two different people might respond differently to the same stressors.

stress
The combination of a stressor, stress reactivity, and strain.

Table 1.2 A Comparison Between Jessie and Rick's Stressful Day

Stressors	Jessie (Stress Profile)	Rick (Healthy Profile)
Alarm clock doesn't go off. Late for class.	*Thoughts:* My professor will be angry with me. I've been late several times already. *Stress Reactivity:* Muscles tension, heart races, start to perspire. *Strain:* Stomach upset, leaves hungry, chooses clothes that do not match.	*Thoughts:* I'll take care of this okay. I will explain and apologize to the professor. *Stress Reactivity:* None *Strain:* None
Burned the toast at breakfast and spilled coffee on the floor.	*Thoughts:* I am such an idiot. I cannot do anything right. *Stress Reactivity:* Breathing rate increases, heart feels like it is pounding in the chest, and feels frustrated. *Strain:* Gets headache, diarrhea, and burns hand on the toaster.	*Thoughts:* Well, I am already late. I'll just toast another slice of bread and clean up the spilled coffee. Then I'll head to class. *Stress Reactivity:* None *Strain:* None
Computer crashes and file for term paper is lost.	*Thoughts:* That's the last straw! Now I'll have to type this whole term paper over. I'll have to stay up late to get it done. *Stress Reactivity:* Feeling frustrated and angry, forehead muscles tense, and can't concentrate. *Strain:* Gets into fight with roommate, develops tension headache, and makes numerous grammatical errors when retyping the paper.	*Thoughts:* Well, things happen. I think I'll have a good lunch to relax in spite of having to redo the paper. It will all get done on time. *Stress Reactivity:* None *Strain:* None
Having difficulty learning the material for an important exam.	*Thoughts:* I'm such a dummy! I'll never learn this material and, as a result, will fail the exam. *Stress Reactivity:* Angry, fists clench, fear of failing, and eyes get tired affecting concentration. *Strain:* Argues with roommate to keep quiet, unable to decide what content is important to learn and what content is not, and considers cutting class so as not to have to take the test.	*Thoughts:* I'll take a short break from studying and come back refreshed. Then I'm sure I will learn what I need to learn and do well on the exam. *Strain Reactivity:* None *Strain:* None

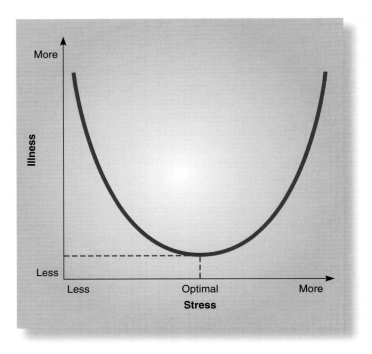

Figure 1.3

The relationship between stress and illness is a complex one. Illness may result from too *little* stress, just as it might from too much stress.

Stress Management Goals

Before concluding this chapter, we should note that the goal of stress management is not to eliminate all stress. Life would certainly be dull without both joyful stressors to which we have to adjust and distressors needing a response. Furthermore, stress is often a motivator for peak performance. For example, when you are experiencing stress about an upcoming test, you will be more likely to study more intensely than if you were not concerned. If you are to speak in front of a group of people and are apprehensive, you probably will prepare a better speech. Stress can be useful, stimulating, and welcome. So, even if it were possible, we should not want to eliminate all stress from our lives.

Our goal should be to limit the harmful effects of stress while maintaining life's quality and vitality. Some researchers have found that the relationship between stress and illness can be plotted on a U-shaped curve, as shown in Figure 1.3. The curve illustrates that, with a great deal of stress, a great deal of illness occurs. However, it also indicates that, with only a minute amount of stress, a great deal of illness can still occur. These researchers found that there is an optimal amount of stress—not too much and not too little—that is healthy and prophylactic.[57] We will keep that important finding to the fore as we proceed toward taking control of our stress.

The Way to Use This Book

Your instructor will help you decide the best way to use this book. There are many options, and he or she is an expert on whom you should rely. Some of these options follow.

Your Personal Stress Profile and Activity Workbook

In my stress management classes, each student completes the accompanying *Your Personal Stress Profile and Activity Workbook*. This is done throughout the semester at the student's own pace. Each student submits a two-page paper when the workbook is turned in near the end of the semester. This paper consists of three paragraphs:

1. A listing of each scale completed and the student's score.

2. An interpretation of the scores (which were satisfactory and which needed improvement).

3. A summary of what was learned by completing the workbook and a plan for remedying those variables on which the student scored low.

My students tell me this is an extremely valuable experience that supplements and complements the content presented in the textbook.

Your instructor may conclude that you, too, would benefit from completing *Your Personal Stress Profile and Activity Workbook*. In the event your instructor makes that decision, we let you know when it is appropriate to go to the workbook at the Online Learning Center for the text (www.mhhe.com/greenberg13e). We do this through the use of a logo alongside content in the textbook that pertains to a section of the workbook. If your instructor decides not to use *Your Personal Stress Profile and Activity Workbook*, you can just ignore this logo.

The Stress Portfolio

In this book, we help you develop a stress portfolio. A portfolio is a grouping of all the material you have produced, similar to an artist's portfolio consisting of drawings and paintings or a model's portfolio composed of past modeling photographs and letters of reference. In your stress portfolio, you will include the results of all of the scales completed in the text or workbook, thoughts you have during particular class sessions or while reading this book, your responses to all of the boxed material in this text, other assignments you may have been expected to complete, the results of all examinations and quizzes in this class, descriptions and accompanying materials that show any ways you have taught others how to manage stress, and any other materials that relate to you and your expertise in stress and stress management (e.g., stress workshops you took outside of this class). By the end of this course, then, you will have a complete summary of how you have come to interact with stress, how much expertise you have developed in managing stress, and evidence to demonstrate this to others (e.g., future employers and graduate or professional schools to which you may apply).

Materials that should be included in your stress portfolio are identified by this logo and should be removed or photocopied from the text or printed from the online workbook. Then these materials should be placed in a folder in which you will add other material throughout this course. At the end of this class, you might want to share your portfolio with several of your classmates. That might give you additional ideas on how to expand your own portfolio and thereby make it even more impressive to anyone who might see it.

"Getting Involved in Your Community" Boxes

We all live in several different communities that can be envisioned as concentric circles. In the middle circle stand you and your immediate family. In the next circle is your extended family. As the circles expand, we find your campus, then your city or county, next the state, then the country, and eventually the world. It is my belief that all of us, in addition to intervening in our own stress, have an obligation to respond to the stress our communities experience. To encourage you to contribute to the health of the communities in which you live, a box entitled "Getting Involved in Your Community" appears in most chapters. It is suggested that you use the knowledge, attitudinal development, skills, and behaviors learned in each chapter not only to limit the stress you experience but also to help your family, friends, classmates, neighbors, and others to be less stressed. Your instructor may suggest still other ways for you to contribute to your community.

Health, Wellness, and Stress[a]

What is the difference between health and wellness? **Health** consists of seven dimensions: physical health, social health, mental health, emotional health, spiritual health, environmental health, and occupational health.

- **Physical health**—the ability of the body to function daily with energy remaining to respond to emergencies; the absence of disease; the level of physical fitness.
- **Social health**—the ability to interact well with people and the environment, to have satisfying interpersonal relationships.
- **Mental health**—the ability to learn and grow intellectually.
- **Emotional health**—the ability to control emotions so that you feel comfortable expressing them and can express them appropriately.
- **Spiritual health**—a belief in some unifying force, which varies from person to person but has the concept of faith at its core. Faith is feeling connected to other humans, believing one's life has purpose and meaning.
- **Environmental health**—a healthy, supportive setting in which to function. It includes the quality of the air you breathe, the purity of the water you drink, the amount of noise to which you are subjected, and the amount of space in which you are able to function. Environmental health also includes the effectiveness of the institutions with which you interact regularly: Schools, health care facilities, recreational facilities, and others.
- **Occupational health**—having a job that is satisfying, doing meaningful work, working with people who value your contributions and who value you as a person, and earning enough money to support your lifestyle.

The extent and degree to which you possess these components of health determine how healthy you are. **Wellness** is the degree to which these components of health are *in balance*. Imagine meeting a friend you haven't seen in some time. You ask how he has been, and he tells you that he never felt better. He started running marathons and devotes most of his day to training and reading about running. His blood pressure is down, his heart rate is lower, he has more stamina, and his blood cholesterol is even better than normal. He appears to be healthy.

Then you ask about his family, and he tells you that he is divorced. He spent so much time running that he had little left for his family (poor social health). Next, you ask about his job, and he tells you that he was fired because he did not spend enough time learning new skills to do the job better (poor mental health). When you ask about his work with the charitable organization he was devoted to, he tells you that he gave that up when he got into running seriously (poor spiritual health). Do you get the point? Your friend may be more physically healthy, but he developed that degree of physical health by ignoring other aspects of his health.

When you achieve wellness, you have the components of health in balance. Imagine *health* as a tire divided into segments, the components of health. If one segment of that tire is too large and others are too small, the tire is out-of-round and will not provide a smooth ride. If your health segments are "out-of-round," you will not have a smooth ride down the road of life, and stressful consequences are likely to occur.

Both *health* and *wellness* are important considerations in the management of stress, and we will refer to them in various ways throughout this book.

[a]Jerrold S. Greenberg, George B. Dintiman, and Barbee Myers Oakes, *Physical Fitness and Wellness*, 3rd ed. (Champaign, IL: Human Kinetics, 2004).

The interesting thing about helping others is that you cannot but help yourself in the process. As Ralph Waldo Emerson wrote, "It is one of the most beautiful compensations of this life that no man can sincerely try to help another without helping himself." If you get involved in your community, you, too, will learn the truth of Emerson's observation. My students have. They participated in a service-learning project in which they used what they learned in their stress management class to help others to be less stressful. One group of students worked with several cancer patients to help them better manage the stress associated with their illness. Other students worked with children in local schools to help them manage the stress of moving from one level of schooling to another (e.g., from middle school to senior high school). Still others worked with volunteer firefighters, nursery school teachers, elderly residents of nursing homes, and youths in local community centers. The interesting thing is that even those students who did not initially want to engage in this assignment reported tremendous benefits at the conclusion of the course. It was not unusual for my students to have stated that they learned more about stress by having to teach the course content to others, that they felt good about helping other people, and that they now wanted to contribute to their communities in still other ways.

Now, you may decide not to contribute to your community. That is your option (unless, like me, your instructor decides this is such a valuable experience that enhances learning and has other benefits that it becomes a course requirement). Before you make that decision, however, remember the words of Marion Wright Edelman, the executive director of the Children's Defense Fund:

> Service is the rent we pay for living. If you see a need, don't ask, "Why doesn't someone do something?" Ask, "Why don't I do something?" . . . We are not all equally guilty but we are all equally responsible.[58]

These volunteers are performing an important community service by helping clean up and improve the environment.

You are naturally concerned with your own health. When you experience stress, you want to know how to alleviate it. This book is devoted to helping you intervene between stress and its negative consequences, yet you not only "receive" stress but you also "emit stress." When you are unnecessarily argumentative or intolerant, for example, others with whom you interact may experience stress from your behavior. When you drive aggressively, other drivers may get "all stressed out." And when you make too much noise or play your stereo too loudly, students in your dormitory, who may require quiet to study, may develop a stress response. Of course, they need not necessarily feel stressed. As we have discussed, that is up to them. Still, when we present them with stressors, it is more likely that they will develop a stress reaction.

To limit the stressors you create for others in your community (your campus, your home, your city), list three people about whom you care and the ways in which you present them with stressors. Next, list three ways you can present each of these people with fewer stressors. Then commit yourself to following through on some of these ways to present others with fewer stressors.

Stressors I present to three people:

1. A relative:
   a. _____
   b. _____
   c. _____

2. A friend:
   a. _____
   b. _____
   c. _____

3. Someone else:
   a. _____
   b. _____
   c. _____

How I can present these people fewer stressors:

1. A relative:
   a. _____
   b. _____
   c. _____

2. A friend:
   a. _____
   b. _____
   c. _____

3. Someone else:
   a. _____
   b. _____
   c. _____

I commit to make the following changes to present people with fewer stressors:

Coping in Today's World

We have become a society that increasingly expresses its stress through anger. The American Automobile Association's Foundation for Traffic Safety reported that aggressive driving increased 7 percent in the 1990s. Airlines report more outbursts of sky rage than before. And we have all read of parents who go "berserk" on the sidelines as their children are playing soccer or baseball. In fact, rough play during his son's ice hockey practice at a Massachusetts ice rink led a father to beat another father to death, as their children looked on. Not even celebrities are immune to this phenomenon. Sean "P. Diddy" Combs and Courtney Love have both been sentenced by a judge to attend anger management programs.

The reasons for Americans becoming so angry are complicated. Certainly, the fact that we are always moving quickly, available 24/7 on our smart phones or iPads, and striving for more and more make us extraordinarily tense and impatient. That can manifest itself in anger and rage. Technology contributes to these feelings as well. Technology was supposed to make our lives more relaxing, more efficient, and easier. Tell that to anyone whose computer has crashed or whose cell phone is repeatedly ringing.

Having recognized all of these stressful influences that result in anger, we need to embrace the realization that no one forces anyone else to be angry. People choose to be angry and, therefore, can choose not to be. This book will teach you how much you can be in control of your life and, unfortunately, how often you give up that control. For example, too many of us respond to someone who yells at us by yelling right back. That is dysfunctional. It is unhealthy. It is stressful. Whereas you cannot control someone else's behavior, you can control your own.

summary

- Physiologist Walter Cannon first described the stress response. Cannon called this the fight-or-flight response.

- Endocrinologist Hans Selye was able to specify the changes in the body's physiology that resulted from stress.

- Selye found rats that he stressed developed substantial enlargement of the adrenal cortex; shrinkage of the thymus, spleen, lymph nodes, and other lymphatic structures; a disappearance of the eosinophil cells; and bleeding ulcers in the lining of the stomach and duodenum.

- Selye summarized stress reactivity as a three-phase process: alarm reaction, stage of resistance, and stage of exhaustion. He defined stress as the nonspecific response of the body to any demand made upon it.

- Cardiologist Herbert Benson studied transcendental meditation and developed a similar meditative technique

that he successfully employed to help reduce his patients' levels of high blood pressure.

- A stressor is a stimulus with the potential of triggering the fight-or-flight response. Stressors can be biological, psychological, sociological, or philosophical in origin. Strain is the outcome of stress reactivity and may be physical, psychological, or behavioral.

- The longer one's physiology varies from its baseline measures (duration) and the greater the variance (degree), the more likely one is to experience ill effects (strains) from stress reactivity.

- Stress has been defined differently by different experts. Some define stress as the stimulus, others as the response, and still others as the whole spectrum of interacting factors. This book defines stress as the combination of a stressor, stress reactivity, and strain.

internet resources

The American Institute of Stress **www.stress.org** *The AIS is a nonprofit organization that is committed to helping advance knowledge of the role of stress in health and disease. It is a clearinghouse for information on all stress-related subjects.*

HELPGUIDE **www.helpguide.org/mental/stress _signs.htm.** *A site devoted to helping people understand, prevent, and resolve life's challenges. HELPGUIDE seeks to empower people with knowledge and hope. Their goal is to give people the information* *and encouragement they need to take charge of their health and well-being and make healthy choices. Among these is the management of stress.*

Stress Education Center **www.dstress.com** *A site devoted to stress management and information*

to enhance health/wellness and productivity. A resource for tapes, books, seminars, and online classes.

references

1. Walter B. Cannon, *The Wisdom of the Body* (New York: W. W. Norton, 1932).

2. Kenneth R. Pelletier, *Mind as Healer, Mind as Slayer* (New York: Dell Publishing, 1977), 71.

3. Hans Selye, *The Stress of Life* (New York: McGraw-Hill, 1956).

4. Hans Selye, *Stress Without Distress* (New York: J. B. Lippincott, 1974), 14.

5. A. T. W. Simeons, *Man's Presumptuous Brain: An Evolutionary Interpretation of Psychosomatic Disease* (New York: E. P. Dutton, 1961).

6. Harold G. Wolff, *Stress and Disease* (Springfield, IL: Charles C. Thomas, 1953).

7. Stewart Wolf, *The Stomach* (Oxford: Oxford University Press, 1965).

8. Lawrence LeShan, "An Emotional Life-History Pattern Associated with Neoplastic Disease," *Annals of the New York Academy of Sciences,* 1966, 780–93.

9. George L. Engel, "Studies of Ulcerative Colitis—III: The Nature of the Psychologic Processes," *American Journal of Medicine,* August 1955, 649–61.

10. Meyer Friedman and Ray H. Rosenman, *Type A Behavior and Your Heart* (Greenwich, CT: Fawcett, 1974).

11. H. Bosma, M. G. Marmot, H. Hemingway, A. C. Nicholson, E. Brunner, and S. A. Stansfeld, "Low Job Control and Risk of Coronary Heart Disease in Whitehall II (Prospective Cohort) Study," *British Medical Journal* 314(1997): 558–65.

12. S. A. Everson, et al., "Interaction of Workplace Demands and Cardiovascular Reactivity in Progression of Carotid Atherosclerosis: Population Based Study," *British Medical Journal* 314(1997): 553–58.

13. C. M. Stoney, R. Niaura, and L. Bausserman, "Temporal Stability of Lipid Responses to Acute Psychological Stress in Middle-Aged Men," *Psychophysiology* 34(1997): 285–91.

14. C. M. Stoney, "Plasma Homocysteine Levels Increase in Women During Psychological Stress," *Life Sciences* 64(1999): 2359–65.

15. C. M. Stoney, R. Niaura, L. Bausserman, and M. Matacin, "Lipid Reactivity to Stress: I. Comparison of Chronic and Acute Stress Responses in Middle-Aged Pilots," *Health Psychology* 18(1999): 241–50.

16. C. M. Stoney, L. Bausserman, R. Niaura, B. Marcus, and M. Flynn, "Lipid Reactivity to Stress: II. Biological and Behavioral Influences," *Health Psychology* 18(1999): 251–61.

17. T. G. Plante and M. Ford, "The Association Between Cardiovascular Stress Responsivity and Perceived Stress Among Subjects with Irritable Bowel Syndrome and Temporomandibular Joint Disorder: A Preliminary Analysis," *International Journal of Stress Management* 7(2000): 103–19.

18. Stewart Wolf and Harold G. Wolff, *Headaches: Their Nature and Treatment* (Boston: Little, Brown, 1953).

19. Carl O. Simonton and Stephanie Matthews-Simonton, "Belief Systems and Management of the Emotional Aspects of Malignancy," *Journal of Transpersonal Psychology* 7(1975): 29–48.

20. Thomas Budzynski, Johann Stoyva, and C. Adler, "Feedback-Induced Muscle Relaxation: Application to Tension Headache," *Journal of Behavior Therapy and Experimental Psychiatry* 1(1970): 205–11.

21. Robert Keith Wallace, "Physiological Effects of Transcendental Meditation," *Science* 167(1970): 1751–54.

22. Herbert Benson, Miriam Z. Klipper, *The Relaxation Response* (New York: HarperCollins, 2000).

23. R. K. Peters, Herbert Benson, and John Peters, "Daily Relaxation Response Breaks in a Working Population: II. Effects on Blood Pressure," *American Journal of Public Health* 67(1977): 954–59.

24. Aggie Casey and Herbert Benson, *The Harvard Medical School Guide to Lowering Your Blood Pressure* (New York: McGraw-Hill, 2005).

25. Aggie Casey, Herbert Benson, and Ann MacDonald, *Mind Your Heart: A Mind/Body Approach to Stress Management, Exercise, and Nutrition for Heart Health* (New York: Simon & Schuster, 2004).

26. Johannes Schultz, *Das Autogene Training* (Stuttgart, Germany: Georg-Thieme Verlag, 1953).

27. Wolfgang Luthe, ed., *Autogenic Training* (New York: Grune and Stratton, 1965).

28. Edmund Jacobson, *Progressive Relaxation,* 2nd ed. (Chicago: University of Chicago Press, 1938).

29. Therese Brosse, "A Psychophysiological Study of Yoga," *Main Currents in Modern Thought* 4(1946): 77–84.

30. B. K. Anand, et al., "Studies on Shri Ramananda Yogi During His Stay in an Air-Tight Box," *Indian Journal of Medical Research* 49(1961): 82–89.

31. A. Kasamatsu and T. Hirai, "Studies of EEG's of Expert Zen Meditators," *Folia Psychiatrica Neurologica Japonica* 28(1966): 315.

32. Daniel J. Goleman and Gary E. Schwartz, "Meditation as an Intervention in Stress Reactivity," *Journal of Consulting and Clinical Psychology* 44(1976): 456–66.

33. Thomas H. Holmes and Richard H. Rahe, "The Social Readjustment Rating Scale," *Journal of Psychosomatic Research* 11(1967): 213–18.

34. Richard S. Lazarus, "Puzzles in the Study of Daily Hassles," *Journal of Behavioral Medicine* 7(1984): 375–89.

35. Anita DeLongis, James C. Coyne, Gayle Dakof, Susan Folkman, and Richard Lazarus, "Relationship of Daily Hassles, Uplifts, and Major Life Events to Health Status," *Health Psychology* 1(1982): 119–36.

36. Robert Ader and N. Cohen. "Behaviorally Conditioned Immunosuppression," *Psychosomatic Medicine* 37(1975): 333–40.

37. J. K. Kiecolt-Glaser and R. Glaser, R. "Psychoneuroimmunology and Cancer: Fact or Fiction?" *European Journal of Cancer* 35(1999): 1603–607.

38. Candice Pert, M. R. Ruff, R. J. Weber, and M. Herkenham. "Neuropeptides and Their Receptors: A Psychosomatic Network," *Journal of Immunology* 135(1985): 820s–26s.

39. Shelly Taylor, et al., "Biobehavioral Response to Stress in Females: Tend-and-Befriend, Not Flight-or-Flight," *Psychological Review* 107(2000): 411–29.

40. Johan Denollet. "DS14: Standard Assessment of Negative Affectivity, Social Inhibition, and Type D Personality," *Psychosomatic Medicine* 67(2005): 89–97.

41. E. L. Worthington. *Handbook of Forgiveness* (New York: Brunner-Routledge, 2005).

42. Holmes and Rahe, "The Social Readjustment Rating Scale."

43. DeLongis, et al., "Relationship of Daily Hassles."

44. B. S. McEwen, "Protective and Damaging Effects of Stress Mediators," *New England Journal of Medicine* 338(1998): 171–79.

45. B. S. McEwen and E. Stellar, "Stress and the Individual: Mechanisms Leading to Disease," *Archives of Internal Medicine* 153(1993): 2093–101.

46. G. W. Evans, P. Kim, A. H. Ting, H. B. Tesher, and D. Shannis, "Cumulative Risk, Maternal Responsiveness and Allostatic Load among Young Adolescents," *Developmental Psychology* 43(2007): 341–51.

47. D. A. Glover, M. Stuber, and R. E. Poland, "Allostatic Load in Women with and without PTSD Symptoms," *Psychiatry* 69(2006): 191–203.

48. M. Shannon, T. L. King, and H. P. Kennedy, "Allostasis: A Theoretical Framework for Understanding and Evaluating Prenatal Health Outcomes," *Journal of Obstetric, Gynecologic, & Neonatal Nursing* 36(2007): 125–34.

49. Lis Nielsen and Teresa Seeman, "Background Statement for NIA Exploratory Workshop on Allostatic Load," in Lis Nielsen, Teresa Seeman, and Anneliese Hahn, *NIA Exploratory Workshop on Allostatic Load* (Washington, DC: Behavioral and Social Research Program, National Institute on Aging, National Institutes of Health, 2007), 3.

50. Suzanne C. Kobasa, et al., "Effectiveness of Hardiness, Exercise, and Social Support as Resources Against Illness," *Journal of Psychosomatic Research* 29(1985): 525–33.

51. B. Ditzen, I. D. Neumann, G. Bodenmann, B. von Dawans, R. A. Turner, U. Ehlert, and M. Heinrichs, "Effects of Different Kinds of Couple Interaction on Cortisol and Heart Rate Responses to Stress in Women," *Psychoneuroendocrinology* 32(2007): 565–74.

52. Alfred A. Keltner and Paul M. B. Young, "Control and Maintenance Effects of Long-Term Relaxation Training in a Case of Hypertension," *International Journal of Stress Management* 1(1994): 75–79.

53. Shelly E. Taylor, Laura Copusino Klein, Brian P. Lewis, Tara L. Gruenewald, Regan A. Gurung, and John A. Updegraff, "Biobehavioral Response to Stress in Females: Tend-and-Befriend, Not Fight-or-Flight," *Psychological Review* 107(2000): 411–29.

54. Richard S. Lazarus, *Psychological Stress and the Coping Process* (New York: McGraw-Hill, 1966).

55. James W. Mason, "A Historical View of the Stress Field," *Journal of Human Stress* 1(1975): 22–36.

56. Robert Dato, "Letter to the Editor: The Law of Stress," *International Journal of Stress Management* 3(1996): 181–82.

57. Clinton G. Weiman, "A Study of Occupational Stressors and the Incidence of Disease/Risk," *Journal of Occupational Medicine* 19(1977): 119–22.

58. Marion Wright Edelman, *The Measure of Our Success: A Letter to My Children and Yours* (Boston: Beacon Press, 1992).

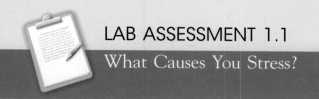

LAB ASSESSMENT 1.1

What Causes You Stress?

To determine what causes you stress and how you react, first list your major stressors. For example, finances, academics, relationships with family and friends, or speaking in front of your class.

Major Stressors

1. _____
2. _____
3. _____
4. _____
5. _____

Your Reactions

To determine how you respond to stress, follow the instructions below.

1. Take your resting pulse rate (see instructions in figure 1.2 on page 11) and record that number in the space provided. _____
2. Next, choose the stressor that is most stressful for you. Close your eyes and imagine experiencing that stressor. Imagine it in all its details for three minutes: the people involved, the place in which it occurs, the challenges it presents, etc.
3. After three minutes, take your pulse rate again and place that number in the space provided. _____
4. List other physical and psychological reactions that occurred when you imagined this stressor. For example, perspiration, muscle tension, anxiety, nervousness, etc.

1. _____
2. _____
3. _____
4. _____
5. _____

How You Can Use This Information

Throughout this book, and in your course, you will learn more about what causes you stress, how you react to stressors, and how you can better manage stress in your life. As you read through this book and learn more about stress and stress management in your course, periodically refer back to this Lab Assessment and try to apply the knowledge and skills you learn to your major stressors.

LAB ASSESSMENT 1.2

Why Do Some of Your Stressors Result in a Stress Response?

You, as the rest of us, have experienced stressors with the potential to elicit a stress reaction. Some of these stressors have resulted in an increased heart rate, tense muscles, perspiration, and other stress reactions. Other stressors, though, seem not to produce those effects. Have you ever wondered why some stressors elicit a stress response while others do not? To explore this question, start by listing three stressors you have encountered that have resulted in a stress reaction:

1. _____
2. _____
3. _____

Now list three stressors you have encountered that did not result in a stress reaction:

1. _____
2. _____
3. _____

What did the stressors that did lead to a stress reaction have in common? Were they all threats to your self-esteem? Were they all threats to your physical health? List three commonalities among these stressors:

1. _____
2. _____
3. _____

What did the stressors that did not lead to a stress reaction have in common? Did they all involve some-one whose opinion of you was unimportant to you? Was the threat minimal? Did you perceive the threat differently? List three commonalities among these stressors:

1. _____
2. _____
3. _____

Now, describe how you can use this insight to respond to stressors/threats in ways that minimize the likelihood they will result in a stress reaction:

_____
_____
_____
_____

Stress Psychophysiology

Whenever I walk through a large shopping mall with my children, Todd and Keri, my shrewdness is put to the test. I kid them by saying that I should have had two more children so I could have named them "the four me's": Buy Me, Give Me, Take Me, and Show Me. If it isn't a soft pretzel they want, it's a new baseball bat, or a new doll, or a new doll holding a new baseball bat. Before leaving our neighborhood shopping mall, we are bombarded by a cacophony of noise (bings, bongs, rings, buzzes, and crashes) and a rainbow of colors and lights. If you haven't guessed yet, our mall is "blessed" with an arcade. Arcade games were probably invented by a malicious child who was punished so often that revenge was foremost in his or her mind. The object of this revenge was parents; the means of revenge was the arcade.

As we walk past the arcade, I start talking about the last soccer game my daughter played in or one she is anticipating. Sometimes I'll discuss a movie they both enjoyed or a vacation we're planning. Do you get the picture? Anything to divert their attention from the arcade and those money-hungry machines. I know my diversion has been successful when I have left the mall without having my arm tugged out of its socket or my pants yanked below my waist. More often than not, I leave the mall with fewer dollars than when I entered.

Computer games are the most popular at these arcades. There are several reasons for this: The sounds and noises are rewarding, and the player can fantasize a trip or battle in space and vent some aggression in a socially acceptable manner. There are probably other reasons as well, and I'm willing to bet one of these has to do with the future and the influence of the computer on that future. Little do we realize, though, that in a sense, we have always had computers. You and I even program computers. Our programs instruct our computers to bing, bong, ring, buzz, and crash and to project rainbows and lights. We have, in other words, our own arcade!

Our computers are our brains, our programs are our minds, and our arcades are our bodies. Enter this arcade with us now and learn how our machines operate, especially when stressed.

The Brain

When we are talking about stress management, we are really talking about managing psychological or sociological stressors. Although stress can be caused by biological agents (e.g., viruses), the environment (e.g., temperature), and other sources, the focus of this book is on threats to our self-esteem, the loss of a loved one and the resultant loneliness, and other such stressors. These psychological and sociological stressors are perceived by the mind and translated by the brain. The brain, in turn, instructs the rest of the body how to adjust to the stressor.

When a stressor occurs, such as having to make a speech in front of your class, you are probably aware of the fear and nervousness you feel. In addition to these feelings, your heart pounds in your chest and your muscles tense up. How does this whole process occur? What is going on here? It all starts with your senses (for

Labels (top to bottom, left side): Skull, Meninges, Cerebrum, Diencephalon, Midbrain, Brain stem { Pons, Medulla oblongata

Labels (right side): Convolution, Sulcus, Corpus callosum, Cerebellum, Spinal cord

Figure 2.1

The brain.

cerebral cortex

The upper part of the brain responsible for thinking functions.

subcortex

The lower part of the brain responsible for various physiological processes necessary to stay alive.

cerebellum

Part of the subcortex responsible for coordination.

medulla oblongata

Part of the subcortex responsible for the regulation of the heartbeat and breathing.

pons

Part of the subcortex responsible for regulating sleep.

diencephalon

Part of the subcortex responsible for regulation of the emotions.

thalamus

Part of the diencephalon that relays sensory impulses to the cerebral cortex.

example, sight and sound) passing along information to your brain, which, in turn, changes your body to be better able to cope with the stressor. Let's now explore the brain's function in this process.

The brain includes two major components: the **cerebral cortex** (the upper part) and the **subcortex** (the lower part). Figure 2.1 shows the structures of the brain and their locations. The subcortex includes the **cerebellum** (coordinates body movements), the **medulla oblongata** (regulates heartbeat, respiration, and other such basic physiological processes), the **pons** (regulates the sleep cycle), and the **diencephalon.** The diencephalon has many purposes, including the regulation of the emotions. It is made up of the **thalamus** and **hypothalamus.** The thalamus relays sensory impulses from other parts of the nervous system to the cerebral cortex. The hypothalamus, a key structure in stress reactivity, is the

Stress and Your Memory[a]

The next time you do poorly on an exam, you might be able to blame it on stress. Researchers have found that, in stressful situations, when an individual perceives a lack of control, an enzyme—protein kinase C (PKC)—is produced by the brain. PKC interferes with the functioning of the prefrontal cortex of the brain, which regulates thoughts, behavior, and emotions. The result is that PKC impairs short-term memory and other functions of the prefrontal cortex. So, instead of saying the dog ate your homework, try the stress excuse the next time.

[a]S. G. Birnbaum, et al., "Protein Kinase C Overactivity Impairs Prefrontal Cortical Regulation of Working Memory," *Science* 306(2004): 882–84.

Table 2.1 Structures of the Brain and their Functions

Cerebral Cortex (Gray Matter)	Cerebral Subcortex

• *Frontal Lobe:* associated with reasoning, planning, parts of speech, movement, emotions, and problem solving
 	
• *Parietal Lobe:* associated with movement, orientation, recognition, perception of stimuli
 	
• *Occipital Lobe:* associated with vision
 	
• *Temporal Lobe:* associated with perception and recognition of sounds, memory, and speech
	• *Cerebellum:* coordinates body movements
	
	• *Medulla Oblongata:* regulates heartbeat, breathing, and other similar physiological processes
	
	• *Pons:* regulates sleep
	
	• *Diencephalon:* regulates emotions and includes the thalamus and hypothalamus
	
	  • *Thalamus:* relays sensory impulses from other parts of the nervous system to the cerebral cortex
	
	  • *Hypothalamus:* activates the autonomic nervous system

primary activator of the **autonomic nervous system,** which controls basic body processes such as hormone balance, temperature, and the constriction and dilation of blood vessels. (See Table 2.1.)

The **limbic system,** called the "seat of emotions," consists of the thalamus and hypothalamus (the diencephalon) and other structures important in stress physiology. The limbic system is connected to the diencephalon and is primarily concerned with emotions and their behavioral expression. The limbic system is thought to produce such emotions as fear, anxiety, and joy in response to physical and psychological signals. As you might expect, since emotions play a big role in the stress response, the limbic system is an important structure when discussing stress psychophysiology.

The cerebral cortex (called the **gray matter**) controls higher-order abstract functioning, such as language and judgment. The cerebral cortex can also control more primitive areas of the brain. When the diencephalon recognizes fear, for instance, the cerebral cortex can use judgment to recognize the stimulus as nonthreatening and override the fear.

Last, there is the **reticular activating system (RAS).** In the past, cortical and subcortical functions were considered dichotomized—that is, human behavior was thought to be a function of one area of the brain or the other. Now, brain researchers believe that neurological connections between the cortex and subcortex feed information back and forth. This network of nerves, the RAS, can be considered the connection between mind and body. The RAS is a complex collection of neurons serving as a point of convergence for signals from the outside world and the internal environment. In other words, it is the part of the brain where the world outside, and thoughts and feelings from inside, meet. When functioning normally, it provides the neural connections that are needed for the processing and learning of information and the ability to pay attention to the correct task. If the RAS doesn't excite the neurons of the cortex as much as it ought to, then an underaroused cortex results in such effects as difficulty in learning, poor memory, and little self-control. If, on the other hand, the RAS is too excited and arouses the cortex too much, we would see stressful responses such as being easily startled, hypervigilance, restlessness, and hyperactivity. Consequently, the RAS needs to be activated to normal levels for the rest of the brain to function as it should.[1]

Now that the brain's key structures have been outlined, let's see how a stressor affects the brain and how the brain functions to prepare the rest of the body to react. When we encounter a stressor, the body part (eyes, nose, muscles, etc.) that first notes the stressor passes a message along nerves to the brain. These messages pass through the reticular activating system either from or to the limbic system and the thalamus. The limbic system is where emotion evolves, and the thalamus

hypothalamus
Part of the diencephalon that activates the autonomic nervous system.

autonomic nervous system
Controls such body processes as hormone balance, temperature, and width of blood vessels.

limbic system
Produces emotions; the "seat of emotions."

gray matter
The cerebral cortex.

reticular activating system (RAS)
A network of nerves that connects the mind and the body.

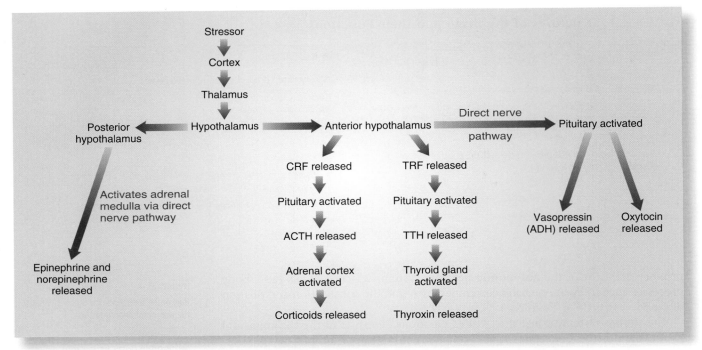

Figure 2.2

Stress and its pathways.

endocrine system

Comprised of hormones that regulate physiological functions.

corticotropin releasing factor (CRF)

Released by hypothalamus and results in the release of adrenocorticotropic hormone.

adrenocorticotropic hormone (ACTH)

Activates the adrenal cortex to secrete corticoid hormones.

thyrotropic hormone releasing factor (TRF)

Released by hypothalamus and stimulates the pituitary gland to secrete thyrotropic hormone.

thyrotropic hormone (TTH)

Stimulates the thyroid gland to secrete thyroxin.

serves as the switchboard, determining what to do with the incoming messages. The hypothalamus then comes into play.

When the hypothalamus experiences a stressor, it activates the two major stress reactivity pathways: the **endocrine system** and the autonomic nervous system. To activate the endocrine system, the anterior portion of the hypothalamus releases **corticotropin releasing factor (CRF),** which instructs the pituitary gland at the base of the brain to secrete **adrenocorticotropic hormone (ACTH).** ACTH then activates the adrenal cortex to secrete corticoid hormones. To activate the autonomic nervous system, a message is sent by the posterior part of the hypothalamus via a nerve pathway to the adrenal medulla. Figure 2.2 diagrams stress's pathways in the body.

The hypothalamus performs other functions as well. One of these is the releasing of **thyrotropic hormone releasing factor (TRF)** from its anterior portion, which instructs the pituitary to secrete **thyrotropic hormone (TTH).** TTH then stimulates the thyroid gland to secrete the hormone thyroxin. The anterior hypothalamus also

Evolution of the Brain

Eons ago, the brain stem was quite primitive. It governed decisions and actions. Eventually, the brain evolved to create the limbic system and the cerebral cortex, which is unique to human beings. Unlike fish, which developed a new appendage or component—fins and gills—the brain developed by laying one evolutionary structure over another. That is why we sometimes have conflicting feelings about stress. When we experience little or no stress, the cerebral cortex is in charge. When we experience significant amounts of stress, the limbic system is interpreting what is happening. And when stress is perceived to be especially significant, even life threatening, the brain stem is dominant. The way the human brain evolved accounts for many of our stress responses.

stimulates the pituitary gland to secrete **oxytocin** and **vasopressin (ADH)**.[2] The functions of these hormones (adrenal medulla and cortex secretions, thyroxin, oxytocin, and vasopressin) are discussed in the next section.

Now that you have an understanding of the relationship between stress and the brain, you might be interested in some research that indicates stress may result in irreversible brain damage.[3,4] Several pieces of information are important to know to understand these findings. First, you need to know that the **hippocampus** is the part of the brain that "sounds the alarm" that stress is present. Next you need to know that glucocorticoids are hormones released by the adrenal glands. The presence of these glucocorticoids is detected by receptors on the cells of the hippocampus. Prolonged stress has been found to damage these receptors and the cells of the hippocampus themselves. Brain cells do not regenerate, so their death means we have lost these cells forever; that is, irreversible brain damage occurs. The net effects of this process are not completely understood, but it probably means we do not respond as well to stress, since we do not have as many glucocorticoid receptors. Research is being done to better understand this process and its implications.

The Endocrine System

One of the most important systems of the body that is related to stress is the endocrine system. The endocrine system includes all the glands that secrete hormones. These hormones alter the function of other bodily tissues and are carried through the circulatory system to various targets. The endocrine system includes the pituitary, thyroid, parathyroid, and adrenal glands, as well as the pancreas, ovaries, testes, pineal gland, and thymus gland. The locations of these endocrine glands are shown in Figure 2.3.

oxytocin
A hormone secreted by the pituitary gland.

vasopressin (ADH)
A hormone secreted by the pituitary gland.

hippocampus
The part of the brain that "sounds the alarm" that stress is present.

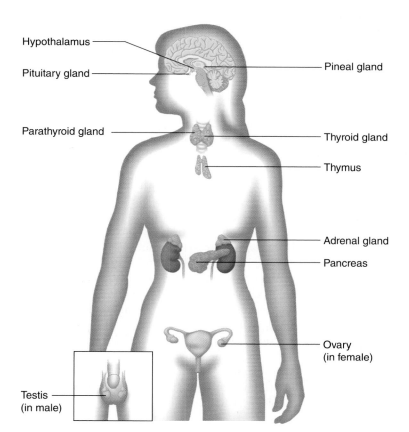

Figure 2.3

Locations of major endocrine glands.

Figure 2.4

An adrenal gland consists of an outer cortex and an inner medulla, which secrete different hormones.

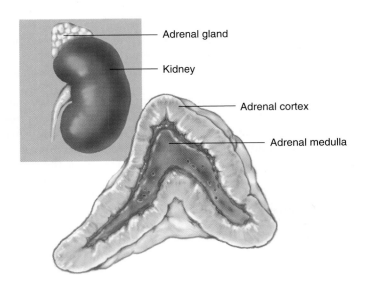

- Adrenal gland
- Kidney
- Adrenal cortex
- Adrenal medulla

adrenal cortex
The part of the adrenal gland that secretes corticoids.

glucocorticoids
Regulate metabolism of glucose.

mineralocorticoids
Regulate the balance between sodium and potassium.

cortisol
The primary glucocorticoid secreted from the adrenal cortex that is responsible for an increase in blood glucose.

aldosterone
The primary mineralocorticoid secreted from the adrenal cortex that is responsible for an increase in blood pressure.

gluconeogenesis
The production of glucose from amino acids by the liver.

When the anterior hypothalamus releases CRF, and the pituitary then releases ACTH, the outer layer of the adrenal glands, the **adrenal cortex,** secretes **glucocorticoids** and **mineralocorticoids** (see Figure 2.4). Chemically classified as steroid molecules, glucocorticoids regulate metabolism of glucose, and mineral corticoids regulate the balance between sodium and potassium. The primary glucocorticoid is the hormone **cortisol,** and the primary mineralocorticoid is **aldosterone.**

Cortisol provides the fuel for battle (fight-or-flight). Its primary function is to increase the blood glucose so we have the energy for action. It does this by the conversion of amino acids to glycogen, which occurs in the liver. When glycogen is depleted, the liver can produce glucose from amino acids. This process is termed **gluconeogenesis.** In addition, cortisol mobilizes free fatty acids from fat (adipose) tissue, breaks down protein, and increases arterial blood pressure. All of this is designed to prepare us to fight or run from the stressor. Cortisol also causes other physiological changes. One of the more significant changes is the decrease of lymphocytes released from the thymus gland and lymph nodes. The lymphocytes, in their role of destroying invading substances (e.g., bacteria), are important for the effectiveness of the immunological system. Consequently, an increase in cortisol decreases the effectiveness of the immune response, and we are more likely to become ill. Salivary cortisol increases have been found within 30 minutes of waking in people who are under considerable stress because of work or family concerns[5] and in female college soccer players experiencing the stress of competition.[6]

Aldosterone also prepares us for action. Its major purpose is to increase blood pressure so we can transport food and oxygen to the active parts of our bodies—limbs as well as organs. The manner in which aldosterone raises blood pressure is to increase blood volume. This is accomplished in two ways: a decrease in urine production and an increase in sodium retention. Both of these mechanisms result in less elimination of body fluids, greater blood volume, and a subsequent increase in blood pressure.

Blood pressure is measured as systolic and diastolic. Systolic blood pressure is the amount of pressure on the arterial walls when blood is pumped from the heart. Diastolic blood pressure is the pressure of blood against the walls of the arteries when the heart is relaxed. An average blood pressure for a young adult is 120/80; the higher number is the systolic reading (120mm Hg), and the lower is the diastolic reading (80mm Hg). Aldosterone can raise systolic blood pressure 15mm–20mm Hg. Although health scientists are not in total agreement regarding the point at which hypertension (high blood pressure) begins, generally a systolic reading consistently above 140 or a diastolic reading consistently above 90 is considered harmful.

In addition to the involvement of the adrenal cortex in stress reactivity, the **adrenal medulla** (the inner portion of the adrenal gland) is activated through a direct nerve connection from the posterior portion of the hypothalamus. The adrenal medulla then secretes the catecholamines **epinephrine** (commonly called *adrenaline*) and **norepinephrine** (commonly called *noradrenaline*). These hormones lead to various changes within the body, which remain ten times longer than the effects of adrenal corticoids,[7] including the following:

adrenal medulla
The inner portion of the adrenal gland that secretes catecholamines.

epinephrine
A catecholamine secreted by the adrenal medulla.

norepinephrine
A catecholamine secreted by the adrenal medulla.

1. Acceleration of heart rate.
2. Increase in force at which blood is pumped out of the heart.
3. Dilation (widening) of coronary arteries.
4. Dilation of bronchial tubes (through which air passes to and from the lungs).
5. Increase in the basal metabolic rate (i.e., most body processes speed up).
6. Constriction (narrowing) of the blood vessels in the muscles and skin of the arms and legs.
7. Increase in oxygen consumption.

The **thyroid gland** is also involved in the stress reaction. Activated by TTH from the pituitary, it secretes thyroxin, which performs the following functions:

thyroid gland
An endocrine gland that secretes the hormone thyroxin.

1. Increases the basal metabolic rate.
2. Increases free fatty acids.
3. Increases rate of gluconeogenesis.
4. Increases gastrointestinal motility (often resulting in diarrhea).
5. Increases the rate and depth of respiration.
6. Accelerates the heart rate.
7. Increases blood pressure.
8. Increases anxiety.
9. Decreases feelings of tiredness.

In addition, through a direct nerve pathway, the hypothalamus instructs the pituitary to secrete vasopressin, also known as antidiuretic hormone (ADH), and oxytocin. Vasopressin acts on the kidneys to promote water retention, which in turn decreases urine production, resulting in more water being retained in the blood. Oxytocin secretion results in contraction of the walls of the blood vessels. Taken together, the physiological changes resulting from the secretion of vasopressin and

Table 2.2 Stress-Related Hormones

Pituitary Gland	Adrenal Gland: Cortex	Adrenal Gland: Medulla	Thyroid Gland
• *Adrenocorticotropic hormone (ACTH):* activates the autonomic nervous system • *Vasopressin (ADH):* instructs the kidneys to retain water • *Oxytocin:* contracts the walls of the blood vessels	• *Glucocorticoids (primarily cortisol):* increases blood glucose for energy, prepares the body for flight or fight • *Mineralocorticoids (primarily aldosterone):* increases blood pressure by increasing sodium retention and decreasing urine production	• *Epinephrine (adrenaline):* increases heart rate, muscle tension, and how hard the heart pumps blood • *Norepinephrine (noradrenaline):* increases heart rate and constricts blood vessels, thereby increasing blood pressure	• *Thyroxin:* increases metabolic rate, breathing, heart rate, blood pressure, and provides energy

oxytocin help explain the relationship between stress and high blood pressure. (See Table 2.2.)

To sum up so far, during stress the hypothalamus activates the adrenal and thyroid glands (either through the pituitary or direct nerve innervation), which in turn secrete cortisol, aldosterone, epinephrine, norepinephrine, and thyroxin. These hormones affect numerous body processes to prepare the stressed person to respond in a physically active manner. The secretion and production of other substances are also involved in the stress response. Among these are leptin, cytokines, insulin, TH1, and TH2.[8–10] These hormones, too, affect the immune system and, thereby, susceptibility to illness and disease.

Using Lab 2.1, at the end of the chapter, assess how much you now know about stress psychophysiology.

Why Men and Women Handle Stress Differently

Men and women respond to stress differently.[a] Men's responses to stress can be characterized by a fight-flight response, whereas women's responses tend to be more of a tend-and-befriend type. Although social learning is certainly a part of this difference, another part relates to different levels of hormones in men and women. In particular, men and women differ in levels of testosterone, oxytocin, and estrogen.

Levels of cortisol and epinephrine are similar in males and females during stressful events. However, in males, testosterone levels increase significantly with acute stress, and that increase is associated with greater hostility.[b] Females, on the other hand, produce more oxytocin and estrogen to stress than do males. These hormones mediate the effects of cortisol and epinephrine, resulting in nurturing and relaxing emotions. Instead of responding aggressively, women respond to stress by enhancing relationships and seeking greater social support. This response has been called tend-and-befriend. This is discussed in greater detail in the Social Support Networking section in Chapter 7.

[a]Shelly E. Taylor, et al., "Biobehavioral Responses to Stress in Females: Tend-and-Befriend, Not Fight-or-Flight," *Psychological Review* 107(2000): 411–29.
[b]S. S. Gidler, L. D. Jamner, and D. Shapiro, "Hostility, Testosterone, and Vascular Reactivity to Stress," *International Journal of Behavioral Medicine* 4(1997): 242–63.

The Autonomic Nervous System

Some people have suggested that you've been feeling terrible for several centuries. Well, maybe not you personally, but the collective you (us)—that is, human beings. The argument goes that human beings viewed themselves as having major importance until Copernicus demonstrated that the earth is but one of many planets revolving about the sun rather than being the center of the universe. We could no longer command the "center of attention" (get it?). Another major blow to *Homo sapiens* was Darwin's theory of evolution. Darwin's ideas became widely accepted, and human beings were relegated to just one rung on the ladder of life. Lastly, when Galen, da Vinci, and other notables described the structure and function of the human body, it became apparent that much of that function was involuntary—beyond our control. Here was one more blow to our self-esteem; we had less free will than we previously believed.

Hearken, brothers and sisters, good news is just ahead. As we shall see, stress research has demonstrated that we are in greater control than we thought. The involuntary functions of the body are controlled by the autonomic (involuntary) nervous system. A general view of the nervous system appears in Figure 2.5. Examples of involuntary functions are heart rate, blood pressure, respiratory rate, and body fluid regulation. This control is maintained by the two components of the autonomic nervous system: the sympathetic and the parasympathetic nervous systems (see Figure 2.6). Generally, the **sympathetic nervous system** is in charge of expending energy (e.g., increasing respiratory rate), and the **parasympathetic nervous system** is in charge of conserving energy (e.g., decreasing respiratory rate).

When you encounter a stressor, the sympathetic nervous system, activated by the hypothalamus, regulates the body to do the following:

1. Increase heart rate.
2. Increase force with which heart contracts.
3. Dilate coronary arteries.
4. Constrict abdominal arteries.
5. Dilate pupils.
6. Dilate bronchial tubes.
7. Increase strength of skeletal muscles.
8. Release glucose from liver.
9. Increase mental activity.

sympathetic nervous system
Part of the autonomic nervous system responsible for expending energy.

parasympathetic nervous system
Part of the autonomic nervous system responsible for conserving energy.

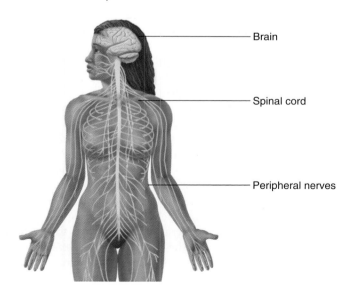

Brain

Spinal cord

Peripheral nerves

Figure 2.5

The nervous system consists of the brain, spinal cord, and numerous peripheral nerves.

Figure 2.6

Visceral organs are usually innervated from fibers from both the parasympathetic and sympathetic divisions.

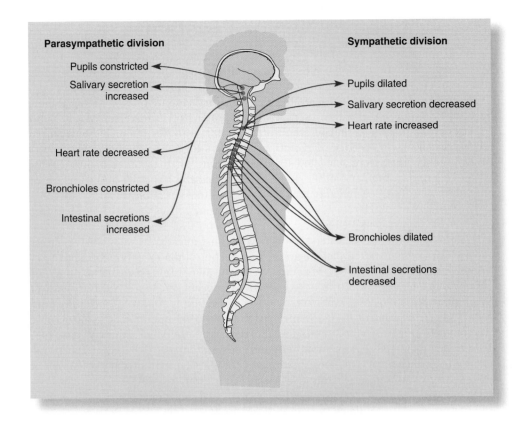

Parasympathetic division
- Pupils constricted
- Salivary secretion increased
- Heart rate decreased
- Bronchioles constricted
- Intestinal secretions increased

Sympathetic division
- Pupils dilated
- Salivary secretion decreased
- Heart rate increased
- Bronchioles dilated
- Intestinal secretions decreased

10. Dilate arterioles deep in skeletal muscles.
11. Increase basal metabolic rate significantly.

Because of these physiological changes, people have been able to perform incredible feats in emergencies. A relatively frail person who pulls a car off a child pinned beneath it is an example of the power of this fight-or-flight response. The parasympathetic nervous system is generally responsible for returning us to a relaxed state when the stressor has passed.

Now to my earlier promise of better things to come. It has been suggested that the first major scientific finding that improves, rather than diminishes, the self-esteem of human beings is the discovery that the involuntary functions of the human body are not totally involuntary. The development of biofeedback equipment, which instantaneously measures and reports what is occurring in the body, has allowed research studies of the voluntary control of "involuntary" body processes. For instance, people have been taught to control their blood pressure, to regulate their heart and respiratory rates, to emit particular brain waves, and to dilate and constrict blood vessels in various parts of their bodies. In other words, people now know they can be more in control of themselves (and their bodies) than they ever believed possible. It is suggested that this knowledge is a major influence on the level of esteem in which people hold themselves.

What some consider to be even more significant is the understanding that we often control our physiology and often allow ourselves to become ill. Once we understand that, we can stop viewing ourselves as helpless and hopeless victims of illnesses and diseases; we can consider ourselves capable of preventing them.

Here is one last word about the sympathetic and parasympathetic nervous systems. Although these two systems are generally counteractive, this is not always the case. Certain things are influenced by the sympathetic system only (e.g., sweat glands and blood glucose), and others are influenced by the parasympathetic system alone (e.g., the ciliary muscles of the eye). Generally, however, the parasympathetic nervous system is responsible for the relaxation response.

Stress Phrases

The stress reaction, as we have come to realize, results in numerous changes in our physiology. These physiological changes often lead to emotional interpretations, as witnessed by our use of phrases such as *cold feet.* We get cold feet when we are stressed because there is a constriction of blood vessels in the arms and legs. When we are stressed we may feel *uptight.* Of course, we do! We have increased muscle tension. Can you think of other "stress phrases" that have a physiological basis? Write them below.

Phrase	Physiological Basis
1.	1.
2.	2.
3.	3.
4.	4.
5.	5.

The Cardiovascular System

When my family and I moved into a new house, we experienced a most frustrating situation. It seems that every few weeks I had to dismantle the faucet to clean out debris. The builder told me this was to be expected in a new house, but I've had a house built before and never experienced that problem. You can imagine the discussions we had over this situation! In any case, every few weeks the screen in the faucet got clogged, and I had to take it out and clean it.

The reason I relate this story is that my problem is analogous to that of your body's fluid system, which includes your heart, blood, and blood vessels (see Figure 2.7). This circulatory system can also become clogged—although this takes a lot of years. When your blood vessels get clogged (not at one end—more like rusting throughout), several things may happen: Organs awaiting the oxygen and food in the blood may die if not enough of these substances is received; blood vessels may burst due to increased pressure on their walls; or other blood vessels may sprout to provide alternative routes to the waiting organs and cells.

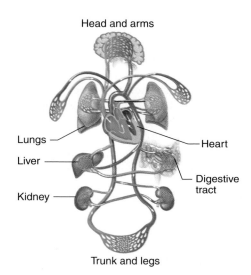

Figure 2.7

The cardiovascular system transports blood between the body cells and organs that communicate with the external environment.

The effects of stress upon the circulatory system are pronounced. When the hypothalamus reacts to a stressor, it signals the pituitary to release oxytocin and vasopressin. Both of these hormones cause contraction of the smooth muscles, resulting in constriction in the walls of the blood vessels. Vasopressin also increases the permeability of the kidney's blood vessels to water, resulting in greater blood volume. Coupled with the sodium retention brought about by aldosterone, the constriction of blood vessels and the increased permeability to water result in an increase in blood pressure caused by stress. Normal systolic blood pressure is 120 and normal diastolic blood pressure is 80. A systolic blood pressure greater than 140 and/or a diastolic blood pressure greater than 90 are classified as high blood pressure (hypertension). Systolic blood pressure between 120 and 139 and/or a diastolic blood pressure between 80 and 89 are considered prehypertension.[11]

In addition, the heart itself is affected by stress. It increases its force of contraction and pumps out more blood when stressed due to the effects of the sympathetic nervous system and the aforementioned hormones. Further, serum cholesterol and other free fatty acids increase during stress. This increases the possibility of clogging of the arteries supplying the heart and death of a part of the heart resulting from a lack of blood supply to that part. Total cholesterol is recommended to be less than 200 mg/dl. Total cholesterol between 200 and 239 mg/dl is considered borderline high, and above 240 is classified as high.[12] Last, severe stressors can shock the heart to such an extent that sudden death occurs.

The Gastrointestinal System

I began this book by describing myself vomiting by the side of a road. You now know that my condition was a function of stress overload. It is obvious, then, that the **gastrointestinal (GI) system** is a component of the stress response.

Some years back, Woody Allen made a movie titled *Everything You Wanted to Know About Sex but Were Afraid to Ask.* In that movie, a scene of the inside of a male's reproductive system includes actors as sperm. Let's use a similar approach in describing the structure and function of the GI system. The purpose of this system is to accept, break down, and distribute food and to eliminate waste products resulting from this process.

"Hey, Harry, here comes another shipment," says Joe *Saliva* to his brother. The Salivas live in the mouth and, when food enters, they help break it down to small, manageable pieces. These pieces are then mailed by pneumatic tube (the *esophagus*) to Phil *Hydrochloric Acid,* who lives in *Stomach*ville. Hydrochloric acid (HCl) activates enzymes that break the food down even further so it can pass into the small intestine. Another town, *Liver,* sends Bobby *Bile* to help break down the fatty shipments. Once these shipments (food) are made small, they can be placed in local post offices for delivery to various other cities (body parts). The pieces without zip codes are unusable and are discarded by being sent via the large intestine through the anus into space (i.e., flushed into another galaxy).

To make sure my attempt at levity hasn't been more confusing than motivating, let me summarize: Food enters the mouth, where it is broken down by chewing and **saliva.** It then passes down the food pipe (the **esophagus**) into the *stomach,* where a number of substances break the food down further. Two of these substances are **hydrochloric acid** and protein-splitting enzymes. The food substances then pass into the **small intestine,** where they are broken down further. The usable food then passes through the walls of the small intestine into the bloodstream for passage to various body parts. The unusable food substances (waste) are transported through the small intestine to the **large intestine,** finally making their way out of the body through the **anal opening.**

Stress has a very significant effect upon the GI system. Because stress decreases the amount of saliva in the mouth, people are often so nervous before speaking

gastrointestinal (GI) system
The body system responsible for digestion.

saliva
Substance in the mouth that starts to break down food.

esophagus
The food pipe.

hydrochloric acid
A substance found in the digestive system that helps break down food for digestion.

small intestine
Part of the digestive system into which the esophagus empties.

large intestine
Part of the digestive system that receives unusable food substances from the small intestine.

anal opening
The exit point for unusable food substances.

in public that their mouths are too dry to speak. Because stress may result in uncontrollable contractions of the muscles of the esophagus, swallowing may be difficult. Because stress increases the amount of hydrochloric acid in the stomach, constricts blood vessels in the digestive tract, and reduces the gastric mucus that protects the lining of the stomach, ulcers (small fissures in the stomach wall) may develop. Because stress may alter the rhythmic movements (*peristalsis*) of the small and large intestines necessary for the transport of food substances, diarrhea (if peristalsis is too fast) or constipation (if peristalsis is too slow) may result. Even irritable bowel syndrome has been associated with stress.[13–15]

The Muscles

To hold yourself in a certain posture or position, or to move, you send messages to your muscles. These messages result in muscular contraction. The absence of these messages results in muscular relaxation. Interacting systems in your body feed back the results of muscular contraction to the brain so you don't contract a muscle group too much or too little for your purposes. To demonstrate this point, place an empty gallon paint can on the floor and tell someone it is full of paint and very heavy. Then ask that person to pick up the "full" can. You will notice how quickly and how high the can is lifted before the muscles adjust to a lighter load. What really happened is that the brain perceived a can full of paint and sent that message to the muscles. Based on past experience, the muscles were instructed that x amount of contraction was needed to lift the full can. When the can was lifted, a message (visual and kinesthetic) was sent to the brain ("Hey, dummy, this can ain't full; it's empty!"), which resulted in an adjustment to make the amount of muscular contraction more appropriate to the task.

Stress results in muscles contracting—tensing. Some people appear as if they are always ready to defend themselves or to be aggressive. They seem "at the ready." This type of muscle tension is called **bracing.** As we shall discuss in the next chapter, this muscular bracing can lead to numerous states of poor health, such as tension headaches and backaches. How many times have you heard someone say, "I've got a knot in my shoulders"? When people say they are "uptight," they mean their muscles are bracing and fatiguing.

bracing
Unnecessary muscle tension.

Many of us never realize our muscles are tensed. We squeeze our pens when writing letters of complaint. We sit on the edges of our chairs ("on edge") during a scary movie. We hold our steering wheels more tightly than necessary during a traffic jam. Or we clench our jaws when angered. Intermittent muscle tension is not the problem; it is the frequent stressor to which we react with bracing that is harmful. When a new stressor is introduced while muscle tension is present, even greater muscle tension is the result.

The previous examples involved **skeletal muscles**—muscles attached to bones. In addition, we have **smooth muscles** that control the contraction of the internal organs. The stress response results in these muscles being contracted as well. For example, when we experience a stressor, the pituitary hormones oxytocin and vasopressin result in increased blood pressure due to their contracting the smooth muscles in the walls of the blood vessels. No wonder that chronic stress can lead to hypertension. When the smooth muscles in the stomach walls contract, we might get stomachaches; when the smooth muscles of the intestines contract, we might wind up with diarrhea; and so on throughout the body.[16]

skeletal muscles
Muscles attached to bones.

smooth muscles
Muscles that control the contraction of internal organs.

In addition, the heart (cardiac muscle) is itself affected by stress. Researchers have found that persistent stress results in the death of cardiac muscle cells and a loss of contractility of the heart.[17] This irreversible deterioration of cardiac function may eventually result in death.

The Skin

Linda was a doctoral student advisee of mine several years ago. One September, she surprised me by saying, "This year I'm not breaking out." When asked to explain what she meant, she told me that each summer she would leave campus and return home to a relatively unstressful existence. During the summer, her skin was very smooth, but when September rolled around and school began, she "broke out" with acne. Linda was telling me several things besides "You guys put too much pressure on us students." She was saying that she manifested her stress in "the window to her body"—her skin—and that she believed she could control that response.

Although there is no definitive relationship between stress and acne, the skin is involved in our stress response. The skin's ability to conduct electrical currents and the skin's temperature are both affected. During stress, perspiration increases. Even though this increased perspiration may be imperceptible, it will increase electrical conductance and can be measured by a galvanometer. This measure is called your **galvanic skin response (GSR)**—sometimes referred to as the electrodermal response—and is a major part of the lie detector test. One of the reasons that the lie detector test is not infallible and is viewed with caution is that people can control their nervousness (and, therefore, their level of skin moisture), thereby affecting their GSR. A good liar may have a lower GSR than a nervous innocent suspect, although a well-trained, experienced lie detector administrator will often (but not always) be able to distinguish between the two.

During stress, the surface temperature of the skin decreases. Because norepinephrine constricts the blood vessels of the skin of the arms and legs, for example, fingers and toes feel colder during stress than otherwise. The skin may also appear pale due to this vasoconstriction. We often hear of people described as appearing "white as a ghost." Now you know why the skin of nervous, anxious, stressed people is described as cold, clammy, and pale.

galvanic skin response (GSR)
The electrodermal response or the electrical conductance of the skin.

Symptoms, Stress, and You

Now that you have an idea of how your body reacts to stress, you are in a better position to be more specific. Using Lab 2.2, at the end of this chapter, assess how often each of the physical symptoms happens to you. If you score between 40 and 75, the chances of becoming physically ill as a result of stress are minimal. If you score between 76 and 100, you have a slight chance of becoming physically ill from the stress in your life. If you score between 101 and 150, it is likely you will become ill from the stress you experience. If you score over 150, you may very well already be ill from the stress you have experienced. Luckily, you are reading this book and will find out how to better manage the stress you encounter and how to eliminate some stressors in the first place.

Coping in Today's World

Do you or someone you know live near an airport? Do you or someone you know live in or near a flight path to the airport with planes flying overhead frequently? These conditions can lead to physiological arousal and a stress response. Some people are fearful of a plane crashing into their neighborhood, as occurred in 2001 in Queens, New York, killing 260 people, 5 of whom were on the ground. That fear is accompanied by increased heart rate, blood pressure, and muscle tension; perspiration; and other evidence of physiological arousal and a stress response. Others are affected by the noise of planes flying in and out throughout the day. A study[a] of the environmental effects of airport noise found that 80 percent of people who lived near the airport were more likely to have high blood pressure than those who did not. Researcher Mats Rosenlund and colleagues hypothesized that the erratic cycle of take-offs and landings affected cognitive functions, caused emotional arousal, and interfered with sleep and relaxation. As a result, those who live in flight paths should regularly be checked for hypertension.

[a]M. Rosenlund, N. Berglind, G. Pershagen, L. Jarup, and G. Bluhm, "Increased Prevalence of Hypertension in a Population Exposed to Aircraft Noise." *Occupational and Environmental Medicine* 58(2001):769–73.

summary

- The brain includes two major components: the cerebral cortex and the subcortex. The subcortex includes the cerebellum, medulla oblongata, pons, and diencephalon. The diencephalon is made up of the thalamus and the hypothalamus.

- When the hypothalamus experiences a stressor, it releases corticotropin releasing factor, which instructs the pituitary to secrete adrenocorticotropic hormone. In addition, the hypothalamus directly activates the adrenal medulla.

- Once instructed by the hypothalamus and pituitary, the adrenal cortex secretes glucocorticoids and mineralocorticoids. The primary glucocorticoid is cortisol, and the primary mineralocorticoid is aldosterone. In addition, the hypothalamus instructs the adrenal medulla to secrete the catecholamines epinephrine and norepinephrine.

- Adrenal hormones cause a number of physiological changes that include accelerated heart rate, dilation of coronary arteries, dilation of bronchial tubes, increased basal metabolic rate, constriction of blood vessels in the limbs, increased oxygen consumption, increased blood sugar, and increased blood pressure.

- In addition to the adrenal gland response to stress, the thyroid gland releases thyroxin, and the pituitary secretes oxytocin and vasopressin. These hormones also help prepare the body for a physical response to the stressor.

- Stress results in secretions of oxytocin and vasopressin, which cause contractions of smooth muscles (such as in the walls of the blood vessels). Therefore, blood vessel constriction occurs. Vasopressin secretion also results in a greater blood volume. The combination of these effects leads to increased blood pressure, which can threaten the cardiovascular system.

- The autonomic nervous system is made up of the sympathetic nervous system (generally in charge of expending energy—such as during stress) and the parasympathetic nervous system (generally in charge of conserving energy—such as during relaxation).

- Stress decreases the amount of saliva in the mouth, leaving a feeling of cotton mouth. It may also lead to uncontrollable contractions of the esophagus, making swallowing difficult. Stress also causes greater secretions of hydrochloric acid, which can result in ulcers.

- The contraction of skeletal muscle that results from stress can lead to tension headaches, backaches, and fatigue. The smooth muscle contractions of the walls of blood vessels can lead to hypertension.

- The skin's ability to conduct electrical currents and the skin's temperature are both affected by stress.

internet resources

Job Stress Network **www.workhealth.org** *Information related to job strain and work stress, by the Center for Social Epidemiology, a private nonprofit foundation whose purpose is to promote public awareness of the role of environmental and occupational stress in the etiology of cardiovascular disease.*

The Medical Basis of Stress, Depression, Anxiety, Sleep Problems, and Drug Use **www.teachhealth.com** *An easy-to-understand presentation of how the brain responds to stress.*

references

1. The ADHD Information Library, "Reticular Activating System and ADHD," *ADHD Neurology*, 2008. Available at: http://newideas.net/adhd/neurology/reticular-activating-system

2. Rod R. Seeley, Trent D. Stephens, and Philip Tate, *Anatomy and Physiology*, 8th ed. (New York: McGraw-Hill, 2008), 773.

3. M. Lippmann, A. Bress, C. B. Nemeroff, P. M. Plotsky, and L. M. Monteggia, "Long-term Behavioural and Molecular Alterations Associated with Maternal Separation in Rats," *European Journal of Neuroscience* 25(2007): 3091–98.

4. N. Maggio and M. Segal, "Striking Variations in Corticosteroid Modulation of Long-Term Potentiation Along the Septotemporal Axis of the Hippocampus," *Journal of Neuroscience* 27(2007): 5757–65.

5. Bruce S. McEwen, "Protective and Damaging Effects of Stress Mediators," *The New England Journal of Medicine* 338(1998): 171–78.

6. K. Haneishi, A. C. Fry, C. A. Moore, B. K. Schilling, Y. Li, and M. D. Fry, "Cortisol and Stress Responses During a Game and

Practice in Female Collegiate Soccer Players," *Journal of Strength and Conditioning Research* 21(2007): 583–88.

7. Stuart Ira Fox, *Human Physiology,* 10th ed. (New York: McGraw-Hill, 2008), 328–29.

8. I. J. Elenkov and G. P. Chrousos, "Stress System—Organization, Physiology and Immunoregulation," *Neuroimmunomodulation* 13(2006): 257–67.

9. I. J. Elenkov and G. P. Chrousos, "Stress Hormones, TH1/TH2 Patterns, Pro/Anti-Inflammatory Cytokines and Susceptibility to Disease," *Trends Endocrinology and Metabolism* 10(1999): 359–68.

10. D. A. Sandoval and S. N. Davis, "Leptin: Metabolic Control and Regulation," *Journal of Diabetes Complications* 17(2003): 108–13.

11. National Library of Medicine, "High Blood Pressure," *Medline Plus,* 2009. Available at: www.nlm.nih.gov/medlineplus /highbloodpressure.html

12. National Heart, Lung and Blood Institute, "How Is High Blood Cholesterol Diagnosed," *High Blood Cholesterol,* 2008. Available at: www.nhlbi.nih.gov/health/dci/Diseases/Hbc/ HBC_Diagnosis.html

13. A. O. Chan, C. Cheng, W. M. Hui, W. H. Hu, N. Y. Wong, K. F. Lam, W. M. Wong, K. C. Lai, S. K. Lam, and B. C. Wong,

"Differing Coping Mechanisms, Stress Level and Anorectal Physiology in Patients with Functional Constipation," *World Journal of Gastroenterology* 11(2005): 5362–66.

14. S. A. Walter, E. Aardal-Eriksson, L. H. Thorell, G. Bodemar, and O. Hallböök, "Pre-experimental Stress in Patients with Irritable Bowel Syndrome: High Cortisol Values Already Before Symptom Provocation with Rectal Distensions," *Neurogastroenterology and Motility* 18(2006): 1069–77.

15. Thomas G. Plante and Maire Ford, "The Association Between Cardiovascular Stress Responsivity and Perceived Stress Among Subjects with Irritable Bowel Syndrome and Temperomandibular Joint Disorder: A Preliminary Study," *International Journal of Stress Management* 7(2000): 103–19.

16. A. D. Heymann, Y. Shilo, A. Tirosh, L. Valinsky, and S. Vinker, "Differences Between Soldiers, with and without Emotional Distress, in Number of Primary Care Medical Visits and Type of Presenting Complaints," *Israel Medical Association Journal* 9(2007): 90–93.

17. Yibin Wang, Shuang Huang, Valerie P. Sah, John Ross, Jr., Joan Heller Brown, Jiahuai Han, and Kenneth R. Chien, "Cardiac Muscle Cell Hypertrophy and Apoptosis Induced by Distinct Members of the p38 Mitogen-activated Protein Kinase Family," *The Journal of Biological Chemistry* 273(1998): 2161–68.

LAB ASSESSMENT 2.1

How Much Do You Know About Stress Psychophysiology?

Directions: Stop for a moment to test your recall of the stress psychophysiology presented so far. See if you can match the numbered items in the column on the left with the lettered items in the column on the right.

_____ 1. Limbic system	a. Thalamus and hypothalamus
_____ 2. Subcortex	b. Upper part of brain
_____ 3. Diencephalon	c. Activated by ACTH
_____ 4. Cerebral cortex	d. "Seat of emotions"
_____ 5. Adrenal medulla	e. Cerebellum, medulla oblongata, pons, and diencephalon
_____ 6. Adrenal cortex	f. Secreted by adrenal cortex
_____ 7. Hypothalamus	g. Activated by nerves from hypothalamus
_____ 8. Aldosterone	h. Releases ACTH
_____ 9. Pituitary	i. Gluconeogenesis
_____ 10. Norepinephrine	j. Releases CRF
	k. Vasopressin
	l. Secreted by adrenal medulla

Check your answers with the key below. If you didn't answer at least seven correctly, you might be wise to review the beginning of this chapter before proceeding further.

Answer key: 1. d, 2. e, 3. a, 4. b, 5. g, 6. c, 7. j, 8. f, 9. h, 10. l

What Are Your Physiological Reactions to Stress?

Directions: Circle the number that best represents the frequency of occurrence of the following physical symptoms, and add up the total number of points.

	Never	Infrequently (More Than Once in Six Months)	Occasionally (More Than Once per Month)	Very Often (More Than Once per Week)	Constantly
1. Tension headaches	1	2	3	4	5
2. Migraine (vascular) headaches	1	2	3	4	5
3. Stomachaches	1	2	3	4	5
4. Increase in blood pressure	1	2	3	4	5
5. Cold hands	1	2	3	4	5
6. Acidic stomach	1	2	3	4	5
7. Shallow, rapid breathing	1	2	3	4	5
8. Diarrhea	1	2	3	4	5
9. Palpitations	1	2	3	4	5
10. Shaky hands	1	2	3	4	5
11. Burping	1	2	3	4	5
12. Gassiness	1	2	3	4	5
13. Increased urge to urinate	1	2	3	4	5
14. Sweaty feet/hands	1	2	3	4	5
15. Oily skin	1	2	3	4	5
16. Fatigue/exhausted feeling	1	2	3	4	5
17. Panting	1	2	3	4	5
18. Dry mouth	1	2	3	4	5
19. Hand tremor	1	2	3	4	5
20. Backache	1	2	3	4	5
21. Neck stiffness	1	2	3	4	5
22. Gum chewing	1	2	3	4	5
23. Grinding teeth	1	2	3	4	5
24. Constipation	1	2	3	4	5
25. Tightness in chest or heart	1	2	3	4	5
26. Dizziness	1	2	3	4	5
27. Nausea/vomiting	1	2	3	4	5
28. Menstrual distress	1	2	3	4	5
29. Skin blemishes	1	2	3	4	5
30. Heart pounding	1	2	3	4	5
31. Colitis	1	2	3	4	5
32. Asthma	1	2	3	4	5
33. Indigestion	1	2	3	4	5
34. High blood pressure	1	2	3	4	5
35. Hyperventilation	1	2	3	4	5
36. Arthritis	1	2	3	4	5
37. Skin rash	1	2	3	4	5
38. Bruxism/jaw pain	1	2	3	4	5
39. Allergy	1	2	3	4	5

Source: H. Ebel, et al., eds., *Presidential Sports Award Fitness Manual*, 197–98. Copyright © 1983 FitCom Corporation, Havertown, PA.

Interpretation

40–75	Low physiological symptoms of stress response	101–150	High physiological symptoms of stress response
76–100	Moderate physiological symptoms of stress response	Over 150	Excessive physiological symptoms of stress response

Stress and Illness/Disease

If stress were only discomforting—that is, if it led only to increased muscle tension, perspiration, rapid and shallow breathing, or a general psychological state of uneasiness—it would be bad enough. Unfortunately, chronic stress also leads to poor health. Numerous examples of the relationship between stress and ill health abound. Perhaps among the more dramatic examples is the breakup of the Soviet Union. During that stressful period, cardiovascular disease was a major contributor to an almost 40 percent increase in the death rate among Russian men.[1] We all have also heard of traumatic events (e.g., war experiences, traffic accidents, or sexual assaults) resulting in ill health (both psychological and physiological) for many years after the event itself. As a result, stress researchers have recommended that physicians and other health care providers help patients "learn coping skills, recognize their own limitations, and relax."[2]

Hot Reactors

Are you a hot reactor? Some people tend to react to stressors with an all-out physiological effort that takes a toll on their health.[3,4] In a sense, their bodies are overreacting to the stressful situation. We call these people **hot reactors.**[5] There is some evidence that nearly 20 percent of the population are hot reactors, who respond to stressors with dramatic increases in blood pressure. Hot reactors tend to suffer from chronic anger or anxiety, which leads to the high blood pressure. The high blood pressure, in turn, is associated with susceptibility to heart attacks. As a result, some experts refer to heart attacks as *hate attacks.*[6] If you notice you anger easily, you are often anxious or depressed, you urinate frequently, you experience constipation or diarrhea more than usual, or you experience nausea or vomiting, you may be a hot reactor. In that case, you may want to obtain regular medical examinations to identify illnesses when they can be easily cured or contained and learn and use stress management techniques and strategies such as those in this book. This chapter presents the body's responses to stress, and you should therefore be better able to understand why it is so important to learn to cope with stress. We identify specific illnesses, diseases, and other negative consequences that are stress related and discuss ways to prevent these from developing.

hot reactors

People who react to stress with an all-out physiological reaction.

Psychosomatic Disease

Bill's wife died last year, and Bill grieved long and hard over her death. He felt it unfair (she was such a kind person), and a sense of helplessness crept over him. Loneliness became a part of his every day, and tears became the companions of his late evening hours. There were those who were not even surprised at Bill's own death just one year after his wife's. They officially called it a heart attack, but Bill's friends, to this day, know he died of a "broken heart."

You probably know some Bills yourself—people who have died or have become ill from severe stress, with seemingly little physically wrong with them. Maybe you have even been guilty of telling these people, "It's all in your mind," or at least

Doctors can go a long way in helping people respond to illness and disease, but approximately half of all deaths in the United States are a result of poor lifestyle choices such as poor nutrition, lack of physical activity, smoking, and the inability to manage stress.

psychosomatic
Conditions that have both a mind and body component.

psychophysiological
Synonymous with psychosomatic.

psychogenic
A physical disease caused by emotional stress without a microorganism involved.

somatogenic
A psychosomatic disease that results from the mind increasing the body's susceptibility to disease-causing microbes or natural degenerative processes.

psychoneuroimmunology
The study of the illness-causing and healing effects of the mind on the body.

thinking that. Well, in Bill's case it was not "all in his mind"—it was, obviously, partially in his heart. Some illnesses are easily seen as being physical (e.g., a skin rash), while others are assuredly recognized as being mental (e.g., neuroses), yet it is impossible to deny the interaction between the mind and the body and the effects of one upon the other.

Why is it, for example, that when we are infected with a cold-causing virus we do not always come down with the common cold? We shall soon discuss numerous diseases and illnesses to which the mind makes the body susceptible. These conditions are called **psychosomatic** (*psyche* for mind; *soma* for body). Psychosomatic disease is not "all in the mind" but involves both mind and body. In fact, the term **psychophysiological** is now sometimes used in place of psychosomatic. Psychosomatic disease is real, can be diagnosed, and is manifested physically. However, it also has a component in the mind, although it is not easily measured. That common cold may be a function of psychological stress, which decreases the effectiveness of the immunological system and results in the body being more vulnerable to cold viruses. That cold may also be caused by psychological stress using up particular vitamins in the body and leading to decreased effectiveness in combating cold viruses.

Psychosomatic disease may be psychogenic or somatogenic. **Psychogenic** refers to a physical disease caused by emotional stress. Asthma is an example of a psychogenic psychosomatic disease. In this case, there is no invasion of disease-causing microorganisms; the mind changes the physiology so that parts of the body break down. **Somatogenic** psychosomatic disease occurs when the mind increases the body's susceptibility to some disease-causing microbes or some natural degenerative process. Examples of diseases suspected of being somatogenic are cancer and rheumatoid arthritis, although there are other causes of these conditions as well.

Stress and the Immunological System

There is a field of scientific inquiry that studies the chemical basis of communication between the mind and the body—in particular, the link between the nervous system and the immune system.[7,8] In 1980, psychologist Robert Ader of the University of Rochester medical school named this scientific field **psychoneuroimmunology**. The focus of researchers in this field is on both the illness-causing and the healing effects the mind can have upon the body. Robert Ornstein and David Sobel summarized data linking the social world to a decrease in the effectiveness of the immunological system.[9] They cite studies that have found the following: Bereaved people have immunological systems functioning below par; rats exposed to stress develop larger cancerous tumors than other rats; West Point cadets who develop mononucleosis come disproportionately from families with fathers who were overachievers; and reoccurrences of oral herpes simplex are associated with stress and the person's emotional reaction to the disease.

On the other hand, you may be able to enhance the functioning of your immunological system by becoming less stressed. College students who watched humorous videotapes,[10] corporate employees who listened to relaxing recreational music,[11] women with breast cancer who were taught to be more optimistic and use social support,[12] and anxious women who experienced acupuncture[13] were found to have a strengthened immune response (e.g., greater natural killer cell activity—NKA).

To understand the relationship between stress and these findings requires an understanding of the immunological system. The most important component of this system is the white blood cell; we each have about 1 trillion of these cells. White

College Students and Stress-related Illnesses

Stress-related conditions are prevalent among Americans, and college students are no exception. The American College Health Association conducted a survey of college students' health. During their last school year, ACHA found that

- 15 percent were diagnosed with depression
- 14 percent felt depressed that it was difficult to function
- 17 percent felt overwhelming anxiety
- 23 percent experienced sleep difficulties
- 39 percent experienced more than average stress and another 9 percent experienced tremendous stress
- 22 percent were treated for allergies
- 3 percent were diagnosed with hypertension

Furthermore, the percentages of students reporting that their academic performance was affected during the last school year were:

- 3 percent by allergies
- 16 percent by anxiety
- 10 percent by depression
- 9 percent by relationship difficulties
- 18 percent by sleep difficulties
- 25 percent by stress

Source: American College Health Association. *American College Health Assessment—National College Health Assessment II. Fall 2010 Reference Group Data Report.* Linthicum, MD: American College Health Association, 2011.

blood cells fall into three groups: the **phagocytes** and two kinds of lymphocytes— **T cells** and **B cells.** These three groups all share one function—to identify and destroy all substances foreign to the body.

When a foreign substance (pathogen)—for example, a virus—invades your body, some of it is initially consumed by the most important phagocytes—the *macrophages.* Macrophages surround and engulf invading substances while summoning *helper T cells.* Helper T cells identify the invader and stimulate the multiplication of *killer T cells* and *B cells.* Killer T cells puncture the membranes of body cells invaded by the foreign substance, thereby killing the cell and the substance. B cells produce antibodies that travel to the site of invasion and either neutralize the enemy or tag it for attack by other cells and chemicals. As the invasion becomes contained, **suppressor T cells** are produced that halt the immune response and **memory T and B cells** are left in the bloodstream and in the lymphatic system to recognize and respond quickly to a future attack by the same invader. Anything that decreases your number of white blood cells, or any of their component parts, threatens your health. Stress has that effect. (See Table 3.1.)

Several researchers have studied personality and health status and have concluded that stress and related constructs can indeed lead to ill health.[14,15] In an interesting article entitled "The 'Disease-Prone Personality,'" researchers Howard Friedman and Stephanie Booth-Kewley[16] cite evidence that a disease-prone personality exists that involves depression, anger/hostility, and anxiety. Psychologist

phagocytes
A type of white blood cell whose purpose is to destroy substances foreign to the body.

T cells
A type of lymphocyte whose purpose is to destroy substances foreign to the body by puncturing invaded body cells and killing the cells and the foreign substances.

B cells
A type of lymphocyte that produces antibodies.

suppressor T cells
Cells whose purpose is to halt the immune response.

memory T and B cells
Cells left in the bloodstream and the lymphatic system to recognize and respond to future attacks to the body by the same invader.

Table 3.1 **Components of the Immunological System**

White Blood Cells

Phagocytes

  Macrophages: surround and engulf invading substances and summon helper T cells

Lymphocytes

  T cells: identify the invading substance and destroy it

  Helper T cells: stimulate the production of killer T cells and B cells

  Killer T cells: puncture membrane of invaded body cells; kill cells and the invader

  B cells: produce antibodies that neutralize the invading substance or tag it for attack by other cells

  Suppressor T cells: halt the immune response when the invasion becomes contained

  Memory T and *Memory B cells:* remain in the bloodstream and lymphatic system to respond quickly to future attacks by the invading substance

Hans Eysenck,[17] entitling his article "Health's Character," presents evidence for a cancer-prone personality (unassertive, overpatient, avoiding conflicts, and failing to express negative emotions) and a coronary heart disease–prone personality (angry, hostile, and aggressive).

The specific effects of stress on immunity have also been researched. In one study,[18] college students' levels of an antibody that fights infections (salivary IgA) were tested five days before, on the day of, and two weeks after their final exams. As expected, S-IgA levels were lowest during the exam period, the most stressful time tested. This result has since been validated in subsequent studies.[19] In another interesting study,[20] positive moods were induced in subjects by asking them to "experience care and compassion." When the researchers measured S-IgA levels during these positive states, they found them to be increased. The researchers concluded that, whereas negative moods (stress) could decrease S-IgA levels thereby making people more susceptible to disease, positive moods could increase S-IgA levels and, consequently, enhance immunosuppressive effects.

Dr. Candace Pert, a neuroscientist and the former section chief of brain biochemistry at the National Institute of Mental Health, has investigated chemicals that send messages between cells to various parts of the brain and between the brain and other parts of the body. Hundreds of these brain message transmitters (called *neuropeptides*) have been found that are produced by the brain itself. The aspect pertinent to our discussion of the mind-body connection is that Pert believes some of these neuropeptides are also produced in small amounts by the macrophages—white blood cells that ingest and destroy bacteria and viruses.[21] In addition, the macrophages are attracted to neuropeptides produced by the brain. If neuropeptides are produced by the brain to fight off an invasion of bacteria, for instance, macrophages will also travel to help combat the invasion. Since relaxation and some forms of visualization result in the production of neuropeptides (e.g., beta-endorphins), it may be possible to purposefully cause the brain to produce more of these substances, thereby making the immunological system more effective. The result may be less disease.

Other evidence of the importance of the mind to physical illness also exists. For example, emotional stress induced by life events such as the birth of another sibling, the influence of a stepparent, serious illness of the mother, marital separation or divorce of parents, or a change in parent's financial status are associated with the onset of childhood diabetes.[22] Even the stress associated with a hostile marriage has been found to lower the effectiveness of the immune system, as evidenced by it taking longer for wounds to heal.[23] Furthermore, stress experienced by pregnant women can affect the fetus, resulting in premature or low-birth-weight babies.[24] Some experts have even suggested that no illness is completely free from the influence of stress.[25]

Stress and Serum Cholesterol

Cholesterol roaming about your blood can accumulate on the walls of your blood vessels, blocking the flow of blood to various parts of your body. When it is the heart that is blocked, you may develop coronary heart disease or die of a heart attack caused by an insufficient supply of oxygen to the heart. When it is the brain that is blocked, you may develop a stroke or die from an insufficient supply of oxygen to the brain.

Hypercholesterolemia is a condition characterized by very high levels of cholesterol in the blood. Cholesterol is a waxy, fat-like substance that is produced in the body and obtained from foods that come from animals (particularly egg yolks, meat, poultry, fish, and dairy products). The body needs this substance to build cell membranes, make certain hormones, and produce compounds that aid in fat digestion. Too much cholesterol, however, increases a person's risk of developing heart disease.

The abnormal buildup of cholesterol forms clumps (plaque) that narrow and harden artery walls. As the clumps get bigger, they can clog the arteries and restrict the flow of blood to the heart. The buildup of plaque in coronary arteries causes a form of chest pain called *angina* and greatly increases a person's risk of having a heart attack.[26]

Blood is watery, and cholesterol is fatty. Just like oil and water, the two do not mix. To travel in the bloodstream, cholesterol is carried in small packages called *lipoproteins*. The small packages are made of fat (lipid) on the inside and proteins on the outside. Two kinds of lipoproteins carry cholesterol throughout your body. It is important to have healthy levels of both:

- **Low-density lipoprotein (LDL)** cholesterol is sometimes called *bad cholesterol*. High LDL cholesterol leads to a buildup of cholesterol in arteries. The higher the LDL level in your blood, the greater chance you have of getting heart disease.

- **High-density lipoprotein (HDL)** cholesterol is sometimes called *good cholesterol*. HDL carries cholesterol from other parts of your body back to your liver. The liver removes the cholesterol from your body. The higher your HDL cholesterol level, the lower your chance of getting heart disease.[27]

The categorization of cholesterol levels appears in Table 3.2.

Hypercholesterolemia
High levels of cholesterol in the blood.

Low-density lipoprotein (LDL)
Sometimes termed *bad cholesterol*, too much LDL leads to a clogging of the arteries and, therefore, is related to the development of coronary heart disease.

High-density lipoprotein (HDL)
Sometimes termed *good cholesterol*, HDL helps to remove cholesterol from the body thereby lowering the chances of developing coronary heart disease.

Table 3.2 Categorization of Cholesterol Levels

Total Cholesterol Level	Total Cholesterol Category
Less than 200 mg/dL	Desirable
200–239 mg/dL	Borderline high
240 mg/dL and above	High

LDL Cholesterol Level	LDL Cholesterol Category
Less than 100 mg/dL	Optimal
100–129 mg/dL	Near optimal/above optimal
130–159 mg/dL	Borderline high
160–189 mg/dL	High
190 mg/dL and above	Very high

HDL Cholesterol Level	HDL Cholesterol Category
Less than 40 mg/dL	A major risk factor for heart disease
40–59 mg/dL	The higher, the better
60 mg/dL and above	Considered protective against heart disease

Source: National Heart, Lung and Blood Institute, "How Is High Blood Cholesterol Diagnosed," *High Blood Cholesterol*, 2008. Available at: www.nhlbi.nih.gov/health/dci/Diseases/Hbc/HBC_Diagnosis.html

Psychoneuroimmunology: Evidence from Viral Challenge

In a unique and classic study, researchers found a direct relationship between the amount of stress and development of the common cold.[a] After completing questionnaires assessing degrees of psychological stress, 394 healthy subjects were given nasal drops containing a respiratory virus. Other subjects were merely given harmless saline nasal drops. The subjects were then quarantined and monitored for the development of evidence of infection and symptoms. The rates of both respiratory infection and colds increased in a dose-response manner; the more psychological stress, the increased rate of infection. Behaviors, such as smoking, drinking alcohol, exercise, or diet did not explain the association between stress and infection. Neither did personality variables, such as self-esteem, sense of personal control, or introversion or extraversion. The researchers concluded that psychological stress was associated with an increased risk of acute infectious respiratory illness.

In a follow-up study,[b] 55 subjects were experimentally infected with influenza A virus after completing a measurement of psychological stress. Subjects were then monitored in quarantine. Higher psychological stress assessed before the *viral challenge* was associated with greater symptom scores. The researchers concluded that their results were consistent with those of earlier studies documenting that persons with higher levels of psychological stress express more symptoms and signs of upper respiratory infectious illness.

[a]S. Cohen, D. A. Tyrrell, and A. P. Smith, "Psychological Stress and Susceptibility to the Common Cold," *New England Journal of Medicine* 325(1991): 606–12.
[b]S. Cohen, W. J. Doyle, and D. P. Skoner, "Psychological Stress, Cytokine Production, and Severity of Upper Respiratory Illness," *Psychosomatic Medicine* 61(1999): 175–80.

Researchers have attempted to determine the causes of increased levels of serum cholesterol so they can help people avoid this condition; they have found stress to be one of the culprits. Friedman, Rosenman, and Carroll conducted one of the early investigations of the relationship between stress and serum cholesterol.[28] They studied accountants during times of the year when they had deadlines to meet—for example, when tax returns had to be prepared—and found average serum cholesterol increased dramatically. Other researchers have verified these results. One interesting study[29] looked at the death rates in Los Angeles during that city's football team's participation in the Super Bowl. Death rates were compared between the year that Los Angeles won the Super Bowl and the year they lost. The death rates from heart disease and heart attacks were significantly higher in the year that the L.A. team lost. The authors attribute this difference to the emotional stress of losing. Other researchers have found that when heart disease patients participated in a program that included stress management as a component, they increased HDL and decreased LDL and total cholesterol.[30,31] Numerous other investigators concur with these findings supporting the relationship between stress and cholesterol and heart disease and stroke.[32,33]

Specific diseases and illnesses are discussed next, but the important concept here is that a person is an interconnected whole. A separation, even just for discussion or research purposes, of the mind from the body is inappropriate. The mind is ultimately affected by what the body experiences, and the body is ultimately affected by what the mind experiences.

Specific Conditions

Now that you understand the concept of psychosomatic disease, we can look at specific diseases and their relationship to stress. As you will discover, stress can lead to both psychogenic and somatogenic psychosomatic diseases.

Hypertension

Hypertension (high blood pressure) is excessive and damaging pressure of the blood against the walls of the arterial blood vessels. Blood pressure is measured with a **sphygmomanometer,** an instrument consisting of an inflatable cuff placed around the upper arm and a stethoscope. The cuff cuts off the blood flow in the brachial artery until it is deflated to the point where the blood pressure forces the blood through. That measure is called the **systolic blood pressure,** and 120mm Hg is considered average (normal). At the point where the cuff is deflated further and the blood is not impeded at all, another measure is taken. That measure is termed the **diastolic blood pressure,** and 80mm Hg is considered average. The total blood pressure is given in this formula: systolic/diastolic (120/80). Systolic blood pressure represents the force against the arterial blood vessel walls when the left ventricle contracts and blood is pumped out of the heart. Diastolic blood pressure represents the force against the arterial walls when the heart is relaxed.

High blood pressure is a relative term. Health scientists disagree as to its exact beginning, but generally a systolic pressure greater than 140mm Hg or a diastolic pressure greater than 90mm Hg is considered hypertension.[34] Because average blood pressure tends to be higher in the elderly than in others, measures slightly above 140/90 are not unusual for this age group. However, that is not to say they are inevitable. Increased blood pressure may be related more to lifestyle than to age.

There are several causes of hypertension. Excessive sodium (salt) intake may cause hypertension in those genetically susceptible. Since we can't determine who is genetically susceptible, dietary guidelines in the United States suggest no more than a 5,000mg daily ingestion of salt. The average diet has been estimated to consist of 10g–20g (10,000mg–20,000mg) of salt daily. The problem with monitoring salt in our diets is that it is hidden in many processed foods. Those who just eliminate the saltshaker may still be ingesting too much salt.

Hypertension may also be caused by kidney disease, too narrow an opening in the aorta (main blood vessel through which blood exits the heart), Cushing's syndrome (oversecretion of cortisol hormones), obesity, and the use of oral contraceptives. However, these conditions cause only an estimated 10 percent of all hypertension. Approximately 90 percent of hypertension is termed **essential hypertension** and has no known cause.

Forty-one percent of the United States population aged 20 to 74 is hypertensive, although many of these people do not even know it, since hypertension occurs without signs and symptoms. Even though many people believe high blood pressure is a condition that affects only older adults, in actuality, slightly over 16 percent of 20- to 24-year-olds are hypertensive. More men than women are hypertensive, and the likelihood of developing hypertension increases with age. Proportionately more blacks than whites are hypertensive. The lowest incidence is found in white women and the highest incidence in black women.

Imagine, for a moment, the Alaska pipeline. Through that tube, oil is pumped that passes through Alaska. When that pipeline works correctly, oil is provided in sufficient quantity without any breaks in the pipeline. What would happen, though, if so much oil were pumped through that it created too great a pressure against the metal tube? The tube would probably rupture. The same thing happens with blood, blood pressure, and blood vessels. Blood is analogous to oil, and blood vessels (in particular, arteries) are analogous to the pipeline. If blood creates too great a pressure upon the arterial walls, they will rupture, and the blood intended for some destination beyond the point of rupture will not reach its goal. If the

sphygmomanometer
An instrument used to measure blood pressure.

systolic blood pressure
The pressure of the blood as it leaves the heart.

diastolic blood pressure
The pressure of the blood against the arterial walls when the heart is relaxed.

essential hypertension
Hypertension with no known cause.

cerebral hemorrhage
A rupture of a blood vessel in the brain.

myocardial infarction
When a part of the heart dies because of a lack of oxygen.

plaque
Debris that clogs coronary arteries.

rupture is in the brain, we call that a **cerebral hemorrhage.** If a coronary artery ruptures, and part of the heart dies from lack of oxygen usually transported to it by the blood, we call that a **myocardial infarction.** Blood can also be prevented from reaching its destination by a blockage of the blood vessels or a narrowing of the vessels by debris (**plaque**) collecting on their inner walls.

Since blood pressure, as well as serum cholesterol, increases during stress (plaque is made up of cholesterol), the relationship between stress and hypertension has long been suspected. Emotional stress is generally regarded as a major factor in the etiology of hypertension.[35] Recognizing this relationship, educational programs for hypertensives have included stress management.[36,37] Although hypertension can be controlled with medication, the possibility of disturbing side effects from these drugs has led to attempts to control hypertension in other ways. Since obesity, cigarette smoking, and lack of exercise are correlates to hypertension, programs involving weight control, smoking withdrawal, and exercise, as well as decreased ingestion of salt, have all been used to respond to high blood pressure.

Stress management has also been employed to control high blood pressure. Unfortunately, too many health care providers tell a hypertensive person that he or she needs to "relax" without providing instruction in how to do so. A notable exception is Dr. Herbert Benson, a cardiologist who has used meditation to reduce blood pressure in hypertensive patients. His patients are instructed in how to meditate and do so in the clinical setting with instructions to meditate between hospital visits. Described in his books *The Relaxation Response,*[38] *Beyond the Relaxation Response,*[39] *Timeless Healing,*[40] and *The Wellness Book,*[41] Dr. Benson's technique has been quite successful.[42]

Further evidence of the relationship between stress and essential hypertension appears in the classic study of 1,600 hospital patients by Flanders Dunbar in the 1940s.[43] Dunbar found that certain personality traits were characteristic of hypertensive patients. For example, they were easily upset by criticism or imperfection, possessed pent-up anger, and lacked self-confidence. One can readily see the role stress might play in "setting off" these susceptible people.

Stroke

apoplexy
A lack of oxygen to the brain resulting from a blockage or rupture of a blood vessel; also called stroke.

stroke
A lack of oxygen to the brain resulting from a blockage or rupture of a blood vessel; also called apoplexy.

Apoplexy (also termed **stroke**) is a lack of oxygen in the brain resulting from a blockage or rupture of one of the arteries that supply it. Depending on the exact location of the brain tissue dying from this lack of oxygen and the amount of time oxygen was denied, paralysis, speech impairment, motor-function impairment, or death may result. Signs and symptoms of stroke are:

- *Trouble with walking:* stumbling or sudden dizziness, loss of balance, or loss of coordination.
- *Trouble with speaking:* slurred speech or not being able to come up with words to explain what is happening (aphasia).
- *Paralysis or numbness on one side of the body:* sudden numbness, weakness, or paralysis on one side of the body.
- *Trouble with seeing:* blurred or blackened vision, or seeing double.
- *Headache:* sudden, severe, or an unusual headache, which may be accompanied by a stiff neck, facial pain, pain between the eyes, vomiting, or altered consciousness.

For most people, a stroke gives no warning. But one possible sign of an impending stroke is a transient ischemic attack (TIA). A TIA is a temporary interruption of blood flow to a part of the brain. The signs and symptoms of TIA are the same as for a stroke, but they last for a shorter period—several minutes to 24 hours—and then disappear, without leaving apparent permanent effects. Some people may have more than one TIA, and the recurrent signs and symptoms may be similar or different. A TIA may indicate that you're at risk of a full-blown stroke. People who have had a TIA are much more likely to have a stroke than are those who haven't had a TIA.[44]

Stroke is related to hypertension, which may also result in a cerebral hemorrhage (rupture of a major blood vessel supplying the brain). Cardiovascular disorders, of which apoplexy is one, kill more Americans each year than any other disorder. Stroke has been related to high blood pressure, diet, and stress.[45]

Coronary Heart Disease

Heart attacks kill more Americans than any other single cause of death. That stress is related to coronary heart disease is not surprising when we consider the physiological mechanisms that stress brings into play: accelerated heart rate, increased blood pressure, increased serum cholesterol, and fluid retention resulting in increased blood volume. Further, the stereotypical heart attack victim has been the highly stressed, overworked, overweight businessman with a cigarette dangling from his lips and a martini in his hand.

Coronary heart disease has been associated with diets high in saturated fats, a lack of exercise, obesity, heredity, and even maleness and baldness. However, the three major risk factors generally agreed to be most associated with coronary heart disease are *hypercholesterolemia* (high serum cholesterol), hypertension, and cigarette smoking; and yet, two researchers state:

> Largely unquestioned, however, has been the repeated finding that these factors are completely absent in more than half of all the new cases of coronary heart disease encountered in clinical practice. Indeed, most patients do not have high blood cholesterol, and only a fraction have high blood pressure. Data from pooled prospective studies in the United States actually show that of men with two or more of these alleged risks, only about 10 percent develop coronary heart disease over a ten-year period, while the remainder do not. . . . Almost twenty years ago we discovered that young coronary patients could be differentiated from healthy control subjects far more readily by the dimensions of occupational stress than by differences in heredity, diet, obesity, tobacco consumption, or exercise. In our study it was found that at the time of their attack 91 percent of 100 patients as compared with only 20 percent of healthy controls had been holding down two or more jobs, working more than sixty hours per week, or experiencing unusual insecurity, discontent, or frustration in relation to employment.[46]

Those researchers go on to present data from studies in which various professionals ranked the specialties within their professions by stress level. Next, the prevalence of coronary heart disease by specialty was determined. The more stressful the specialty, the more prevalent was coronary heart disease. For example, within the practice of medicine, dermatology was found to be the least stressful specialty and the general medical practice the most stressful. Consistent with the theory that stress is related to coronary heart disease, dermatologists had a lower prevalence of heart disease than general practitioners during their younger years (40–49) as well as later in life (60–69). Similarly, periodontists were the least stressed of the dentists, with general practitioner dentists being the most stressed. As with the physicians, the least stressed dentists (periodontists) had a lower prevalence of coronary heart disease than the most stressed dentists (the general practitioners). The same held true for attorneys. The least stressed (patent attorneys) had the lowest prevalence of coronary heart disease, and the most stressed (the general practice attorneys who handle a variety of cases) had the highest rate of coronary heart disease. When we add to this our knowledge that heart attack deaths for men in the United States are most prevalent on Mondays and least prevalent on Fridays, we can consider stress in general, and occupational stress in particular, a major cause of coronary heart disease.

Further evidence of the relationship between stress and coronary heart disease was presented in the studies of Meyer Friedman and Ray Rosenman. These two cardiologists and their work are discussed in more detail in Chapter 8. For purposes of this discussion, suffice it to say that Friedman and Rosenman identified a **Type A** behavior pattern disproportionately represented among heart attack patients. These patients were aggressive, competitive, time-urgent, and hostile; often found themselves doing things

Type A
A behavior pattern associated with the development of coronary heart disease.

quickly; were overly concerned with numbers (quantity rather than quality); and often did more than one thing at a time (e.g., read the newspaper over breakfast).[47] A comprehensive review of studies of the Type A behavior pattern has verified the relationship between these stress-related behaviors and coronary heart disease;[48] however, other researchers have found conflicting results, some finding hostility to be the prime culprit.[49] We discuss the Type A behavior pattern in greater detail in Chapter 8.

The physiological mechanisms that appear to lead from chronic stress down the road to coronary heart disease seem to be related to the increased serum cholesterol, blood pressure, blood volume, and accelerated heart rate associated with stress reactivity. The last three make the heart work harder, and the first (hypercholesterolemia) leads to clogging of arteries (**atherosclerosis**) and eventual loss of elasticity of the coronary and other arteries (**arteriosclerosis**). Both of these conditions also result in an excessive workload for the heart muscle, as well as a decreased supply of oxygen to the heart itself. Not to be disregarded, however, is the interaction between other coronary risk factors and stress. One might expect a person who is overstressed not to have time to exercise, to overeat as a reward for "hard work," or to smoke cigarettes to relax (actually, nicotine is physiologically a stimulant). Consequently, the negative effects of stress upon the heart are often multiplied by the introduction of other heart-damaging behaviors.

Another physiological mechanism explaining the relationship between stress and coronary heart disease relates to production of plasma homocysteine. Homocysteine is an amino acid formed during the metabolism of plasma methionine, an amino acid derived from dietary proteins. Increased levels of homocysteine have been associated with an increased risk of coronary heart disease.[50] In a study of the effects of anger and hostility on homocysteine levels, Stoney[51] found a positive association between these variables. As anger and hostility increased, so did the level of homocysteine in the blood. Stoney concluded that "it is possible that one mechanism for the increased risk of CHD as a function of psychological stress is through a stress-associated elevation in homocysteine."[52]

Other researchers have found additional factors explaining the relationship between stress and coronary heart disease. For example, Everson and her colleagues found stress to exacerbate the effects of socioeconomic status on carotid artery atherosclerosis.[53] As one stress investigator put it:

> . . . low SES may have indirect influence on lipid and hemostatic profiles through smoking and lack of exercise. For example, the neuroendocrine response to a stressful psychosocial environment may be determined by the person's cognitive appraisal of the severity of environmental demands in relation to his or her own coping resources. A lack of balance between demands (e.g., job stress) and buffering resources (e.g., social network) evokes negative emotions (such as hopelessness). Negative emotions may lead to smoking, lack of exercise, and poor diet, which may in part be reflected by obesity and poor lipid and hemostatic profiles. Another hypothesis is that psychosocial stress may have direct effects on physiological systems independent of effects on health behaviors. For example, psychosocial stress may result in pathogenic physiological mechanisms, through nervous and endocrine processes. Stress hormones, including catecholamines, have pronounced effects on hemodynamics, lipid metabolism, hemostasis, and other aspects of metabolism.[54]

Hostility may be one of these psychosocial stressors changing physiological mechanisms resulting in heart disease. A study by Iribarren and his colleagues demonstrated a two times greater prevalence in coronary calcification in young adult subjects who scored above the median in hostility.[55] Iribarren concludes that "Our results are consistent with the hypothesis that hostility might contribute to the development of coronary atherosclerosis not only through poor health habits . . . but via other physiological mechanisms." He then goes on to cite some possible physiological mechanisms such as cardiovascular reactivity, blood pressure morning surge, increased platelet activation, increased catecholamine levels, and prolonged neuroendocrine responses.

atherosclerosis
Clogging of the coronary arteries.

arteriosclerosis
Loss of elasticity of the coronary arteries.

Characteristics of Cardiac Muscle

Cardiac muscle has some unique characteristics. One such characteristic is larger diameter *transverse tubules* (T tubules) than other striated muscle. The wider tubules result in a slow onset of contraction and a prolonged contraction phase not characteristic of other striated muscle. In addition, calcium enters cardiac muscle from the T tubules and from outside the muscle fibers. Calcium affects cardiac contraction rhythm and is more slowly diffused in cardiac muscle than in other muscle tissue. That is why some patients are prescribed medications called calcium channel blockers to decrease the affects of calcium on heart muscle contractions.

Another important difference between cardiac muscle and other striated muscle relates to *Adenosine triphosphate* (ATP). ATP provides the energy for the heart to contract, but ATP production depends on an adequate supply of oxygen. Not enough oxygen means not enough ATP. That is why cardiac muscle cannot develop a large oxygen debt as can other muscles. Development of a large oxygen debt, which could be caused by a blockage of blood vessels to the heart, would result in muscular fatigue and a cessation of heart contractions. That is why patients who have blocked coronary arteries need to have those arteries either opened (*angioplasty*) or bypassed (*coronary bypass surgery*) in order for adequate oxygen to be supplied to the cardiac muscle.

Another physiological mechanism that researchers have found related to stress and coronary heart disease pertains to the heart's rhythm. McCraty and colleagues conducted studies of the variability in heart rhythm and concluded that it is modified by the autonomic nervous system and emotional state. The heart beats faster and less rhythmically during stress and "when a person is in a state of deep peace and inner harmony the heart shifts to a very regular and coherent rhythm."[56]

Ulcers

Ulcers are fissures or cuts in the wall of the stomach, duodenum, or other parts of the intestines. Over 15 million American adults have been diagnosed with ulcers. That is almost 7 percent of the population.[57] For many years, it was thought that stress led to the production of excessive amounts of hydrochloric acid in the stomach and the intestines. There was ample evidence for this conclusion. Selye reported that ulcers developed in the stomach and duodenum of rats exposed to stress.[58] When studying grief reactions, Lindemann reported 33 out of 41 ulcer patients "developed their disease in close relationship to the loss of an important person."[59] Others have noted a sense of utter helplessness among ulcer patients and believe this feeling preceded, rather than resulted from, the development of ulcers.

One theory explaining the effects of stress on the development of ulcers pertains to the mucous coating that lines the stomach. The theory states that, during chronic stress, norepinephrine secretion causes capillaries in the stomach lining to constrict. This, in turn, results in a shutting down of mucosal production, and the mucous protective barrier for the stomach wall is lost. Without the protective barrier, hydrochloric acid breaks down the tissue and can even reach blood vessels, resulting in a bleeding ulcer.

However, it has since been discovered that many cases of ulcers—in particular, peptic ulcers—are caused by a bacteria called *Helicobacter pylori* (or *H. pylori*). Although the exact mechanism by which it causes ulcers is unknown, it is believed that *H. pylori* inflames the gastrointestinal lining, stimulates acid production, or both. A panel convened by the National Institutes of Health has advised doctors to treat ulcers with a two-week course of antibiotics in combination with nonprescription bismuth. This is in contrast to the long-standing treatment by costly drugs used to block acid secretion. These drugs—called histamine blockers, or H2 blockers, such as Tagamet, Zantac, and Pepcid—are no longer deemed necessary in many ulcer cases, although they are still helpful when ulcers are caused by something other than *H. pylori*.

Another major cause of ulcers is the ingestion of aspirin and other nonsteroidal anti-inflammatory drugs (*ibuprofen* such as in brand names Advil, Motrin, and Nuprin; *naproxen* such as in the brand name Naprosyn; and *piroxicam* such as in the brand name Feldene). These drugs promote bleeding in the stomach and can wear away its protective lining.

Still, stress can exacerbate the conditions in the digestive tract to make ulcers more likely to occur. Stress results in an increase in hydrochloric acid in the intestinal tract and stomach, and a decreased effectiveness of the immunological system that is marshaled to combat the invasion by *H. pylori*.

Migraine Headaches

Terry was a very busy and productive woman. She had two adorable boys and an equally adorable dentist husband (whom the boys greatly resembled). Because she felt her roles as mother and wife were not fulfilling enough, and because she had a special talent, Terry painted most afternoons and eventually entered a master's degree program in art. She did so well in her graduate work that, upon the awarding of her master's degree, she was asked to join the faculty. All of this wasn't enough, so she served on committees for local museums and civic organizations.

It was clear to everyone but Terry herself that she was doing too much. She had been having headaches. Soon, the headaches came more frequently and became more severe. Many a time Terry's neighbors had to watch her children while her husband drilled teeth and she hibernated in a bedroom darkened by drawn shades, waiting out the migraine. I know because I was one of Terry's neighbors.

Migraine headaches are the result of a constriction and dilation of the carotid arteries of one side of the head. The constriction phase, called the **preattack** or **prodrome,** is often associated with light or noise sensitivity, irritability, and a flushing or pallor of the skin. When the dilation of the arteries occurs, certain chemicals stimulate adjacent nerve endings, causing pain.

Over the years, extreme measures have been taken to treat migraines. Among these "treatments" are tiny holes bored into the skull, bleeding of the scalp, and the ingestion of mercury (which cured the headache by killing the patient). English physicians even applied a mixture of dried houseflies and hot vinegar to the scalp and, when blisters appeared, punctured them in the hopes of finding an outlet for the pain.

The migraine is not just a severe headache. It is a unique type of headache with special characteristics, and it usually involves just one side of the head. The prodrome consists of warning signs, such as flashing lights, differing patterns, or some dark spaces. The prodrome usually occurs one or two hours prior to the headache itself. The actual headache usually involves a throbbing pain that lasts approximately six hours (although this varies greatly from person to person). An interesting point about migraine attacks is that they usually occur after a pressure-packed situation is over, rather than when the pressure is being experienced. Consequently, attacks often occur on weekends. Many of Terry's weekends were spent waiting out a migraine.

Migraines are quite prevalent. In 2004, the percentage of U.S. adults who experienced a severe headache or migraine during the preceding three months decreased with age, from 18 percent among persons aged 18 to 44 years to 6 percent among persons aged 75 years or older. In every age group, the proportion of women who experienced severe headache or migraine was greater than that of men.[60] Approximately

preattack
Synonymous with prodrome.

prodrome
The constriction phase of a migraine headache; also called preattack.

30 million Americans have one or more migraines a year.[61] Migraine is also common worldwide. Prevalence has been reported to be between 5 and 25 percent in women and 2 and 10 percent in men.[62] Migraines can also be quite costly to employers when their workers are prone to them. It is estimated that migraines cost businesses $24 billion a year.[63]

Diet may precipitate migraine headaches for some people. Chocolate, aged cheese, and red wine are implicated culprits. However, predominant thought on the cause of migraine focuses on emotional stress and tension. People often have migraines during times of increased emotional or physical stress.[64]

Although migraines most often occur between the ages of 16 and 35 and are greatly reduced in frequency by age 50, migraine sufferers aren't willing to wait years for relief. Medications of various sorts are available for migraine sufferers, most of which contain ergotamine tartrate and are taken during the prodrome to constrict the carotid arteries. Migraine medication, however, may produce side effects: weakness in the legs, muscle pain, numbness, and heart-rate irregularity.

Other relief that does not produce disturbing side effects is available to sufferers of migraine headaches. Since the major problem is the dilation of blood vessels in the head, any method of preventing an increased blood flow to the head would help prevent or treat migraine. Relaxation techniques that are discussed later in this book (biofeedback, meditation, and autogenic training) result in an increased blood flow in the peripheral blood system (arms and legs). This increased flow comes from several areas, of which the head is one. As you might imagine, these techniques have been found successful in the prevention and treatment of migraine.[65]

An important point needs to be made here. Migraines are a sign and symptom of a lifestyle gone awry. Treating signs and symptoms with either medication or meditation without eliminating the underlying cause (one's lifestyle) is probably not the best strategy. Rather than care for the migraine after it occurs or during the prodrome, why not prevent it in the first place by changing your lifestyle? Help in doing that is available in subsequent chapters of this book.

Tension Headaches

Headaches are serious business—yes, business. Not only do many pharmaceutical companies and health care providers make a good deal of money treating headache sufferers, but businesses also suffer their consequences. Pain from headaches can affect a worker's ability to do physical work (e.g., lift, walk, or even sit) and his or her cognitive work performance (e.g., ability to think, concentrate, or effectively interact with others). One study found that 36 percent of people who suffered from moderate to severe headache pain were unable to obtain or keep full-time work at some time during the three-year study period.[66]

Headaches may be caused by muscle tension accompanying stress. This muscle tension may affect the forehead, jaw, or neck. I'm often amazed at the numbers of students who come to my classes, especially the early or late evening ones, with tension headaches. Perhaps a whole day of work or school is the instigator, but we all have control over our own muscles. If we only knew how to relax them prior to the onset of a tension headache! Once the headache occurs, it tends to fuel itself. It is difficult to relax when you're in pain.

Treatment for tension headaches may include medication (aspirin or a tranquilizer), heat on tense muscles, or massage. However, just as I'm amazed at the number of students entering my classes with tension headaches, I'm also amazed (actually, I've long since stopped being amazed about the potency of stress management) at the numbers of students who leave my classes without headaches when we've been practicing a relaxation technique. Others have also reported on the effectiveness of relaxation training (in particular, biofeedback) for control and prevention of tension headaches.[67-69] As with migraines, however, an ounce of prevention is worth a pound of cure.

Stress can lead to tension headaches, which can be quite debilitating.

Cancer

Although many people do not realize it, both the prevention and the treatment of cancer are suspected of being related to stress. Cancer is really several diseases, some of which may be caused by ingested **carcinogens** (cancer-causing agents), some by inhaled carcinogens (in the environment or in cigarette smoke), and some by viruses. In any case, cancer is the unbridled multiplication of cells that leads to tumors and, eventually, organ damage.

When a viral cancer occurs, the immunological system—particularly its lymphocytesis—is called into play. The number of **T-lymphocytes** that normally destroy mutant cells prior to their multiplying and causing damage is reduced during stress. Consequently, some researchers believe that chronic stress results in a chronic inability of the immune response to prevent the multiplication of mutant cells, which some believe are present but normally controlled in most people.

The role of stress in the development of cancer is still being debated, but because cancer is the second leading cause of death in the United States, research in this area has been and is presently being conducted. Some support has been provided for a cancer-prone personality type. The cancer-prone person has been described as (1) holding resentment, with the inability to forgive; (2) using self-pity; (3) lacking the ability to develop and maintain meaningful interpersonal relationships; and (4) having a poor self-image.[70] The classic study by Lawrence LeShan in the 1950s of the psychological characteristics of cancer patients found that these patients differed from healthy controls. The patients more frequently

1. Reported a lost relationship prior to the cancer diagnosis.
2. Were unable to express hostility in their own defense.
3. Felt unworthy and disliked themselves.
4. Had a tense relationship with one or both parents.[71]

More recent studies, though, have not found an association between personality and the development of cancer or the effectiveness in treating cancer.[72-74] Consequently, this remains an area of some controversy.

Even the treatment of cancer has included the recognition that the mind can affect the body. Cancer patients have been taught to imagine the T-lymphocytes attacking the cancerous cells. These visualization skills and other relaxation techniques are utilized because it seems sensible to conclude that if T-lymphocytes are decreased during the stress response, they will be increased during the relaxation response. The immunological system will then be more potent in controlling the cancerous cells. It should be recognized, however, that this type of treatment for cancer is controversial and experimental. Further, visualization therapy always includes more treatment modalities as well—for example, X-ray, chemical, and surgical methods.

Allergies, Asthma, and Hay Fever

Allergies—asthma and hay fever are but two examples—are the body's defense against a foreign, irritating substance called an **antigen**. In response to this antigen, the body produces **antibodies**. Among their other functions, antibodies stimulate the release of chemicals. Histamine, one of these chemicals, causes tissues to swell, mucous secretions to increase, and air passages in the lungs to constrict. Now you know why the drug of choice for allergy sufferers is an antihistamine.

Some medical scientists, unable to identify any antigen in many asthmatics, have argued that allergies are emotional diseases. Supporting this theory is the result of an experiment in which a woman who was allergic to horses began to

carcinogens
Cancer-causing agents.

T-lymphocytes
A part of the immune system that destroys mutant cells.

antigen
A foreign substance irritating to the body.

antibodies
Substances produced by the body to fight antigens.

Figure 3.1

Stress and the immune response.

wheeze when shown only a picture of a horse; another woman who was allergic to fish had an allergic reaction to a toy fish and empty fishbowl; and others reacted to uncontaminated air when suspecting it contained pollen.[75]

In support of the relationship between emotional factors (in particular, stress) and allergic reactions, recall the decrease in the effectiveness of the immunological system discussed previously. The reduced number of T-lymphocytes that results during stress means decreased effectiveness in controlling antigens, since it is these T-cells that destroy the antigens (either by direct contact or by secreting toxins). Further, we know that the cortisol secreted by the adrenal cortex during the stress response decreases the effectiveness of histamine.

Some have concluded, therefore, that the effects of stress on the immunological system either decrease our ability to withstand an antigen (meaning a decreased allergic threshold) or, even in the absence of an antigen, can lead to an allergiclike response (see Figure 3.1). Some allergy sufferers—in particular, asthmatics—are being taught relaxation techniques and breathing-control exercises to enable them to control their physiology during allergic reactions. As you will learn in the next chapter, such an approach to stress management is incomplete if it doesn't also include adjustments in the life situation to avoid stressors in the first place or change our perceptions of the stressors we encounter.

Rheumatoid Arthritis

Rheumatoid arthritis afflicts a large number of U.S. citizens (three times as many women as men) with inflammation and swelling in various body joints, which may proceed developmentally to be extremely painful and debilitating. The exact cause of this condition is unknown, though it is suspected of being related to the faulty functioning of the immune response.

The normal joint is lined with a synovial membrane, which secretes fluid to lubricate the joint. In rheumatoid arthritis, this synovial membrane multiplies exceedingly fast and creates swelling. This swelling can cause the membrane to enter the joint itself, eventually to deteriorate the cartilage covering the ends of the bones, and perhaps even to erode the bone itself. The last stages of this disease process may be the development of scar tissue that immobilizes the joint and makes for knobbiness and deformity. The beginning of rheumatoid arthritis may be an infection of the synovial cells. For some reason, antibodies produced to fight this infection may attack healthy as well as unhealthy cells, leading to multiplication to replace the healthy cells. Then the process described above occurs.

It also appears that some people are hereditarily susceptible to rheumatoid arthritis. Approximately half of the sufferers of this condition have a blood protein called the **rheumatoid factor,** which is rare in nonarthritic people.

Since rheumatoid arthritis involves the body's turning on itself (an **autoimmune response**), it was hypothesized that a self-destructive personality may manifest itself through this disease. Although the evidence to support this hypothesis is not conclusive, several investigators have found personality differences between rheumatoid arthritis sufferers and others. Those afflicted with this disease have been found to be perfectionists who are self-sacrificing, masochistic, self-conscious, shy, and inhibited. It has been suggested that people with the rheumatoid factor who experience chronic stress become susceptible to rheumatoid arthritis.[76] Their immunological system malfunctions, and their genetic predisposition to rheumatoid arthritis results in their developing the condition. We know, for instance, that stress can precipitate arthritic attacks. Because the standard treatment of cortisone brings with it the possible side effects of brittle bones, fat deposits, loss of muscular strength, ulcers, and psychosis, it would be very significant if stress management techniques were found to be effective in reducing the amount of cortisone needed.

Backache

The National Institutes of Health reports that back pain affects an estimated 80 percent of people. They describe back pain as one of society's most common medical problems.[77] Like headaches, backaches affect people's abilities to do physical and cognitive work. Stang and his colleagues found that 48 percent of people who suffered from moderate-to-severe back pain were unable to obtain or keep full-time work at some time during the three-year study period.[78] The estimated annual cost of Workmen's Compensation insurance for back pain is $20 billion to $50 billion.[79] Lumbar back injuries result in approximately 149 million lost work days per year.[80] Millions of people suffer backache and erroneously bemoan their posture or jobs. Certainly, backache may result from lifting a heavy object incorrectly or from structural problems.[81] The vast majority of backache problems, however, are the result of muscular weakness or muscular bracing.

As with tension headaches, bracing causes muscle to lose its elasticity and fatigue easily. Bracing may lead to muscle spasms and back pain. This constant muscular contraction is found in people who are competitive, angry, and apprehensive. Backaches have been found more frequently in people who have experienced a good deal of stress.[82] For example, 100 people with lower back pain

---

rheumatoid factor

A blood protein associated with rheumatoid arthritis.

autoimmune response

A physiological response in which the body turns on itself.

were studied for five years.[83] At the conclusion of the five years, the researchers concluded that psychosocial factors contributed more to subjects' back pain than did structural factors. Other researchers found that nursing students with significant low back pain had higher stress scores than other students.[84] These findings pertain to populations in other countries as well. For example, 1,600 employees in six hospitals in Turkey were studied for nine months.[85] Perceived work stress was found to be a statistically significant risk factor for low back pain. In delving further into the relationship between stress and back pain, researchers have consistently found that mental distress and depression are associated with low back pain.[86,87] An explanation for this relationship was offered in a summary of related research.[88] This summary reports on an early study in which workers who reported such signs of stress as dissatisfaction, worry, and fatigue were more likely to experience back pain than those who had physical stressors such as a lot of lifting. Workers who had higher stress levels tended to lift objects more quickly and used their back muscles in a way that made them susceptible to injury.

TMJ Syndrome

The temporomandibular joint, which connects the upper to the lower jaw, is a complex structure requiring the coordination of five muscles and several ligaments. When something interferes with the smooth operation of this joint, **temporomandibular (TMJ) syndrome** may develop (see Figure 3.2). TMJ syndrome sufferers may have facial pain, clicking or popping sounds when they open or close their mouths, migraine headaches, earaches, ringing in the ears, dizziness, or sensitive teeth. It is most often women between the ages of 20 and 40 who develop TMJ syndrome, although estimates vary widely as to how many in the population experience this condition (from 28 percent to 86 percent—obviously, it is difficult to diagnose). TMJ syndrome has many causes. It can develop as a result of malocclusion of the teeth, a blow to the head, gum chewing, nail biting, or jaw jutting. However, the most common cause is clenching or grinding of the teeth (termed *bruxism*) due to stress.[89] Treatment often consists of wearing an acrylic mouthpiece (an orthodontic splint)—either 24 hours a day or only while asleep—the dentist adjusting the bite by selectively grinding the teeth, using crowns and bridges, or orthodontia. In addition, stress reduction techniques such as biofeedback are taught to TMJ sufferers to relax the jaw and to limit teeth grinding (especially when done during the waking hours).[90]

temporomandibular (TMJ) syndrome
The interference with the smooth functioning of the jaw.

Figure 3.2

The disc separating the bones of the temporomandibular joint may pop loose, causing discomfort. Grinding the teeth as a result of stress can also lead to muscular pain and/or misalignment of the upper and lower jawbones.

It seems clear from the research literature that illness and disease may be stress related. Such conditions as TMJ syndrome, hypertension, stroke, heart disease, ulcers, migraines, tension headaches, cancer, allergies, asthma, hay fever, rheumatoid arthritis, and backache may develop because the body has changed its physiology because of what the mind has experienced. Recognizing the vast physiological changes associated with the stress response, it should not be surprising that poor health can result from stress. Likewise, that poor health is itself stressful and further aggravates the condition is only common sense. The conclusion that can be drawn from all of this is that managing stress can help prevent disease and illness and can be a valuable adjunct to therapy once they have developed. The wonders of the mind-body relationship are only beginning to be realized. The fruits of this knowledge are only beginning to be harvested. There are, though, some insights that you can use immediately to improve the quality of your life. These are presented in Part 2 of this book.

Obesity

Obesity is defined as a body mass index (see Chapter 6) of 30 or higher.[91] A molecule called neuropeptide Y (NPY) has been shown to increase angiogenesis (the growth of the blood vessels) necessary to support new tissue growth.[92] We also know that NPY is released from certain nerve cells during stress. Other research has also shown that NPY and its receptors seem to play a role in appetite and obesity. Putting these results together, it was thought that NPY might be involved in new fat growth during stressful situations. Consequently, researchers tested the effects of chronic stress on fat growth in mice. They compared the effects of stress when the mice were fed a normal diet and when they were fed a diet high in fat and sugar to reflect the comfort foods many people eat when they're stressed.

These researchers found that stress (in the form of making the mice stand in cold water or exposing them to an aggressive mouse for 10 minutes a day) led to the release of NPY from nerves.[93] For the mice eating the normal diet, stress had little effect on body fat. For those mice eating the high–fat and sugar diet, however, stress led to a significant increase in belly fat over a two-week period.

In the presence of the high-fat and sugar diet, the researchers found, abdominal fat produced more NPY along with its receptor, NPY2R. This stimulated angiogenesis (growth of blood vessels) in fat tissue and the proliferation of fat cells, resulting in more belly fat. Eventually, after three months of stress and a high-fat and sugar diet, the mice developed a metabolic syndrome-like condition. Metabolic syndrome in people is linked to abdominal obesity and increases the chance of developing heart disease, diabetes, and other health problems.

The researchers then tested whether they could use NPY to manipulate fat levels. They put a pellet under the animals' skin that released NPY over a period of 14 days. The pellet increased the amount of fat tissue in both genetically obese and genetically lean mice by 50 percent. By contrast, injections with a molecule that blocks NPY2R decreased the amount of fat tissue in both obese and lean mice by 50 percent. The NPY2R-blocking molecule, the researchers found, decreased the number of blood vessels and fat cells in abdominal fat pads. NPY, then, acting through NPY2R, stimulates angiogenesis and fat tissue growth.

The researchers showed that NPY and its receptor also play a role in the growth of human fat cells. One of the leading experts in the study of the link between stress and obesity is "hopeful that these findings might eventually lead to the control of metabolic syndrome, which is a huge health issue for many Americans."[94] It seems that managing stress would have to be a central component of any such effort.

Current Research in Complementary and Alternative Medicine

In 1993, Congress created the Office of Alternative Medicine within the National Institutes of Health to explore the value of unconventional modalities in the treatment of illness and disease. The rationale behind funding such an office was related to the large number of Americans who were turning to these treatments. The government decided to fund the testing of these unconventional medical treatments to provide guidance regarding which ones were effective and which were a waste of money or, worse, unsafe. In 2007, approximately 38 percent of Americans used these forms of therapy. In recognition of this increasing trend, the government elevated the office, creating the National Center for Complementary and Alternative Medicine (NCCAM). In 2008, the NCCAM reported:

- Between 2002 and 2007, the use of acupuncture, deep breathing exercises, massage therapy, meditation, naturopathy, and yoga increased.

- American Indians and Alaska Natives (50 percent) and white adults (43 percent) were more likely to use CAM than Asian Americans (40 percent), African Americans (26 percent), or Hispanics (24 percent).

- CAM methods were used for a variety of reasons: to treat back pain or back problems, head or chest colds, neck pain and neck problems, joint pain or stiffness, and anxiety and depression.

- CAM use was more prevalent among women than men.

- Adult CAM users had higher educational attainment than nonusers.

- CAM users had one or more existing health conditions and made more frequent medical visits than nonusers.

Percent of Americans Who Have Used CAM:

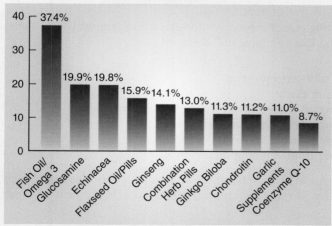

Source: Patricia M. Barnes, Barbara Bloom, and R. L. Nahin, "Complementary and Alternative Medicine Use among Adults and Children: United States, 2007," *CDC National Health Statistics Report*, No.12 (Hyattsville, MD: National Center for Health Statistics, 2008).

Posttraumatic Stress Disorder

Posttraumatic stress disorder (PTSD) is a condition that develops in people who have experienced an extreme psychological or physical event that is interpreted as particularly distressing. The American Psychiatric Association's *Diagnostic and Statistical Manual*, 4th ed.,[95] describes PTSD as involving

1. A threat to one's life or serious injury or being subject to horror with intense fear and helplessness.

2. Recurrent flashbacks, repeated memories and emotions, dreams, nightmares, illusions, or hallucinations related to traumatic events from which one is often amnesic.

PTSD first appeared as a diagnosis in the American Psychiatric Association's *Diagnostic and Statistical Manual* in 1980. The diagnosis was revised in 1987 and appears in the latest version of the *Manual* (1994). The *International Classification of Disease,* published by the World Health Organization, added PTSD in 1992.[96]

Symptoms of PTSD

PTSD can occur at any age, and although we associate PTSD with soldiers returning from war zones, it can be triggered by any number of traumatic events such as assault; domestic abuse; rape; terrorism; or a train, automobile, or airplane accident. Symptoms of PTSD fall into three main categories:[97]

1. "Reliving" the event, which disturbs day-to-day activity.
    *   Flashback episodes, where the event seems to be happening again and again.
    *   Repeated upsetting memories of the event.
    *   Repeated nightmares of the event.
    *   Strong, uncomfortable reactions to situations that remind you of the event.

2. Avoidance
    *   Emotional "numbing," or feeling as though you don't care about anything.
    *   Feeling detached.
    *   Being unable to remember important aspects of the trauma.
    *   Having a lack of interest in normal activities.
    *   Showing less of your moods.
    *   Avoiding places, people, or thoughts that remind you of the event.
    *   Feeling like you have no future.

3. Arousal
    *   Difficulty concentrating.
    *   Startling easily.
    *   Having an exaggerated response to things that startle you.
    *   Feeling more aware (hypervigilance).
    *   Feeling irritable or having outbursts of anger.
    *   Having trouble falling or staying asleep.

Symptoms typical of anxiety, stress, and tension may also occur such as agitation or excitability, dizziness, fainting, feeling the heart beat in one's chest, and headache.

Treatment of PTSD

PTSD affects about 7.7 million American adults in a given year.[98] PTSD is more prevalent than many of us realize. Epidemiologists report that most people will experience a traumatic event and that up to 25 percent of them will develop PTSD.[99,100] Some experts believe PTSD is as prevalent as any other mental disorder, yet only a minority of people obtain treatment.[101] Although the cause of PTSD is not known, a history of mental illness in oneself or one's family seems to increase the likelihood of developing PTSD.[102] Being prone to anxiety attacks or depression also increases this likelihood.[103] However, not everyone who experiences trauma develops posttraumatic stress disorder. Furthermore, if you can anticipate a traumatic event, you can decrease the likelihood of that event's resulting in PTSD. This was demonstrated in a study of 106 British soldiers returning from United Nations peacekeeping duties in the former Yugoslavia.[104] In anticipation of the trauma they would experience, they received an Operational Stress Training Package. As a result, very low rates of PTSD were experienced by these soldiers. The researchers concluded that "a high incidence of psychiatric morbidity is not an inevitable consequence of military conflict."

Among the characteristics of those who have successfully managed PTSD are that they had supportive relationships with family and friends, they did not dwell on the trauma, they had personal faith/religion/hope, and they had a sense of humor.[105]

Treatment consists of several approaches that may include talk therapy, medication, and exposure therapy. The most common *talk therapy* is cognitive behavior therapy, the goal of which is for the patient to perceive the fear more realistically and as less of a threat. *Medications* such as antidepressants (for example, Zoloft and Paxil), anti-anxiety medications, and sleep medicines have also been used to treat PTSD. *Exposure therapy* is designed to expose the patient to the event that precipitated PTSD, in small doses—such as remembering and discussing the event—until the actual event seems less frightening and symptoms subside. Systematic desensitization, discussed in chapter 8, is a form of exposure therapy. With technological advances, *virtual reality exposure therapy,* in which immersive technology

Soldiers returning from war experience post-traumatic stress disorder, but anyone who experiences a traumatic event (such as a rape or car accident) may also have PTSD symptoms.

can recreate a multisensory experience—sight, sound, smell, and touch—in the comfort of a therapist's office, has recently been added to PTSD treatment modalities.

Stress is associated with a variety of psychosocial illnesses besides posttraumatic stress disorder. Anxiety and depression are two of the most common. They are discussed in detail in Chapter 8. However, mention is made of them here so that you are not left with the impression that it is only the physical health consequences of stress with which we need be concerned. In fact, it is nearly impossible to separate physical consequences from psychological or sociological ones. We know this from research involving placebos.

A placebo is a substance that looks like a medication but is not. A placebo has no effect on the condition that a researcher is studying. Still, people who are told that a placebo is a drug that will improve their health often report feeling better. Why? The only explanation is that their minds perceive a benefit and convince their bodies that the substance is working. So it is with many other conditions.

Earlier in this chapter we discussed the relationship between stress, the immune system, and allergies. If we assume that allergies interfere with your ability to be productive at work—not an unrealistic assumption—we have a sociological effect of stress to add to its physical and psychological effects.

Stress and Other Conditions

Stress has been shown to affect other health conditions as well. For example, stress can lead pregnant women to miscarry. In one study, 70 percent of women who had a miscarriage had at least one stressful experience four to five months before the miscarriage, as compared with 52 percent of women who did not have a miscarriage.[106] One explanation for this finding is offered by another researcher who found that women with PTSD entering pregnancy are at increased risk for engaging in high-risk health behaviors, such as smoking, alcohol consumption, substance use, poor prenatal care, and excessive weight gain.[107]

Even sports injuries can be caused by stress.[108] It has been known for some time that sports injuries occur more frequently in athletes who have experienced recent stressors and who do not have the resources and skills to cope well with stress. One explanation for this observation is the stress-injury model first described by Anderson and Williams way back in 1988.[109] According to this model, during sports events that are inherently stressful, the athlete's history of stressors, personality characteristics, and coping resources contribute interactively to the stress response. With high stress and poor coping resources, the result is increased muscle tension and attention redirected toward the stress and away from the event. Anderson and Williams hypothesized that increases in muscle tension, narrowing of the field of vision, and increased distractibility were the primary causes of sports injury.

Anderson and Williams[110] further investigated the causes of athletic injuries and determined that negative life events were the best predictors of injury. Those with the most negative life events had the most injuries. Furthermore, those athletes who had the least social support experienced the most injuries. Interestingly, other researchers[111] found that athletes who were optimistic, had high hardiness scores (see Chapter 8), and had higher self-esteem experienced the fewest injuries. Anxiety has also been found to relate to muscle tension and increased chance of athletic injury.[112] Recognizing that these variables are associated with athletic injury, programs have been developed to intervene in these variables and thereby reduce such injuries. One of these programs involved collegiate soccer players who were trained to feel more confident, to feel less anxious, and to have greater self-esteem, among other variables.[113] This program did indeed prevent injuries. When you are engaging in athletic activities, it would behoove you to use the skills presented in this book to manage anxiety, improve self-esteem, acquire social support, and manage stress. Doing so will lessen your chance of being injured.

Coping in Today's World

Being ill is not funny! Especially if you are a kid. Then why are there so many clowns roaming around hospitals throughout the United States? There they are, dressed in their clown outfits, with bulbous noses and clown makeup. They suddenly appear in sick children's rooms blowing bubbles, singing songs, and showing up with irremovable bandages and invisible strings to pull. At Children's Hospital in Washington, DC, they are members of the *Clown Care Unit,*[a] which originated with the Big Apple Circus in New York in 1986. There are 17 hospitals around the United States that are affiliated with the Clown Care Unit. In these 17 hospitals, there are more than 90 clowns who make 250,000 visits to sick children each year. These clowns are the same ones who perform at children's birthday parties, magic shows, and other such events. Yet, when they are performing in hospitals, the only pay they receive is the reward of knowing they made a child feel better, even if for only a short period of time.

After having read this chapter and learning about the mind-body connection, it should not be surprising that clowns can not only make children feel better but may also be contributing to the health of the children for whom they perform. We would expect positive changes in the immunological system, and in emotional and mental health, when children laugh and forget about their illnesses for a while. What other health benefits do you think result from visits of members of the Clown Care Unit?

Hospitals are always looking for volunteers. Are you interested in offering your services to make children or other patients feel better? Perhaps you can be trained to become a clown. Check with your local hospital if you are interested in helping to alleviate some of the stress experienced by its patients.

[a]"Is There a Clown in the House? The Art of Medical Slapstick." *Washington Post Magazine,* May 9, 2004: 13.

summary

- Psychosomatic disease involves the mind and the body; it is a real disease and not "just in the mind."

- Psychogenic psychosomatic disease is a physical disease caused by emotional stress. There is no invasion of disease-causing microorganisms; the mind changes the physiology so that parts of the body break down.

- Somatogenic psychosomatic disease occurs when the mind increases the body's susceptibility to disease-causing microbes or a natural degenerative process.

- Stress-related diseases include hypertension, stroke, coronary heart disease, ulcers, migraine headaches, tension headaches, cancer, allergies, asthma, hay fever, rheuma-

- toid arthritis, backache, TMJ syndrome, and posttraumatic stress disorder.

- Stress increases blood pressure and serum cholesterol, so it is no surprise that studies have found it associated with hypertension, stroke, and coronary heart disease.

- Stress decreases the effectiveness of the immunological system by decreasing the number of T-lymphocytes. A less effective immunological system is suspected of resulting in allergic reactions, asthma attacks, and even cancer.

- Stress results in increased muscle tension and bracing. It is this phenomenon that is thought to be the cause of tension headaches, backaches, and neck and shoulder pain.

internet resources

NIOSH Safety and Health Topic: Traumatic Incident Stress **www.cdc.gov/niosh/topics/traumaticincident/** *Examines the symptoms of traumatic stress (physical symptoms, cognitive symptoms, emotional symptoms, and behavioral symptoms) and provides recommendations for maintaining health following the incident.*

National Center for Post Traumatic Stress Disorder **www .ptsd.va.gov** *This website provides information on the science, diagnosis, and treatment of PTSD and stress-related disorders.*

Stress Management for Patient and Physician **www.mental health.com/mag1/p51-str.html** *An article that lists 10 practical techniques for reducing stress.*

references

1. M. Bobak and M. Marmot, "East-West Mortality Divide and Its Potential Explanations: Proposed Research Agenda," *British Medical Journal* 312(1996): 421–25.

2. Bruce S. McEwen, "Protective and Damaging Effects of Stress Mediators," *The New England Journal of Medicine* 338(1998): 171–78.

3. M. R. Bhattacharyya and A. Steptoe, "Emotional Triggers of Acute Coronary Syndromes: Strength of Evidence, Biological Processes, and Clinical Implications," *Progress in Cardiovascular Diseases* 49(2007): 353–65.

4. D. S. Krantz, M. B. Olson, J. L. Francis, C. Phankao, C. N. Bairey Merz, G. Sopko, D. A. Vido, L. J. Shaw, D. S. Sheps, C. J. Pepine, and K. A. Matthews, "Anger, Hostility, and Cardiac Symptoms in Women with Suspected Coronary Artery Disease: The Women's Ischemia Syndrome Evaluation (WISE) Study," *Journal of Women's Health* 15(2006): 1214–23.

5. Cleveland Clinic Heart Center, "Angry Young Men Become Angry Old Men—With Heart Attacks," *Health Extra.* November 2002. www.clevelandclinic.org/heartcenter/ pub/guide/prevention/stress/anger.htm

6. Andrews, John. Are heart attacks hate attacks? *activemeditation .com.* undated. Available at: www.activemeditation.com/ Research/MedicalArticles/HeartAttacks.html

7. A. E. Ganesh-Kumar, J. Bienenstock, Edward J. Goetzl, and Michael G. Blennerhassett, *Autonomic Neuroimmunology* (London: Taylor & Francis, 2003).

8. R. Ader, D. L. Felten, and N. Cohen, eds., *Psychoneuro-immunology,* 3rd ed. (San Diego: Academic Press, 2001).

9. Robert Ornstein and David Sobel, *The Healing Brain: A New Perspective on the Brain and Health* (New York: Simon & Schuster, 1987).

10. K. M. Dillon, F. Minchoff, and K. H. Baker, "Positive Emotional States and Enhancement of the Immune System," *International Journal of Psychiatry in Medicine* 15(1985): 13–18.

11. M. Wachiuli, M. Koyama, M. Utsuyama, B. B. Bittman, M. Kitagawa, and K. Hirokawa, "Recreational Music-Making Modulates Natural Killer Cell Activity, Cytokines, and Mood States in Corporate Employees," *Medical Science Monitor* 13(2007): CR57–CR70.

12. D. V. Ah, D. H. Kang, and J. S. Carpenter, "Stress, Optimism, and Social Support: Impact on Immune Responses in Breast Cancer," *Research in Nursing and Health* 30(2007): 72–83.

13. L. Arranz, N. Guayerbas, L. Siboni, and M. De la Fuente, "Effect of Acupuncture Treatment on the Immune Function Impairment Found in Anxious Women," *American Journal of Chinese Medicine* 35(2007): 35–51.

14. Gatt, Justine Megan. The personality-disease link: An evaluation of a predictive personality measure, the mediating mechanisms of the personality-disease link and a preventative intervention. *The University of Sydney, Sydney eScholarship Repository.* 2005. Available at: http://ses.library.usyd.edu.au/handle/2123/915

15. Disease-prone personality. *Mind Body Health.* 2008. Available at: http://byumindbodyhealth.blogspot.com/2008/11/disease-prone-personality.html

16. Howard S. Friedman and Stephanie Booth-Kewley, "The 'Disease-Prone Personality': A Meta-Analytic View of the Construct," *American Psychologist* 42(1987): 539–55.

17. Hans J. Eysenck, "Health's Character," *Psychology Today,* December 1988, 28–35.

18. "Princeton Study: Student Stress Lowers Immunity," *Brain Mind Bulletin* 14(1989): 1, 7.

19. S. Chandrashekara, K. Jayashree, H. B. Veeranna, H. S. Vadiraj, M. N. Ramesh, A. Shobha, Y. Sarvanan, and Y. K. Vikram, "Effects of Anxiety on TNF-Alpha Levels During Psychological Stress," *Journal of Psychosomatic Research* 63(2007): 65–69.

20. Glen Rein, Mike Atkinson, and Rollin McCraty, "The Physiological and Psychological Effects of Compassion and Anger: Part 1 of 2," *Journal of Advancement in Medicine* 8(1995): 87–105.

21. Sally Squires, "The Power of Positive Imagery: Visions to Boost Immunity," *American Health,* July 1987, 56–61.

22. T. Djarova and N. Dube, "Influence of Stressful Life Events on the Onset of Type 1 Diabetes in Childhood," *African Journal of Health Sciences* 5(1998): 190–97.

23. J. K. Kiecolt-Glaser, T. J. Loving, J. R. Stowell, W. B. Malarkey, S. Lemeshow, S. L. Dickenson, and R. Glaser, "Hostile Marital Interactions, Proinflammatory Cytokine Production, and Wound Healing," *Archives of General Psychiatry* 62(2005): 1377–84.

24. M. A. Diego, N. A. Jones, T. Field, M. Hernandez-Reif, S. Schanberg, C. Kuhn, and A. Gonzalez-Garcia, "Maternal Psychological Distress, Prenatal Cortisol, and Fetal Weight," *Psychosomatic Medicine* 68(2006): 747–53.

25. C. A. Paternak, "Molecular Biology of Environmental Stress," *Impact of Science on Society* 41(1991): 49–57.

26. National Library of Medicine, "Hypercholesterolemia," *Genetics Home Reference*, 2009. Available at: http://ghr.nlm.nih.gov/condition=hypercholesterolemia

27. National Heart, Lung and Blood Institute, "How Is High Blood Cholesterol Diagnosed," *High Blood Cholesterol*, 2008. Available at: www.nhlbi.nih.gov/health/dci/Diseases/Hbc/HBC_Diagnosis.html

28. Meyer Friedman, Ray Rosenman, and V. Carroll, "Changes in the Serum Cholesterol and Blood Clotting Time in Men Subjected to Cycle Variation of Occupational Stress," *Circulation* 17(1958): 852–64.

29. R. A. Kloner, S. McDonald, J. Leeka, and W. K. Poole, "Comparison of Total and Cardiovascular Death Rates in the Same City During a Losing Versus Winning Super Bowl Championship," *American Journal of Cardiology* 103(2009): 1647–50.

30. S. R. Govil, G. Weidner, T. Merritt-Worden, and D. Ornish, "Socioeconomic Status and Improvements in Lifestyle, Coronary Risk Factors, and Quality of Life: The Multisite Cardiac Lifestyle Intervention Program," *American Journal of Public Health* 99(2009):1263–70.

31. J. J. Daubenmier, G. Weidner, M. D. Sumner, N. Mendell, T. Merritt-Worden, J. Studley, and D. Ornish, "The Contribution of Changes in Diet, Exercise, and Stress Management to Changes in Coronary Risk in Women and Men in the Multisite Cardiac Lifestyle Intervention Program," *Annals of Behavioral Medicine* 33(2007): 57–68.

32. A. Rozanski, J. A. Blumenthal, K. W. Davidson, P. G. Saab, and L. Kubzansky, "The Epidemiology, Pathophysiology, and Management of Psychosocial Risk Factors in Cardiac Practice: The Emerging Field of Behavioral Cardiology," *Journal of the American College of Cardiology* 45(2005): 637–51.

33. V. M. Figueredo, "The Time Has Come for Physicians to Take Notice: The Impact of Psychosocial Stressors on the Heart," *American Journal of Medicine* 122(2009): 704–12.

34. National Heart, Lung and Blood Institute, "High Blood Cholesterol: What Is Cholesterol?" *High Blood Cholesterol*, 2008. Available at: www.nhlbi.nih.gov/health/dci/Diseases/Hbc/HBC_WhatIs.html

35. Eric R. Braverman, *The Amazing Way to Reverse Heart Disease: Beyond the Hypertension Hype: Why Drugs Are Not the Answer* (North Bergen, NJ: Basic Health Publications, 2004).

36. N. A. Khan, et al., "The 2007 Canadian Hypertension Education Program Recommendations for the Management of Hypertension: Part 2—Therapy," *Canadian Journal of Cardiology* 23(2007): 539–50.

37. G. Y. Yeh, R. B. Davis, and R. S. Phillips, "Use of Complementary Therapies in Patients with Cardiovascular Disease," *American Journal of Cardiology* 98(2006): 673–80.

38. Herbert Benson and Miriam Z. Klipper, *The Relaxation Response* (New York: William Morrow, 2000).

39. Herbert Benson and William Proctor, *Beyond the Relaxation Response* (East Rutherford, NJ: Berkley Publishing Group, 1985).

40. Herbert Benson and Marg Stark, *Timeless Healing: The Power and Biology of Belief* (New York: Simon & Schuster, 1996).

41. Herbert Benson and Eileen M. Stuart, *The Wellness Book: The Comprehensive Guide to Maintaining Health and Treating Stress-Related Illness* (New York: Simon & Schuster, 1992).

42. Ruanne K. Peters, Herbert Benson, and John M. Peters, "Daily Relaxation Response Breaks in a Working Population: II. Effects on Blood Pressure," *American Journal of Public Health* 67(1977): 954–59.

43. Flanders Dunbar, *Psychosomatic Diagnosis* (New York: Harper, 1943).

44. Mayo Clinic Staff, "Stroke: Symptoms," *MayoClinic.com*, 2008. Available at: www.mayoclinic.com/health/stroke/DS00150/DSECTION=symptoms

45. G. L. Bakris, "Current Perspectives on Hypertension and Metabolic Syndrome." *Journal of Managed Care Pharmacy* 13(2007): 3–5.

46. Henry I. Russek and Linda G. Russek, "Is Emotional Stress an Etiological Factor in Coronary Heart Disease?" *Psychosomatics* 17(1976): 63.

47. Meyer Friedman and Ray H. Rosenman, *Type A Behavior and Your Heart* (Greenwich, CT: Fawcett, 1974).

48. Jack Sparacino, "The Type A Behavior Pattern: A Critical Assessment," *Journal of Human Stress* 5(1979): 37–51.

49. J. C. Richards, A. Hof, and M. Alvarenga, "Serum Lipids and Their Relationships with Hostility and Angry Affect and Behaviors in Men," *Health Psychology* 19(2000): 393–98.

50. H. Turhan, A. R. Erbay, A. S. Yasar, A. Bicer, O. Sahin, N. Basar, and E. Yetkin, "Plasma Homocysteine Levels in Patients with Isolated Coronary Artery Ectasia," *International Journal of Cardiology* 104(2005): 158–62.

51. Catherine M. Stoney, "Plasma Homocysteine Levels Increase in Women During Psychological Stress," *Life Sciences* 64(1999): 2359–65.

52. Catherine M. Stoney and Tilmer O. Engebretson, "Plasma Homocysteine Concentrations Are Positively Associated with Hostility and Anger," *Life Sciences* 66(2000): 2267–75.

53. Susan A. Everson, George A. Kaplan, Riitta Salonen, and Jukka T. Salonen, "Does Low Socioeconomic Status Potentiate the Effects of Heightened Cardiovascular Responses to Stress on the Progression of Carotid Atherosclerosis?" *American Journal of Public Health* 88(1998): 389–94.

54. Sarah P. Wamala, Murray A. Mittleman, Karen Schenck-Gustafson, and Kristina Orth-Gomer, "Potential Explanations for the Educational Gradient in Coronary Heart Disease: A Population-Based Case-Control Study of Swedish Women," *American Journal of Public Health* 89(1999): 315–21.

55. Carlos Iribarren, Stephen Sidney, Diane E. Bild, Kiang Liu, Jerome H. Markovitz, Jeffrey M. Roseman, and Karen Matthews, "Association of Hostility with Coronary Artery Calcification in Young Adults," *Journal of the American Medical Association* 283(2000): 2546–51.

56. Rollin McCraty, Mike Atkinson, and William A. Tiller, "New Electrophysiological Correlates Associated with Intentional Heart Focus," *Subtle Energies* 4(1995): 251–62.

57. Centers for Disease Control and Prevention, *Summary Health Statistics for U.S. Adults: National Health Interview Survey, 2005* (Atlanta, GA: Centers for Disease Control and Prevention, 2006, tables 7, 8).

58. Hans Selye, *The Stress of Life* (New York: McGraw-Hill, 1956).

59. Erich Lindemann, "Symptomatology and Management of Acute Grief," in *Stress and Coping: An Anthology,* Alan Monet and Richard S. Lazarus, eds. (New York: Columbia University Press, 1977), 342.

60. "QuickStats: Percentage of Persons Aged ≥ 18 Years Reporting Severe Headache or Migraine During the Preceding 3 Months, by Sex and Age Group—United States, 2004," *Morbidity and Mortality Weekly Report* 55(2006): 77.

61. Chawla, Jasvinder, et al. Migraine headache. *Medscape.* 2011. Available at: http://emedicine.medscape.com/article/1142556-overview

62. Luis E. Morillo, "Migraine Headache," *American Family Physician*, May 2002. Available at: www.aafp.org/afp/20020501/british.html

63. Thomson Medstat, The Thomson Corporation, "New Data Estimate Migraine Headaches Cost U.S. Employers More Than $24 Billion Annually," Press Release, June 27, 2006. Available at: www.medstat.com/news/newsdetail.aspx?id=545

64. United States Department of Health and Human Services. "Migraine: Frequently Asked Questions," Womenshealth.gov.2008. Available at: www.womenshealth.gov/faq/migraine.cfm#c

65. P. S. Sandor and J. Afra, "Nonpharmacologic Treatment of Migraine," *Current Pain and Headache Report* 9(2005): 202–5.

66. Paul Stang, Michael Von Korff, and Bradley S. Galer, "Reduced Labor Force Participation Among Primary Care Patients with Headache," *Journal of General Internal Medicine* 13(1998): 296–302.

67. N. Kanji, A. R. White, and E. Ernst, "Autogenic Training for Tension Type Headaches: A Systematic Review of Controlled Trials," *Complementary Therapies in Medicine* 14(2006): 144–50.

68. D. M. Biondi, "Physical Treatments for Headache: A Structured Review," *Headache* 45(2005): 738–46.

69. B. Larsson, J. Carlsson, A. Fichtel, and L. Melin, "Relaxation Treatment of Adolescent Headache Sufferers: Results from a School-Based Replication Series," *Headache* 45(2005): 692–704.

70. Carl O. Simonton and Stephanie Simonton, "Belief Systems and Management of the Emotional Aspects of Malignancy," *Journal of Transpersonal Psychology* 7(1975): 29–48.

71. Lawrence LeShan and R. E. Worthington, "Some Recurrent Life-History Patterns Observed in Patients with Malignant Disease," *Journal of Nervous and Mental Disorders* 124(1956): 460–65.

72. N. Nakaya, Y. Tsubono, T. Hosokawa, Y. Nishino, T. Ohkubo, A. Hozawa, D. Shibuya, S. Fukudo, A. Fukao, I. Tsuji, and S. Hisamichi, "Personality and the Risk of Cancer," *Journal of the National Cancer Institute* 95(2003): 1638.

73. M. A. Price, C. C. Tennant, R. C. Smith, P. N. Butow, S. J. Kennedy, M. B. Kossoff, and S. M. Dunn, "The Role of

Psychosocial Factors in the Development of Breast Carcinoma: Part I. The Cancer Prone Personality," *Cancer* 91(2001): 679–85.

74. Hyphantis, T., Paika, V., Almyroudi, A., Kampletsas, E. O., and Pavlidis, N. Personality variables as predictors of early non-metastatic colorectal cancer patients' psychological distress and health-related quality of life: a one-year prospective study. *Journal of Psychosomatic Research* 270(2011): 411–21.

75. Walter McQuade and Ann Aikman, *Stress* (New York: Bantam Books, 1974), 69.

76. R. Geenen, H. Van Middendorp, and J. W. Bijlsma, "The Impact of Stressors on Health Status and Hypothalamic-Pituitary-Adrenal Axis and Autonomic Nervous System Responsiveness in Rheumatoid Arthritis," *Annals of the New York Academy of Sciences* 1069(2006): 77–97.

77. National Institutes of Health, National Institute of Arthritis and Musculoskeletal and Skin Diseases, "Back Pain," 2009. Available at: www.niams.nih.gov/Health_Info/Back_Pain/default.asp

78. Paul Stang, Michael Von Korff, and Bradley S. Galer, "Reduced Labor Force Participation Among Primary Care Patients with Headaches," *Journal of General Internal Medicine* 13(1998): 296–302.

79. Pai, S. and Sundaram, L. J. Low back pain: An economic assessment in the United States. *Orthopedic Clinics of North America* 35(2004): 1–5.

80. Maetzel, A. and Li, L. The economic burden of low back pain: A review of studies published between 1996 and 2001. *Best Practice and Research Clinical Rheumatology* 16(2002): 23–30.

81. L. R. Prado-Leon, A. Celis, and R. Avila-Chaurand, "Occupational Lifting Tasks as a Risk Factor in Low Back Pain: A Case-Control Study in a Mexican Population," *Work* 25(2005): 107–14.

82. F. S. Violante, F. Graziosi, R. Bonfiglioli, S. Curti, and S. Mattioli, "Relations between Occupational, Psychosocial and Individual Factors and Three Different Categories of Back Disorder among Supermarket Workers," *International Archives of Occupational and Environmental Health* (2005): 1–12.

83. E. J. Carragee, T. F. Alamin, J. L. Miller, and J. M. Carragee, "Discographic, MRI and Psychosocial Determinants of Low Back Pain Disability and Remission: A Prospective Study in Subjects with Benign Persistent Back Pain," *The Spine Journal* 5(2005): 24–35.

84. T. Mitchell, P. B. O'Sullivan, A. Smith, A. F. Burnett, L. Straker, J. Thornton, and C. J. Rudd, "Biopsychosocial Factors Are Associated with Low Back Pain in Female Nursing Students: A Cross-Sectional Study," *International Journal of Nursing Studies* 46(2009): 678–88.

85. A. Karahan, S. Kav, A. Abbasoglu, and N. Dogan, "Low Back Pain: Prevalence and Associated Risk Factors among Hospital Staff," *Journal of Advanced Nursing* 65(2009): 516–24.

86. D. Christiansen, K. Larsen, Jensen O. Kudsk, and Nielsen C.Vinther, "Pain Responses in Repeated End-Range Spinal Movements and Psychological Factors in Sick-Listed Patients with Low Back Pain: Is There an Association?" *Journal of Rehabilitation Medicine* 7(2009): 545–49.

87. T. Pincus, A. K. Burton, S. Vogel, and A. P. Field, "A Systematic Review of Psychological Factors as Predictors of Chronicity/Disability in Prospective Cohorts of Low Back Pain," *The Spine Journal* 5(2002): E109–20.

88. Richard Laliberte, "Is Stress Making You Ache? It Can Be the Overlooked Cause of Headaches, Back Pain, Neck Aches and More. How to Ease the Tension," *Shape*, June, 2002. Available at: http://findarticles.com/p/articles/mi_m0846/is_10_21/ai_86035122/

89. T. Fujii, T. Torisu, and S. Nakamura, "A Change of Occlusal Conditions after Splint Therapy for Bruxers with and without Pain in the Masticatory Muscles," *Craniology* 23(2005): 113–18.

90. K. Wahlund, T. List, and B. Larsson, "Treatment of Temporomandibular Disorders among Adolescents: A Comparison between Occlusal Appliance, Relaxation Training, and Brief Information," *Acta Odontology Scandinavia* (2003): 203–11.

91. Harrison Wein, "Stress, Obesity Link Found," *Research Matters*, July 9, 2007. Available at: www.nih.gov/news/research_matters/july2007/07092007stress.htm

92. Zofia Zukowska and Giora Z. Feuerstein, "The NPY Family of Peptides: From Neurotransmitters and Hormones to Immune Modulators, Cytokines and Growth Factors," In Zofia Zukowska, and Giora Z. Feuerstein (Editors), *The NPY Family of Peptides in Immune Disorders, Inflammation, Angiogenesis and Cancer* (Boston: Birkhauser Verlag, 2005), xiii–xv.

93. Lydia E. Kuo, Joanna B. Kitlinska, Jason U. Tilan, Lijun Li, Stephen B. Baker, Michael D. Johnson, Edward W. Lee, Mary Susan Burnett, Stanley T. Fricke, Richard Kvetnansky, Herbert Herzog, and Zofia Zukowska, "Neuropeptide Y Acts Directly in the Periphery on Fat Tissue and Mediates Stress-Induced Obesity and Metabolic Syndrome," *Nature Medicine* 13(2007): 803–11.

94. National Heart, Lung and Blood Institute, "Overweight and Obesity: How Are Overweight and Obesity Diagnosed?" *Diseases and Conditions Index*, 2009. Available at: www.nhlbi.nih.gov/health/dci/Diseases/obe/obe_diagnosis.html

95. American Psychiatric Association, *Diagnostic and Statistical Manual of Mental Disorders,* 4th ed. (Washington, DC: American Psychiatric Association, 1994).

96. G. J. Turnbull, "A Review of Post-Traumatic Stress Disorder. Part I: Historical Development and Classification," *Injury* 29(1998): 87–91.

97. Post-traumatic stress disorder. *PubMed Health*. 2011. Available at: www.ncbi.nlm.nih.gov/pubmedhealth/PMH0001923/

98. National Institutes of Health. Post-Traumatic Stress Disorder (PTSD). *NIH Fact Sheets*. 2011. Available at: http://report.nih.gov/NIHfactsheets/ViewFactSheet.aspx?csid=58&key=P#P

99. R. B. Hidalgo and J. R. Davidson, "Posttraumatic Stress Disorder: Epidemiology and Health-Related Considerations," *Journal of Clinical Psychiatry* 61(2000): 5–13.

100. D. J. Nutt, "The Psychobiology of Posttraumatic Stress Disorder," *Journal of Clinical Psychiatry* 61(2000): 24–29.

101. R. C. Kessler, "Posttraumatic Stress Disorder: The Burden to the Individual and to Society," *Journal of Clinical Psychiatry* 61(2000): 4–12.

102. Hidalgo and Davidson, "Posttraumatic Stress Disorder."

103. G. C. Davis, "Post Traumatic Stress Disorder in Victims of Civilian Trauma and Criminal Violence," *Psychiatric Clinics of North America* 17(1994): 289–99.

104. M. Deahl, M. Srinivasan, N. Jones, J. Thomas, C. Neblett, and A. Jolly, "Preventing Psychological Trauma in Soldiers: The Role of Operational Stress Training and Psychological Debriefing," *British Journal of Medical Psychology* 73(2000): 77–85.

105. E. Eliot Benezra, "Personality Factors of Individuals Who Survive Traumatic Experiences Without Professional Help," *International Journal of Stress Management* 3(1996): 147–53.

106. R. Neugebauer, et al., "Association of Stressful Life Events with Chromosomally Normal Spontaneous Abortion," *American Journal of Epidemiology* 143(1996): 588–96.

107. L. Morland, D. Goebert, J. Onoye, L. Frattarelli, C. Derauf, M. Herbst, C. Matsu, and M. Friedman, "Posttraumatic Stress Disorder and Pregnancy Health: Preliminary Update and Implications," *Psychosomatics* 48(2007): 304–8.

108. S. A. Galambos, P. C. Terry, G. M. Moyle, S. A. Locke, and A. M. Lane, "Psychological Predictors of Injury among Elite Athletes," *British Journal of Sports Medicine* 39(2005): 351–54.

109. M. B. Anderson and J. M. Williams, "A Model of Stress and Athletic Injury: Prediction and Prevention," *Journal of Sport Psychology of Injury* 10(1988): 294–306.

110. Mark B. Anderson and Jean M. Williams, "Athletic Injury, Psychosocial Factors and Perceptual Change During Stress," *Journal of Sports Sciences* 17(1999): 735–41.

111. Ian W. Ford, Robert C. Eklund, and Sandy Gordon, "An Examination of Psychosocial Variables Moderating the Relationship Between Life Stress and Injury Time-Loss Among Athletes of a High Standard," *Journal of Sports Sciences* 18(2000): 301–12.

112. Richard M. Suinn, "Behavioral Intervention for Stress Management in Sports," *International Journal of Stress Management* 12(2005): 343–62.

113. Urban Johnson, Joan Ekengren, and Mark B. Anderson, "Injury Prevention in Sweden: Helping Soccer Players at Risk," *Journal of Sport and Exercise Psychology* 27(2005): 32–38.

LAB ASSESSMENT 3.1

Do You Know What to Do for Posttraumatic Stress Disorder?

Many of us have experienced a traumatic event. For some, it is an automobile accident, and they report seeing their lives flash before their eyes. For others, it is the sudden death of a loved one, and the memory of how they were told is forever etched in their minds. For still others, it is a sexual assault by a stranger, relative, or date/acquaintance, and the violation seems as if it occurred yesterday, even though it was some time ago. Many of these traumatic events will manifest themselves in symptoms of posttraumatic stress disorder such as fear, nightmares, limitation on where one goes or what one does, or impaired relationships. If you have experienced a traumatic event with the potential to elicit these symptoms, describe that event here. If you have not, describe a traumatic event that someone you know has experienced.

_____

_____

_____

What were/are the symptoms that resulted from this event? Be sure to list physical, psychological, and social/relationship symptoms.

1. _____

2. _____

3. _____

4. _____

5. _____

6. _____

How can you or this other person receive help with these symptoms? Cite *from whom* help should be solicited and *what type* of help that source can provide. Include family members, professionals, and others such as professors/teachers, coaches, friends, and clergy.

1. _____

2. _____

3. _____

4. _____

Of course, just listing sources will not help with these symptoms. These sources actually have to be accessed for assistance to be provided. If it is you who experienced the traumatic event, write in your calendar when you will contact each source, and adhere to that schedule. If it is someone else who experienced the traumatic event, encourage that person to specify when assistance will be sought, and offer to help that person to remember to do so.

LAB ASSESSMENT 3.2

Why Did You Get Sick as a Result of Stress?

Stress changes many of your body's and mind's parameters. Heart rate, blood pressure, breathing, and serum cholesterol increase, as do anxiety and muscle tension. Stress also affects the ability to concentrate, decreases the number of T-lymphocytes, and speeds food through the digestive tract. As a result, illnesses and disease can develop. To determine how stress has affected your health, list three stressful events you experienced and the ill health that followed.

Stressful Event

1. _____

2. _____

3. _____

Illness/Disease

1. _____

2. _____

3. _____

For each illness/disease you listed above, describe the stress-related changes in your body and mind that led to these conditions. Try to list as many stress-related body and mind changes as you can that were associated with the subsequent illness/disease you developed.

1. _____

2. _____

3. _____

4. _____

5. _____

As you have read in this and the previous chapter, stress results in several physiological and emotional changes with the potential for the development of associated illnesses and diseases. To assess your biomedical indices related to stress and identify the stress-related illnesses and diseases you experience, provide the information requested below. To obtain several of these biomedical indices requires seeing a physician or other medical care provider. In any case, it is good to have a baseline of these measures to identify changes that may occur over time and, thereby, obtain treatment early so it is more likely to be effective.

Your Blood Pressure

_____ Systolic   _____ Diastolic

Your Blood Chemistry

_____ Total Cholesterol   _____ HDL

_____ LDL   _____ Triglyceride

Your Stress-Related Illnesses and Diseases

There are many conditions which are caused or exacerbated by stress. Some are physical diseases, some emotional illnesses, and others are behavioral manifestations of stress. Check any of these conditions you experience.

Physical Diseases

_____ hypertension   _____ stroke

_____ coronary heart disease   _____ headaches

_____ cancer   _____ allergies, asthma, and hay fever

_____ common colds

Emotional Illnesses

_____ anxiety   _____ depression

_____ panic attacks   _____ posttraumatic stress disorder

Behavioral Manifestations

_____ increased arguments   _____ increased conflict and aggressiveness

_____ inability to concentrate and   _____ social withdrawal
be productive

If you find that your biomedical measures are out of the normal range, or that you are experiencing an inordinate amount of stress-related illnesses or diseases (physical, emotional, or behavioral), consult with your instructor about ways to become healthier. You might also want to speak with your health care provider or someone at the campus health center for advice on how to be healthier and less negatively affected by stress. Lastly, reading this book and participating in the course in which this book is assigned should be a big help.

Stress and the College Student

4

Jack's best friend put a gun to his own head and pulled the trigger. Aside from feeling a deep sense of loss, Jack was angry and disappointed. "I was his best friend. Why didn't he talk with me about this? Why did he have to kill himself?" It seemed that much of Jack's day was preoccupied by such questions. His schoolwork and his job outside of school were both affected.

Kim was a student from Taiwan who was sent, at great expense to her family, to the United States to attend college. With the difficulty she had with studying in a second language and the pressure she felt to succeed in school (her parents sacrificed to send her to school in the United States), she was just keeping her head above water. She barely passed several courses and had to take incompletes in others. Her concern and frustration about her schoolwork overflowed into her social life. She found herself being angry and argumentative with friends and devoting so much time to her studies that she soon had no friends. Alone and lonely in a foreign country, not doing well in school, Kim was experiencing a great deal of stress.

Bill was a mail carrier who was attending college at night to prepare for another career when he retired from the postal service. He was having problems with his marriage, his job, and his schooling. There never seemed enough time for any of these. His wife and daughter complained that with being at work and school he was seldom home, and, when he was, he was always doing schoolwork. His supervisor at the post office claimed he always seemed tired and grouchy, and this was affecting his job performance. His professors told Bill that he was not turning in his work on time, nor was it of sufficient quality to pass his courses. When Bill finally left his family (his domestic problems became more and more serious), he brooded so much that he had less time, instead of more, to concentrate on the other aspects of his life.

These are but a few of the students enrolled in my stress management classes during *one semester*. They came to me to discuss these problems and to get guidance regarding how to manage them. Too often the life of the college student is depicted as "rah-rah," fraternity row, and football games. These are carefree and fun years for many students. For many others, though, college is just another life change to which they must adapt. They may be young and experiencing the growing and developing pains of youth; they may be older students with too many other responsibilities to enjoy their schooling; or they may experience unique situations during the time they are supposed to be concentrating on their studies. In any case, college is very stressful for a large number of students.

There is plenty of evidence that chronic stress is often a companion of college students. As they observed college students, researchers concluded that college students are particularly prone to chronic stress as a result of their experiencing and having to manage developmental transitions.[1,2] To make matters worse, the stress experienced by college students can interfere with the learning processes necessary for academic success.[3] Having difficulties academically then feeds back into the stress loop as a life-situation stressor to create even more stress. Other stress researchers have noted students' concerns such as finances,[4] living arrangements,[5] safety,[6] and their weight[7] to be significant stressors. On my own campus, a survey of the top health issues found stress to be second only to fitness and exercise. What do you

Table 4.1
Top-Ten Reported Negative Influences on Students' Academic Performance

Rank	Negative Influence	Influence Percentage (%)
1	Stress	28.6%
2	Sleep difficulties	20.4
3	Anxiety	20.0
4	Cold/flu/sore throat	14.7
5	Internet use/computer games	11.9
6	Depression	11.9
7	Concern for troubled friend or family member	10.8
8	Relationship difficulty	9.8
9	Sinus infection/ear infection/bronchitis/strep throat	5.7
10	Death of friend/family member	5.4

Source: American College Health Association. *American College Health Association National College Health Assessment II: Reference Group Report Spring 2011.* Hanover, MD: American College Health Association, 2011. Available at: www.acha-ncha.org/docs/ACHA-NCHA-II_ReferenceGroup_DataReport_Fall2011.pdf

think students on your campus would rate as the top-three health issues? I'll bet stress is one of them. (see Table 4.1)

The Younger College Student

The younger college student—one who enters college from high school or shortly thereafter—experiences stressors such as the dramatic lifestyle change from high school to college, grades, course overload, managing finances, making friends, love and sex stressors, shyness, jealousy, and breakups.

Lifestyle Change

The more life changes you experience, the more stress you will feel and the more likely it is that illness and disease will result. Just imagine all the life changes associated with attending college for the first time!

You attend high school while living at home, under the supervision of your parents, and usually without the need to work. There is plenty of time to meet friends after school, to do homework, and to relax. After all, the laundry is done by someone else, the meals are prepared by someone else, and the car may even be filled with gas by someone else. Food somehow, miraculously, appears in the refrigerator and cupboards, and the dust on the furniture and floors periodically vanishes.

Although many high school students do take on household responsibilities and do have jobs, generally the high school years are comfortable ones. When college begins, however, a dramatic change takes place. Time must be set aside for shopping, cooking, cleaning, doing the laundry, and myriad other routine chores. For the first time in many students' lives, they must assume responsibilities they never had to assume before. Further, no one keeps asking if they've done their homework. They must remember to fit this in between all their other activities.

However, in addition to all of these, other changes are dictated by college life. Usually it requires finding an apartment or choosing a dormitory in which to live. A whole new network of same-sex and opposite-sex friends must be established. Schoolwork seems excessive, and it seems that not enough time is available to accomplish it. The fear of flunking permeates the air.

As though all of this weren't enough, the younger college student is confronted with several important tasks during that time of his or her life:

1. Achieving emotional independence from family.
2. Choosing and preparing for a career.

College students have a lot of stressors in their lives, only one of which relates to their schoolwork.

Although college is fraught with stress, many students believe the reward at the end makes it all worthwhile. What do you believe?

3. Preparing for emotional commitment and family life.

4. Developing an ethical system.[8]

Managing these transitional changes requires college students to develop new roles and modify old ones, and that can result in a great deal of stress.[9]

Considering all these changes and the effects of stress on the immunological system, it is no small wonder that influenza epidemics and bouts of mononucleosis are frequent visitors to college campuses. Of course, the close living quarters exacerbate this situation. We also should not be surprised to learn that suicide is the second leading cause of death on college campuses (accidents being number one).

Grades

The old story of the college professor who tossed the term papers down the stairs and graded those landing on the top three steps an A, those on the next three steps a B, and so on emphasizes the confusion about grading. Grades—students have to get them and professors have to give them. Unfortunately, both groups seem to gear too much of their behavior toward them. Students see their goal as getting good grades instead of learning as much as they can. Professors see their goal as accurately differentiating between an A student and a B student rather than teaching as much as they can. As with all such generalizations, there are numerous exceptions. However, I think anyone associated with a college campus will agree that too much emphasis is placed upon grades.

Students may even link their self-worth with their grades—for example, "Boy, am I dumb. I flunked English." Instead, they'd be better off saying, "Boy, I guess I didn't study long enough or well enough. I'll have to remember that for the next test."

Let's not kid ourselves, though. Grades are very important. They are important to students who want to go to graduate school or whose prospective employers consider them prior to hiring. They are also important to the university that wants its graduates considered competent and well educated. The university will use grades to weed out those who will not reflect well upon it. However, I have seen students so preoccupied by grades that they have let their physical health deteriorate. They give up exercise, don't have enough time to prepare balanced meals, or pull "all-nighters" so frequently that they walk around with bags under their eyes. I have seen other students so grade-conscious that they don't have a social life—they're always studying.

The life of the typical college student may be quite hectic. For this reason, it is very important that students make time for relaxation; that is, relaxation in a healthy way such as regularly employing a relaxation technique, exercising, and using the social support of family and friends.

course overload
Having too many courses or courses too difficult to complete well during one semester.

Course Overload

Related to the issue of grades is **course overload.** Course overload is having too many courses or courses that are too difficult to do well during any one semester. In today's goal-oriented, rush-rush society, the more you accomplish in the shortest period of time, the better. The result is people rushing through their lives and experiencing very little. They achieve a lot of goals but don't enjoy the trip to those goals.

Course overload results in a similar predicament. If I had a dollar for every student who, upon graduation, told me "I wish I had taken more courses I enjoyed" or "I wish I had devoted more time to my studies" or "I wish I had taken fewer courses each semester and learned more in the ones I did enroll in," I'd be wealthy today. Hoping to graduate in the shortest time possible, too many students overload themselves and suffer physically, psychologically, socially, and educationally for it.[10] In a study of American college freshmen, 29 percent reported feeling frequently overwhelmed by all they had to do; 18 percent of males and 39 percent of females.[11] They may get physically ill, their emotions may be ready to explode, they may not have time for friends, and while taking more courses, they actually learn less. In this case, more is less.

Finances

Some of the most significant stressors that college students experience relate to money. To begin with, paying for college is a challenge for many students and their families. As can be seen in Figure 4.1, when tuition and fees, room and board, books and supplies, and other expenses (such as travel) are added up, college is beyond the reach of many students. In fact, the Advisory Committee on Student Financial Assistance estimates costs prevent 3.2 million college-qualified high school graduates from attending any college at all,[12] and 62 percent of entering freshmen stated that their financial situation led to them to not attend their first-choice college.[13]

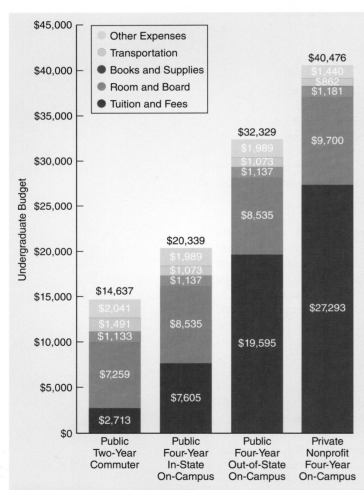

Figure 4.1

Average Estimated Undergraduate Budgets, 2010–2011

Source: Trends in College Pricing. © 2010 The College Board. www.collegeboard.org. Reproduced with permission.

Type of College	% with Student Loan Debt	Amount Owed
Public Universities	62%	$20,200
Private Nonprofit Universities	72%	$27,650
Private For-Profit Universities	96%	$33,050

Table 4.2
Graduating College Students' Loan Debt, 2008

Source: Project on Student Debt, *Quick Facts about Student Debt, 2010*. Available at http://projectonstudentdebt.org/Files/File/Debt_Facts_and_Sources.pdf

Education Loans for College Students

There are several sources of loans for college students and their parents to help pay for the costs associated with attending college. Some of these sources are sponsored by the federal government whereas others are private.

Federal Loans

- Federal *Stafford loans* are fixed-rate, low-interest loans available to at least half-time students attending schools that participate in the federal financial aid system. There are two types of Stafford loans: *Subsidized Stafford* loans are need-based, and interest does not accrue while students are still in school. *Unsubsidized Stafford* loans are not need-based, and interest that accrues on the loan is due even while attending school.

- Federal *Perkins loans* are low-interest (5 percent) loans for undergraduate and graduate students with exceptional financial need. Perkins loans have no fees and offer a longer grace period for repayment than do Stafford loans.

- Federal *Parent PLUS* loans are low-interest student loans for parents of undergraduate, dependent students. With a Parent PLUS loan, families can fund the entire cost of a child's education (less other financial aid).

- Federal *Graduate PLUS* loans are federally sponsored loans for students attending graduate school. With a Grad PLUS loan, students may borrow up to the full cost of their education, less other financial aid received.

Private Loans

- With the Sallie Mae *Smart Option Student Loan,* students can borrow up to the full cost of a college education, less other aid received. The Smart Option Student Loan requires making interest-only payments while in school. A creditworthy cosigner can help students qualify and/or receive a lower interest rate.

- There are grants, scholarships, and work-study programs that provide financial assistance for college. A financial aid advisor on campus can help direct students toward these sources of funding.

Given these figures, it is no surprise that many students graduate with a good deal of debt. As shown in Table 4.2 and the box entitled "Facts About College Student Debt," not only do students incur loan debt from public sources, but many need to get financial assistance from private sources as well. In addition, many students have to work while attending school to afford their college education. Forty-six percent of all full-time working students work 25 or more hours per week, with 42 percent reporting that working hurt their grades. One in five full-time

College Students and Credit Card Statistics

- Eighty-four percent of the student population overall have credit cards, an increase of approximately 11 percent since the fall of 2004.

- Undergraduates are carrying record-high credit card balances. The average (mean) balance grew to $3,173, the highest in the years the study has been conducted. Median debt grew from $946 in 2004 to $1,645 currently. Twenty-one percent of undergraduates had balances of between $3,000 and $7,000, also up from the last study.

- Half of college undergraduates had four or more credit cards in 2008. That's up from 43 percent in 2004 and just 32 percent in 2000.

- Since 2004, the percentage of students who arrived on campus as freshmen with a credit card already in hand have increased from 23 percent to 39 percent.

- In the spring of 2008, only 15 percent of freshmen had a zero balance, down dramatically from 69 percent in the fall of 2004. The median debt freshmen carried was $939, nearly triple the $373 in 2004.

- Seniors graduated with an average credit card debt of more than $4,100, up from $2,900 almost four years ago. Close to one-fifth of seniors carried balances greater than $7,000.

- Sixty percent of undergrads experienced surprise at how high their balance had reached, and 40 percent said they have charged items knowing they didn't have the money to pay the bill.

- Only 17 percent said they regularly paid off all cards each month, and another 1 percent had parents, a spouse, or other family members paying the bill. The remaining 82 percent carried balances and thus incurred finance charges each month.

- The average college graduate has nearly $20,000 in debt; average credit card debt has increased 47 percent between 1989 and 2004 for 25-to 34-year-olds and 11 percent for 18- to 24-year-olds. Nearly one in five 18- to 24-year-olds is in "debt hardship," up from 12 percent in 1989.

Source: Woolsey, Ben and Schulz, Matt. Credit card statistics, industry facts, debt statistics: Demographics. *CreditCards.com.* 2011. Available at: www.creditcards.com/credit-card-news/credit-card-industry-facts-personal-debt-statistics-1276 .php#Young-adults.

working students actually hold a full-time job, working 35 or more hours per week. Fifty-three percent of all full-time working students who work 25 or more hours per week report that employment limits their class schedule, and 38 percent said that work limits their class choice.[14] Furthermore, 64 percent of students who work while attending school report they frequently or occasionally overslept or missed classes or appointments, and 45 percent did not have time to study due to job responsbilities.[15] However, 63 percent of all full-time working students who work 25 or more hours per week state that they would not be able to afford college if they did not work.

Of course, that is not the only debt college students incur. In addition to student loans, credit card debt plagues many college students.

As shown in the box entitled "College Students and Credit Card Statistics," college students incur an excessive amount of credit card debt, and that situation has gotten worse over the years.

Facts About College Student Debt

- By the time they graduate, 67 percent of students at four-year colleges and universities have student loan debt. In 1993, fewer than half of graduating students had loan debt.

- From 2004 to 2008, graduating seniors' student loans were up 24 percent.

- The average debt for a college graduate in 2007–2008 was $20,098. Forty-one percent had no debt, 20 percent had less than $10,000 debt, 18 percent had between $10,000 and $19,999 debt, and one-third had more than $20,000 debt.

- In 2008, 59 percent of undergraduate students had an education loan. Fifty-five percent had a federal loan averaging $5,100 per borrower, and 30 percent had a private loan averaging $6,522 per borrower.

- In 1993, approximately 32 percent of undergraduate students borrowed to attend college. From 1993 through 2008, the average yearly debt load increased by 50 percent.

- In 1993, private student loans barely existed. Federal loans provided adequate financial support to attend college. In 2008, private companies aggressively market college loans, often with steep interest rates (some as high as 18 percent).

- Regarding full-time students, 16 percent took out private loans in 2004. In 2008, that number nearly tripled to 43 percent.

Sources: Advisory Committee on Student Financial Assistance, *Condition of Access and Persistence Study*, 2009. Available at: www.ed.gov/about/bdscomm/list/acsfa/edlite-caps.html
Steele, Patricia and Sandy Baum, "How Much are College Students Borrowing?" *College Board Policy Brief*, August 2009. Available at: http://professionals.collegeboard.com/profdownload/cb-policy-brief-college-stu-borrowing-aug-2009.pdf
Dillon, Erin and Kevin Carey, "Drowning in Debt: The Emerging Student Loan Crisis," *Charts You Can Trust*, July 9, 2009. Available at: www.educationsector.org/usr_doc/CYCT_Student_Aid.pdf

To better manage their use of credit cards, the College Board recommends students adhere to the following:

- Consider using a debit card instead of a credit card. Money is deducted directly from your checking account, so you can't spend more than you actually have.

- Read all application materials carefully—especially the fine print. What happens after the "teaser rate" expires? What happens to your interest rate if you're late with a payment or fail to make a payment? What's the interest rate for a cash advance?

- Pay bills promptly to keep finance and other charges to a minimum; pay the balance off if you can.

- Use credit only if you're certain you are able to repay the debt.

- Avoid impulse shopping on your credit card.

- Save your credit card for a money emergency.

How to use a credit card appropriately is not the only financial skill that gets college students into financial hot water and thereby causes them stress. In a study of more than 1,000 college students from 27 universities in 19 states,[16] it was found that 92 percent knew how to balance a checkbook but only 62 percent actually did it. Developing a budget and adhering to it would help these students a great deal. Yet only 38 percent prepared a monthly budget, and only 28 percent of those that did so stuck to it. To develop a budget for the semester, complete Lab 4.1.

The Credit Card Accountability, Responsibility, and Disclosure (CARD) Act of 2009

The Credit Card Accountability, Responsibility, and Disclosure (CARD) Act of 2009 took effect in 2010. The law is designed to help consumers avoid unfair fees, penalties, interest rate increases, and other unwarranted changes from credit card companies, and includes provisions aimed at protecting students. It also imposes new requirements on colleges and alumni groups that offer credit cards.

The student-focused provisions in the Credit CARD Act include the following:

1. **Restriction on credit cards for those under 21.** The law prohibits issuing credit cards to individuals under 21 unless they have a cosigner or they demonstrate a financial ability to repay.

2. **Protection from prescreened offers.** The law prohibits issuers from sending prescreened credit offers to individuals under 21. (Issuer would need to get consent to send these offers.)

3. **Disclosure of contracts.** Colleges and universities must publicly disclose any contracts made with creditors for the "purpose of marketing a credit card."

4. **Gifts/inducements prohibited.** The law prohibits credit issuers from offering inducements to get students to apply for a credit card if the offer is made on campus, near campus, or at an event sponsored by or related to a college or university. (Here the burden is on the credit card company.)

5. **Sense of Congress resolution on institution of higher education policies.** Each institution should consider adopting the following policies: (a) requiring card issuers to notify the institution of any location they will market credit cards on campus; (b) limiting the number of locations on campus where marketing of credit cards may take place; and (c) offering credit card and debt education sessions as a regular part of new student orientation programs.

6. **College affinity card provisions/reports by creditors.** Each creditor must submit an annual report to the Federal Reserve Board containing the terms and conditions for all college affinity card agreements. The law specifies the information in the report, including the amount of any payments from the creditor to the institution and the total number of credit card accounts covered by the agreement, and that the report will be organized according to institution, organization or foundation. Note that there is no obligation on the part of institutions to report to the Board on their affinity card agreements (however, see provision number 3 above).

Source: American Council on Education. *Credit CARD Law Includes Provisions to Protect College Students. 2010.* Available at: www.acenet.edu/AM/Template.cfm?Section=Search&template=/CM/HTMLDisplay.cfm&ContentID=35559.

Friendship

Giving up or changing old friendships and developing new ones is often a stressful activity associated with college life. Will people like me? Will I find someone with similar interests? How about boyfriends and girlfriends? Will people want to date me? All of these questions and many others are of concern during this phase of life. Old friends were accompanied by old routines—you knew just how much you could tell whom. Since friendship is a function of the degree of self-disclosure friends are

Attending college brings the opportunity of making new friends.

willing to share, new friends require a period of testing to see just how much self-disclosure feels comfortable with this new person. To demonstrate this point, complete Lab 4.2 (at the end of this chapter) on friendship and "acquaintanceship."

Love

With old friends and family back home, many students fill the void with new love relationships. These relationships themselves, however, may create new stresses. Any new relationship requires a new set of rules and standards. How often do we see each other? How often do we telephone? Where should we go on dates? Who should pay? With whose friends should we hang out?

In addition, some love relationships involve two people who are different types of lovers. To understand this point better, complete Lab 4.3 at the end of this chapter. If you are now involved in a love relationship, perhaps you'll want your lover to complete Lab 4.3 as well.

Erotic love (eros) is a passionate, all-enveloping love. The heart races, a fluttering appears in the stomach, and there's a shortness of breath when erotic lovers meet. **Ludic love (ludus)** is a playful, flirtatious love. It involves no long-term commitment and is basically for amusement. Ludic love is usually played with several partners at once. **Storgic love (storge)** is a calm, companionate love. Storgic lovers are quietly affectionate and have goals of marriage and children for the relationship. **Manic love (mania)** is a combination of erotic and ludic love. A manic lover's needs for affection are insatiable. He or she is often racked with highs of irrational joy, lows of anxiety and depression, and bouts of extreme jealousy. Manic attachments seldom develop into lasting love.

Imagine that a ludic lover is in a love relationship with a storgic lover. One is playing games with no intention of a lasting or exclusive relationship, and the other is thinking marriage and children. Love relationships on college campuses may be stressful because of misunderstandings regarding the types of love involved.

What is your love style? If you are presently in a love relationship, is your love style compatible with that of your lover? Recognizing that love styles may change during different stages of your life, when do you think you will adopt a different love style from the one you have now? Do you look forward to this transition, or not? Why? As with other aspects of your life, you are in control of the types of relationships that

erotic love (eros)
A passionate, all-enveloping type of love recognized by the heart racing and other signs of excitement.

ludic love (ludus)
A playful, flirtatious type of love involving no long commitment.

storgic love (storge)
A calm, companionate type of love conceiving of a long commitment.

manic love (mania)
A combination of passionate love (eros) and flirtatious playing love characterized by jealousy and irrational joy that usually does not result in a long commitment.

you enter, and you can choose compatible ones or ones that can result in stress. Why not ask someone with whom you might have an initial romantic interest to complete Lab 4.3 and see if you are compatible before you become too committed?

There are online "love tests" that match people on a variety of characteristics and personality traits. Some of the variables they measure are adventurousness, communication style, relationship role, temperament, romanticism, importance of wealth, and need for independence. During one month it is estimated approximately 20 million people use online matching services such as Match.com, Americansingles .com, and Date.com.[17] Online personal ads generated over $400 million in 2003, up from $72 million in 2001. It seems that a lot of people are looking for love and are willing to pay for it.

Sex

One of the assignments in my undergraduate stress management class is for students to keep a journal of stressors they encounter. Invariably, several female students describe the pressure they are receiving—from their female friends as well as their boyfriends—to engage in sexual intercourse. It's the talk of the dorm or sorority house. Although no male student has ever described a similar stressor, I'm convinced that the pressure to be sexually active is at least as great for male students as it is for female students. Why else would young males feel compelled to exaggerate their sexual experiences or describe an enjoyable, relaxing evening as a Roman orgy? I believe that males are just less apt to admit that they feel stressed by pressure to be sexually active.

To compound this stressor, the older public looks at college students as a promiscuous, pill-popping, irresponsible group of rascals and tolerates them only because they are young and soon will learn better. At age 19, however, many females have never experienced sexual intercourse, yet even college students tend to exaggerate the sexual experience of their compatriots.

To determine just how much you really know about sexuality and about the sexual behavior of your peers, and how any misconceptions affect the degree of stress you experience, answer the following true/false questions:

    _____ 1. By the time they graduate from college, all students have masturbated.

    _____ 2. Almost all college students have experienced sexual intercourse several times.

    _____ 3. Masturbation is a habit of the young and is eliminated as one becomes an adult.

    _____ 4. As long as "safer sex" is practiced, both pregnancy and sexually transmitted diseases can be prevented.

    _____ 5. Masturbation can result in either physical illness or psychological harm.

    _____ 6. Sexual fantasies are wishes you have for participation in sex.

    _____ 7. Oral-genital sex is abnormal and perverse.

All of the previous statements are false. Let's look more closely at them one at a time.

1. Most researchers have found that approximately 90 percent of men and 60 percent of women have masturbated at some time. Stated another way, approximately 10 percent of men and 40 percent of women have *not* had masturbatory experience. In a landmark study of sex in America, Laumann and his colleagues found that both males and females masturbate, although 85 percent of men as opposed to 45 percent of women masturbated in the year prior to the study.[18]

2. Fifty-one percent of males and 47 percent of females who are 15 to 19 years old have never had sexual intercourse. Twelve percent of males and

13 percent of females who are 20 to 24 years old have never had sexual intercourse. Even 5 percent of males and 3 percent of females who are 24 to 29 years old have never had sexual intercourse.[19] In another study, 53 percent of males and 62 percent of females ages 18 to 19, 63 percent of males and 80 percent of females ages 20 to 24, and 86 percent of males and 87 percent of females ages 25 to 29 engaged in sexual intercourse within the past 12 months.[20] Obviously, not everyone is doing "it," and when they are, it isn't with everyone on campus.

3. Masturbation is engaged in throughout one's life. Whether it's because one's sexual partner is unavailable, pregnant, or ill, or just for the pleasure of it, masturbation is practiced by adults at all ages.

4. We shall discuss sexually transmitted diseases, and AIDS in particular, shortly. For now, you should know that there is no such thing as safe sex. Anytime coitus occurs, for instance, there is the chance of a pregnancy resulting (there is no *100 percent* effective means of birth control) and the possibility of contracting one of several **sexually transmitted infections (STIs)**. However, there are ways to engage in "safer" sex—that is, decreasing the chances of conception or of infection occurring—for example, using a condom.

sexually transmitted infections (STIs)
Diseases such as syphilis, gonorrhea, chlamydia, and genital warts that are transmitted through sexual activity.

5. Experts agree that the only danger of masturbation is the psychological harm resulting from guilt, shame, or embarrassment one associates with it. If people were to learn how prevalent masturbation is, how it doesn't interfere with normal relationships or the ability to later be sexually functional, and that it usually continues throughout one's life (albeit at a lesser frequency), masturbation might not be associated with guilt and other negative feelings and thereby not create any harm at all.

6. Because you fantasize about something doesn't necessarily mean you would actually like to experience that fantasy. For example, when you become angry with a professor, you might dream about slashing the tires on his or her car. However, most of us would not do that even if we knew we wouldn't get caught (at least I hope my students reading this agree). Likewise, sexual thoughts and fantasies may or may not be events we would like to experience. We shouldn't feel guilty or embarrassed about our sexual thoughts; that can only do us harm. However, we should be held accountable for our sexual *behavior*.

7. Many men and women have engaged in oral sex. In a national survey conducted by Michael and his colleagues, they found that 77 percent of men and 68 percent of women reported having given oral sex *to* a partner, and 79 percent of men and 73 percent of women had received oral sex *from* a partner.[21] Whether one chooses to view oral-genital sex as perverse depends on one's values. However, given its frequency, it certainly cannot be considered abnormal.

Does the information regarding sexual myths surprise you? If so, don't worry. You are probably in good company, with significant numbers of your classmates also believing many of the same myths about the sexual behavior of college students. Given the misconceptions you have regarding how sexually active you "would be" if you were "normal," the pressure for you to engage in sex can be intense. This pressure comes from outside yourself and from within. The pressure might lead to stress that interferes with your health, grades, and interpersonal relationships. Hopefully, a more realistic perception of the sexual behavior of your classmates will help you see yourself as not unusual in your own sexual behavior and thereby help you to better deal with the pressure to be sexually active, whether you are sexually experienced or inexperienced. (Remember, in either case you are in the company of a large number of other college students.)

HIV/AIDS

There is a good deal of concern both on and off college campuses regarding the spread of sexually transmitted infections—in particular, **acquired immune deficiency syndrome (AIDS)**. This section describes the causes, treatments, and means of prevention of AIDS, with the hope that knowledge will aid in alleviating undue stress regarding your sexual behavior and will help you prevent AIDS from developing in the first place.

Acquired immune deficiency syndrome is caused by a virus called the **human immunodeficiency virus (HIV)**. AIDS results in an ineffectiveness of the immunological system so that its victims develop opportunistic infections that eventually lead to death. The Centers for Disease Control and Prevention reports that, by 2007, 576,000 Americans died of AIDS. In 2009, there were 42,010 new cases of HIV infection.[22]

There is no known cure for AIDS, although there are some drugs that can slow the course of the disease and prolong the life of the AIDS victim. The most effective of these drugs is azidothymidine (AZT) used in combination with other drugs such as protease inhibitors (called combination therapy or "drug cocktail").

HIV is transmitted through bodily fluids such as blood and semen. High-risk groups are homosexuals, intravenous drug users, and infants born to women with the virus in their bloodstream. However, public health officials would rather direct attention to high-risk *behaviors* than to high-risk *groups,* since membership in the group is immaterial—it's what you *do* that can give you AIDS, not what group you belong to. If you share needles with others (as IV drug users are prone to do), if you engage in oral or genital sex without using a condom or in anal sex even if you do use a condom, or if you have multiple sex partners, you are more likely to contract AIDS than if you don't engage in these high-risk behaviors. In spite of some widespread misconceptions, AIDS is not transmitted casually. It cannot be contracted by touching a person with AIDS, sharing eating utensils, swimming in the same swimming pool, being in the same classroom, being stung by a mosquito, or kissing.[23] You also cannot acquire AIDS by giving blood; since 1985, the blood supply has been screened so that contracting AIDS through a blood transfusion is only a remote possibility. AIDS is classified as a *sexually* transmitted infection, even though it can be transmitted in nonsexual ways (e.g., when a health care worker accidentally comes in contact with HIV-infected blood).

Other Sexually Transmitted Infections

Other sexually transmitted infections include chlamydia, gonorrhea, syphilis, genital herpes, human papillomavirus, pelvic inflammatory infection, trichomoniasis, vaginosis, hepatitis B, and genital warts. These STIs are caused by parasites, bacteria, or viruses, all transmitted through sexual activity. As with HIV infection, the only 100 percent effective prevention involves abstaining from sexual activities that can transmit the causative agent. The prevalence, causes, and treatment for these STIs are presented in Table 4.3.

Prevention of Sexually Transmitted Infections

To alleviate some distress you may have regarding STIs, engage in behaviors that can make you less prone to contracting it. There are several things you can do to protect yourself. The best approach in terms of prevention is to abstain from sex: oral sex, coitus, and anal sex. If you decide that alternative is not acceptable to you, the next best approach is to maintain a monogamous sexual relationship with someone you know to be STI-free. The problem here, though, is determining that someone is STI-free. The test for AIDS, for example, actually tests for the presence of antibodies that you develop after coming in contact with HIV. Since the test

Table 4.3 Sexually Transmitted Infection: Prevalence, Causes, and Treatment

Infection	Prevalence	Cause	Treatment
Chlamydia	In 2007, 1,108,374 cases	Parasite: *Chlamydia trachomatis*	Azithromycin or doxycycline
Gonorrhea	In 2007, 355,991 cases	Bacteria: *Neisseria gonorrhoeae*	Antibiotics: ceftriaxone or spectinomycin
Syphilis	In 2007, 40,920 cases	Bacteria: *Treponema pallidum*	Antibiotic: penicillin
Genital Herpes	In 2007, 317,000 cases	Virus: *Herpes simplex viruses*	No cure. Antiviral medications can shorten and prevent outbreaks during the time medication is taken.
Human Papillomavirus	22.5% of U.S residents are infected	Virus: *Human Papilloma virus*	No cure. A vaccine (*Gardasil*) is available to persons age 9–26.
Pelvic Inflammatory Disease	In 2007, 146,000 cases	Various STIs that are left untreated	Antibiotics, although damage already done to organs cannot be reversed
Trichomoniasis	In 2007, 205,000 cases	Bacteria: *Trichomonas vaginalis*	Antibiotic: metronidazole
Bacterial Vaginosis (*candidiasis* is the most common)	Most common vaginal infection. In 2007, over 3,723,000 cases	Bacteria: *Candida albicans*	Antibiotics: metronidazole and clindamycin
Hepatitis B	In 2007, 43,000 cases	Virus: *Hepatitis B virus*	No cure. Antiviral drugs used to treat chronic hepatitis B.
Genital Warts	In 2007, 312,000 cases	Virus: *Human Papillomavirus*	No cure. Cryotherapy freezes tissue to remove surface wart, or the drug podophyllin serves as a skin irritant to remove surface wart.

Sources: Centers for Disease Control and Prevention, *Sexually Transmitted Disease Surveillance, 2007*, July, 2009. J. S. Greenberg, C. E. Bruess, and S. C. Conklin, *Exploring the Dimensions of Human Sexuality* (Sudbury, MA: Jones and Bartlett, 2007).

may not identify the presence of these antibodies for up to six or eight months after exposure, even if someone has a negative AIDS test today, if that person had sex with someone else within the past eight months, he or she may still possess the virus. What the experts say is really true: When you sleep with someone, you are sleeping with that person's previous sexual partners and those previous partners' sexual partners.

If you engage in sex, always use a condom made of latex rather than animal skin (such as lambskin), since the animal skin condom may be too porous to prevent the disease-causing organism from penetrating. Unfortunately, too many college students do not use condoms, or do not use them often enough, even though they engage in sexual behaviors that put them at risk of contracting an STI. In a study of almost 65,000 sexually active women ages 20 through 44, 22 percent had two or more sexual partners, yet only 19 percent reported always using condoms, and 27 percent never used condoms.[24] In another larger scale study, males who had two or more sexual partners reported using condom only 63 percent of the time.[25] Alarmingly, in a study of adolescents, researchers found condoms were used in only 59 percent of sexual intercourse experiences.[26] Even if these subjects used another method of contraception, they did not get the benefit and protection from sexually transmitted infections that a condom can provide.

Acquaintance Rape

As if the threat of contracting a sexually transmitted infection such as AIDS is not stressful enough, imagine the feelings evoked when sex is forced upon someone. That is precisely what is happening on college campuses. It is most often the male forcing sex on his female date: "She said NO but I knew she really wanted it. It just took a little coercion." Well, that is RAPE! Anytime sex is forced on someone

2020 National Health Objectives Related to Sexually Transmitted Infections

1. *Reduce the proportion of adolescents and young adults with chlamydia trachomatis infections.*
2. *Reduce chlamydia rates among females aged 15 to 44 years.*
3. *Increase the proportion of sexually active females aged 24 years and under enrolled in Medicaid plans who are screened for genital chlamydia infections during the measurement year.*
4. *Increase the proportion of sexually active females aged 24 years and under enrolled in commercial health insurance plans who are screened for genital chlamydia infections during the measurement year.*
5. *Reduce the proportion of females aged 15 to 44 years who have ever required treatment for pelvic inflammatory disease (PID).*
6. *Reduce gonorrhea rates.*
7. *Reduce sustained domestic transmission of primary and secondary syphilis.*
8. *Reduce congenital syphilis.*
9. *Reduce the proportion of females with human papillomavirus (HPV) infection.*
10. *Reduce the proportion of young adults with genital herpes infection due to herpes simplex type 2.*

else, that is legally defined as rape. **Acquaintance rape,** forcible sex between people who know one another (such as dates), occurs more frequently among college students, particularly freshmen, than any other age group. One in four women report being victims of rape; 84 percent of their assailants were dating partners or acquaintances. One in four college men have admitted to using sexual aggression with women. Victims of date rape may feel ashamed, guilty, betrayed, and frightened. The psychological effects can be devastating and last for a long time. Date rape is a serious matter and needs to be prevented.

Interestingly, experts recognize that rape is more about violence and control than it is about sex. Rapists may want to act out violently against the person being raped because of some past experiences. The rapist may believe that a history of rejection or feeling inferior can, for the moment, be forgotten through this violent behavior. Alternatively, the rapist may wish to demonstrate control over someone else in the most intimate part of that person's life.

Not to be lost in this discussion is the role that sex plays in our society. Look at ads in magazines and on television, and you will note that sex is used to sell even the most remote of products. Pay attention in movies, and you will undoubtedly see sex portrayed in one way or another. The Internet makes pornographic images and films readily available. The behavior portrayed in these films is anything but sensitive, romantic, or respectful. It is shameful when people use these actions as models for what they think will be exciting sex. That can lead to forceful sex, which is rape.

Acquaintance Rape and College Students

Women ages 16 to 24 experience rape at rates four times higher than the assault rate of all women, making the college (and high school) years the most vulnerable for women. College women are more at risk for rape and other forms of sexual assault than women the same age but not in college. It is estimated that almost 25 percent of college women have been victims of rape or attempted rape since the age of 14. College women are raped at significantly higher rates than college men.

College men are more likely to report experiencing unwanted kissing or fondling than intercourse. College men who are raped are usually raped by other men. But, since so few men report rape, information is limited about the extent of the problem. However, survey data suggest that up to 10 percent of acquaintance rape victims on campus are men.

Stranger rape of college students is less common than acquaintance rape. Ninety percent of college women who are victims of rape or attempted rape know their assailant. The attacker is usually a classmate, friend, boyfriend, ex-boyfriend, or other acquaintance (in that order). Most acquaintance rapes do not occur on dates; rather they occur when two people are otherwise in the same place (e.g., at a party, studying together in a dorm room). Thus, *date rape* (rape that occurs during or at the end of a date) is not the appropriate term to describe the majority of acquaintance rapes of college women, as date rapes account for only 13 percent of college rapes (although they make up 35 percent of attempted rapes).

Source: Rana Sampson. *Acquaintance Rape of College Students* (Washington, DC: U.S. Department of Justice, Office of Community Oriented Policing Services, 2002).

Below you will read some suggestions for protecting yourself from being forced to engage in sexual activity or from forcing another to do so. As you read these helpful suggestions, keep in mind that it is not your responsibility to prevent yourself from being raped. It doesn't matter what you wear, how you act, or the setting you are in. None of this excuses rape—none of it!

The American College Health Association recommends the following to prevent acquaintance rape:

Think: Think about how you respond to social pressures and ask yourself

- What role does sex play in my life?
- What role do I want it to play?
- How does alcohol affect my sexual decision making?
- How do I learn someone's desires and limits?
- How do I express my own?

Challenge the myths and stereotypes: Challenge your friends who belittle rape or don't understand it, who accept definitions of sex and gender roles that include forcing someone to have sex or getting him or her too drunk to say no. Talk with friends and give one another the opportunity to be assertive, respectful, honest, and caring.

Communicate effectively: Saying no or yes may be difficult, but it's important. Acting sorry or unsure sends mixed messages. The other person can't really know how you feel without hearing it from you.

Trust your instincts: Even if you can't explain why, you have the right to trust your feelings and have them respected. Tell your partner what you want—or don't want—and stick with your decision.

Listen... carefully to what the other person is saying. Are you getting mixed messages? Do you understand him or her? If not—ask.

Ask... rather than assume. Let you and your partner talk about what would be most enjoyable together.

Remember... effective and assertive communication may not always work. Sometimes people simply don't listen. However—NO ONE DESERVES TO BE RAPED![27]

In addition, avoid excessive use of alcohol or other drugs that may cloud your ability to make decisions in your best interest. The American College Health Association reminds us that consenting sex requires sober, verbal communication without intimidation or threats. Many states have laws acknowledging that someone who is drunk is not capable of consenting to sex.

Several colleges have developed guidelines to help limit date rape. Perhaps the most controversial of these was produced at Antioch College. At Antioch, students were required to verbally request permission to proceed sexually. They had to ask if they could kiss their partner, then if they could touch their partner, then if they could sleep with their partner, and so on. Permission had to be explicit. Proceeding without verbal permission placed a student at risk of being accused of date rape. The intent was to prevent miscommunication—that is, a student believing that "no" really means "yes." Some opponents of this policy described it at best as silly, and at worse as interfering with students' private relationships. What do you think of Antioch's policy on date rape? Would you like to see it adopted at your school?

Shyness

Because entering college is a new experience, and the people and surroundings are new, it is not surprising to find many students feeling and acting shy. **Shyness** can

shyness
To be afraid of people and being worried of what strangers and powerful others think of oneself.

be a significant stressor for some college students, but it is one, as we shall see later, that can be effectively responded to.

> To be shy is to be afraid of people, especially people who for some reason are emotionally threatening: strangers because of their novelty or uncertainty, authorities who wield power, members of the opposite sex who represent potential intimate encounters.
>
> Shyness can be a mental handicap as crippling as the most severe of physical handicaps, and its consequences can be devastating.
>
> Shyness makes it difficult to meet new people, make friends, or enjoy potentially good experiences.
>
> It prevents you from speaking up for your rights and expressing your own opinions and values.
>
> Shyness limits positive evaluations by others of your personal strengths.
>
> It encourages self-consciousness and an excessive preoccupation with your own reactions.
>
> Shyness makes it hard to think clearly and communicate effectively.
>
> Negative feelings like depression, anxiety, and loneliness typically accompany shyness.[28]

College students may experience stress due to their shyness with professors, club leaders, or people whom they would like to date. This shyness is uncomfortable and, as cited above, may have severe consequences.

Jealousy

College students need to make new friends—both same-sex and opposite-sex ones. Making new friends is ego-threatening ("What if they don't want to be friends with me?"), requires a risk, takes time, and takes a good deal of energy. After all of that, friendship becomes comfortable. We know with whom we can go places, in whom we can confide, and from whom we can receive love. It is understandable, then, that we should value these friendships greatly and become protective and defensive when they are threatened. Even if the threat is only a perceived one—not a real one—jealousy may result.

jealousy
Fear of losing one's property, such as a lover, friend, status, or power.

Jealousy is the fear of losing our property, whether that be our lover, friend, status, or power. We respond to jealousy by either protecting our egos—for example, arguing with our friends or trying to get even—or trying to improve the relationship. Obviously, the second way is preferable.

Jealousy is a stressor some college students experience. It becomes stressful whether we are jealous ourselves or our friends or lovers are the jealous ones.

Breakups

Breakups can be very stressful, especially for the person not wanting to end the relationship.

Jealousy sometimes becomes so stressful that it results in a breakup of the relationship. Sometimes relationships break up because the partners are too dissimilar (one may be interested in sports and the other in the theater) or because they have different expectations of the relationship (one may be a ludic lover and the other a storgic lover). Younger college students are at a stage of life in which they are experimenting with different kinds of relationships, so it is not surprising that many of these relationships do not become permanent. Younger college students usually experience several breakups of relationships during the college years, and these breakups can be quite stressful.

People tend to maintain romantic relationships when their partners meet their fundamental psychological needs, and break up when they do not.[29] One of the needs found very important in maintaining relationships is called *attachment anxiety,* being dependent on their partners to affirm their worthiness of having their needs met.[30] People with high attachment anxiety seem to be less psychologically willing or able to break up a relationship even when their partners fail to meet their psychological needs. For these people, being in any relationship may be preferable to being alone.[31]

When a breakup does occur, students experiencing the most distress are those who have highly invested in the relationship in terms of time and commitment, whose partners break up with them (being left by the other), whose partner has an interest in other relationships and has more alternatives to pursue that interest, and who are fearful of abandonment in the first place.[32] Since most relationship breakups are nonmutual,[33] and we have already seen that having control of a potentially stressful situation can alleviate some of the stress, it is understandable that many relationships result in distress on the part of the person left.

Eating Disorders

If you were told you could be attractive and feel better about your body but would develop intestinal problems, decayed teeth, malnutrition, dehydration, stomach ruptures, esophagus tears, serious heart, kidney, and liver damage, and death, would you agree to that Faustian bargain? Well, that is exactly what some college students do. They adopt an eating disorder that subjects them to serious health consequences, such as those above, in order to perceive that their bodies look better. Ironically, they usually wind up looking worse: gaunt, hollow faced, thin legged, and appearing fatigued.

The Perfect Body

Many people are dissatisfied with their bodies. Generally, women want to lose weight and men want to gain muscle. Women report concern about their body size, buttocks, breasts, thighs, facial features, and body hair.[34]

What does the perfect body look like? A quick glance at the covers of major fashion and sports magazines, and the ads inside, usually depict men and women with seemingly perfect bodies. The same can often be said about actors in movies. These bodies seem almost too perfect to believe. Can these people really look like this all the time? The answer, of course, is no. To capture this perfect body image, models prepare meticulously for that millisecond when the camera's shutter captures their pose. Movie stars may spend months before shooting begins working with a personal trainer and controlling their diets to sculpt their bodies. Clothes, makeup, and lighting are carefully chosen to create the desired image. Hair styling, body makeup, and skintight outfits further enhance the image. As if that were not enough, after the photo or film is taken, editing refines the image to make it perfect. *Playboy* magazine, for example, regularly slims models' waists and thighs before publishing photos, and *Penthouse* magazine routinely augments breast size. Magazines do the same with male athletes and male models.

The search for that perfect body too often results in people adopting eating habits that are unhealthy and may even be life threatening. Among the more common eating disorders are anorexia nervosa and bulimia.

Anorexia Nervosa

Anorexia nervosa is an eating disorder characterized by emaciation, a relentless pursuit of thinness and unwillingness to maintain a normal or healthy weight, a distortion of body image and intense fear of gaining weight, a lack of menstruation among girls and women, and extremely disturbed eating behavior. Some people with anorexia lose weight by dieting and exercising excessively; others lose weight by self-induced vomiting, or misusing laxatives, diuretics, or enemas.

anorexia nervosa
An eating disorder in which a person takes in so few calories as to potentially starve him- or herself.

Many people with anorexia see themselves as overweight, even when they are starved or are clearly malnourished. Eating and food and weight control become obsessions. People with anorexia typically weigh themselves repeatedly, portion foods carefully, and eat only very small quantities of only certain foods. Some who have anorexia recover with treatment after only one episode. Others get well but have relapses. Still others have a more chronic form of anorexia, in which their health deteriorates over many years as they battle the illness.

People with anorexia are up to ten times more likely to die as a result of their illness compared to those without the disorder. The most common complications that lead to death are cardiac arrest, and electrolyte and fluid imbalances. Suicide also can result.

Many people with anorexia also have coexisting psychiatric and physical illnesses, including depression, anxiety, obsessive behavior, substance abuse, cardiovascular and neurological complications, and impaired physical development. Other symptoms that may develop over time include thinning of the bones (osteoporosis), brittle hair and nails, dry and yellowish skin, growth of fine hair over the body, mild anemia and muscle weakness, severe constipation, low blood pressure, and lethargy.[35]

Treating anorexia involves three components: restoring the person to a healthy weight, treating the psychological issues related to the eating disorder, and reducing or eliminating behaviors or thoughts that lead to disordered eating and preventing relapse. Different forms of psychotherapy, including individual, group, and family-based, can help address the psychological reasons for the illness.

Bulimia

Bulimia nervosa is another eating disorder. It is characterized by recurrent and frequent episodes of eating unusually large amounts of food (binge-eating), and feeling a lack of control over the eating. This binge-eating is followed by a type of behavior that compensates for the binge, such as purging (e.g., vomiting, excessive use of laxatives, or diuretics), fasting, and/or excessive exercise.

Unlike anorexia, people with bulimia can fall within the normal range for their age and weight. But like people with anorexia, they often fear gaining weight, want desperately to lose weight, and are intensely unhappy with their body size and shape. Typically, bulimic behavior is done secretly, because it is often accompanied by feelings of disgust or shame. The binging and purging cycle usually repeats several times a week. Similar to anorexia, people with bulimia often have coexisting psychological illnesses, such as depression, anxiety, and/or substance abuse problems. Many physical conditions result from the purging aspect of the illness, including electrolyte imbalances, gastrointestinal problems, and oral and tooth-related problems. Other symptoms include chronically inflamed and sore throat, swollen glands in the neck and below the jaw, worn tooth enamel and increasingly sensitive and decaying teeth, gastroesophageal reflux disorder, intestinal distress and irritation from laxative abuse, kidney problems from diuretic abuse, and severe dehydration from purging of fluids.[36]

As with anorexia, treatment for bulimia often involves a combination of approaches and depends on the needs of the individual. To reduce or eliminate binge and purge behavior, a patient may undergo nutritional counseling and psychotherapy, especially cognitive behavioral therapy (CBT), or be prescribed medication. Some antidepressants, such as fluoxetine (Prozac), which is the only medication approved by the U.S. Food and Drug Administration for treating bulimia, may help patients who also have depression and/or anxiety. Prozac also appears to help reduce binge-eating and purging behavior, reduces the chance of relapse, and improves eating attitudes.[37]

If you have an eating disorder, consult with your instructor or a health care provider at the campus health center. If you have a friend or classmate who you

bulimia
An eating disorder characterized by binge eating followed by purging of food, such as by inducing vomiting or ingesting a laxative.

think has an eating disorder, let your instructor or a health care provider at the campus health center know. This is not "ratting out" your friend. Quite the contrary. It is demonstrating concern for that person's health and welfare. You might even be saving someone's life.

The Older College Student

Many college students are not in their early twenties. More and more, college student populations include a large percentage of older students. These older students have been in the armed services, have developed careers, have raised families, or were engaged in some other activities that led them to postpone their college educations. Those other responsibilities well managed or completed, they are now entering college. Between 1995 and 2010, college enrollment increased by 44 percent, from 14.3 million to 20.6 million. Although the number of young students has been growing more rapidly than the number of older students, this pattern is expected to shift. Between 1999 and 2009, the enrollment of students under age 25 increased by 14 percent. By 2009, though, persons 25 and over comprised 39 percent of all college students.[38] From 2006 to 2017, the National Center for Education Statistics[39] projects a rise of 10 percent in enrollments of persons under 25, and an increase of 19 percent in the number of those 25 and over (see Table 4.4). The response will be large class sizes and more distance learning using the Internet.[40] This is a trend occurring throughout the United States. Older students experience stressors similar to those experienced by younger college students: grades, course overload, jealousy, and breakups. However, they also experience some stressors that are unique to them. We shall briefly discuss three of these: mixing career and school, handling family and school responsibilities concurrently, and doubting their abilities to do well in college.

Career and School

The year was 1964, and I was teaching in a high school in New York City. The students were from Harlem and had problems that were foreign to me. Still, I was very concerned with responding to their needs and, within the limits that existed, helping them to improve the quality of their lives. In other words, I was committed to my job. As the last period of the school day ended, however, I had to rush

Table 4.4 Total Fall Enrollment in Degree-Granting Institutions, by Age: Selected Years, 1970 Through 2017 (in thousands)

Age	1970	1980	1990	1995	2000	2005	2006	Projected 2008	2012	2017
Males and females	8,581	12,097	13,819	14,262	15,312	17,487	17,759	18,200	19,048	20,080
14 to 17 years old	259	247	177	148	145	199	231	191	190	211
18 and 19 years old	2,600	2,901	2,950	2,894	3,531	3,610	3,769	3,953	3,940	3,960
20 and 21 years old	1,880	2,424	2,761	2,705	3,045	3,778	3,648	3,723	3,993	3,958
22 to 24 years old	1,457	1,989	2,144	2,411	2,617	3,072	3,193	3,289	3,584	3,753
25 to 29 years old	1,074	1,871	1,982	2,120	1,960	2,384	2,401	2,531	2,658	3,035
30 to 34 years old	487	1,243	1,322	1,236	1,265	1,354	1,409	1,434	1,616	1,813
35 years old and over	823	1,421	2,484	2,747	2,749	3,090	3,107	3,080	3,066	3,350

Source: U.S. Department of Education, National Center for Education Statistics, *Digest of Education Statistics, 2008* (Washington, DC: U.S. Department of Education, 2009).

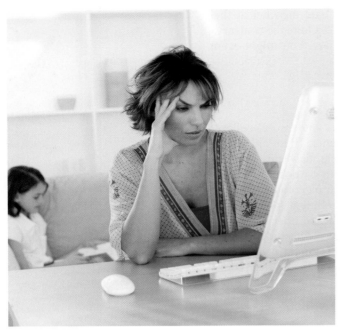

Going to school while raising a family requires creating an effective support system.

to the subway to take a 30-minute train ride to CCNY, where I was taking 12 credits toward my master's degree. My classes were over at about 9:30 p.m., which is when I rushed to the subway to take a one-hour train ride back to my apartment in Brooklyn.

This situation is not unique. Having taught on a college campus, I have seen many students experiencing what I experienced. I recall one student, for example, whose job required her to be in Europe Thursday through Sunday—she was an airline flight attendant—but she was taking several college courses on Monday and Tuesday. Others have had careers that they were committed to—students of mine who were social workers, accountants, and police officers come to mind—but were enrolled in college, too. The need to do well with a career may cause stress, and the need to do well at school may also cause stress. Even though each of these stressors may be manageable alone, when they coexist there may be an overload. The result may be illness or disease.

Family and School

Not only are many older college students working, but many have family responsibilities as well. A number of students have discussed with me the problem of what to do with after-work time. Should they work on their term paper? Study for an exam? Read next week's chapter? Or should they play with their kids or spend time with their spouses? Will the in-laws understand if they don't visit because they're doing schoolwork?

It takes a very understanding spouse to provide psychological support for a student who has family and work responsibilities, too. It is tiring and often frustrating to have so much to do in a day. It is stressful and may be unhealthy as well. A spouse who can provide those extra few minutes with the kids that the student-parent can't, who can take on more than his or her share of the household chores, and who can provide a shoulder to lean on and an ear to listen, can go a long way in intervening between stress and illness for the older college student.

Not to be forgotten in this discussion is the financial investment necessary to attend college. Older students who must support a family must decide if the investment in education is worthwhile. There will be a payoff down the road—either in increased income or in improved lifestyle that a more enjoyable or less demanding job may afford. Often, however, a financial sacrifice is required by the student and his or her family while the schooling takes place. This sacrifice is easier to bear if the whole family believes it worthwhile and is willing to put off immediate pleasures to achieve long-range goals. If the older student continually has to justify the expense of college, or if the family's sacrifice is periodically brought up to make him or her feel guilty, the stress associated with college will be greater than otherwise.

Self-Doubt

Some colleges are recognizing that returning college students—those who dropped out years ago—and older, first-time college students have all sorts of doubts about their ability to be successful in their studies. Consequently, they are offering counseling programs for these students. These self-doubts are understandable, since our society too often perceives learning as a young person's activity. How can I compete with young, bright people? How can I do well when I'm also working full-time?

How can I pass my courses when I need to devote time to my family? How will I be able to spend as much time at the library as students who live on campus? I don't have someone to study with or professors to consult with frequently, as does the student living on campus. I've forgotten how to study. I haven't taken an exam in ages. These are some of the stressful concerns of the older college student.

The Minority College Student

Minority college students face stressors that are similar to those faced by other college students. However, in addition they can experience other stressors that are specific to their minority status. One obvious stressor is racism. Researchers have found racism associated with high blood pressure,[41–43] respiratory illness,[44] body aches and pains,[45] poor self-rated health,[46,47] mental health problems,[48,49] and several chronic health conditions.[50–52]

Racism can also have devastating effects on students' grades. Latino students are less likely to complete college through the traditional path (enroll within one year of high school graduation, and attain a postsecondary credential within the "traditional" time frame). Only 4 percent of Hispanics completed a postsecondary credential through the traditional path, compared to 15 percent of whites and 23 percent of Asians.[53] In 2005–2006, Latino students earned 9 percent of awards conferred in higher education. Of these, 33 percent were in certificates, 23 percent were associate degrees, and 31 percent were bachelor degrees.[54] Latinos have increased their associate degree attainment 125 percent and bachelor degree attainment 88 percent in 10 years (1994–2004). In 2004, Hispanic students earned 11 percent of associate's and 7 percent of bachelor's degrees awarded.[55] A study conducted at the University of Maryland[56] found Hispanic students' grades were lower when they experienced racism. It should be noted, though, that Hispanic students who took advantage of campus minority services were able to handle the racism better and, as a result, their grades were higher than those of other Hispanic students. This is particularly important since the proportion of American college students who are minorities has been increasing. In 1976, some 15 percent were minorities, compared with 34 percent in 2009. Much of the change can be attributed to rising numbers of Hispanic and Asian/Pacific Islander students. The proportion of Asian/Pacific Islander college students rose from 1 percent to 7 percent, and the Hispanic proportion rose from 4 percent to 13 percent during that time period. The proportion of African American students fluctuated during most of the early part of the period, before rising to 14 percent in 2009 from 10 percent in 1976 (see Table 4.5).[57] If you experience racism, consult with your instructor regarding services available on your campus.

Race/Ethnicity	1976	1980	1990	2000	2005	2007	2008	2009
Total	100.0	100.0	100.0	100.0	100.0	100.0	100.0	100.0
White, non-Hispanic	83.4	81.4	77.6	68.3	65.7	64.4	63.3	62.3
Total minority	14.5	16.1	19.6	28.2	30.9	32.2	33.3	34.3
Black, non-Hispanic	9.5	9.2	9.0	11.3	12.7	13.1	13.5	14.3
Hispanic	3.5	3.9	5.7	9.5	10.8	11.4	11.9	12.5
Asian or Pacific Islander	0.8	2.4	4.1	6.4	6.5	6.7	6.8	6.5
American Indian/Alaskan Native American	0.7	0.7	0.7	1.0	1.0	1.0	1.0	1.0
Nonresident alien	2.0	2.5	2.8	3.5	3.3	3.4	3.5	3.4

Table 4.5
Total Fall Enrollment in Degree-Granting Institutions, by Race/Ethnicity of Student: Selected Years, 1976 Through 2009

Source: U.S. Department of Education, National Center for Education Statistics, *Digest of Education Statistics, 2010* (Washington, DC: U.S. Department of Education, 2010).

Staying Safe on Campus[a]

The topic of school-associated violence triggers many emotions: panic, anxiety, fear, stress, shock, apathy, and grief. The rigors of academic life can be stressful enough, let alone the added pressure to mentally embrace the possibility of what, where, why, or when violence might occur. However, school-associated homicides occur very infrequently. Data from the School-Associated Violent Death Study[b] indicate that school-associated homicide rates decreased significantly from 1992 to 2006.

Rarely does an individual just "snap." Rather, it's a series of behavioral indicators over time that may lead to one's physically acting out. Some of the warning signs are

- Withdrawing from classmates and social settings.
- Feeling isolated, lonely, and rejected.
- Being a victim of violence.
- Being bullied and taunted.
- Exhibiting poor academic performance and lack of interest in academics.
- Having unmanageable anger and aggressive behaviors.
- Threatening violence.

Pay attention to a combination of these signs, rather than one in isolation. However, if you observe something that doesn't seem "right," when in doubt report it to a school counselor, official, professor, or mental health professional.

Knowing your surroundings is key to your safety in any situation, be it at school, at home, at the mall, in a parking lot, or at work. Know where exits are—from both the room and the building. Plan out how you would react to an emergency, be it a violent threat or natural disaster.

Many schools have implemented "e-lert" systems for contacting students regarding safety emergencies at school, through e-mail, phone, or text messages. Determine if you need to sign up to be alerted and find our where at school you should go if an emergency does occur.

[a]Ferrett, Sharon K. *Peak Performance: Success in College and Beyond, 7th ed.* (New York: McGraw-Hill, 2010), p. 133.
[b]W. Modzeleski, T. Feucht, J. E. Hall, T. R. Simon, L. Butler, A. Taylor, M. Hunter, M. A. Anderson, L. Barrios, and M. Hertz, "School-Associated Student Homicides—United States, 1992—2006," *MMWR Weekly,* 57(January 18, 2008): 33–36.

Another stressor experienced by minority college students relates to the manner in which college classes are conducted. For example, some classes rely on debate and confrontation to discuss controversial issues. Certain cultural groups' values of politeness and respect for others may be at odds with the type of classroom climate fostered by some college instructors. Furthermore, when accommodations in the classroom are recognized as needed to adjust to the different learning styles of minority students, too often the interpretation results in broad generalizations about the intellectual ability of these students. Rather than the accommodations being considered a flexible approach by the instructor, minority student deficits requiring remediation is the stereotypical conclusion drawn.

In addition, the pressure to perform well academically from well-meaning family members may be very stressful for some minority students. This pressure may stem from a cultural value placed on education, or it may relate to the student being the first one in his or her family to go to college. In either case, the family is invested in the student's success in college.

These are not the only stressful situations encountered by minority college students. Some of these students attended a high school in which they were the majority. Now having minority status requires an adjustment that can be stressful. Other students may not have appropriate role models at their colleges with whom to consult and from whom to receive guidance and encouragement. There is still an under-representation of minority faculty and university administrators on college campuses.

In spite of these unique stressors that minority college students can and often do experience, many do exceptionally well in their studies. If you are a minority on your campus, use the resources available to you to be one of the successful ones. Consult with your instructor for assistance, speak with someone at the counseling center or the campus health center, or seek the help of any campus organizations designed to assist minority students.

Interventions

Interventions can diminish the stress of college for both younger and older students. These interventions can be at the levels of life situation, perception, emotional arousal, or physiological arousal.

Life-Situation Interventions

Students entering college are bombarded with numerous life changes. To prevent adding to these needed adjustments, other aspects of life should be made as routine as possible. More life changes mean more stress; thus, entering college is not the time to take on added job responsibilities, to have a baby, or to break up old relationships. I've long suspected that the large number of college dropouts is more a function of stress than of grades. When we consider that most students enter college, move out of their homes, leave old friends, make new friends, accept new responsibilities, and live in a new town, it is not surprising that all of these life changes are stressful to them. Recognizing this situation, at least two suggestions seem sensible: (1) that high schools teach stress management and (2) that colleges offer stress management workshops during orientation sessions for entering students. More and more of this is occurring, but still not enough. High school graduates are not only entering college; some are entering the military, some are taking full-time jobs, and some are raising families. In spite of what they do when they leave high school, their lives change dramatically and swiftly. They should be helped to deal with this change by managing the stress accompanying it. And they should be taught how to manage their finances during this time of greater independence. This, too, should be a part of orientation programs for students entering college. Some banks also offer this service free of charge for those who open accounts.

Another life-situation intervention responds to the need to make new friends. The more people you meet, the more likely you are to find a new friend. Joining clubs, participating in intramurals, going to parties and dances, and working with other students to improve campus life are all good ways to meet people. Remember, however, that the idea is to improve your health—psychological and physical—so don't engage in unhealthy or dysfunctional activities just to be part of a group. I've had several students talk with me about their problem with abusing alcohol because "all" their friends spend their time drinking at an off-campus hangout. When we looked more closely at the situation, we found that not "all" the friends drank and that friendships could be maintained with those who did drink without having to get drunk oneself. Once students realized that it was they, not their friends, who were responsible for their drinking, they were better able to control it.

To respond to stressors associated with shyness and self-doubt, try some of the following suggestions. These suggestions come from one of the country's authorities on shyness and the director of the Stanford University Shyness Clinic.[58]

Alcohol is sometimes thought of as the answer to all problems. After the alcohol wears off, however, the stressful problems remain or are sometimes made even worse by attempting to cope by drinking.

1. Recognize your strengths and weaknesses and set your goals accordingly.

2. Decide what you value, what you believe in, what you realistically would like your life to be like. Take inventory of your library of stored scripts and bring them up-to-date, in line with the psychological space you are in now, so they will serve you where you are headed.

3. Determine what your roots are. By examining your past, seek out the lines of continuity and the decisions that have brought you to your present place. Try to understand and forgive those who have hurt you and not helped when they could have. Forgive yourself for mistakes, sins, failures, and past embarrassments. Permanently bury all negative self-remembrances after you have sifted out any constructive value they may provide. The bad past lives on in your memory only as long as you let it be a tenant. Prepare an eviction notice immediately. Give the room to memories of your past successes, however minor.

4. Guilt and shame have limited personal value in shaping your behavior toward positive goals. Don't allow yourself to indulge in them.

5. Look for the causes of your behavior in physical, social, economic, and political aspects of your current situation and not in personality defects in you.

6. Remind yourself that there are alternative views to every event. "Reality" is never more than shared agreements among people to call it the same way rather than as each one separately sees it. This enables you to be more tolerant in your interpretation of others' intentions and more generous in dismissing what might appear to be rejections or putdowns of you.

7. Never say bad things about yourself; especially, never attribute to yourself irreversible negative traits such as "stupid," "ugly," "uncreative," "a failure," "incorrigible."

8. Don't allow others to criticize you as a person; it is your specific actions that are open for evaluation and available for improvement—accept such constructive feedback graciously if it will help you.

9. Remember that sometimes failure and disappointment are blessings in disguise, telling you the goals were not right for you, the effort was not worth it, and a bigger letdown later on may be avoided.

10. Do not tolerate people, jobs, and situations that make you feel inadequate. If you can't change them or yourself enough to make you feel more worthwhile, walk on out, or pass them by. Life is too short to waste time on downers.

11. Give yourself the time to relax, to meditate, to listen to yourself, to enjoy hobbies and activities you can do alone. In this way, you can get in touch with yourself.

12. Practice being a social animal. Enjoy feeling the energy that other people transmit, the unique qualities and range of variability of our brothers and sisters. Imagine what their fears and insecurities might be and how you could help them. Decide what you need from them and what you have to give. Then let them know that you are ready and open to sharing.

13. Stop being so overprotective about your ego; it is tougher and more resilient than you imagine. It bruises but never breaks. Better it should get hurt occasionally from an emotional commitment that didn't work out as planned than get numbed from the emotional insulation of playing it too cool.

14. Develop long-range goals in life, with highly specific short-range subgoals. Develop realistic means to achieve these subgoals. Evaluate your progress regularly and be the first to pat yourself on the back or whisper a word of praise in your ear. You don't have to worry about being unduly modest if no one else hears you boasting.

15. You are not an object to which bad things just happen, a passive nonentity hoping, like a garden slug, to avoid being stepped on. You are the culmination

of millions of years of evolution of our species, of your parents' dreams, of God's image. You are a unique individual who, as an active actor in life's drama, can make things happen. You can change the direction of your entire life anytime you choose to do so. With confidence in yourself, obstacles turn into challenges and challenges into accomplishments. Shyness then recedes, because, instead of always preparing for and worrying about how you will live your life, you forget yourself as you become absorbed in the living of it.

For jealousy-related stress, Walster and Walster recommend three steps.[59] The first step involves finding out exactly what is making you jealous. Key questions to ask are "What was going on just before you started feeling jealous?" and "What are you afraid of?" As we discussed earlier, you're probably afraid of losing something (e.g., love, self-esteem, property, status, or power). The second step asks you to put your jealous feeling in proper perspective. Is it really so awful that your friend is interested in someone else? Aren't you interested in other people as well? Is your jealousy irrational? What's the difference between *having* to have this person love you and *wishing* this person loved you? Is it really true that you couldn't stand to lose this person's love? Or is it that you'd *like* not to?

Lastly, you can negotiate a "contract" with the other person. This contract should help you be less jealous but must not be too restrictive on the other person. To expect your friend to lunch only with you might be unfair. To expect your friend to lunch with you on Tuesdays and Thursdays, on the other hand, might ensure you're spending time together while allowing each of you the freedom to spend time with other people.

Other life-situation interventions follow:

1. Limit the courses in which you enroll to a number you can handle without overloading yourself.

2. Improve your communication with a romantic lover so both of you have the same expectations for, and understanding of, the relationship.

3. The best way to manage a breakup is to seek out new relationships. Get involved with other people—and not only romantically.

4. To coordinate family and school responsibilities, schedule each of these. Working out specific times for schoolwork with your family will ensure you're getting your work done and your family is not being disappointed you're not with them. Working out specific times to be with your family will ensure that you do not overlook their needs.

When intervening at the life-situation level, don't forget some obvious resources. You can consult with your professor, seek assistance from personnel at the campus health center, speak with your adviser, or get help from the community health department. These and other resources have proven valuable to many of my students, and I believe they will for you as well. Help is all around you if you look and ask for it.

Perception Interventions

As we've stated many times in this book, as important as external events are in relation to stress, so is your perception of those events. The following are some ways to perceive the stressors of college life as less distressing:

1. To perceive shyness and jealousy as less threatening, questions such as "What am I really afraid of? How probable is it that this thing I fear will happen? How bad is it if it does happen?" will help you view the shyness or jealousy more realistically.

2. Use selective awareness to focus upon the positive aspects of college. The opportunity to learn new things, meet new people, prepare for a

Getting Involved In Your Community

Academic concerns certainly can cause many college students a great deal of stress. After all, in college you are preparing for your future. However, students also experience stress unrelated to their coursework. That is one reason many campuses have a health center.

Of course, campus health centers concern themselves with flu and measles outbreaks and other illnesses and diseases. But they also offer services related to the mental health of the college community. At the health center on my campus, counseling services are available to students who are feeling "stressed out" about their relationships with other students, their girlfriends or boyfriends, or their parents. I have referred more than one student to that health center who was wrestling with feelings associated with the death of a close friend or relative. And, unfortunately, a college, like any other community, has its share of violence and crime, so we also have a rape crisis hotline and sexuality counseling program.

Interestingly, many of these services are offered by students themselves. These are volunteers who go through a fairly extensive training program so as to offer effective service. These peer education and peer counseling programs are highly regarded by our campus community, and they provide an invaluable service.

Does your campus have a health center? Does that health center offer similar programs? If so, perhaps you might consider volunteering to participate in a peer education or counseling program. If such a program does not presently exist on your campus, perhaps you can organize one.

future you are looking forward to, and find out how capable you really are should occupy your thoughts, rather than how difficult or time-consuming it is or how much time it requires away from your family and your job.

3. Smell the roses along the way—literally and figuratively. I love the look and smell of my campus. Whether it be winter or summer, spring or fall, the trees, bushes, buildings, and grounds have a pleasing nature. I sometimes walk off the path to hear the crunch of snow under my feet, and I've been known to walk right up to a flowering crab apple tree to smell its fragrance. Maybe your campus isn't as pretty as mine, or maybe it's prettier. In any case, there are things about your campus that, if you paid attention to them, would make the time you spend there more pleasant.

4. When looking at all of your responsibilities, you might feel overloaded. However, if you were to write a schedule for them, you would probably recognize that you do have enough time for it all. Only when viewed collectively do they appear overwhelming.

Emotional Arousal Interventions

As with other stressors, college-related ones can be managed at the emotional level by regular practice of relaxation techniques. When I mention this to groups of people who have so little time (e.g., students who work full-time and also have family responsibilities), I'm frequently told that there just aren't 40 minutes a day for relaxation. I tell them that if they don't have the time then they, in particular, need the regular relaxation. The paradox is that those without the time probably need the practice more than those who can fit it in. At this point in your reading, you should recognize that we all have the time; we just choose to use it for something else. You can rearrange how you use your time so you can practice a relaxation technique regularly. It's up to you!

Physiological Arousal Interventions

Regular exercise will use the stress products you build up. The body is prepared to do something physical, and exercise will afford it a healthy way to make use of this preparation.

College students are more fortunate than others relative to physiological arousal intervention, since they usually have access to exercise facilities and equipment. They can join intramural teams, participate in recreational sports hours (these usually occur during the noon hour or late afternoon or evening), or do exercise alone (e.g., jog around campus or shoot baskets).

College life can be made less stressful with attention paid to managing college-related stressors. You're probably tired of reading this, *but* whether it's stressful or not is really up to you.

Coping in Today's World

Lisa is so busy she has no time to work on the term paper that is due next week. Since the grade on that paper makes up a significant percent of the grade in that course, Lisa decides to pay a friend to write the term paper for her.

In Juan's stress management course, students are assigned to groups. Each group is expected to develop an outline and conduct a workshop for people, off campus, in need of learning stress management skills. In past semesters, groups have helped cancer patients cope better with their disease, taught elementary school children to manage conflict with classmates less confrontationally, and shown nursing home residents how to communicate more effectively with staff and family members to experience less stressful relationships. However, Juan is studying in preparation to take the MCATs for entrance to medical school. How he does on that exam will determine whether he gets accepted to a medical school and, therefore, whether he can achieve his goal of becoming a physician. So, Juan decides to study for the exam rather than attend planning meetings scheduled by his group or participating in the development of the group's workshop outline. At the end of the semester, Juan asks the group to put his name on their project paper even though he hardly contributed to it. The professor will never know, he argues.

Tonya and Latricia are good friends. Both recognize that Latricia learns more easily and is a more conscientious student. So when it comes to taking the midterm exam in the course for which they are both enrolled, Tonya, relying on their friendship, expects Latricia will let her copy off of her answer sheet.

The situations described above all include ethical violations by college students. They involve taking credit for a paper or group project to which the student made little if any contribution, or relying on cheating on an exam. Ethical behavior, while always important, has recently been highlighted by corporate scandals such as the collapse of large businesses like Enron and World-Com—which resulted from unethical behavior by corporate executives that involved financial lies and "cooking the books." However, the rest of us too often do not realize that some of our common behaviors are also unethical. Forty-four percent of Americans lie about their work history when applying for a job, 25 percent have downloaded music illegally, 30 percent own pirated software, and 75 percent of high school and college students admit to some form of cheating.[a] Furthermore, 79 percent of workers say they would steal from their employers, 17 percent lie on their tax returns, and 3 percent of scientists admit to unethical scientific conduct such as fabricating data.

Imagine the stress associated with behaving unethically. First there is the energy required to engage in the unethical act and then to hide it from others. Then there are the potential consequences if the unethical behavior is uncovered. Many universities and colleges have Honor Codes, and violations can result in suspension, expulsion, and/or notations on violators' permanent records. Embarrassment before one's family and friends is another stressful consequence that can be expected. And, even if one is not caught, the loss of trust and respect among those who do know about the act (e.g., friends and classmates) can be quite stressful. As with other stressors, the best place to set up a roadblock is at the life-situation level of our stress model. In other words, do not act unethically in the first place and none of the potential stress reactions will occur.

[a]"Lies, Damn Lies, and Statistics," *Wired*, March 24, 2004: 60–61.

summary

- College life can be quite stressful because it requires adapting to a dramatic life change. College life involves assuming greater responsibility for one's life, managing finances, making new friends, studying a great deal, and learning about a new environment.

- Specific stressors experienced by college students include striving for good grades, coping with a greater amount of schoolwork, making friends, managing pressure to be sexually active, preventing date rape, being shy, becoming jealous, breaking up with a dating partner, and ethnic and racial discrimination.

- Many college students are over 25 years of age. It is estimated that the number of older college students will increase dramatically in the coming years.

- Older college students experience stressors unique to their situations. They must juggle career, school, and family responsibilities.

- Older college students often doubt their abilities to return to school, to achieve academically, and to interact well with classmates who may be much younger.

- Colleges and high schools need to offer stress management educational experiences to their students to help them manage the degree of change that occurs upon graduating from high school and entering college.

- To manage jealousy-related stress, determine what makes you jealous, put your jealous feelings in proper perspective, or negotiate a contract with the other person.

- Minority college students can face unique stressors. Among these are racism, classrooms conducted in ways that are at odds with cultural values, pressure to succeed in school, minority status in school for the first time, and the lack of role models from whom to seek guidance and encouragement.

internet resources

Stress in College: Common Causes of Stress in College **http://stress.about.com/od/studentstress/a/stress_college.htm** *Description of causes of stress for college students including academic stress, social stress, weight issues, and dropout.*

Managing Stress: A Guide for College Students **www.uhs.uga.edu/stress/** *Produced by the University of Georgia University Health Center, this site places a discussion of stress within a wellness lifestyle view.*

Help Now: Stress Management **http://ub-counseling.buffalo.edu/stressmanagement.shtml** *Managed by the University of Buffalo, this site discusses what stress is, its symptoms, causes of stress, and what to do about it.*

Managing Stress **www.cmhc.utexas.edu/stress.html** *The Counseling & Mental Health Center at the University of Texas at Austin presents signs of stress that include feelings, thoughts, behaviors, and physical signs.*

National Eating Disorders Association **www.nationaleatingdisorders.org/information-resources/** *The National Eating Disorders Association presents information regarding eating disorders including the following topics: general information, audio and videos, women and girls, men and boys, family and friends, educators and coaches, treatment professionals, toolkits, stories of hope, and resources and links.*

references

1. L. J. Friedlander, G. J. Reid, N. Shupak, and R. Cribble, "Social Support, Self-Esteem, and Stress as Predictors of Adjustment to University Among First-Year Undergraduates," *Journal of College Student Development* 48(2007): 259–74.

2. M. J. Fischer, "Settling into Campus Life: Differences by Race/Ethnicity in College Involvement and Outcomes," *Journal of Higher Education* 78(2007): 125–56.

3. S. H. Murff, "The Impact of Stress on Academic Success in College Students," *Abnf Journal* 16(2005): 102–04.

4. The Project on Student Debt, *Quick Facts about Student Debt*, 2007. Available at: http://projectonstudentdebt.org/files/File/Debt_Facts_and_Sources_5_4_07.pdf

5. Elizabeth Scott, "Stress in College: Common Causes of Stress in College. *About.com Guide*, 2008. Available at: http://stress.about.com/od/studentstress/a/stress_college.htm

6. Robin Humphrey, et al., "Stress and the Contemporary Student," *Higher Education Quarterly* 52(1998): 221–42.

7. Elizabeth Scott, "What Causes the Freshman 15?: What's Behind New College Students' Weight Gain," *About.com Guide,* 2007. Available at: http://stress.about.com/od/studentstress/a/freshman15cause.htm

8. A. Chickering and R. Havighurst, "The Life Cycle," in *The Modern American College,* ed. A. Chickering, et al. (San Francisco: Jossey-Bass, 1998).

9. Friedlander, Reid, Shupak, and Cribble, "Social Support, Self-Esteem, and Stress," 259.

10. E. C. Chang, "Perfectionism and Dimensions of Psychological Well-Being in a College Student Sample: A Test of a Stress-Mediation Model," *Journal of Social and Clinical Psychology* 25(2006): 1001–22.

11. J. H. Pryor, H. Hurtado, L. DeAngelo, L. Palucki, and S. Tran Blake, *The American Freshman: National Norms, Fall 2010* (Los Angeles, CA: Higher Education Research Institute, UCLA, 2010).

12. Advisory Committee on Student Financial Assistance, *Condition of Access and Persistence Study,* 2009. Available at: www.ed.gov/about/bdscomm/list/acsfa/edlite-caps.html

13. Scott, "What Causes the Freshman 15?"

14. Higher Education Project, *At What Cost? The Price That Working Students Pay for a College Education,* 2002. Available at: www.calpirgstudents.org/reports/higher education/higher-education-reports/at-what-cost-the-price-that-working-students-pay-for-a-college-education

15. V. B. Saenz and D. S. Barrera, *Findings from the 2005 College Student Survey (CSS): National Aggregates* (Los Angeles: UCLA Higher Education Research Institute, 2007). Available at: www.gseis.ucla.edu/heri/PDFs/2005_CSS_REPORT_FINAL.pdf

16. "Student Finances, by the Numbers," *Chronicle of Higher Education* 49(2002): 13.

17. "Online Dating Magazine Media Center: Abbreviated Online Dating Facts and Stats," *Online Dating Magazine,* 2007. Available at: www.onlinedatingmagazine.com/mediacenter/onlinedatingfacts.html

18. Edward O. Laumann, John H. Gagnon, Robert T. Michaels, and Stuart Michaels, *The Social Organization of Sexuality: Sexual Practices in the United States* (Chicago: University of Chicago Press, 1994).

19. National Center for Health Statistics, "Sexual Behavior and Selected Health Measures: Men and Women 15–44 Years of Age, United States, 2002," *Advance Data* 32(2005): 21–22, 25.

20. National Survey of Sexual Health and Behavior (NSSHB). *Center for Sexual Health Promotion,* 2010. Available at: www.nationalsexstudy.indiana.edu/

21. Robert T. Michael, John H. Gagnon, Edward O. Laumann, and G. Kolata, *Sex in America: A Definitive Survey* (New York: Warner Books, 1995).

22. Centers for Disease Control and Prevention. "Diagnoses of HIV Infection and AIDS in the United States and Dependent Areas," *HIV Surveillance Report* 21(2009).

23. C. Everett Koop, *Understanding AIDS: A Message from the Surgeon General* (Washington, D.C.: Department of Health and Human Services, 1988).

24. L. D. Lindberg and S. Singh, "Sexual Behavior of Single Adult American Women," *Perspectives on Sexual and Reproductive Health* 40(2008): 27–33.

25. Centers for Disease Control and Prevention, "Heterosexual Populations. Section 1: Core Epidemiologic Questions. Direct Measure of Risk Behavior." *Sample: Integrated Epidemiologic Profile for HIV/AIDS Prevention and Care Planning—Louisiana, 2002.* Available at: www.cdc.gov/hiv/topics/surveillance/resources/guidelines/epi-guideline/la_supp/section1q3_heterosexual.htm

26. K. Ford, W. Sohn, and J. Lepkowski, "Characteristics of Adolescents' Sexual Partners and Their Association with Use of Condoms and Other Contraceptive Methods," *Family Planning Perspectives* 33(2001): 101–05, 132.

27. American College Health Association, *Acquaintance Rape* (Baltimore: American College Health Association, 1992).

28. Philip G. Zimbardo, *Shyness: What It Is and What to Do About It* (Reading, MA: Addison-Wesley, 1990), 12, 158–60.

29. H. Patrick, C. R. Knee, A. Canevello, and C. Lonsbary, "The Role of Need Fulfillment in Relationship Functioning and Well-Being: A Self-Determination Theory Perspective," *Journal of Personality and Social Psychology,* 92(2007): 434–56.

30. M. Mikulincer and P. R. Shaver, *Attachment in Adulthood: Structure, Dynamics, and Change* (New York: Guilford, 2007).

31. Erica B. Slotter and Eli J. Finkel, "The Strange Case of Sustained Dedication to an Unfulfilling Relationship: Predicting Commitment and Breakup from Attachment Anxiety and Need Fulfillment within Relationships," *Personality and Social Psychology Bulletin* 35(2009): 85–100.

32. Susan Sprecher, Diane Felmlee, Sandra Metts, Beverley Fehr, and Debra Vanni, "Factors Associated with Distress Following the Breakup of a Close Relationship," *Journal of Social and Personal Relationships* 15(1998): 791–809.

33. Susan Sprecher, "Two Sides of the Breakup of Dating Relationship," *Personal Relationships* 1(1994): 199–222.

34. Laura G. Knapp, Janice E. Kelly-Reid, and Scott A. Ginder, *Enrollment in Postsecondary Institutions, Fall 2009; Graduation Rates, 2003 & 2006 Cohorts; and Financial Statistics, Fiscal Year 2009* (Washington, DC: National Center for Education Statistics, 2009). Available at: http://nces.ed.gov/pubsearch/pubsinfo.asp?pubid=2011230

35. T. J. Hunt, M. D. Thienhaus, and A. Ellwood, "The Mirror Lies: Body Dysmorphic Disorder," *American Family Physician* 78(2008): 217–22.

36. National Institute of Mental Health (a), *Anorexia Nervosa,* 2010. Available at: www.nimh.nih.gov/health/publications/eating-disorders/anorexia-nervosa.shtml

37. National Institute of Mental Health (b), *Bulimia,* 2010. Available at: www.nimh.nih.gov/health/publications/eating-disorders/bulimia-nervosa.shtml

38. Ibid.

39. U.S. Department of Education, National Center for Education Statistics, *Digest of Education Statistics, 2008.* (Washington, D.C.: U.S. Department of Education, 2009).

40. Amy Argetsinger, "Colleges Brace for the Baby Boom," *The Washington Post,* July 8, 2000, B5.

41. E. Brondolo, M. A. Rieppi, K. P. Kelly, and W. Gerin, "Perceived Racism and Blood Pressure: A Review of the Literature and Conceptual and Methodological Critique," *Annals of Behavioral Medicine* 25(2003): 55–65.

42. Clarence C. Gravlee, Amy L. Non, and Connie J. Mulligan, "Genetic Ancestry, Social Classification, and Racial Inequalities in Blood Pressure in Southeastern Puerto Rico," *Plos One,* 2009. Available at: www.plosone.org/article/info%3Adoi%2F10 .1371%2Fjournal.pone.0006821

43. William W. Dressler, Kathryn S. Oths, and Clarence C. Gravlee, "Race and Ethnicity in Public Health Research: Models to Explain Health Disparities," *Annual Review of Anthropology* 34(2005): 231–52.

44. S. Karlsen and J. Y. Nazroo, "Relation Between Racial Discrimination, Social Class, and Health Among Ethnic Minorities," *American Journal of Public Health* 92(2002): 624–31.

45. T. L. Bowen-Reid and J. P. Harrell, "Racist Experiences and Health Outcomes: An Examination of Spirituality as a Buffer," *Journal of Black Psychology* 28(2002): 18–36.

46. A. Schulz, B. Israel, D. Williams, E. Parker, A. Becker, and S. James, "Social Inequalities, Stressors and Self-Reported Health Status Among African American and White Women in the Detroit Metropolitan Area," *Social Science and Medicine* 51(2000): 1639–53.

47. J. Stuber, S. Galea, J. Ahern, S. Blaney, and C Fuller, "The Association Between Multiple Domains of Discrimination and Self-Assessed Health: A Multilevel Analysis of Latinos and Blacks in Four Low-Income New York City Neighborhoods," *Health Services Research* 38(2003): 1735–60.

48. H. Landrine, E. A. Klonoff, I. Corral, S. Fernandez, and S. Roesch, "Conceptualizing and Measuring Ethnic Discrimination in Health Research," *Journal of Behavioral Medicine* 29(2006): 79–94.

49. S. Noh and V. Kaspar, "Perceived Discrimination and Depression: Moderating Effects of Coping, Acculturation, and Ethnic Support," *American Journal of Public Health* 93(2003): 232–38.

50. B. A. Finch, R. A. Hummer, B. Kolody, and W. A. Vega, "The Role of Discrimination and Acculturative Stress in Mexican-Origin Adults' Physical Health," *Hispanic Journal of Behavioral Science* 23(2001): 399–429.

51. G. C. Gee, J. Chen, M. Spencer, et al. "Social Support as a Buffer for Perceived Unfair Treatment Among Filipino Americans: Differences Between San Francisco and Honolulu," *American Journal of Public Health* 96(2006): 677–84.

52. G. C. Gilbert, M. S. Spencer, J. Chen, and D. Takeuchi, "A Nationwide Study of Discrimination and Chronic Health Conditions Among Asian Americans," *American Journal of Public Health* 97(2007): 1275–82.

53. National Center for Health Statistics, *Racial/Ethnic Differences in the Path to a Postsecondary Credential*, July 22, 2003. Available at: http://nces.ed.gov/pubsearch/pubsinfo. asp?pubid=2003005

54. *Excelencia in Education*, 2006. Available at: www.edexcelencia .org/initiatives/examples-of-excelencia/2006

55. National Center for Health Statistics, *Digest of Education Statistics, 2005.* August 10, 2006. Available at: http://nces.ed .gov/pubsearch/pubsinfo.asp?pubid=2006030

56. Martha R. Carkcl, "Grades and Racism Linked in Report," *The Diamondback,* October 11, 1993, 1, 7.

57. Thomas D. Snyder and Sally A. Dillow, *Digest of Education Statistics 2010* (Washington, DC: National Center for Education Statistics, 2011), 331–32.

58. Zimbardo, *Shyness,* 158–60.

59. Elaine Walster and G. William Walster, *A New Look at Love* (Reading, MA: Addison-Wesley, 1978), 91–93.

LAB ASSESSMENT 4.1

Budgeting While in School: Using a Worksheet to Help Manage Your Money

Directions: This worksheet can help you develop a budget for the semester. To do so, fill in the information requested. If you aren't sure about some of the information, find out. For example, call utility companies, contact apartment complexes to find out about the rental fees, or ask your parents about utility bills and deposits.

I. Semester Info

Number of months in semester   _____

II. Semester Expenses

Tuition and fees   _____

Books   _____

Deposits   _____

Transportation/Moving   _____

   Total   _____

   Per month   _____

III. Semester Income

Family Contribution   _____

Student Loans   _____

Other Financial Aid
(Grants/Scholarships/Gifts)   _____

   Total   _____

   Per Month   _____

IV. Monthly Income

Estimated monthly salary   _____

Minus taxes (*approx. 28%*)   _____

Net income   _____

Other income   _____

   Total   _____

V. Monthly Expenses

Rent   _____

Combined utilities   _____

Groceries   _____

Auto expenses   _____

Student loan payment(s)   _____

Other loan payment(s)   _____

Credit cards   _____

Insurance   _____

Medical expenses   _____

Entertainment   _____

Miscellaneous   _____

   Total   _____

VI. Discretionary Income

Total Monthly Income   _____

Total Monthly Expenses   _____

   Monthly Total   _____

   Semester Total   _____

Source: Texas Guaranteed Student Loan Association, "Budgeting While in School," *Adventures in Education, 2009.* Available at www.aie.org/paying-for-college/finance-tools/budgeting-while-in-school.cfm

LAB ASSESSMENT 4.2

How Intimate Are Your Friendships?

Directions: Think of a casual acquaintance and one of your closest friends. First circle the number of the following statements that you discuss with your friends in private conversation. Next, list the set of statements you would discuss with a casual acquaintance.

1. Whether or not I have ever gone to a church other than my own (2.85)

2. The number of children I want to have after I am married (5.91)

3. How frequently I like to engage in sexual activity (10.02)

4. Whether I would rather live in an apartment or a house after getting married (3.09)

5. What birth control methods I would use in marriage (9.31)

6. What I do to attract a member of the opposite sex whom I like (8.54)

7. How often I usually go on dates (5.28)

8. Times that I have lied to my girlfriend or boyfriend (8.56)

9. My feelings about discussing sex with my friends (7.00)

10. How I might feel (or actually felt) if I saw my father hit my mother (9.50)

11. The degree of independence and freedom from family rules that I have (had) while living at home (5.39)

12. How often my family gets together (2.89)

13. Who my favorite relatives (aunts, uncles, and so on) are and why (5.83)

14. How I feel about getting old (6.36)

15. The parts of my body I am most ashamed for anyone to see (8.88)

16. My feelings about lending money (4.75)

17. My most pressing need for money right now (outstanding debts, some major purchases that are needed or desired) (6.88)

18. How much I spend for my clothes (7.17)

19. Laws that I would like to see put in effect (3.08)

20. Whether or not I have ever cried as an adult when I was sad (8.94)

21. How angry I get when people hurry me (5.33)

22. What animals make me nervous (3.44)

23. What it takes to hurt my feelings deeply (9.37)

24. What I am most afraid of (8.25)

25. How I really feel about the people I work for or with (7.29)

26. The kinds of things I do that I don't want people to watch (8.85)

The amount of disclosure is shown by the number of statements circled for each person. Intimacy of disclosure is found by adding up the numbers in parentheses for the circled statements, divided by the total number of statements circled. For instance, if you have circled statements 1, 4, 12, 19, and 22 for an acquaintance, 5 indicates the amount you would disclose, and 3.07 (2.85 + 3.09 + 2.89 + 3.08 + 3.44 = 15.35 ÷ 5) would be the intimacy of disclosure figure—not very much in this case.

As you can see by the results of the friendship and acquaintanceship questionnaire you just completed, self-disclosure is a vital ingredient in friendship. Without self-disclosure of a significant degree, your relationship stops at the acquaintance level. Although acquaintances may help alleviate loneliness, they don't provide the social support that friends do, which we have learned can act as a buffer for our stress.

Source: D. A. Taylor and I. Altman, "Intimacy-Scaled Stimuli for Use in Research on Interpersonal Exchange," *Naval Medical Research Institute Technical Report No. 9,* MF 022, 01.03–1002, May 1966.

LAB ASSESSMENT 4.3

What Type of Lover Are You?

Directions: To find out what type of lover you are, answer each question as it applies to your boyfriends, girlfriends, lovers, or spouse.

A = almost always
U = usually
R = rarely
N = never (or almost never)

_____ 1. You have a clearly defined image of your desired partner.

_____ 2. You felt a strong emotional reaction to him or her on the first encounter.

_____ 3. You are preoccupied with thoughts about him or her.

_____ 4. You are eager to see him or her every day.

_____ 5. You discuss future plans and a wide range of interests and experiences.

_____ 6. Tactile, sensual contact is important to the relationship.

_____ 7. Sexual intimacy was achieved early in the relationship.

_____ 8. You feel that success in love is more important than success in other areas of your life.

_____ 9. You want to be in love or have love as security.

_____ 10. You try to force him or her to show more feeling and commitment.

_____ 11. You declared your love first.

_____ 12. You are willing to suffer neglect and abuse from him or her.

_____ 13. You deliberately restrain frequency of contact with him or her.

_____ 14. You restrict discussion and display of your feelings with him or her.

_____ 15. If a breakup is coming, you feel it is better to drop the other person before being dropped.

_____ 16. You play the field and have several persons who could love you.

_____ 17. You are more interested in pleasure than in emotional attachment.

_____ 18. You feel the need to love someone you have grown accustomed to.

_____ 19. You believe that the test of time is the only sure way to find real love.

_____ 20. You don't believe that true love happens suddenly or dramatically.

Some researchers have identified four basic types of love: erotic, ludic, storgic, and manic. If you answered A or U to 1–8, you are probably an erotic lover. If you answered A or U to 3–4 and 8–12, your love style tends to be manic. If you answered A or U to 13–17 and R or N to the other questions, you are probably a ludic lover. If you answered A or U to 17–20, together with R or N for the other statements, your love style tends to be storgic. Refer back to the section on love for descriptions of these types of lovers.

Source: John Alan Lee, *The Colours of Love* (Toronto: New Press, 1973).

General Applications
Life-Situation and Perception Interventions

Intervention

A young boy asked his older brother where babies come from. The older brother told him that babies come from the stork. Seeking verification of this shocking revelation, the young boy asked his father where babies come from. The father said that babies come from the stork. Not wanting to be impolite but still not completely satisfied, the boy approached the wise old sage of the family, his grandfather, and asked him where babies come from. The grandfather, following the party line, told him that babies come from the stork. The next day in school, the young boy related his conversations with his brother, father, and grandfather to the teacher and his classmates, concluding that there hadn't been normal sexual relations in his family for at least three generations.

Obviously, there was miscommunication in this family. To prevent any miscommunication regarding stress management, Part 1 of this book has provided you with information about the nature of stress, examples of stressors, the manner in which the body reacts to stressors, and illnesses and diseases associated with stress. You are, therefore, more prepared to see stress management as a complex of activities rather than something accomplished simply by following some guru. There are no simple, "stork-like" answers to coping with stress. There is, however, a comprehensive stress management system that you can employ to control stress and tension. This chapter presents a model of stress and its relationship to illness, and stress management techniques are seen as interventions within this model. **Interventions** are activities to block a stressor from resulting in negative consequences, such as psychological discomfort, anxiety, illness, and disease. You'll soon see that comprehensive stress management is sensible, logical, and possible and that you can manage your own stress.

Coping with a Stressor

The most widely accepted notion of coping and stress appraisal was formulated many years ago by Richard Lazarus.[1] Lazarus perceived **stress** to be the result of a determination that a demand exceeds resources available to meet that demand. Consequently, the demand is evaluated as a threat. In that case, some form of coping is needed. **Coping** is engaging in a behavior or thought to respond to a demand. For example, you might have a difficult final exam and perceive that as stressful because it is not one of your better subjects. In response to this demand, you try to find a successful way to cope. That may mean finding a better way to learn the material and earn a good grade on the exam. Lazarus called that *task-oriented coping*. Or it might mean managing your feelings and/or accepting that this is a subject in which you are not particularly talented. Lazarus called that *emotion-focused coping*.

To engage in either coping mechanism requires an appraisal of the demand. Lazarus described three primary categories of appraisal: primary appraisal, secondary appraisal, and reappraisal. **Primary appraisal** involves judging how much of a threat is involved, and how important is the outcome. Once that primary appraisal occurs, you must determine whether you have the resources needed to meet the

Interventions
Activities to prevent a stressor from resulting in negative consequences.

stress
The result of a demand that exceeds resources available to meet that demand.

coping
Engaging in a behavior or thought to respond to a demand.

primary appraisal
Judging how much of a threat is involved, and how important is the outcome.

Figure 5.1   Lazarus' Model of Appraisal

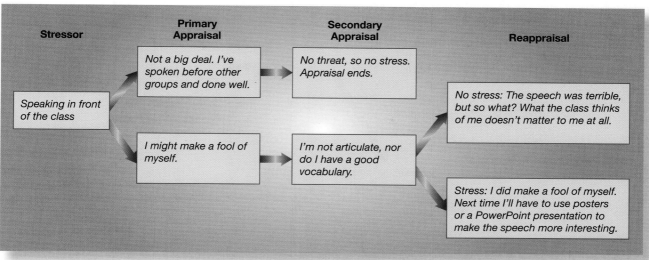

Source: R. Lazarus and S. Folkman, *Stress Appraisal and Coping.* New York: Springer, 1985.

demand. Lazarus called that **secondary appraisal.** Once attempts are made to respond to the threat or to meet the demand, a **reappraisal** occurs to determine whether any further coping is needed.

Lazarus's model then considers stress occurring when we perceive a threat. (See Figure 5.1.) That determination is made by *primary appraisal.* Then a determination is made—*secondary appraisal*—regarding whether we have the resources available to effectively respond to that threat. Once we do respond, we evaluate whether the response was effective, and if not, choose a different response (*reappraisal*).

One important form of appraisal is determining how confident you are in managing the demand/threat. If you are confident, you will engage in behavior or thought to manage the demand/threat since you believe what you do will be effective. If you are not confident, why even attempt to do anything? You don't think it will work. In his classic article, Bandura called this **self-efficacy.**[2,3] Self-efficacy is discussed in more detail in Chapter 14. For now, suffice it to say that there are two forms of self-efficacy: *outcome efficacy* and *personal efficacy.* You might believe that people can engage in a number of strategies to give up cigarette smoking. That is *outcome efficacy.* However, you might also believe that although many people can do this, you will never be successful at giving up cigarette smoking. That is *personal efficacy.* To believe it is worth the effort to attempt to manage a demand/threat, you must believe not only that there is a strategy that can be effective but that you can successfully employ that strategy.

A Model of Stress

Stress begins with a *life situation* that knocks you (gently or abruptly) out of balance. You are nudged or shoved into disequilibrium and need to right yourself. This life situation could be a change in temperature, a threat from another person, the death of a loved one, or some other change in your life to which you need to adapt.

We all know, however, that the same situation presented to different people may result in different reactions. That is because different people will interpret the situation differently. This is termed their **cognitive appraisal** and, as we will see later, it can be controlled.

Some people may view the death of a loved one, for example, as terrible and dwell on that loss. Others may also view the death of a loved one as terrible but think about the nice times experienced with the one who died. A life situation to

secondary appraisal
Determining whether resources needed to meet the demand are available.

reappraisal
Evaluation of whether the response made to a demand/threat was effective.

self-efficacy
Confidence in the ability to manage a demand/threat.

cognitive appraisal
Interpretation of a stressor.

Figure 5.2

Perception of a life situation.

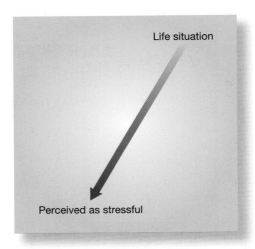

which you must adapt is therefore a necessary but not sufficient component of stress. What is also necessary is your perception of that life situation as stressful.

So far, then, we have a life situation that is *perceived* (or cognitively appraised) as distressing. This is represented in Figure 5.2. What occurs next is *emotional arousal* to the distressing life event. Such feelings as fear, anger, and insecurity or feelings of being rushed, overwhelmed, frustrated, or helpless may be results of perceiving a life situation as stressful.

These feelings lead to *physiological arousal*. As described in detail in Chapter 2, stress reactivity includes increases in serum cholesterol, respiratory and heart rates, muscle tension, blood pressure, and blood glucose, along with decreases in the effectiveness of the immunological system, strength of the cardiac muscle, digestion, and histamine effectiveness. If physiological arousal is chronic or prolonged, illness or disease may result. In addition to illness or disease (be it physical or psychological), stress can lead to other *consequences* (poor performance in school or on the job, poor interpersonal relationships, or other such negative effects). The stress model is now complete and appears in Figure 5.3.

Let's follow a person down this road to the consequences of prolonged stress to demonstrate the functioning of this model. Suppose you work for the automobile industry and are relatively well adjusted. Your job is pleasing, and you've been employed at the same location for eight years. You have become comfortable interacting with your fellow workers, and you know when the coffee breaks occur, the best routes to travel to and from work, and to whom to be especially nice.

Figure 5.3

Stress model.

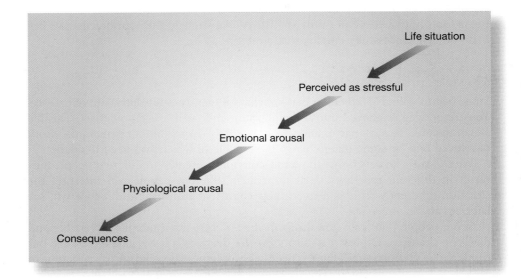

Unfortunately, the economy takes a turn for the worse. Credit becomes tight and interest rates rise. People stop buying cars, and your company decides to lay off several hundred employees. Your pink slip appears in the envelope with your paycheck. Thus, a life situation has presented itself to which you need to adapt.

You consider this situation earth-shattering! How will you pay the rent, buy food, pay medical bills? How will you occupy your time? What will people think of you? Can you get another job? How should you begin to look for one? Questions, questions, concerns, concerns. You have now progressed to the second component of the model: You perceive being fired as distressing. Recognize, though, that not everyone will perceive this same event as distressing. Some of your fellow employees may be saying:

1. It's not good being fired, but I really do need a rest. I've been working too hard lately.
2. I'm going to use this opportunity to spend more time with my children.
3. I think I'll take advantage of this situation by going back to school. I always wanted the time to be able to do that.

These people have set up a roadblock between the life situation and their perceptions of that situation. They have changed their cognitive appraisal of being fired. They are not perceiving the event as a major catastrophe, and therefore it will not become one.

You, however, have perceived being fired as traumatic and subsequently are aroused emotionally. You feel *fear* about the future. You become *unsure* of your self-worth. You are *angry* at the boss for choosing you as one of those fired. You are *frustrated* at the whole situation and *confused* about what to do next. These feelings result in physiological arousal. You wind up with more blood fats roaming within your blood vessels. You perspire more, breathe differently, brace your muscles, secrete more hydrochloric acid in your stomach, and have fewer lymphocytes in your blood to combat infectious agents. If you don't use these built-up stress products in some way, and if this situation and your reaction to it remain the same, you may contract a stress-related illness.

Feedback Loops in the Stress Model

The stress model presented in Figure 5.3 is fairly simple. One part of the model leads to the next, and the next part leads farther down the model. This conceptualization is helpful when we consider how to manage stress better, later in this chapter. In reality, however, stress and our reaction to it are much more complex, and the stress model can have many feedback loops. For example, when an illness results from stress—a negative consequence—that illness is a life situation that starts down the road of stress all over again. If it is perceived as distressing, emotional and physiological arousal result, and still other negative consequences occur. Or emotional arousal, such as anger, may lead to arguing at work. The result may be losing your job. Job loss then becomes a life situation you need to manage. Keep in mind that the way we interact with stressors and stress is quite complicated. Still, the simple conceptualization of the stress model (in Figure 5.3), and of how we can set up roadblocks on that model makes stress management more easily understood.

Setting Up Roadblocks

Once the progression from a life situation through perception, emotion, physiological arousal, and vulnerability to disease and other consequences is understood, it is then possible to intervene short of these consequences. Intervention entails setting up roadblocks at various points on the stress theory model (see Figure 5.4). Because this model includes sequential phases, with each phase dependent upon

Figure 5.4

Think of the stress model as a map that goes through different towns. As with all roads, you can set up roadblocks along the way.

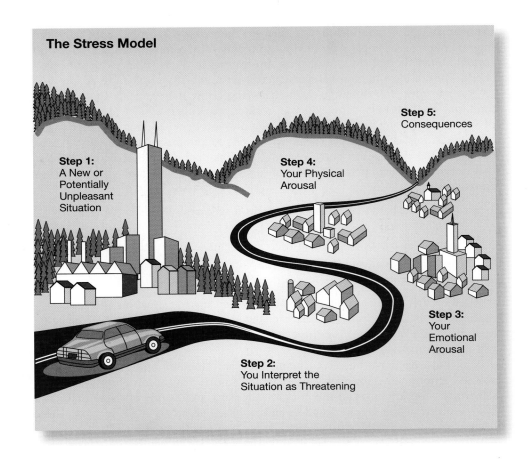

The Stress Model

Step 1: A New or Potentially Unpleasant Situation

Step 2: You Interpret the Situation as Threatening

Step 3: Your Emotional Arousal

Step 4: Your Physical Arousal

Step 5: Consequences

the full development of the previous phase, any interruption of this sequence will short-circuit the process. For example, even though a life situation requiring adaptation presents itself to you, a roadblock between that life situation and the next phase (perceiving it as stressful) could be set up. This roadblock might consist of prescribed medications (sedatives, tranquilizers, depressants), illicit drugs (marijuana, cocaine), or your insistence that you will not allow yourself to view this situation as disturbing. Regarding the last option, you might decide to focus upon the positive aspect of the situation (there is something good about *every* situation, even if that "good" is that things can't get any worse). A roadblock between the perception phase and the emotion phase can also be established. Relaxation techniques are also excellent ways to keep emotional reactions from leading to prolonged physiological arousal. Once physiological arousal occurs, a roadblock between it and poor health must consist of some form of physical activity that uses the built-up stress products. Remember that at the point of physiological arousal your body has prepared itself with the fight-or-flight response. A physical activity (e.g., jogging) will use the body's preparedness rather than allow the state of arousal to lead to poor health.

Comprehensive Stress Management

Some *incomplete* stress management programs teach participants only one or just a few stress management skills. Consequently, they are prepared to set up a roadblock at only one location on the stress theory model. Some programs teach people meditation, yoga, or time management. To understand the reason these programs are incomplete, you must first be introduced to the sievelike aspect of the stress theory model.

Research Identifies the Best Level of the Stress Model in Which to Intervene

Stress researcher Robert Epstein found that there are four trainable skill sets or competencies people can use to effectively manage stress. These include the following:

1. *Source Management*—reducing or eliminating the source of the stress.
2. *Relaxation*—techniques such as meditation or diaphragmatic breathing.
3. *Thought Management*—reinterpreting stressful thoughts to be less stressful.
4. *Prevention*—planning to avoid stressors.

Furthermore, Epstein's research concluded that *prevention* is the most effective of the four. Second is *source management,* with the least effective being *relaxation* and *thought management,* in that order. That is not to say that relaxation and thought management should not be part of a comprehensive program to manage stress. Just that preventing stressful events in the first place is more effective than trying to relax away stress or think differently about stressful events after they occur.

Source: Epstein, Robert. "Fight the Frazzled Mind," *Scientific American Mind* 22(2011): 30–35.

At each level on the model, it is possible to filter out only a portion of the stress experience. Consequently, a roadblock (intervention technique) employed at only one place on the road will not stop *all* the "bad guys" from getting through. Each roadblock will stop some "bad guys," but no *one* roadblock will stop all it encounters. Each roadblock, then, is like a sieve that sifts and filters out some stress but allows some to pass through to the next phase of the stress theory model. It follows, then, that programs teaching only one or just a few stress management skills are helping their participants to some extent but not to the greatest degree possible.

Complete, comprehensive stress management includes intervention at *all* phases of the stress theory model and *several* means of intervening at *each* of these locations. As you can see from the table of contents of this book, Chapters 6 through 15 give us means to do just that. Each of those chapters focuses upon one phase of the stress theory

Getting away from your normal routine and focusing on something other than your stressors can be a very effective roadblock on the stress model.

model and describes several ways to sift out some of the stress experienced at that phase. Your goal, however, will not be to eliminate all of your stress. Remember from our earlier discussion that there is an optimum amount of stress. It is impossible, and undesirable, to eliminate all stress. Complete stress management does not subscribe to that goal but conveys the nature of eustress to its participants.

Eustress and the Model

So far, we have focused upon the negative consequences of stress: illness, disease, poor performance, and impaired interpersonal relationships—that is, **distress.** However, we can use the same stress model to better understand the positive consequences

distress

Stress that results in negative consequences such as decreased performance and growth.

of stress. Stress that results in good consequences, such as producing personal growth, is called **eustress.** Stress that leads to actions that are beneficial to a person is also eustress. And stress that encourages optimum performance is eustress.

An example of eustress will make it more understandable. When I teach stress management, the class is conducted informally but includes most of the topics discussed in this book. A glance at the table of contents will show the array and number of topics studied. It would be easy for these topics to be lost and for their interconnectedness to be overlooked. My dilemma is how to keep the class interesting yet encourage students to study the content so as to realize how, for example, time management and biofeedback (two seemingly unrelated subjects) are cousins in the same stress management family.

I decided on a final examination as the vehicle by which students are required to deal with the array of topics studied as a meaningful whole. The test, then, serves as a eustressor—it leads to stress for the students who seek to do well on the exam and results in more learning than would have otherwise been accomplished. The stress is beneficial and useful (more learning occurs) and is, therefore, positive—eustress.

Using the stress model to explain the positive consequences in this example, the test is the life situation. Next, my students interpret the test as a threat and perceive it as stressful. That perception results in such emotions as fear, self-doubt, and worry, which lead to physiological arousal. However, because of this stress, my students study longer and consequently learn more. The positive outcome is that they know more about stress and how to manage it than they would have known if they hadn't experienced this situation, and they do better on the test than they might have done otherwise. So, you see, the stress model can be used to explain both the negative and the positive consequences of stress.

I'll bet you have experienced stress that, when it was over, made you consider yourself better for the experience. Either it was a positive life event that required significant adjustment (a move to a grass shack in Hawaii) or a more threatening event that led you to make important changes in your life (a brush with death that made you reorganize your priorities). In any case, you were stressed "for the better." That is eustress. The following are some other examples of eustressors:

1. Having to make a presentation before a group of people and preparing better because of the stress.

2. Asking someone out on a date and rehearsing a better way of doing it because of the stress.

3. Having someone you love tell you the things he or she dislikes about you and using that information to make you a better you.

See Figure 5.5.

Taking Control

If there is only one concept by which you remember this book, I'd like it to be that *you are in much greater control over yourself than you have ever realized.* Managing stress is really just exercising that control rather than giving it up to others or to your environment. Let me give you an example of the kind of control you have over yourself. Recall an occasion when you became angry with someone. As vividly as you can, remember what preceded your anger. What happened earlier that day? What was the weather like? What were you anticipating? What was your previous relationship with that person? What did that person do that made you angry? Also recall your angry response in all its detail: How did you feel, what did you want to do, what did you actually do, and how did it all work out?

So often we hear others say, "So-and-so made me angry!" No one can make you angry. Rather, you *allow* yourself to be angered by what so-and-so has said or done. When you describe your behavior as dependent upon another's, you have given

Source: R. M. Yerkes and J. D. Dodson, "The Relation of Strength of Stimulus to Rapidity of Habit Formation," *Journal of Comparative Neurology and Psychology* 18(1908): 459–82.

Figure 5.5

The Yerkes-Dodson Curve

The Yerkes-Dodson Curve is an excellent way to envision the difference between too much stress and too little stress. Stress can be productive and have positive consequences—increase performance, as depicted to the left of the midpoint. However, stress can also have negative consequences—interfere with performance, as depicted to the right of the midpoint. In fact, there is an optimal level of stress that results in maximum performance. For example, a tennis player experiencing too much stress will be too tense to perform well, whereas a tennis player experiencing too little stress may lose focus and not play well. However, a player experiencing an optimal level of stress will be alert and, yet, not too tense. That player's performance will be maximized.

up control of that behavior *to* that other person. To demonstrate this point for yourself, manipulate the variables in the situation you just recalled.

Instead of a rainy day, imagine it to have been warm and sunny. Instead of a person with whom you have had a bad relationship doing or saying the thing about which you became angry, imagine it to have been the person you love most. Further, imagine that you received word of getting straight A's in school, a promotion, a salary raise, or some other nice event just prior to the situation about which you became angered. To summarize: You awakened to a nice, warm, sunny day. When you arrived at work, you were told you were promoted and given a substantial increase in salary. Soon afterward, a person whom you dearly love did or said X (the event about which you became angered).

Responding to the situation as it is now described in the same manner in which you responded to the original situation probably seems incongruous. The point is that the actual event does not necessarily have anger as its consequence. The anger was brought to that situation by you—not by the event or the other person. On some days, the same event would not have resulted in your becoming angry. You may have been having a great day and telling yourself it was so great that nothing was going to ruin it. What's more, nothing did! You are in charge of your behavior. You may not be able to get other people to change what they say or do, but certainly you can change how you react to what they say or do. *You are in charge of you.*

Generalizing this concept of control to stress management, it is your decision whether or not to increase your blood pressure, your heart rate, or your muscle tension. It is your decision whether or not to become frightened or anxious, or to vomit at the side of the road. It is your decision whether or not you will regularly practice relaxation techniques (e.g., meditation). The practice of these techniques is a good example of taking control and assuming responsibility for (owning) your own behavior. Students and participants in workshops I conduct often tell me they would like to meditate but don't have the time. Hogwash. I don't care if you have 10 screaming, unruly teenage werewolves at home and don't think you can find the place, the time, or a quiet-enough environment to meditate. I've heard it all

Demonstrating You Can Take Charge

In the space provided, rewrite each of the statements to indicate that *you* are really in control. The first two statements serve as examples.

1. You make me upset.

   When you do that, I allow myself to become upset.

2. It was my insecurity that forced me to do that.

   When I allow myself to feel insecure, I do things that I later regret

3. I was so frightened, I was helpless.

   _____

4. It's just a rotten habit that I can't break.

   _____

5. I'm just destined to be a failure.

   _____

6. If I were articulate, I'd be better at my job.

   _____

7. I was successful because I work well under pressure.

   _____

8. I'm the way I am because of my upbringing and parents.

   _____

before. The time you already have. You have chosen to use it for something else. The quiet you can get. I recall meditating in a car in the garage of the apartment house in which my parents lived because their two-bedroom apartment with four adults, two children, and several neighbor children creating dissonance (one screeching violin strings and the other hammering the keys of an irreparably out-of-tune piano) was not conducive to relaxation.

The *place* is also available, since you can meditate anywhere. I've meditated on airplanes, under a tree on a golf course in the Bahamas, and once in the front seat of a car my wife was driving at 60 miles per hour on a highway in Florida.

In any case, you are in charge of what you do or do not do to manage your stress. Further, you are responsible for that decision and must accept its consequences. The intervention skills presented in this book can help you to control the stress and tension you experience. Whether they do that depends on whether you learn these skills, practice them, and incorporate them into your daily routine.

It would be dysfunctional to employ stress management techniques in a stressful way—yet that is not uncommon. Trying very hard to control stress will, in and of itself, create stress. If you have not bothered to use comprehensive stress management for the many years of your life, don't rush into it now. Read slowly and carefully. Try the skills; use those that work for you, and discard the others. If you are under medical care, check the appropriateness of these techniques and skills with your physician. You may need less medication, or certain procedures may be contraindicated for someone with your condition. Enjoy managing stress rather than making it one more thing to do. Use comprehensive stress management to free up, rather than clutter up, your day.

Making a Commitment

While you are advised not to rush into this stress management system, a beginning should be made immediately. This beginning may consist only of a commitment to read this book so as to learn more about stress and its control. That first step

Contract of Commitment

I, _____, am concerned about the effects of stress upon my health and have decided to learn how to better manage the stress I encounter. Therefore, I commit myself to completely reading this book, practicing the skills presented, and incorporating at least two of these skills into my daily routine.

If I have met this commitment by _____

(two months from now)

I will reward myself by _____

(buying or doing something out-of-the-ordinary)

_____

If I have not met this commitment by the date above, I will punish myself by

_____

(depriving yourself of something you really enjoy)

_____   _____

(Signature)   (Date)

Getting Involved in Your Community

Are there life situations that occur on your campus that can cause stress? Perhaps there is not a sufficient study period between the end of classes and the beginning of final examinations. Perhaps the library is not open late enough. Maybe because there is no place on campus to gather, students mingle at local bars that serve alcohol. Identify these life situations below.

1. _____
2. _____
3. _____
4. _____
5. _____

What can you do that would result in a change in these life situations? What can you do to either eliminate the stressor altogether or adjust the situation to make it less stressful? List these below.

1. _____
2. _____
3. _____
4. _____
5. _____

Will you commit to work on these changes to make your campus less stressful? If so, remember to be tactful, polite, and cooperative. Belligerence might result only in others being resistant to change.

is significant, however, because subsequent steps depend on it. Since stress reactivity that is chronic or prolonged may result in your becoming ill, the longer you wait to begin controlling your stress, the less healthy you can expect to be. If you're healthy now, you want to maintain that status. If you're presently ill and that illness is exacerbated by stress, you can move toward health by managing that stress. Are you willing to begin? How much are you willing to do? Behaviorists know that behavior that is reinforced is repeated, whereas behavior that is punished tends to be eliminated. Determine your commitment to managing your stress by completing a contract with yourself; you can use the contract presented here. Notice that it contains a reward for accomplishing what you contract to do and a punishment for not living up to the contract.

Be realistic and don't make this contract too stressful. Some examples of rewards you might use include tickets to the theater, a new coat or shoes, a restrung tennis racket, or a day of pampering. Some possible punishments include no television for a week, sweets for three weeks, or nights out with friends for a month.

There's no time like the present to get started . . . *the sooner the better*!

Coping in Today's World

Researchers have found that humor has significant healthful effects. For example, when 52 healthy men viewed a humorous video for one hour, they produced increased levels of natural killer cells, immunoglobulin, T-cells, and other changes that lasted 12 hours.[a] In a similar study,[b] 27 healthy volunteers watched a cheerful, comical video for 30 minutes. It was found that their levels of free radical-scavenging capacity significantly increased, indicating better health. Recognizing these healthful effects, those in stressful jobs are particularly advised to use humor as a eustressor. For example, this advice has been recommended to nurses[c] and, in particular, to nurses who work in the operating room.[d] When nurses used humor, their

bodies reacted in ways that indicated they were healthier. So, make a point of smiling, finding the humor in situations, and clowning it up. You will be happier and healthier if you embrace eustress.

[a]L. S. Berk, D. L. Felton, S. A. Tan, B. B. Bittman, and J. Westengard, "Modulation of Neuroimmune Parameters During the Eustress of Humor-Associated Mirthful Laughter," *Alternative Therapies in Health and Medicine* 7(2001): 62–72, 74–76.
[b]T. Atsumi, S. Fujisawa, Y. Nakabayashi, T. Kawarai, T. Yasui, and K. Tonosaki, "Pleasant Feeling from Watching a Comical Video Enhances Free Radical-Scavenging Capacity in Human Saliva," *Journal of Psychosomatic Research* 56(2004): 377–79.
[c]B. A. D'Anna, "Nurse Clowns in the OR: An Interview with Barbara D'Anna," *Today's OR Nurse* 15(1993): 25–27.
[d]B. L. Simmons and D. L. Nelson, "Eustress at Work: The Relationship between Hope and Health in Hospital Nurses," *Health Care Management Review* 26(2001): 7–18.

summary

- Interventions are activities designed to block a stressor from resulting in negative consequences such as illness or disease. Stress management consists of the use of these interventions.

- Stress begins with a life situation that knocks you out of balance. However, for the stress response to develop, this situation has to be perceived and cognitively appraised as distressing.

- When life situations are perceived and cognitively appraised as distressing, emotional reactions such as fear, anger, and insecurity develop. These emotional reactions then lead to physiological arousal.

- Physiological arousal that is chronic or prolonged can lead to negative consequences such as illness or disease, poor performance, and impaired interpersonal relationships.

- Stress management involves "setting up roadblocks" on the road leading from life situations through perception, emotional arousal, and physiological arousal and ending at negative consequences.

- Incomplete stress management programs teach only one or a few stress management skills. Comprehensive programs teach means of intervening at each level of the stress model.

- Stress that leads to positive consequences is called eustress. Eustress involves change that still requires adaptation but is growth producing and welcome. A test can be an example of a eustressor when concern for a good grade results in your studying and learning more.

- You are in much greater control of yourself than you have ever realized. Managing stress is really just exercising that control, rather than giving it up to others or to your environment.

internet resources

MEDLINE Plus—Stress **www.nlm.nih.gov/medlineplus/ stress.html** *A National Institutes of Health site that provides links to stress-related sites.*

How to Master Stress **www.mindtools.com/smpage.html** *A "how to" site on understanding stress and its effects, with stress management techniques.*

Stress Cure **www.stresscure.com** *Contains a Health Resource Network for general stress information as well as strategies for coping with stress.*

references

1. Richard Lazarus and Susan Folkman, *Stress, Appraisal, and Coping* (New York: Springer, 1984).

2. Albert Bandura, "Self-Efficacy: Toward a Unifying Theory of Behavioral Change," *Psychological Review* 84(1977): 191–215.

3. Albert Bandura, *Self-Efficacy: The Exercise of Control* (New York: W. H. Freeman, 1997).

LAB ASSESSMENT 5.1

What Eustressors Have You Experienced?

Eustress is the result of a threat that is encountered, that elicits a response, and that results in beneficial outcomes. For example, the fear of failing an exam results in your studying extra long, and the result is an "A" on the exam. Or, the fear of approaching your boss for a raise in salary leads you to prepare extra well for that discussion, and the result is your getting the raise. List three occasions when you experienced eustress:

1. _____

2. _____

3. _____

Why did you classify those instances as eustress? What were the beneficial outcomes? For the three eustress occasions above, list three of these beneficial outcomes:

1. _____

2. _____

3. _____

What did you do that resulted in eustress on these occasions, when it could have turned out badly and resulted in distress? In these examples, the student studied longer than otherwise, and the worker prepared for a discussion he or she might not have prepared for otherwise. For each of the eustress occasions listed, identify what you did that resulted in eustress instead of distress:

1. _____

2. _____

3. _____

What can you learn from this insight about managing stressors? Draw three conclusions:

1. _____

2. _____

3. _____

Life-Situation Interventions: Intrapersonal

A t the end of the semester, the professor wrote on the chalkboard, "Which of the required readings in this course did you find least interesting?" Students engaged in a lively and animated discussion, citing several readings as of particularly little interest. Then the professor wrote the second question on the chalkboard, "To what defect in yourself do you attribute this lack of interest?"

Now, I am not so confident as to profess every word in this chapter is a gem, nor that if you disagree, there is something wrong inside of you. But there is much included that has implications for how you can better manage stress by managing that which is within you. In other words, this chapter discusses the life-situation phase of the stress model—in particular, intrapersonal matters. We focus on what is between you and you, rather than between you and others.

It has been said that the difference between a smart person and a wise one is that a smart person can work his or her way out of a difficulty that a wise person will not get into in the first place. In this chapter we help you to be *wise*—that is, prevent stress in the first place—but recognizing that stress is unavoidable, we also help you be *smart*—that is, cope better with the stress you do encounter.

Eliminating Unnecessary Stressors

The higher on the stress theory model you can siphon off stressors, the more likely it is that you will be able to manage the stress in your life. For example, if you experience stress when you drive on a major, crowded road in your town or city, you could perceive it as less stressful by focusing on the nice scenery (perception level). Or, you could engage in relaxation techniques, such as meditation, to manage your feelings of frustration and anger (emotional arousal level). Or, you could exercise daily to deplete the built up stress by-products such as high blood pressure and muscle tension. However, it would be even better if you would choose another road on which to drive (life situation level) so you do not start down the stress model road in the first place. You would think that if you could eliminate all stressors from your life, you would never experience stress and therefore would never become ill from it. Because that goal is both impossible and undesirable, your attempt at stress management at the top level of the model (life situation) should be to eliminate as many distressors as is feasible. To accomplish this end, this chapter presents you with introspective activities for identifying unnecessary stressors in your life and eliminating them.

In my course "Controlling Stress and Tension," students keep a diary for three weeks. Why don't you keep a diary as well? A sample page appears in Figure 6.1. This diary must include seven components for each day:

1. Stressors for that day:
   a. Routine stressors (experienced often).
   b. Unique stressors (seldom encountered).

Figure 6.1

The stress diary.

Responses	Means of Coping			Means of	Coping Better
	Psychological	Physiological	Behavioral		
1. *Routine*					
a. Taking tests	anxious	headache	eat quickly	pull an "all nighter"	study with classmate
b.					
c.					
2. *Unique*					
a. Get the flu	frustrated	tired	stay in bed	drink fluids/sleep	go to campus health center
b.					
c.					

Relaxation techniques tried	Effectiveness of technique
1. Meditation	Helps me relax and learn faster
2.	
3.	

Sensations

Body Sensations	Mind Sensations

2. Reactions to *each* stressor encountered:
   a. Psychological reactions (e.g., fear, anxiety, confusion).
   b. Physiological reactions (e.g., perspiration, increased pulse rate, muscle tension).
   c. Behavioral reactions (e.g., became aggressive, called a friend).
3. Means of coping with *each* stressor.
4. Better means of coping that might have been attempted.
5. Relaxation techniques tried that day.
6. Effectiveness of these relaxation techniques.
7. Sensations during that day:
   a. Bodily sensations (e.g., headache, stomach discomfort, backache).
   b. Mind sensations (e.g., anxiety attack, feelings of insecurity, sense of being rushed).

In addition to reporting how tedious it becomes to keep a diary for three weeks, students say they value this learning experience highly among others with which they have ever been presented. To understand this reaction requires an explanation of how we use the diary once the three-week period is concluded. The contents of the diary are considered data from which generalizations (or patterns) about each student and each student's life can be gleaned. Rather than focusing on one occurrence or even one day, we try to identify consistent features that will provide insight into how each student interacts with the stress of his or her life. To accomplish this end, we ask the following questions:

1. What stressors do you frequently experience?
2. Which routine stressors can you eliminate? How?
3. How does your body typically respond to stressors?

4. How does your psyche typically respond to stressors?

5. What do you typically do when confronted with a stressor?

6. Are there any coping techniques that you use more than others?

7. Do these techniques work for you or against you?

8. Are there any coping techniques that you believe would be helpful but you don't use often enough?

9. Are any particular relaxation techniques more effective for you than others?

10. Summarize what you will *do* as a result of recording and analyzing this diary. Be as specific as you can; for example, rather than state that you will relax more, describe the time of day, place, and method of relaxation.

After three weeks, ask and answer the previous 10 questions. You will probably gain much insight into your stress experience and be able to adjust your life to experience fewer stressors. What you will be doing is taking charge of your life to prevent stressors from leading to poor health by eliminating unnecessary stressors before they even begin their journey down the stress road. The more stressors you can eliminate in this fashion, the less likely it is that stress will cause illness or disease for you. The importance of eliminating unnecessary stressors will become even more evident in the next section.

Nutrition and Stress

The relationship between nutrition and stress remains unclear. This is definitely one stress-related area fertile for research. However, we do know that certain food substances can produce a stresslike response, that other substances provided by foods can be depleted by stress, and that certain stress-related illnesses can be exacerbated by dietary habits. We also know that feelings of stress can lead to poor nutritional habits. People who have low self-esteem—in particular, those who feel badly about their physical selves—may take drastic measures to improve their bodies. Some of these measures turn into eating disorders, such as **anorexia nervosa** and **bulimia**, and cause stress in and of themselves. *Anorexia nervosa* is a condition in which a person takes in so few calories as to basically starve him- or herself. *Bulimia* is binge eating followed by the purging of consumed foods by induced vomiting, use of laxatives, or some other method. Both of these eating disorders are discussed in Chapter 4 and in detail later in this section. For now, recognize that they sometimes result when a person feels distressed about his or her body.

Before ways to eliminate nutrition stressors are recommended, a discussion of nutrition per se seems in order. To be nutritionally healthy, you need to maintain a balanced diet. A balanced diet is one that contains a variety of foods that will provide you with a variety of nutrients (proteins, carbohydrates, fats, minerals, vitamins, and water). To ensure that you get the appropriate variety of foods, you should eat foods in the amounts consistent with the food pyramid described in Figure 6.2. The pyramid is designed to be used by individuals via the Internet. If you go to www.mypyramid.gov, you will be able to find your recommended balance between food and physical activity, learn how to make smart choices in every food group, and see how to get the most nutrition out of your calories. After all, no one wants to be *malnourished*. Being malnourished means you eat either too little or too much of the recommended foods, or you ingest some nutrients in inappropriate amounts.

Although following the food pyramid guidelines is appropriate for many people, there are exceptions. For example, vegetarians may not want to eat meat; some people may be lactose intolerant and cannot drink milk; others may come from cultures that make following the general pyramid impractical. For this reason, food pyramids, based on the original food guide pyramid, have been devised to reflect individual concerns. For example, there are food pyramids for elders

anorexia nervosa

An eating disorder in which a person takes in so few calories as to potentially starve him- or herself.

bulimia

An eating disorder characterized by binge eating followed by purging of food, such as by inducing vomiting or ingesting a laxative.

Figure 6.2

MyPyramid
STEPS TO A HEALTHIER YOU
MyPyramid.gov

1% MILK

GRAINS	VEGETABLES	FRUITS	MILK	MEAT & BEANS
Make half your grains whole	Vary your veggies	Focus on fruits	Get your calcium-rich foods	Go lean with protein
Eat at least 3 oz. of whole-grain cereals, breads, crackers, rice, or pasta every day	Eat more dark-green veggies like broccoli, spinach, and other dark leafy greens	Eat a variety of fruit	Go low-fat or fat-free when you choose milk, yogurt, and other milk products	Choose low-fat or lean meats and poultry
1 oz. is about 1 slice of bread, about 1 cup of breakfast cereal, or ½ cup of cooked rice, cereal, or pasta	Eat more orange vegetables like carrots and sweet potatoes Eat more dry beans and peas like pinto beans, kidney beans, and lentils	Choose fresh, frozen, canned, or dried fruit Go easy on fruit juices	If you don't or can't consume milk, choose lactose-free products or other calcium sources such as fortified foods and beverages	Bake it, broil it, or grill it Vary your protein routine — choose more fish, beans, peas, nuts, and seeds

For a 2,000-calorie diet, you need the amounts below from each food group. To find the amounts that are right for you, go to MyPyramid.gov.

Eat 6 oz. every day	Eat 2½ cups every day	Eat 2 cups every day	Get 3 cups every day; for kids aged 2 to 8, it's 2	Eat 5½ oz. every day

Find your balance between food and physical activity
- Be sure to stay within your daily calorie needs.
- Be physically active for at least 30 minutes most days of the week.
- About 60 minutes a day of physical activity may be needed to prevent weight gain.
- For sustaining weight loss, at least 60 to 90 minutes a day of physical activity may be required.
- Children and teenagers should be physically active for 60 minutes every day, or most days.

Know the limits on fats, sugars, and salt (sodium)
- Make most of your fat sources from fish, nuts, and vegetable oils.
- Limit solid fats like butter, stick margarine, shortening, and lard, as well as foods that contain these.
- Check the Nutrition Facts label to keep saturated fats, *trans* fats, and sodium low.
- Choose food and beverages low in added sugars. Added sugars contribute calories with few, if any, nutrients.

MyPyramid.gov
STEPS TO A HEALTHIER YOU

U.S. Department of Agriculture
Center for Nutrition Policy and Promotion
April 2005
CNPP-15

USDA is an equal opportunity provider and employer

MyPlate and How to Create a Healthy Diet

The U.S. Department of Agriculture developed a website entitled *ChooseMyPlate.gov*—www.choosemyplate.gov/—to help people learn more about what types of foods they should eat and in what amounts, and which foods they should avoid. On that website is an illustration of a plate (see below). Clicking on a part of the plate brings up information about that part of the diet.

Below are some of the recommendations on that website which are based on the U.S. Department of Agriculture's *Dietary Guidelines for Americans, 2010*.

Healthy foods are low in saturated fat, *trans* fat, cholesterol, sodium (salt), and added sugar. Healthy foods include:

- Fat-free and low-fat milk and milk products, such as low-fat yogurt, cheese, and milk.
- Lean meat, fish, poultry, cooked beans, and peas.
- Whole-grain foods, such as whole-wheat bread, oatmeal, and brown rice. Other grain foods include pasta, cereal, bagels, bread, tortillas, couscous, and crackers.
- Fruits, which can be canned (in juice or water), fresh, frozen, or dried.
- Vegetables, which can be canned (without salt), fresh, frozen, or dried.
- Canola and olive oils, and soft margarines made from these oils, which are heart healthy. Consume these in small amounts since they are high in calories.
- Unsalted nuts, like walnuts and almonds, as long as you limit the amount you eat (nuts also are high in calories).

Foods to Limit

Foods that are high in saturated and *trans* fats and cholesterol raise blood cholesterol levels and also may be high in calories. These fats raise the risk of heart disease and stroke, so they should be limited. Saturated fat mainly is found in:

- Fatty cuts of meat, such as ground beef, sausage, and processed meats (e.g., bologna, hot dogs, and deli meats).

(continued)

- Poultry with the skin.
- High-fat milk and milk products like whole-milk cheeses, whole milk, cream, butter, and ice cream.
- Lard, coconut, and palm oils, which are found in many processed foods.
- *Trans* fat mainly found in foods with partially hydrogenated oils, such as many hard margarines and shortening.
- Baked products and snack foods, such as crackers, cookies, doughnuts, and breads.
- Foods fried in hydrogenated shortening, such as french fries and chicken.

Also, limit foods and drinks with added sugars, such as high-fructose corn syrup.

Sources: National Heart, Blood and Lung Institute, Diseases and Conditions Index, *How Can Overweight and Obesity be Prevented?* 2011. Available at: www.nhlbi.nih.gov/health/dci/Diseases/obe/obe_prevention.html

U.S. Department of Agriculture, *ChooseMyPlate.gov,* 2011. Available at: www.choosemyplate.gov/

U.S. Department of Agriculture and U.S. Department of Health and Human Services. *Dietary Guidelines for Americans,* 2010, 7th ed. (Washington, DC: U.S. Government Printing Office, December 2010).

(http://fitnessandfreebies.com/seniors/fgp4seniors.html) as well as for children (www.mypyramid.gov/kids/). Figure 6.3 provides an example, a pyramid for vegetarians. Ethnic food pyramids can be found in the "Ethnic Food Pyramids" box.

In addition to resulting in malnourishment, ingesting too much or too little of particular nutrients can lead to illnesses that in and of themselves can cause a great

Figure 6.3

A food pyramid for vegetarians.

Vegetarian Pyramid Food Guide
© 1994 New York Medical College

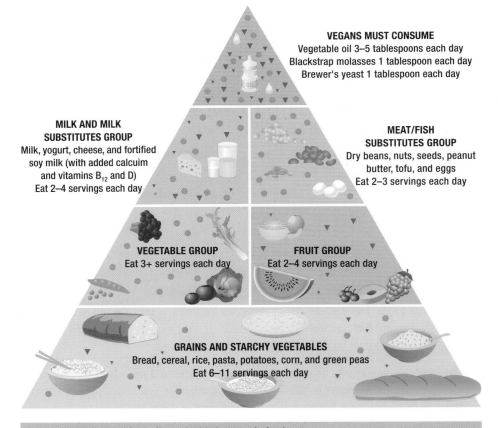

VEGANS MUST CONSUME
Vegetable oil 3–5 tablespoons each day
Blackstrap molasses 1 tablespoon each day
Brewer's yeast 1 tablespoon each day

MILK AND MILK
SUBSTITUTES GROUP
Milk, yogurt, cheese, and fortified soy milk (with added calcuim and vitamins B$_{12}$ and D)
Eat 2–4 servings each day

MEAT/FISH
SUBSTITUTES GROUP
Dry beans, nuts, seeds, peanut butter, tofu, and eggs
Eat 2–3 servings each day

VEGETABLE GROUP
Eat 3+ servings each day

FRUIT GROUP
Eat 2–4 servings each day

GRAINS AND STARCHY VEGETABLES
Bread, cereal, rice, pasta, potatoes, corn, and green peas
Eat 6–11 servings each day

These symbols show fats, oils, and added sugars in foods.
- Fat (naturally occurring and added)
▼ Sugars (added)

Ethnic Food Pyramids

1. *Food Guide Pyramid with a Mexican Flavor.* University of California Agriculture and Natural Resources. (800) 994-8849.

2. *Puerto Rican Food Guide Pyramid.* Hispanic Health Council, the University of Connecticut Department of Nutrition, the COOP Extension, and the Connecticut State Department of Social Services.

3. *East African Eating Guide for Good Health, Native American Food Guide, Southeast Asian Food Guide, Pacific Northwest Native American Food Guide.* Washington State Department of Health Warehouse Materials Management. (360) 664-9046 or fax: (360) 664-2929.

4. *Multicultural Pyramid Packet* from the Penn State Nutrition Center, with eight different cultural pyramids: African American, Chinese, Jewish, Puerto Rican, Navajo, Mexican, Indian, and Vietnamese for $10 at (814) 865-6323 or fax: (814) 865-5870; Penn State Nutrition Center, 5 Henderson Building, University Park, PA 16802.

5. *Asian, Latin American, Mediterranean, and Vegetarian Pyramids.* Oldways Preservation & Exchange Trust, 25 First Street, Cambridge, MA 02141. (617) 621-3000; fax: 617-621-1230; www.oldways@tiac.net.

6. Other international food guide pyramids are available at J. Painter, J. Rah, and Y. Lee, "Comparison of International Food Guide Pictorial Representations," *Journal of the American Dietetic Association* 102 (2002): 483–89.

deal of stress. The relationship of nutrition to heart disease and cancer are discussed as examples here because of the prevalence of those conditions in our society. However, many other illnesses are also related to nutrition.

Coronary heart disease results when the arteries supplying the heart with oxygen are so clogged that blood cannot pass through and the heart does not get needed oxygen. As a result, parts of the heart may die, and if those parts are in certain places in the heart or are extensive throughout the heart, the victim may die. Over time, diets high in saturated fats (derived from red meats, whole milk, butter) increase the amount of cholesterol in the blood. The cholesterol then accumulates on the walls of the arteries, and coronary heart disease develops. That is why the amount of saturated fats in a person's diet should be restricted. One way to do this is to substitute monounsaturated fats (e.g., peanut and olive oils) or polyunsaturated fats (e.g., liquid vegetable oils such as corn, soybean, or safflower oils) for saturated fats.

Cancer has also been associated with diet. The data indicate that people are more prone to developing certain cancers if their diets are low in fiber (e.g., whole-grain bread, cereal, and flour; fruits; vegetables; nuts; and popcorn) or high in saturated fats. To prevent certain cancers, the American Cancer Society recommends diets low in fats (to prevent breast, colon, and prostate cancers), high in fiber (to prevent colon cancer), and high in vitamins A and C (to prevent larynx, esophagus, stomach, and lung cancers). The American Cancer Society also recommends eating five or more servings of a variety of vegetables and fruits each day, choosing whole grains over processed (refined) grains, and limiting the intake of processed and red meats.[1] In addition, body fat has been clearly linked to six cancers. Carrying excess body fat increases the risk for cancer of the colon, kidney, pancreas, esophagus, and endometrium as well as postmenopausal breast cancer.[2]

The Heavy Toll of Diet-Related Chronic Diseases

What you eat is related to your health—today and in the years to come. Below are some examples of how diet affects health.

Cardiovascular Disease

- 81.1 million Americans—37 percent of the U.S. adult population—have cardiovascular disease. Major risk factors include high levels of blood cholesterol and other lipids, type 2 diabetes, hypertension (high blood pressure), metabolic syndrome, overweight and obesity, physical inactivity, and tobacco use.
- 16 percent of the U.S. adult population has high total blood cholesterol.

Hypertension

- 74.5 million Americans—34 percent of U.S. adults—have hypertension.
- Hypertension is a major risk factor for heart disease, stroke, congestive heart failure, and kidney disease.
- Dietary factors that increase blood pressure include excessive sodium and insufficient potassium intake, overweight and obesity, and excess alcohol consumption.
- 36 percent of American adults have prehypertension—blood pressure numbers that are higher than normal, but not yet in the hypertension range.

Diabetes

- Nearly 24 million people—almost 11 percent of the population—ages 20 years and older have diabetes. The vast majority of cases are type 2 diabetes, which is heavily influenced by diet and physical activity.
- About 78 million Americans—35 percent of the U.S. adult population ages 20 years or older—have pre-diabetes. Pre-diabetes (also called impaired glucose tolerance or impaired fasting glucose) means that blood glucose levels are higher than normal, but not high enough to be called diabetes.

Cancer

- Almost one in two men and women—approximately 41 percent of the population—will be diagnosed with cancer during their lifetime.
- Dietary factors are associated with risk of some types of cancer, including breast (postmenopausal), endometrial, colon, kidney, mouth, pharynx, larynx, and esophagus.

Osteoporosis

- One out of every two women and one in four men ages 50 years and older will have an osteoporosis-related fracture in their lifetime.
- About 85 to 90 percent of adult bone mass is acquired by the age of 18 in girls and the age of 20 in boys. Adequate nutrition and regular participation in physical activity are important factors in achieving and maintaining optimal bone mass.

Source: U.S. Department of Agriculture and U.S. Department of Health and Human Services, *Dietary Guidelines for Americans*, 2010, 7th ed. (Washington, DC: U.S. Government Printing Office, December 2010).

Table 6.1 Behavioral Principles of Weight Loss

Principles	

I. STIMULUS CONTROL
  A. Shopping
    1. Shop for food after eating.
    2. Shop from a list.
    3. Avoid ready-to-eat foods.
    4. Don't carry more cash than needed for items on shopping list.
  B. Plans
    1. Plan to limit food intake.
    2. Substitute exercise for snacking.
    3. Eat meals and snacks at scheduled times.
    4. Don't accept food offered by others.
  C. Activities
    1. Store food out of sight.
    2. Eat all food in the same place.
    3. Remove food from inappropriate storage areas in the house.
    4. Keep serving dishes off the table.
    5. Use smaller dishes and utensils.
    6. Avoid being the food server.
    7. Leave the table immediately after eating.
    8. Don't save leftovers.
  D. Holidays and Parties
    1. Drink fewer alcoholic beverages.
    2. Plan eating habits before parties.
    3. Eat a low-calorie snack before parties.
    4. Practice polite ways to decline food.
    5. Don't get discouraged by an occasional setback.
 	
II. EATING BEHAVIOR
    1. Put fork down between mouthfuls.
    2. Chew thoroughly before swallowing.
    3. Prepare foods one portion at a time.
    4. Leave some food on the plate.
    5. Pause in the middle of the meal.
    6. Do nothing else while eating (read, watch television).
	III. REWARD
	    1. Solicit help from family and friends.
	    2. Help family and friends provide this help in the form of praise and material rewards.
	    3. Utilize self-monitoring records as basis for rewards.
	    4. Plan specific rewards for specific behaviors (behavioral contracts).
	
	IV. SELF-MONITORING
	  Keep diet diary that includes
	    1. Time and place of eating.
	    2. Type and amount of food.
	    3. Who is present/how you feel.
	
	V. NUTRITION EDUCATION
	    1. Use diet diary to identify problem areas.
	    2. Make small changes that you can continue.
	    3. Learn nutritional values of foods.
	    4. Decrease fat intake; increase complex carbohydrates.
	
	VI. PHYSICAL ACTIVITY
	  A. Routine Activity
	    1. Increase routine activity.
	    2. Increase use of stairs.
	    3. Keep a record of distance walked each day.
	  B. Exercise
	    1. Begin a very mild exercise program.
	    2. Keep a record of daily exercise.
	    3. Increase the exercise very gradually.
	
	VII. COGNITIVE RESTRUCTURING
	    1. Avoid setting unreasonable goals.
	    2. Think about progress, not shortcomings.
	    3. Avoid imperatives such as "always" and "never."
	    4. Counter negative thoughts with rational restatements.
	    5. Set weight goals.

Source: Reprinted with permission from *American Journal of Clinical Nutrition* 41(1985): 823. Copyright © 1985, American Society for Clinical Nutrition, Inc.

Although it is desirable to control your body weight, an overemphasis on dieting can itself be unhealthy. Sometimes, for example, obesity can be in the mind of the beholder. We are bombarded with media images of the ideal body type as being thin with all the curves in the right places. Consequently, when our bodies differ from this ideal, we become distressed and vow to diet that extra weight off. As the results of several Gallup polls[3,4] found, approximately 50 percent of Americans worry about their weight either *all the time* (15 percent) or *some of the time* (34 percent). Furthermore, when asked how many different times they seriously tried to lose weight, 24 percent of Americans answered *once or twice,* 28 percent answered *three or more times,* and 11 percent answered that they seriously tried to lose weight *more than 10 times.* The popularity and abundance of diet books also attests to our desire to lose weight. Unfortunately, some diets are unhealthy and therefore can lead to even more stress. Table 6.1 presents what we know about how to lose weight effectively and also healthfully.

Nutrition experts now recommend paying more attention to body mass than to weight alone. This gauge seems to more accurately reflect a person's risk of ill

Table 6.2 Body Mass Index Table

To use this table, find the appropriate height in the left-hand column. Move across to a given weight. The number at the top of the column is the BMI at the height and weight. Pounds have been rounded off.

Height (inches)	19	20	21	22	23	24	25	26	27	28	29	30	31	32	33	34	35	36
											Body Weight (pounds)							
58	91	96	100	105	110	115	119	124	129	134	138	143	148	153	158	162	167	172
59	94	99	104	109	114	119	124	128	133	138	143	148	153	158	163	168	173	178
60	97	102	107	112	118	123	128	133	138	143	148	153	158	163	168	174	179	184
61	100	106	111	116	122	127	132	137	143	148	153	158	164	169	174	180	185	190
62	104	109	115	120	126	131	136	142	147	153	158	164	169	175	180	186	191	196
63	107	113	118	124	130	135	141	146	152	158	163	169	175	180	186	191	197	203
64	110	116	122	128	134	140	145	151	157	163	169	174	180	186	192	197	204	209
65	114	120	126	132	138	144	150	156	162	168	174	180	186	192	198	204	210	216
66	118	124	130	136	142	148	155	161	167	173	179	186	192	198	204	210	216	223
67	121	127	134	140	146	153	159	166	172	178	185	191	198	204	211	217	223	230
68	125	131	138	144	151	158	164	171	177	184	190	197	203	210	216	223	230	236
69	128	135	142	149	155	162	169	176	182	189	196	203	209	216	223	230	236	243
70	132	139	146	153	160	167	174	181	188	195	202	209	216	222	229	236	243	250
71	136	143	150	157	165	172	179	186	193	200	208	215	222	229	236	243	250	257
72	140	147	154	162	169	177	184	191	199	206	213	221	228	235	242	250	258	265
73	144	151	159	166	174	182	189	197	204	212	219	227	235	242	250	257	265	272
74	148	155	163	171	179	186	194	202	210	218	225	233	241	249	256	264	272	280
75	152	160	168	176	184	192	200	208	216	224	232	240	248	256	264	272	279	287
76	156	164	172	180	189	197	205	213	221	230	238	246	254	263	271	279	287	295

health as a result of too much weight. Table 6.2 helps you calculate your body mass. The desirable body mass index (BMI) is between 18.5 and 24.9.[5] Recognize, though, that people with high muscle mass—such as weight trainers—may have a BMI out of range but actually be the right weight and have a healthy percentage of body fat. Lab 6.1 (at the end of this chapter) presents another way to determine how much weight you should lose.

BMI is not the only measure of obesity. In a study involving almost 17,000 subjects,[6] obesity was measured by different methods (body mass index [BMI], waist circumference, and waist/height ratio). An association between all of these different obesity measures and cardiac artery disease was found. In another study,[7] waist-hip ratio was used as a measure of obesity and was related to the development of hypertension.

For some people, the obsession with being thin takes the form of excessive weight loss through self-imposed starvation (anorexia nervosa) or binge eating followed by purging through self-induced vomiting, fasting, abuse of laxatives, diuretics or enemas, or excessive exercise (bulimia). The prevalence of anorexia nervosa, bulimia, and binge eating disorder are 0.9 percent, 1.5 percent, and 3.5 percent among females; and 0.3 percent, 0.5 percent, and 2.0 percent among males.[8] People with eating disorders often have obsessional, perfectionistic, and anxious personality styles[9] that lead them to want to maintain total control over what they perceive to be ideal weight.

Table 6.2 (continued)

To use this table, find the appropriate height in the left-hand column. Move across to a given weight. The number at the top of the column is the BMI at the height and weight. Pounds have been rounded off.

Height (inches)	37	38	39	40	41	42	43	44	45	46	47	48	49	50	51	52	53	54
									Body Weight (pounds)									
58	177	181	186	191	196	201	205	210	215	220	224	229	234	239	244	248	253	258
59	183	188	193	198	203	208	212	217	222	227	232	237	242	247	252	257	262	267
60	189	194	199	204	209	215	220	225	230	235	240	245	250	255	261	266	271	276
61	195	201	206	211	217	222	227	232	238	243	248	254	259	264	269	275	280	285
62	202	207	213	218	224	229	235	240	246	251	256	262	267	273	278	284	289	295
63	208	214	220	225	231	237	242	248	254	259	265	270	278	282	287	293	299	304
64	215	221	227	232	238	244	250	256	262	267	273	279	285	291	296	302	308	314
65	222	228	234	240	246	252	258	264	270	276	282	288	294	300	306	312	318	324
66	229	235	241	247	253	260	266	272	278	284	291	297	303	309	315	322	328	334
67	236	242	249	255	261	268	274	280	287	293	299	306	312	319	325	331	338	344
68	243	249	256	262	269	276	282	289	295	302	308	315	322	328	335	341	348	354
69	250	257	263	270	277	284	291	297	304	311	318	324	331	338	345	351	358	365
70	257	264	271	278	285	292	299	306	313	320	327	334	341	348	355	362	369	376
71	265	272	279	286	293	301	308	315	322	329	338	343	351	358	365	372	379	386
72	272	279	287	294	302	309	316	324	331	338	346	353	361	368	375	383	390	397
73	280	288	295	302	310	318	325	333	340	348	355	363	371	378	386	393	401	408
74	287	295	303	311	319	326	334	342	350	358	365	373	381	389	396	404	412	420
75	295	303	311	319	327	335	343	351	359	367	375	383	391	399	407	415	423	431
76	304	312	320	328	336	344	353	361	369	377	385	394	402	410	418	426	435	443

Source: National Heart, Lung and Blood Institute. Body Mass Index Table. 2009. Available at: www.nhlbi.nih.gov/guidelines/obesity/bmi_tbl.htm

Since anorexia nervosa and bulimia can eventually lead to severe illness or death, if you know someone with one of these conditions, you ought to encourage him or her to seek professional help as soon as possible. If you find you are obsessive about your own weight and you really needn't be, you might want to consult with a counselor at your campus health center or with your personal physician.

Furthermore, certain food *substances* have particular relationships with stress. For example, a group of food substances can actually produce a stresslike response. These substances are called **pseudostressors,** or **sympathomimetics.** They mimic sympathetic nervous system stimulation. Colas, coffee, tea, and chocolate that contain caffeine are examples of sympathomimetic agents. Tea also contains theobromine and theophylline, which are sympathomimetics. These substances increase metabolism, make one highly alert, and result in the release of stress hormones, which elevate the heart rate and blood pressure. In addition to creating a pseudostress response, sympathomimetics make the nervous system more reactive and thereby more likely to have a stressor elicit a stress response. Nicotine (found in tobacco) is also a sympathomimetic agent.

Another way nutrition is related to stress is by the effect of stress on *vitamins.* The production of cortisol (the stress hormone produced by the adrenal cortex)

pseudostressors
Food substances that produce a stresslike response; also called sympathomimetics.

sympathomimetics
Synonymous with pseudostressors.

requires the use of vitamins.[10] Consequently, chronic stress can deplete the vitamins we take into our bodies. In particular, the B complex vitamins (thiamine, riboflavin, niacin, pantothenic acid, and pyridoxine hydrochloride) and vitamin C seem to be the most affected. A deficiency in these vitamins can result in anxiety, depression, insomnia, muscular weakness, and stomach upset. Not only may stress deplete these vitamins, but because these vitamins are used to produce adrenal hormones, their depletion makes one less able to respond satisfactorily to stress. Thereby, a vicious cycle develops. Vitamin B can be obtained by eating cereals, green leafy vegetables, liver, and fish. Vitamin C is contained in citrus fruits, tomatoes, cabbage, and potatoes.

In addition, stress can interfere with calcium absorption in the intestines and can increase calcium excretion, as well as increase the excretion of potassium, zinc, copper, and magnesium. This is of particular concern to women who are trying to prevent the development of osteoporosis (a condition in which the bones become weak and brittle and the woman is at increased risk of fractures), since osteoporosis is a result of a decalcification of the bones.[11] Although postmenopausal women are most prone to osteoporosis (decalcification is related to decreased levels of estrogens), it appears that long-term lifestyle habits (diet and exercise, in particular) affect one's susceptibility to this condition. Eating a diet sufficient in calcium, exercising regularly, and managing stress—all begun at a young age—are the best ways to prevent or postpone the development of osteoporosis.

Sugar is another stress culprit. To break down sugar, the body must use some of its B complex vitamins. We now know what that means. This results in the symptoms described previously and a diminished ability to produce adrenal hormones in response to stressors. *Processed flour* also requires the body to use B complex vitamins (as well as other nutrients) and, unless enriched with vitamins and minerals, can have the same effect as sugar.

Sugar ingestion has other stress implications. Ingestion of a large amount of sugar in a short period of time or missing meals and then ingesting sugar over a period of time can result in a condition called **hypoglycemia** in susceptible individuals. Hypoglycemia is low blood sugar that is preceded by elevated levels of blood sugar. This condition may be accompanied by symptoms of anxiety, headache, dizziness, trembling, and irritability. Subsequent stressors are likely to provoke an unusually intense stress response.

Furthermore, the stress response and accompanying cortisol production cause an elevation in the level of blood glucose. To respond to the blood glucose, the beta cells of the islets of Langerhans produce insulin. Stress that is chronic can burn out these beta cells. These cells are not replaceable; thus, the body's ability to produce insulin is compromised. The result might be the development of diabetes in genetically susceptible individuals.

Another food substance that has a relationship to stress is *salt*. Some people are genetically susceptible to sodium and develop high blood pressure when they ingest too much of it. The federal government recommends no more than 5,000 milligrams of salt (sodium chloride), which translates to 2,000 milligrams of sodium, daily. On a short-term basis, sodium ingestion can raise blood pressure by causing the retention of body fluids. When a person whose blood pressure is elevated encounters stress, his or her blood pressure may be further elevated to a dangerous level.

Now that you have an appreciation for the relationship of nutrition to stress, it is time to study ways of using this information to manage stress better. Here are some ways to reduce stressors in your diet:

1. Eat a balanced diet that includes the amounts recommended in the food pyramid.

2. Limit the amount of saturated fats in your diet, and increase the amount of fiber.

3. Add cruciferous vegetables (such as broccoli, cauliflower, and brussels sprouts) to your diet, and limit the amount of alcohol you ingest.

hypoglycemia
A condition of low blood sugar.

4. Be more realistic about your weight. Lose weight if you need to, but don't expect to measure up to the ideal projected by the media. Remember, obsession about weight can lead to anorexia nervosa or bulimia.

5. Limit your intake of cola, coffee, tea, and chocolate and other products containing caffeine. Also, do not smoke cigarettes or use other tobacco products (snuff, chewing tobacco).

6. During particularly stressful times, you might want to consider supplementing your diet with vitamins. In particular, focus on vitamin C and the B complex vitamins. However, many experts believe that eating a balanced diet that includes a wide variety of foods will ensure a sufficient amount of vitamins.

7. Limit foods containing sugar. If ingesting sugar, do not take in large amounts in a short period of time, and do not skip meals.

8. Limit intake of processed flour. However, some experts believe that if the flour is enriched with vitamins and minerals, it need not be avoided.

9. Limit your intake of sodium.

Part of eliminating unnecessary stressors includes eliminating those food substances that either make us more prone to stress or create a stresslike response. This is another area of our lives we need to take charge of.

Noise and Stress

Anyone who has roomed with a noisy person, worked in a noisy office, or tried to study with a party going on in the next room can attest to the effect of noise on one's level of stress. Noise can raise blood pressure, increase heart rate, and lead to muscle tension. Noise has been found to be related to job dissatisfaction and to result in irritation and anxiety.[12] Noise can result in sleep disturbance, headaches, and hypertension.[13]

Most disturbing is noise that constantly changes in pitch, intensity, or frequency. We may become used to more common and stable noise and almost ignore it. People who live near airports, for example, seem not to hear the planes after a while. However, just because you become accustomed to a noise or are able to tune it out doesn't mean you are not being affected by it.

Noise is measured in decibels. At 85 decibels, stress responses usually develop, and prolonged exposure to sounds above 90 decibels can result in hearing damage. Of course, depending on one's level of concentration and the task being performed, even low levels of noise can be bothersome. Figure 6.4 lists decibel ratings for some common sounds. To reduce noise levels, you can

1. Use cotton or ear plugs if your job requires constant exposure to loud noises.
2. Sit as far away as possible from the performers at loud rock, symphony, or band concerts.
3. Learn to enjoy listening to music at home at a moderate volume.
4. Put drapes over windows to reduce street noise.
5. Choose acoustical tile for ceilings and walls when building a house or adding a room.
6. Use carpeting or select an apartment with carpeting in all rooms adjacent to other units.
7. Keep noise-making appliances away from bedrooms, den, and living room.
8. Select home sites or apartments away from truck routes, airports, businesses, and industrial areas.

In spite of its potential for stress, noise can at times be soothing. In fact, on many stress management audiotapes, you will find noise to help you relax. This is called "white noise," and its purpose is to drown out other sounds that may interfere with relaxation. Sounds such as the surf rolling onto the shore, birds

When using devices such as an iPod, follow the 60/60 rule: no more than 60% volume for no more than 60 minutes at a stretch.

Figure 6.4

Common sounds and their decibel ratings.

Source: National Institute on Deafness and Other Communication Disorders, National Institutes of Health, 2009. Availabel at: www.nidcd.nih.gov/health/hearing/ruler/asp

HOW LOUD IS TOO LOUD?

DECIBELS	COMMON SOUNDS
150	Firecracker
120	Ambulance siren
110	Chainsaw, rock concert
105	Personal stereo system at maximum level
100	Wood shop, snowmobile
95	Motorcycle
90	Power mower
85	Heavy city traffic
60	Normal conversation
40	Refrigerator humming
30	Whispered voice

chirping, or the wind rustling through the leaves can serve as comforting sounds. In addition, some sounds are used to focus upon to bring about relaxation. For example, some forms of meditation use a word (called a **mantra**) for focusing, and other methods of relaxation employ chanting.

So you can see that *noise* can be stressful but certain *sounds* can be relaxing. You can take greater control of your life by limiting disturbing noises and seeking out relaxing sounds. Walk through the woods; recline on a beach. Noise or relaxing sound—it's up to you.

Life Events and Stress

The information in this section will have more meaning for you if you follow these instructions: If you are presently a college student, determine which events you have experienced by completing Lab 6.2, a life-events scale developed by G. E. Anderson.

If you are older than the typical college student, assess the amount of life events you have experienced within the past year by completing Lab 6.3, a life-events scale developed by Thomas Holmes and Richard Rahe.

Labs 6.2 and 6.3 will help you assess the amount of significant changes in your life to which you have had to adjust. In other words, your life-change units (LCU)

mantra

A word that is the focus of meditation.

is a measure of the stressors you encountered this past year. The original research in this field was conducted by Holmes and Rahe, who developed the *Social Readjustment Rating Scale* appearing in Lab 6.3. They argued that if stress results in illness and disease, then people experiencing a great deal of stress should report more illness than people reporting only a little stress. Their theory was subsequently supported by their research. Lab 6.2 is an adaptation of the Social Readjustment Rating Scale specific to college students.

Many other researchers have supported the findings of Holmes and Rahe.[14–17] However, not all studies measuring life-change units have been so supportive of this theory. The inconsistency of these research findings should not be surprising. If you'll recall the stress theory model, all that these life-events scales measure is the top phase (life situation). We know, though, that changes in life situations alone are not enough to cause illness and disease. These changes must be perceived as distressing and result in emotional and, subsequently, physiological arousal that is chronic, prolonged, or unabated. We also now know that it is possible to establish roadblocks (intervention techniques) to inhibit the development of illness or disease from stressors we experience. Researchers have found one such roadblock to be **social support**.[18] People who experienced a great deal of life change but had family or friends with whom to discuss their problems contracted no more illness than people who experienced less life change. However, people who experienced a great deal of life change but *did not* have family or friends with whom to discuss their problems contracted much more illness than the others. Suffice it to say that life change does not, in and of itself, lead to poor health.

social support
The presence of significant others with whom to discuss stressors.

What should you do if your score on the life-events scale concerns you? First, let's look at how people typically react to a stressful period of time. We often hear people say, "I've been under a lot of stress lately. I need a vacation." If you have too many life-change units, why add more? Vacation is worth 13 points! Rather than add to your stress, you'd be better advised to make your life more routine to reduce your need to adapt to changes. Rather than taking a vacation, maintain your daily routine (perhaps eliminating some events but *not* substituting others). I'm often asked how such pleasant events as a vacation and Christmas or Hanukkah can be stressors. Remember that stress occurs when we are knocked out of balance. We are in equilibrium when suddenly something occurs requiring us to use energy to adapt. All of the adjustments required prior to, during, and returning from a vacation are the reasons why a vacation can be a stressor.

Another interesting revelation can be inferred from the Holmes and Rahe scale. If you have a marital separation, you accumulate 65 stressor points. That event requires you to adjust from being married and the routines you have established within your marriage to being single again. The functions your spouse performed now need your attention. The time you spent together now needs to be used for another purpose. You need to adjust to aloneness or loneliness or both. You need to spend time meeting new people. It is evident that this separation requires a great deal of adaptation energy and can be quite stressful. Let's assume that you have spent six months adjusting to your marital separation and have finally adapted to your new routines and way of living. Lo and behold, the old flame flickers once again, and you and your spouse decide to try a reconciliation. Notice, though, that marital reconciliation is worth 45 stressor points. Once again, you are requiring yourself (mind and

It's the daily hassles that might be more threatening to your health than major life events. Having a parking meter expire or getting a traffic ticket, or searching for a job, can create chronic stress and its accompanying negative consequences.

body) to adapt to being married just after you have finally adapted to being single. Your daily routines need changing, your associations and affiliations may need to be readjusted, and you must develop your marital relationship more effectively than before.

The moral of this story is to be sure of your need for marital separation (and other breaks in your relationships with loved ones) prior to the separation and, once you have made that decision, do not easily revert to that old relationship. Of course, there are intervening variables associated with these decisions. For some people, the separation can be so stressful and the adaptation so difficult that the stress associated with reconciliation would be less than the stress of continuing the separation. Others may be willing to tolerate the threat to their health in order to reestablish their marriage (or other relationship). You can probably think of other considerations that enter into this decision. However, recognize that the more your life situation requires adaptation, the more likely you are to become ill. Some stressors you may not be able to eliminate (e.g., the death of a spouse or close friend), but others you can control. You can, therefore, decide that they will no longer be a part of your life; to do so would be to improve your health.

Hassles and Chronic Stress

Carrying the life change–stress relationship further, Kanner[19] and colleagues hypothesized that everyday **hassles** would be even more detrimental to health than major life events. They defined hassles as daily interactions with the environment that were essentially negative and, because of their chronic nature, could take a significant toll on health. Losing a wallet, smoking too much, and having troublesome neighbors are examples of these hassles. Furthermore, Lazarus[20] proposed that the absence of **uplifts**—positive events we interpret in ways that make us feel good—would also be related to ill health.

Although the absence of uplifts has not been found to be related to ill health, the presence of hassles has. Hassles have been shown to be predictive of psychological distress[21] and the dynamics of stress and aging[22] and to be related to poorer mental and physical health.[23,24] In general, Lazarus's theory has been shown to be correct in asserting that hassles are related to subsequent illness and disease to a greater degree than are major life events.[25,26] One major difference between these scales is that the hassles scale asks respondents to judge the severity of the event. This is important because an event can occur but be perceived as inconsequential. In that case, it might not have much effect on the respondent's health.

You can assess the amount and intensity of the hassles you experience by completing Lab 6.4. When a group of adults completed the hassles scale,[27] they reported experiencing a mean of 20.6 hassles per month over a nine-month period of time. The mean intensity of these hassles was 1.47. In a study of college students, the most frequent hassles experienced were time pressures, finances, and those related to relationships in that order. The hassles rated as most severe were time pressures, traffic, finances, employment, and physical appearance.[28] Once you have identified your hassles, try to eliminate as many of them as you can while recognizing that many others will either take a long time to change or are unchangeable (you will have to learn to live with these).

Success Analysis

A while ago a friend of mine wrote a book that I was most impressed with. Its title reflects both her personality and her reality: *Success: You Can Make It Happen.*[29] You really can make it happen. Success need not be left to chance. As

Age	Success Experience		Reasons It Was a Success
1.			
2.			
3.			
1.			
2.			
3.			
1.			
2.			
3.			
Most Successful Experience			**Reason**
Least Successful Experience			**Reason**

Table 6.3
Your Success Chart

Source: From Lila Swell, *Success: You Can Make It Happen.* © 1976 by Lila Swell. Reprinted by permission of Lila Swell.

gambling casinos give themselves an edge to ensure a profit, you can give yourself an edge to ensure being successful. Giving yourself success (don't miss the importance of this phrasing) will result in your thinking better of yourself. Stated more academically, success will lead to improved self-esteem. The converse, of course, is that lack of success (failure) will lead to diminished self-esteem, resulting in a very significant stressor.

At this point, you need some information about yourself to infer personal meaning from our discussion. Complete the success chart shown in Table 6.3. Divide your life into three equal time periods, beginning at age 5. If you are 50 years old, your three time periods will be 5 to 20, 21 to 35, and 36 to 50; if you are 20 years old, they'll be 5 to 10, 11 to 15, and 16 to 20. Next, think of three of your successes during each period and the reasons you consider these experiences successes. Place these successes and reasons within the success chart. Lastly, write in what you consider to be the most successful experience of your life and the least successful one, along with the reasons you consider them such. The last part of this data-gathering procedure requires you to list, on a separate sheet of paper, 10 strengths of yours—your most positive characteristics and talents. Please do this before reading further.

Success is multifaceted and, like beauty, is in the eyes of the beholder. What you view as successful, others might not. Some consider themselves successful when they achieve independence, and their success charts reflect this viewpoint, with successes such as owning their first car, getting their first job, or moving into their own apartment. Their reasons for regarding these as successes might be "Didn't have to rely on others" or "Now I had money to do my own thing."

Others view success as competing and winning. Their success charts include successes such as playing on a championship team, winning a trophy, and competing with other students and winning a scholarship to college. The reasons given might be "The competition was intense" or "A lot of people tried to do this, but only I succeeded." Still others define success in other ways:

1. Being chosen (or elected) by others.
2. Pleasing others (parents, teachers, friends).
3. Being helpful.
4. Achieving academically.
5. Achieving in sports activities.

6. Being the best.
7. Achieving in spite of great obstacles and difficulty (if too easy, the achievement is not viewed as a success).
8. Learning a skill.
9. Getting recognition from others.
10. Being happy.

How do you define success? Scan your success chart and list at least four patterns that emerge. Make sure that your patterns are just that—patterns. They must appear several times within the chart. You should conclude with a sentence that begins "Success to me is . . . ."

Now that you know your own view of success, how can you achieve it? The best way is to use the strengths you listed previously. Try to maximize those strengths and minimize any weaknesses you have in order to "fix the deck" and increase your chances of being successful. Prescribe life experiences for yourself that use those strengths; shy away from experiences that rely on talents, skills, or characteristics that you lack. For example, if you perceive success as achieving independence, don't seek success occupationally by working on an assembly line. If you don't have the "gift of gab," you should not become a salesperson. You might try to be successful as an author if you view success as recognition from others and have a talent for writing. If you also have *helping others* as a component of your success definition, the books you write should present information that can be used to help others.

With the data you have acquired regarding your definition of success and your list of strengths, you are now able to give *yourself* success. You are now in control of one more possible stressor. You are now better able to maintain your health and improve the quality of your life. *But* you will do this only if you use this information to make your life situation consistent with what you have learned.

Coping in Today's World

Researchers have uncovered some interesting findings regarding the life event they define as marital discord.[a] Married couples were admitted twice to a hospital research unit for twenty-four hours each admission. During the first admission, couples had a social support interaction that would result in greater marital accord. During the second hospital admission, couples discussed marital disagreement and how to resolve several marital problems. During each admission, researchers inflicted blister wounds on the subjects and measured the pace at which these wounds healed. They also measured the level of cytokine production since cytokine facilitates healing. Researchers found that wounds healed more slowly, and local cytokine production was lower at wound sites, following marital conflicts than after social support interactions. Furthermore, couples who demonstrated consistently high levels of hostile behaviors healed 60 percent more slowly than low-hostility couples. It seems that supporting one another and limiting hostility is not only emotionally healthy but also physically healthy. And, this is probably true in other relationships as well.

[a]J. K. Kiecolt-Glaser, T. J. Loving, J. R. Stowell, W. B. Malarkey, S. Lemeshow, S. L. Dickinson, and R. Glaser, "Hostile Marital Interactions, Proinflammatory Cytokine Production, and Wound Healing," *Archives of General Psychiatry* 62(2005):1377–84.

summary

- Good nutrition may help in managing stress. Foods should be eaten from a variety of sources. Eating the recommended amounts of foods from the food pyramid groups is one way of ensuring that you eat a balanced diet.

- Maintaining nutritional health by practices such as consuming less saturated fat and alcohol and eating more fiber and cruciferous vegetables may also reduce stressors in your diet.

- Food substances that produce a stresslike response are called pseudostressors or sympathomimetics, since they mimic sympathetic nervous system stimulation. Foods containing caffeine are examples of these substances.

- Stress may deplete the B complex and C vitamins; in the case of chronic stress, the diet may require supplementation with vitamins and minerals. Ingestion of sugar and processed flour may make this situation even worse, since both of these use up valuable nutrients when the body metabolizes them.

- To manage stress better, limit intake of caffeine, sugar, and foods containing processed flour that has not been enriched. During stressful times, consider vitamin supplementation.

- Noise can be either distressing or relaxing. Noises louder than 85 decibels usually elicit a stress response, and prolonged exposure to sounds above 90 decibels can result in hearing damage. White noise is used to drown out disturbing noises while one is trying to relax.

- Thomas Holmes and Richard Rahe found that the more significant changes a person has in his or her life, the greater is the chance that he or she will contract some physical or psychological illness. Since they conceptualized stress as adapting to change, Holmes and Rahe viewed more change as equivalent to more stress and, consequently, to more illness and disease.

- Richard Lazarus found that the daily hassles a person experiences are more harmful to his or her health than are the significant life changes that concerned Holmes and Rahe. Lazarus believed these daily events are so damaging to health because of how frequently they occur, as compared with the major life events that Holmes and Rahe researched, which were usually encountered only rarely.

internet resources

Medline Plus **www.nlm.nih.gov/medlineplus/tutorials/managingstress/htm/index.htm** *Provides tutorials for managing stress.*

Food and Nutrition Information Center **www.fnic.nal.usda.gov/nal_display/index.php?info-center=4&tax_level=1** *A USDA site that provides access to a variety of nutrition-related databases.*

Stress Less **www.stressless.com** *Offers a wide selection of stress reduction products and programs for use in coping with the effects of excess stress.*

references

1. Lawrence H. Kushi, Tim Byers, Colleen Doyle, Elisa V. Bandera, Marji McCullough, Ted Gansler, Kimberly S. Andrews, and Michael J. Thun, "American Cancer Society Guidelines on Nutrition and Physical Activity for Cancer Prevention: Reducing the Risk of Cancer with Healthy Food Choices and Physical Activity," *CA: A Cancer Journal for Clinicians* 56(2006): 254–81.

2. American Institute for Cancer Research, "Landmark Report: Excess Body Fat Causes Cancer," *AICR Annual Research Conference.* Washington, DC: November 3–4, 2011.

3. Joseph Carroll, "Six in 10 Americans Have Attempted to Lose Weight: Women More Likely Than Men to Diet," *Gallup Poll,* August 16, 2005. Available at: www.gallup.com/poll /content/default.aspx?ci=17890

4. Joseph Carroll, "Who's Worried About Their Weight?" *Gallup Poll,* August 9, 2005. Available at: www.gallup.com/poll/ content/default.aspx?ci=17752

5. Centers for Disease Control and Prevention, "About BMI for Adults," *Healthy Weight—It's Not a Diet, It's a Lifestyle! 2009.* Available at: www.cdc.gov/healthyweight/assessing/bmi/ adult_bmi/index.html#Interpreted

6. Bernhard M. Kaess, Jacek Jozwiak, Miroslaw Mastej, Witold Lukas, Wladyslaw Grzeszczak, Adam Windak, Wieslawa Piwowarska, Andrze Tykarski, Ewa Konduracka, Katarzyna Rygiel, Ahmed Manasar, Nilesh J. Samani, and Maciej Tomaszewski, "Association Between Anthropometric Obesity Measures and Coronary Artery Disease—A Cross-Sectional Survey of 16,657 Subjects from 444 Polish Cities," *Heart,* published online: August 2, 2009. Available at: http://heart .bmj.com/cgi/content/abstract/hrt.2009.171520v1

7. C. A. Feldstein, M. Akopian, A. O. Olivieri, A. P. Kramer, M. Nasi, and D. Garrido, "A Comparison of Body Mass Index and Waist-to-Hip Ratio as Indicators of Hypertension Risk in an Urban Argentine Population: A Hospital-Based Study," *Nutrition, Metabolism and Cardiovascular Disease* 15(2005): 310–15.

8. James I. Hudson, Eva Hiripi, Harrison G. Pope, Jr., and Ronald C. Kessler, "The Prevalence and Correlates of Eating Disorders in the National Comorbidity Survey Replication," *Biological Psychiatry* 61(2007): 348–58.

9. W. H. Kaye, K. L. Klump, G. K. Frank, and M. Strober, "Anorexia and Bulimia Nervosa," *Annual Review of Medicine* 51(2000): 299–313.

10. David Shier, Jackie Butter, and Ricki Lewis, *Hole's Human Anatomy and Physiology,* 12th ed. (New York: McGraw-Hill, 2009).

11. Rod R. Seeley, Trent D. Stephens, and Philip Tate, *Anatomy & Physiology* (New York: McGraw-Hill, 2008), 196.

12. M. Boudarene, J. J. Legros, and M. Timsit-Berthier, "Study of the Stress Response: Role of Anxiety, Cortisol and DHEAs," *Encephale* 28(2002): 139–46.

13. G. Bluhm, E. Nordling, and N. Berglind, "Road Traffic Noise and Annoyance—An Increasing Environmental Health Problem," *Noise Health* 6(2004): 43–49.

14. D. J. Lynch, A. McGrady, E. Alvarez, and J. Forman, "Recent Life Changes and Medical Utilization in an Academic Family Practice," *Journal of Nervous and Mental Disorders* 193(2005): 633–35.

15. A. J. Costa, S. Labuda Schrop, G. McCord, and C. Ritter, "Depression in Family Medicine Faculty," *Family Medicine* 37(2005): 271–75.

16. D. Clarke and R. Singh, "Life Events, Stress Appraisals, and Hospital Doctors' Mental Health," *New Zealand Medical Journal* 117(2004): U1121.

17. Y. Yamada, K. Tatsumi, T. Yamaguchi, N. Tanabe, Y. Takiguchi, T. Kuriyama, and R. Mikami, "Influence of Stressful Life Events on the Onset of Sarcoidosis," *Respirology* 8(2003): 186–91.

18. G. I. Ringdal, K. Ringdal, M. S. Jordhoy, and S. Kaasa, "Does Social Support from Family and Friends Work as a Buffer Against Reactions to Stressful Life Events Such as Terminal Cancer?" *Palliative and Supportive Care* 5(2007): 61–69.

19. A. D. Kanner, et al., "Comparison of Two Modes of Stress Management: Daily Hassles and Uplifts Versus Major Life Events," *Journal of Behavioral Medicine* 4(1981): 1–39.

20. Richard S. Lazarus, "Puzzles in the Study of Daily Hassles," *Journal of Behavioral Medicine* 7(1984): 375–89.

21. C. K. Holahan, C. J. Holahan, and S. S. Belk, "Adjustment in Aging: The Roles of Life Stress, Hassles, and Self-Efficacy," *Health Psychology* 3(1984): 315–28.

22. Richard S. Lazarus and A. DeLongis, "Psychological Stress and Coping in Aging," *American Psychologist* 38(1983): 245–54.

23. Kanner, et al., "Comparison of Two Modes," 1–39.

24. J. J. Zarski, "Hassles and Health: A Replication," *Health Psychology* 3(1984): 243–51.

25. S. Jain, P. J. Mills, R. von Kanel, S. Hong, and J. E. Dimsdale, "Effects of Perceived Stress and Uplifts on Inflammation and Coagulability," *Psychophysiology* 44(2007): 154–60.

26. E. Newman, D. B. O'Connor, and M. Connor, "Daily Hassles and Eating Behaviour: The Role of Cortisol Reactivity Status," *Psychoneuroendocrinology* 32(2007): 125–32.

27. Anita DeLongis, James C. Coyne, Gayle Dakof, Susan Folkman, and Richard S. Lazarus, "Relationship of Daily Hassles, Uplifts, and Major Life Events to Health Status," *Health Psychology* 1(1982): 119–36.

28. Marjorie A. Pett and Mary Jayne M. Johnson, "Development and Psychometric Evaluation of the Revised University Student Hassles Scale," *Educational and Psychological Measurement* 65(2005): 984–1010.

29. Lila Swell, *Success: You Can Make It Happen* (New York: Simon & Schuster, 1976).

LAB ASSESSMENT 6.1

What Is Your Resting Metabolic Rate (RMR)?

Everyone's caloric needs are determined by the calories expended during physical activities, as well as during nonactivity. Approximately one-third of calories burned each day are a result of regular metabolic activity. This includes calories to maintain body temperature, heartbeat, breathing, organ repair, and basic chemical reactions. This is your Resting Metabolic Rate, or RMR. The other two-thirds of the calories expended each day are a function of activities engaged in that particular day. It stands to reason that if you desire to lose weight, you want to keep your RMR high and increase your other activities (assuming your caloric intake remains constant). One way to keep RMR high is to maintain a high level of physical fitness. A physically fit body burns more calories at rest than does an unfit one. RMR also decreases with age, about 2 percent per decade, because of muscle loss. Therefore, to keep RMR high, weight training is recommended.

If you want to lose weight, a first step might be to calculate your RMR. The formula to do so is one that was developed many years ago but is still the preferred method, short of laboratory procedures. It was developed in 1919 by Francis G. Benedict and J. Arthur Harris and is called the Harris-Benedict equation.

Directions: Calculate your RMR by completing the sections below, depending on whether you are female or male.

Women		Men	
1. Begin with a base of 655 calories.	655	1. Begin with a base of 655 calories.	655
2. Multiply your weight in pounds by 4.3.	____	2. Multiply your weight in pounds by 6.3.	____
3. Multiply your height in inches by 4.7.	____	3. Multiply your height in inches by 12.7.	____
4. Add the totals from #1, #2, #3.	____	4. Add the totals from #1, #2, #3.	____
5. Multiply your age by 4.7.	____	5. Multiply your age by 6.8.	____
6. Subtract #5 from #4 to find your RMR.	____	6. Subtract #5 from #4 to find your RMR.	____
7. To maintain your current weight, multiply #6 by your Physical Activity Factor (see below).	____	7. To maintain your current weight, multiply #6 by your Physical Activity Factor (see below).	____
8. For a weight-loss diet, subtract 250 calories.	____	8. For a weight-loss diet, subtract 250 calories.	____

Physical Activity Factor: 1.2 for low activity (sedentary); 1.4 for moderate activity (light exercise); 1.6 for high levels of activity.

LAB ASSESSMENT 6.2

What Stressful Events Do You Experience?

Directions: Determine which events you have experienced in the past year.

Mean Value	Event
(50)	Entered college
(77)	Married
(38)	Had either a lot more or a lot less trouble with your boss
(43)	Held a job while attending school
(87)	Experienced the death of a spouse
(34)	Experienced a major change in sleeping habits (sleeping a lot more or a lot less, or a change in part of the day when asleep)
(77)	Experienced the death of a close family member
(30)	Experienced a major change in eating habits (a lot more or a lot less food intake, or very different meal hours or surroundings)
(41)	Made a change in or choice of a major field of study
(45)	Had a revision of your personal habits (friends, dress, manners, associations, etc.)
(68)	Experienced the death of a close friend
(22)	Have been found guilty of minor violations of the law (traffic tickets, jaywalking, etc.)
(40)	Have had an outstanding personal achievement
(68)	Experienced pregnancy or fathered a child
(56)	Had a major change in the health or behavior of a family member
(58)	Had sexual difficulties
(42)	Had trouble with in-laws
(26)	Had a major change in the number of family get-togethers (a lot more or a lot less)
(53)	Had a major change in financial state (a lot worse off or a lot better off than usual)
(50)	Gained a new family member (through birth, adoption, older person moving in, etc.)
(42)	Changed your residence or living conditions
(50)	Had a major conflict in or change in values
(36)	Had a major change in church activities (a lot more or a lot less than usual)
(58)	Had a marital reconciliation with your mate
(62)	Were fired from work
(76)	Were divorced
(50)	Changed to a different line of work
(50)	Had a major change in the number of arguments with spouse (either a lot more or a lot less than usual)
(47)	Had a major change in responsibilities at work (promotion, demotion, lateral transfer)
(41)	Had your spouse begin or cease work outside the home
(74)	Had a marital separation from your mate
(57)	Had a major change in usual type and/or amount of recreation
(52)	Took a mortgage or loan *less* than $10,000 (such as purchase of a car, TV, school loan, etc.)
(65)	Had a major personal injury or illness
(46)	Had a major change in the use of alcohol (a lot more or a lot less)
(48)	Had a major change in social activities
(38)	Had a major change in the amount of participation in school activities
(49)	Had a major change in the amount of independence and responsibility (for example, for budgeting time)
(33)	Took a trip or a vacation
(54)	Were engaged to be married
(50)	Changed to a new school
(41)	Changed dating habits
(44)	Had trouble with school administration (instructors, advisors, class scheduling, etc.)
(60)	Broke or had broken a marital engagement or a steady relationship
(57)	Had a major change in self-concept or self-awareness

Source: G. E. Anderson, "College Schedule of Recent Experience." *Master's thesis*, North Dakota State University, 1972.

Scoring: Multiply the number of times an event occurred by its mean value. Then total all of the scores. The result is your life-change unit (LCU) score. Although there are no norms for scoring this scale as there are for Lab 6.3, the greater the number of LCUs, the greater is the chance of a resulting illness or disease. Based on research of the *Social Readjustment Rating Scale* (presented in Lab 6.3), LCUs between 150 and 199 lead to a 37 percent chance of these stressors leading to illness or disease, LCUs between 200 and 299 lead to a 51 percent chance, and LCUs over 300 increase the chance to 79 percent.

LAB ASSESSMENT 6.3

Are Your Life Events Unhealthy?

Directions: Determine which events you have experienced in the past year.

Mean Value	Event
(100)	Death of spouse
(73)	Divorce
(65)	Marital separation
(63)	Jail term
(63)	Death of close family member
(53)	Personal injury or illness
(50)	Marriage
(47)	Fired at work
(45)	Marital reconciliation
(45)	Retirement
(44)	Change in health of family member
(40)	Pregnancy
(39)	Sex difficulties
(39)	Gain of new family member
(39)	Business readjustment
(38)	Change in financial state
(37)	Death of close friend
(36)	Change to different line of work
(35)	Change in number of arguments with spouse
(31)	Mortgage or loan for major purchase (home, etc.)
(30)	Foreclosure of mortgage or loan
(29)	Change in responsibilities at work
(29)	Son or daughter leaving home
(29)	Trouble with in-laws
(28)	Outstanding personal achievement
(26)	Spouse begins or stops work
(25)	Change in living conditions
(24)	Revision of personal habits
(23)	Trouble with boss
(20)	Change in work hours or conditions
(20)	Change in residence
(19)	Change in recreation
(19)	Change in church activities
(18)	Change in social activities
(17)	Mortgage or loan for lesser purchase (car, TV, etc.)
(16)	Change in sleeping habits
(15)	Change in number of family get-togethers
(15)	Change in eating habits
(13)	Vacation
(12)	Christmas or Hanukkah
(11)	Minor violations of the law

Reprinted from "The Social Readjustment Rating Scale" by Thomas H. Holmes and Richard H. Rahe. *Journal of Psychosomatic Research* 11(1967): 213–18 with permission from Elsevier.

Scoring: Multiply the number of times an event occurred by its mean value. Then total all of the scores. The result is your life-change unit (LCU) score. If you scored between 150 and 199, there is a 37 percent chance of these stressors leading to illness or disease. If you scored 200–299, there is a 51 percent chance of these stressors leading to illness or disease. Over 300, and the chance increases to 79 percent.

LAB ASSESSMENT 6.4

What Hassles Do You Encounter?

Directions: Hassles are irritants that can range from minor annoyances to major pressures, problems, or difficulties. They can occur few or many times. Listed here are ways in which a person can feel hassled. First, circle the hassles that have happened to you in the past month. Then look at the numbers to the right of the items you circled. Indicate by circling 1, 2, or 3 how often each of the circled hassles has occurred in the past month. If a hassle did not occur in the past month, do not circle it.

Hassles	How Often: 1 = Somewhat Often, 2 = Moderately Often, 3 = Extremely Often	Hassles	How Often: 1 = Somewhat Often, 2 = Moderately Often, 3 = Extremely Often	Hassles	How Often: 1 = Somewhat Often, 2 = Moderately Often, 3 = Extremely Often
Misplacing or losing things	1 2 3	Unexpected company	1 2 3	Financial dealing with friends or acquaintances	1 2 3
Troublesome neighbors	1 2 3	Too much time on hands	1 2 3	Job dissatisfactions	1 2 3
Social obligations	1 2 3	Having to wait	1 2 3	Worries about decisions to change jobs	1 2 3
Inconsiderate smokers	1 2 3	Concerns about accidents	1 2 3	Trouble with reading, writing, or spelling abilities	1 2 3
Troubling thoughts about your future	1 2 3	Being lonely	1 2 3	Too many meetings	1 2 3
Thoughts about death	1 2 3	Not enough money for health care	1 2 3	Problems with divorce or separation	1 2 3
Health of a family member	1 2 3	Fear of confrontation	1 2 3	Trouble with arithmetic skills	1 2 3
Not enough money for clothing	1 2 3	Financial security	1 2 3	Gossip	1 2 3
Not enough money for housing	1 2 3	Silly practical mistakes	1 2 3	Legal problems	1 2 3
Concerns about owing money	1 2 3	Inability to express yourself	1 2 3	Concerns about weight	1 2 3
Concerns about getting credit	1 2 3	Physical illness	1 2 3	Not enough time to do the things you need to do	1 2 3
Concerns about money for emergencies	1 2 3	Fear of rejection	1 2 3	Television	1 2 3
Someone owes you money	1 2 3	Difficulties with getting pregnant	1 2 3	Not enough personal energy	1 2 3
Financial responsibility for someone who doesn't live with you	1 2 3	Sexual problems that result from physical problems	1 2 3	Concern about inner conflicts	1 2 3
Cutting down on electricity, water, etc.	1 2 3	Concerns about health in general	1 2 3	Feel conflicted over what to do	1 2 3
Smoking too much	1 2 3	Not seeing enough people	1 2 3	Regrets over past decisions	1 2 3
Use of alcohol	1 2 3	Friends or relatives too far away	1 2 3	Menstrual (period) problems	1 2 3
Personal use of drugs	1 2 3	Preparing meals	1 2 3	The weather	1 2 3
Too many responsibilities	1 2 3	Wasting time	1 2 3	Nightmares	1 2 3
Decisions about having children	1 2 3	Auto maintenance	1 2 3	Concerns about getting ahead	1 2 3
Nonfamily members living in your home	1 2 3	Filling out forms	1 2 3	Hassles from boss or supervisor	1 2 3
Care for pet	1 2 3	Neighborhood deterioration	1 2 3	Difficulties with friends	1 2 3
Planning meals	1 2 3	Financing children's education	1 2 3	Not enough time for family	1 2 3
Concerned about the meaning of life	1 2 3	Problems with employees	1 2 3	Transportation problems	1 2 3
Trouble relaxing	1 2 3	Problems on job due to being a woman or a man	1 2 3	Not enough money for transportation	1 2 3
Trouble making decisions	1 2 3	Declining physical abilities	1 2 3	Not enough money for entertainment and recreation	1 2 3
Problems getting along with fellow workers	1 2 3	Being exploited	1 2 3	Shopping	1 2 3
Customers or clients give you a hard time	1 2 3	Concerns about bodily functions	1 2 3	Prejudice and discrimination from others	1 2 3
Home maintenance (inside)	1 2 3	Rising prices of common goods	1 2 3	Property, investments, or taxes	1 2 3
Concerns about job security	1 2 3	Not getting enough rest	1 2 3	Yard work or outside home maintenance	1 2 3
Concerns about retirement	1 2 3	Not getting enough sleep	1 2 3	Concerns about news events	1 2 3
Laid-off or out of work	1 2 3	Problems with aging parents	1 2 3	Noise	1 2 3
Don't like current work duties	1 2 3	Problems with your children	1 2 3	Crime	1 2 3
Don't like fellow workers	1 2 3	Problems with persons younger than yourself	1 2 3	Traffic	1 2 3
Not enough money for basic necessities	1 2 3	Problems with your lover	1 2 3	Pollution	1 2 3
Not enough money for food	1 2 3	Difficulties seeing or hearing	1 2 3		
Too many interruptions	1 2 3	Overload with family responsibilities	1 2 3		
		Too many things to do	1 2 3		
		Unchallenging work	1 2 3		
		Concerns about meeting high standards	1 2 3		

Source: With kind permission from Springer Science+Business Media: "Comparison of Two Modes of Stress Management: Daily Hassles and Uplifts Versus Major Life Events," Allan D. Kanner, *Journal of Behavioral Medicine* 4(1981): 1–39.

Scoring: The mean score is 20.6 hassles per month. The mean intensity of these hassles is 1.47. If your scores are higher, you experience more hassles, or more intense hassles, than the average person. If that is the case, you are more susceptible than is the average person to negative consequences, such as illness and disease, because of this increased level of stress.

Life-Situation Interventions: Interpersonal

While some life-situation interventions can be successfully employed when no one else is directly involved, this chapter presents life-situation interventions that are useful when the situation involves other people as well as yourself. The topics we will consider include assertiveness; resolving conflicts; communicating effectively with others; emotional intelligence; technostress; and managing time wisely and coordinating it with coworkers, family, and friends. We will also consider how to develop a network of supporters to serve as a buffer between stress and its negative consequences.

Because other people are involved, you might want to consider teaching these stress management techniques to the people you interact with often. In that way, when a situation presents itself that calls for one of the stress management strategies discussed in this chapter and you forget to use it, the other person might remember. The result can be more effective interactions for you, and that can only mean less stress.

Asserting Yourself

> Ring! Gladys picks up the telephone to hear the dulcet voice of her friend Sue. "Gladys, I have an appointment for lunch. Can you watch Billy from noon until three?"
>
> "Sure, Sue. Take your time and enjoy yourself. I'll expect you at noon." But in Gladys' mind another conversation is being recorded: "I don't believe that Sue! She's always asking me to watch her kid. What am I, a babysitter? I was looking forward to scheduling a tennis match with Joan today. Well, there goes that idea."

This scenario is not atypical and not exclusive to women. Men and women who find it difficult to say no when asked by the boss if they can handle one other chore or responsibility and youths who can't say no to friends when teased into trying a mood-altering substance (alcohol or other drugs) have the same problem as Gladys does. Training programs have been mushrooming throughout the country and world to help people say no when they should, say yes when they want to, and generally behave in a self-actualizing manner. These training programs teach assertive behavior. Several definitions are necessary at this point:

1. *Assertive behavior:* Expressing yourself and satisfying your own needs. Feeling good about this and not hurting others in the process.
2. *Nonassertive behavior:* Denying your own wishes to satisfy someone else's. Sacrificing your own needs to meet someone else's needs.
3. *Aggressive behavior:* Seeking to dominate or to get your own way at the expense of others.

To assess your general pattern of behavior regarding assertiveness, complete Lab 7.1 at the end of this chapter.

In the phone conversation just described, Gladys's response was **nonassertive.** She gave up her need for scheduling recreation time and did not express her feelings of being used and taken advantage of by Sue. If she had been **aggressive,**

nonassertive
Giving up what one is entitled to, one's rights, in order not to upset another person.

aggressive
Acting in a way to get what one is entitled to, one's rights, but at the expense of someone else's rights.

Gladys might have said, "How dare you ask me to watch that brat of yours? I have more important things to do. You're selfish and self-centered. You never even asked if you could watch my children." Acting aggressively, Gladys would have denied Sue's right to ask a favor of her. Gladys would have gone about fulfilling her needs, but she would have done so in a manner that was unfair to Sue. Sue has the right to ask, and Gladys should not deny her that right. However, Gladys owns her own behavior. She has the right to say no. In a more **assertive** response to Sue's request, Gladys might have replied, "I can appreciate your need for someone to watch Billy, but I've been so busy lately that I promised myself today I wouldn't take on any such commitments. I really need some recreation time, so I'm going to play tennis with Joan. Perhaps Mary is free to watch Billy. Do you have her phone number?" It would also be appropriate during this response, or sometime soon after, for Gladys to express to Sue her feelings of being used. If these feelings are expressed, they can be dealt with, and Sue will have the information she needs to change her behavior. However, if Gladys never lets Sue know how she feels, Sue will continue to make the same request, and Gladys's feelings will persist, diminishing the quality of their relationship. Soon we will discuss how Gladys can express these feelings assertively—both verbally and nonverbally.

Assertiveness has several health implications. For example, assertive college students are more likely to employ safer sex practices[1] and help anticipate and respond to sexual assault.[2] Assertive women are also more likely to communicate better with their physicians, view their physicians as health advisors, and obtain a mammogram.[3,4] And assertive people are better able to resolve conflicts and communicate more effectively in response to verbal abuse.[5]

The relationship of assertive behavior to stress lies in satisfaction of needs. If you generally act assertively, you are usually achieving your needs while maintaining effective interpersonal relationships. If you generally act nonassertively, you are not satisfying your needs, and those unsatisfied needs will become stressors. If you generally behave aggressively, your needs are met but at the expense of your relationships with others. Poor interpersonal relationships will become stressors. You can see that, to siphon off stressors at the life-situation level, you need to learn, practice, and adopt assertive behavior as your general pattern of satisfying needs.

You may understand that you have a right to act assertively, and even know how to do so, but decide not to. There could be several reasons for that decision. You might decide that acting nonassertively in a particular situation is in your best interest. Or you might decide to act nonassertively because you lack confidence and have low self-esteem. Self-esteem, discussed in detail in Chapter 8, is regard for oneself. Do you think you are smart enough to make good decisions? Do you believe you are worthy of being treated with respect and dignity? If you have low regard for yourself—low self-esteem—you might not believe you are worthy of having your rights met, and you might decide not to act assertively. If this is the case, the recommendations for improving self-esteem in Chapter 8 should help.

Assertion theory is based on the premise that every person has certain basic rights. Unfortunately, we are often taught that acting consistently with these rights is socially or morally unacceptable. We are taught some traditional assumptions as children—which stay with us as adults—that interfere with basing our behavior on these basic rights. These assumptions violate our rights, and we need to dispense with them.

Nonverbal Assertiveness

Unwilling to deny your basic human rights, you may choose to become more assertive. Behaving assertively is more difficult for some than others, but the hints in this section should allow everyone to begin moving in the assertive direction. Assertiveness is not only a matter of *what* you say but also a function of *how* you say it.[6] Even if you make an assertive verbal response, you will not be believed if your body's response is nonassertive. Those who express themselves assertively

1. Stand straight, remain steady, and directly face the people to whom they are speaking, while maintaining eye contact.
2. Speak in a clear, steady voice, loud enough for the people to whom they are speaking to hear them.
3. Speak fluently, without hesitation and with assurance and confidence.

In contrast, nonassertive body language includes

1. Lack of eye contact; looking down or away.
2. Swaying and shifting of weight from one foot to the other.
3. Whining and hesitancy when speaking.

Aggressive behavior can also be recognized without even hearing the words; it includes

1. Leaning forward, with glaring eyes.
2. Pointing a finger at the person to whom you are speaking.
3. Shouting.
4. Clenching the fists.
5. Putting hands on hips and wagging the head.

   If you want to act assertively, then you must pay attention to your body language. Practice and adopt assertive nonverbal behavior while concentrating on eliminating signs of nonassertive and aggressive behavior.

Verbal Assertiveness

A formula I have found effective in helping people verbally express themselves assertively is the **DESC form**. The verbal response is divided into four components:

1. *Describe:* Paint a verbal picture of the other person's behavior or the situation to which you are reacting: "When . . . "
2. *Express:* Express your feelings (such as anger or frustration) regarding the other person's behavior or the situation you have just described. Use "I" statements here: "I feel . . . "
3. *Specify:* Be specific by identifying several ways you would like the other person's behavior or the situation to change. Rather than saying, "You should . . . ," use "I" statements: "I would prefer . . . ," "I would like . . . ," "I want . . ."
4. *Consequence:* Select the consequences you have decided to apply to the behavior or situation. What will you do if the other person's behavior or the situation changes to your satisfaction? "If you do _____, I will . . . " What will be the consequences if nothing changes, or if the changes do not meet your needs? "If you don't _____, I will . . . "*

   To demonstrate the DESC form of organizing assertive responses, let's assume Jim and Kathy are dating. Jim wants Kathy to date him exclusively. Kathy believes she's too young to eliminate other men from her love life. Jim's assertive response to this situation might take this form:

> (Describe) When you go out with other men, (Express) I feel very jealous and have doubts about the extent of your love for me. (Specify) I would prefer that we date only each other. (Consequence) If you date only me, I'll make a sincere effort to offer you a variety of experiences so that you do not feel you've missed anything. We'll go to nice restaurants, attend plays, go to concerts, and whatever else you'd like that

DESC form

A formula for verbally expressing assertiveness consisting of a description of the situation, expression of feelings, specification of preferred change, and consequences of whether or not a change is made.

*Source: S. Bower and G. A. Bower, *Asserting Yourself,* 2nd ed. (p. 126). © 1976 by Susan Anthony Bower and Gordon A. Bower. Reprinted by permission of Perseus Book Publishers, a member of Perseus Books, L.L.C.

I can afford and that is reasonable. If you do not agree to date me exclusively, I will not date you at all. The pain would just be more than I'm willing to tolerate.

A woman in my class whose boss required that she work Monday through Friday *and* Saturdays organized the following DESC form assertive response:

(Describe) When I am expected to work six days a week, (Express) I feel tired and abused. (Specify) I would prefer working only Monday through Friday. (Consequence) If I can work only those five days, I will be conscientious about doing all my work well and on time. If need be, I'll work through some lunch hours, stay later when necessary, or even be willing to take some work home. However, if I'm required to work on Saturdays, I will resign and look for another job. That is how strongly I feel about my right to have a total weekend for myself.

Organize your own assertive response! Think of a situation that has been of concern to you for which an assertive response would be helpful. For example, one of my students recalled having invited a friend to dinner. While dinner was cooking, the friend received a call from a man she was longing to see. Before the telephone conversation was too old, he asked her out for dinner that night, and she accepted. Upon hanging up, this "friend" apologized to my student as she left to have dinner with her male acquaintance. Another student was anticipating her son's return from college with his girlfriend for a Christmas vacation. She knew he would want to sleep in the same room as his girlfriend, since they shared a room while away at school. Believing that these sleeping arrangements would violate her rights, she chose to prepare an assertive response to convey to her son. She prepared a response, stated it to her son and his girlfriend, and reported that things worked out marvelously.

Is there a situation in your life crying out for assertive behavior? Can you give up the assumptions preventing you from claiming your basic human rights in this situation? Write what you would say if you responded assertively.

_____

_____

_____

How does that feel to you? Will you do it? If so, remember to use assertive body language as well.

Conflict Resolution

If you become effective in resolving conflict, your interpersonal relationships will be improved. The result of this improvement will be a decrease in the number of stressors you experience. Less conflict of shorter duration resolved to your satisfaction will mean a less-stressed and healthier you.

Before we proceed with suggestions for effectively resolving conflict, you might be interested in an identification of your typical modus operandi—that is, how you usually deal with conflict situations. To make this determination, complete Lab 7.2 at the end of this chapter.

Resolving conflict can be relatively simple. What confounds the situation are usually a lack of listening, an attempt at winning, an inability to demonstrate an understanding of the person with whom you are in conflict, and a rigidity that prevents you from considering alternative solutions. Consider the following extended example from *Sexuality Education: Theory and Practice* (Bruess and Greenberg, 2004).*

*Source: Clint E. Bruess and Jerrold S. Greenberg, *Sexuality Education: Theory and Practice*, 4th ed. 107–8, 2004: Jones & Bartlett Learning, Burlington, MA.

Paul: Well, Barbara, as you know, Thanksgiving vacation is soon, and I'd like you to come home with me and spend it with my family.

Barbara: Now you ask! I've already told my folks to expect us for Thanksgiving dinner!

Paul:	You've got some nerve! You didn't even ask me if I wanted to go to your house for Thanksgiving.
Barbara:	Ask you? You've been hitting the books so much lately that I've hardly seen you long enough to say hello, much less ask you to Thanksgiving dinner.
Paul:	What would you rather I do, fail my courses? You're pretty selfish, aren't you?
Barbara:	I've had it! Either we're going to my house for Thanksgiving or you can say goodbye right now.
Paul:	In that case, GOODBYE!

In this situation, both Paul and Barbara are trying to win. Each is trying to get the other to spend Thanksgiving vacation at the family home. However, neither Paul nor Barbara can win! You see, there are several choices presented by them, either overt or implied:

1. Spend the vacation at Paul's house.

2. Spend the vacation at Barbara's house.

3. Break up their relationship.

If they decide to spend the vacation at Paul's, Barbara will be required to cancel her plans with her family and put up with the hassle that would entail. Further, she will feel that her wishes are not very important in the relationship. The bottom line is that she will resent being at Paul's for Thanksgiving. But if they spend the vacation at Barbara's house, Paul will resent having to be *there*. He might feel that, since he asked first, they should be at his house. Further, he objects to Barbara's assuming she can make plans that include him without even bothering to consult him. It becomes evident, then, that regardless of whose house they visit for the vacation, one or the other will be resentful. This resentment will probably result in the Thanksgiving vacation being uncomfortable and unenjoyable for all concerned. In other words, no matter who wins, both really lose. They both wind up with a miserable vacation. The third possibility, dissolving the relationship, is also obviously a no-win solution.

How might the issue be better decided? Consider the following communication.

Paul:	Well, Barbara, as you know, Thanksgiving vacation is soon, and I'd like you to come home with me and spend it with my family.

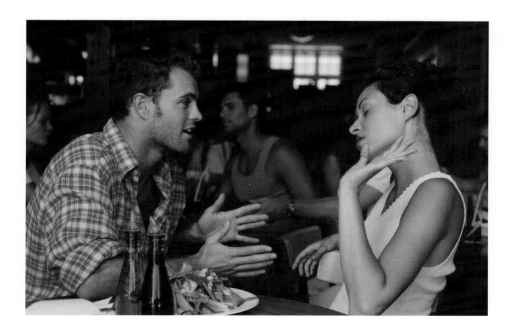

Some arguments could be avoided if couples would listen to each other.

Barbara: Now you ask! I've already told my folks to expect us for Thanksgiving dinner!

Paul: You thought we would go to your house for Thanksgiving vacation?

Barbara: Yes, and my parents have made preparations already.

Paul: Your parents would be upset if we canceled Thanksgiving dinner with them?

Barbara: You bet! And I wouldn't want to be the one to have to tell them either!

Paul: You think that your parents would really hassle you if you didn't spend Thanksgiving with them?

Barbara: Yes.

Paul: Would you also feel some embarrassment in having to change plans that your parents thought were definite?

Barbara: Yes, I guess I would.

Paul: It sounds like you were really looking forward to our being together at your house and with your family this vacation.

Barbara: Yes, I really was.

Paul: I'm glad that you included me in your Thanksgiving plans, but I really was looking forward to spending this vacation together with you and with my family. I haven't seen my family for a while and, further, I know that they would really like you. And I'm a little bothered that you didn't consult me before making plans for the vacation.

Barbara: Gee, I guess you have some rights, too. I'm sorry.

Paul: Well, let's see if there are some alternatives that we haven't considered.

Barbara: Maybe we could spend half the vacation at my house and half at yours.

Paul: Or perhaps we could invite your family to my house.

Barbara: How about staying here and not spending Thanksgiving with either of our families?

Paul: It seems like we have several possibilities. We could divide the vacation in half at each of our houses, but that would mean that we waste a good part of the vacation in travel.

Barbara: It's not very realistic, either, to expect that my whole family could cancel their plans to go to your house.

Paul: At the same time, if we stayed here, both sets of parents and family would be disappointed. That would be cutting off our noses to spite our faces.

Barbara: Would it make sense to agree to spend Thanksgiving vacation at one of our houses and the next vacation at the other's?

Paul: That seems sensible, and since you've already made plans, let's spend Thanksgiving at your house.

Barbara: Okay. Remember, though, the next vacation will be at your house.

In this example, Paul followed a simple procedure to resolve interpersonal conflict. The steps of this communication process consist of the following:

1. Active listening (reflecting back to the other person his or her *words* and feelings).

2. Identifying your position (stating your *thoughts* and *feelings* about the situation).

3. Exploring alternative solutions (brainstorming other possibilities).

Paul began by employing a technique known as **active listening,**[7,8] or **reflective listening.** This technique requires the listener to paraphrase the speaker's words

active listening
Paraphrasing the speaker's words and feelings; also called reflective listening.

reflective listening
Paraphrasing the speaker's words and feelings; also called active listening.

so the speaker knows that his or her meaning has been received. Further, it requires the listener to go beyond the speaker's words to paraphrase the *feelings* left unspoken. Note that Paul understood Barbara would be embarrassed to have to cancel Thanksgiving vacation with her family, even though she never explicitly stated that she would. By reflecting the speaker's *words* and *thoughts,* the listener creates an awareness on the speaker's part that the listener cares enough to really understand his or her views. Once the speaker appreciates this fact, he or she is more receptive to hearing and understanding the listener's viewpoint. The net result will be both people understanding each other's point of view better; each will also be less insistent that his or her way is the only way.

The next step is to explore alternative solutions by "brainstorming"—that is, listing all possible solutions prior to evaluating their appropriateness. Once all possible solutions are listed, evaluate each proposed solution until both people agree upon one. With this technique, it initially appears that no one wins. However, in fact, everyone wins. In the previous example, Paul will accompany Barbara to her house for Thanksgiving without being resentful. He will know that she now understands his need to be involved in their planning and that the next vacation is going to be spent with his family. Consequently, he will be better able to enjoy being with Barbara and her family. The vacation will be fun, and everyone will win.

I can tell you that many people to whom I have taught this technique have dealt with their conflicts more successfully. Remember, though, that the purpose of this technique is *not* to convince someone that your point of view is correct. It is not a technique to manipulate anyone. The intention is to end up at an *alternative* solution that makes both you and the other person happy. If you are not willing to end up at some solution other than the one you had in mind, do not use this method of resolving conflict. If you are not willing to give up your power over the other person (e.g., parent over child or boss over employee), then don't use this technique.

A student of mine asked, "What happens if I use the steps you outlined and my daughter says, 'There you go with that psychology crap again.' What do I do then?" I told her to tell her daughter, "You're right. This is something I learned at school to help resolve conflict. I love you so much and place such a high value on our relationship that I felt I would try this technique. I hope we can both use it so, when we disagree, we come to a solution both of us are happy with. Would you like me to teach it to you?" How can anyone object to the use of a system designed to help them arrive at a solution satisfactory to them both and maintain their relationship?

I'll bet there are some conflicts that you can anticipate. Why not try achieving a positive resolution of those conflicts rather than generally giving in or being so stubborn that, although you get your way, you're not happy? Why not try a system that lets both you and the other person win? Try it; you'll like it.

Communication

In addition to learning to be more assertive and to resolve conflicts well, other communication skills will help you get along better with friends, family, and coworkers, with the result being less stress.

There several components of any communication. As depicted in Figure 7.1, these include a *sender* who conveys a *message* through some *medium* to the *receiver*

Figure 7.1

A Model of Communication

Sender   Exercise   Medium   Receiver

of the message. Using this book as an example, the author (*sender*) relates how managing stress can improve health and quality of life (*message*) through the written page (*medium*) to the reader (*receiver*). To communicate effectively requires attention to each of these components of communication.

- Senders must be knowledgeable about the topic. They must also be believable and trusted. Studies have found that people similar to the people to whom the message is directed are most effective. That is why peer education programs are offered on many campuses.
- The message must also be credible. One way to assure credibility is to include evidence as part of the message.
- The medium through which the message is communicated also should be effective. For example, when working out a disagreement with someone, it is best to communicate in person rather than through e-mail.
- For the message to be received as intended the sender should know a lot about the receiver. What does that person value? How does that person prefer to receive messages? Whom does that person trust? Answers to these questions and others will allow the sender to create a message specific to those to whom the sender wishes to communicate.

Nonverbal Communication

We also communicate with our bodies. Notice the body posture of your classmates. During an interesting lecture or activity, most of them will probably be leaning or looking toward the lecturer or the center of the group, indicating that they are involved in what is going on. During a boring class, they will probably be leaning away from the lecturer or group. We call this physical behavior *body language*. Communication by body posture often says as much as the spoken word. When people feel uncomfortable about expressing their thoughts or feelings verbally, body language is sometimes the only form of communication they participate in.

We all recognize the importance of communicating nonverbally, since we smile when we say hello, scratch our heads when perplexed, and hug a friend to show affection. We also have an array of body terms to describe our nonverbal behavior: "Keep a stiff upper lip," "I can't stomach him," "She has no backbone," "I'm tongue-tied," "He caught her eye," "I have two left feet," and "That was spine-tingling." We show appreciation and affection, revulsion, and indifference with expressions and gestures. We tell people we are interested in them by merely making eye contact and, like the male peacock displaying his feathers, we display our sexuality by the way we dress, by the way we walk, and even by how we stand.[9]

Verbal Communication

Unfortunately, the nonverbal expression of feelings and thoughts is easy to misinterpret. Consequently, depending on nonverbal communication alone to express yourself is to risk being misunderstood. Furthermore, if another person is depending on nonverbal communication to express feelings to you, it is up to you to ask—verbally—whether you are getting the right message. Without such a *reality check*, the other person, while totally failing to connect, might assume that he or she is communicating effectively. For example, imagine that a man and woman on their first date begin hugging, kissing, and caressing each other after a movie. The woman's breathing speeds up and the man, taking this as a sign of sexual arousal and interest, presses onward. When the woman suddenly pushes free and complains that the man is too impatient, he is confused. The problem here is one of interpretation rather than incompatibility. The rapid breathing that the man took as a sign of arousal was really a sign of nervousness. If these people had been more effective verbal communicators, they would have been able to clarify the situation in the beginning. Instead, they reached a silent impasse, with him confused and her resentful. Check out your impressions of someone's nonverbal communication, and improve your communication by making your nonverbal and verbal messages as consistent as you can.

Planning Time to Talk

One common barrier to communication is the television set. We are often so busy watching it that we don't take the time to talk with those around us. To improve your communication with others, you may need to plan time for discussions. In setting up such times, it is wise to do the following:

1. Make sure you allow sufficient time to have a meaningful discussion.
2. Disconnect the phone and don't allow other people to barge in on you.
3. Accept all feelings and one's right to the verbal expression of these feelings. For example, it is just as appropriate to say, "I feel angry when . . . " as it is to say, "I feel terrific when. . . . "
4. Take a risk and really describe your thoughts and feelings. Don't expect the other person to guess what they are.
5. Approach your discussions with both of you understanding that the goal is to improve your relationship.

Listening

This hint seems obvious, yet as demonstrated in our discussion of conflict resolution, it is often ignored. Listening and paraphrasing (active or reflective listening) are effective in regular conversation as well as during conflict. All of us can do a better job at listening. Try to pay more attention to this aspect of your communications.

Beginning with Agreement

You would be surprised at how much better you can communicate with someone with whom you disagree if you start your message with a point on which you do agree. Of course, this requires you to listen carefully so you can identify something with which you can agree. For example, if you are disagreeing about who should do the dishes, you might begin by saying, "I agree that it is important the dishes be cleaned." If you look and listen intently, you can always find a point of agreement.

"And," Not "But"

The word "but" is like an eraser; it erases everything that precedes it. When someone says, "Yes, your needs are important but . . . " they are saying, "Your needs may be important, but let's forget about them because I'm about to tell you what's *really* important." In other words, the importance of your needs is being erased and now we can focus on the real issue. Listen to how people use the word "but" and you will get a real insight into how people communicate. Listen to how *you* use "but"!

Substituting the word "and" for "but" is so simple yet so significant. "And" leaves what preceded it on the table and *adds* something to it. "Your needs are important and . . . " means that we will not discount (erase) your needs; we will consider them in addition to considering what will be presented next. Use more "ands" and fewer "buts."

"I" Statements

Too often we try to get other people to behave or believe as we do. Others naturally resent that, just as we resent it when others try to get us to behave or believe as they do. Part of this problem relates to the words we use when communicating. Remember the DESC form example of the student who was expected to work on Saturdays? If not, reread it now and notice that the wording of her assertive response includes many "I" statements. For example, she doesn't say, "When *you* expect me to work on Saturdays. . . . " She says, "When *I* am expected to work on Saturdays. . . . " In this manner, she places the focus not on the boss's behavior but on the situation. Consequently, the boss need not get defensive, and they can better discuss and resolve the situation. When we say "you," we are making the other person feel that he or she is being criticized and needs to defend himself or herself. When we say "I," we are focusing on our feelings, beliefs, and interpretations. Feeling less defensive, the other person is more likely to listen to us, and the result is more effective communication.

Avoid "Why" Questions

As with statements that include "you" instead of "I," questions that begin with "why" make the other person defensive. "Why did you leave so early?" makes the other person have to justify leaving early. In addition, "why" questions are often veiled criticisms. "Why don't you spend more time with me?" may be asked to get an answer, but more often than not, it is a statement ("You don't spend enough time with me!") rather than a question. Avoid "why" questions.

Emotional Intelligence

emotional intelligence
Perceiving feelings, using them appropriately, and managing emotions.

One contributor to preventing and to resolving conflict well is emotional intelligence. Intelligence can be more than just having knowledge. It can also relate to emotions and the way we use these emotions. That form of intelligence is called emotional intelligence. **Emotional intelligence** is "the ability to accurately identify and understand one's own emotional reactions and those of others, and to regulate one's emotions and to use them to make good decisions and act effectively."[10]

Daniel Goleman was the first person to define and popularize emotional intelligence.[11] Goleman's model included more than 25 characteristics of emotional intelligence including emotional self-awareness, teamwork and collaboration, service orientation, initiative, and achievement motivation—all of which are important in developing and maintaining human relationships.

Goleman's model of emotional intelligence has been condensed into the four branch model:[12]

1. Accurately perceive emotions in oneself and others.
2. Use emotions to facilitate thinking.
3. Understand emotional meanings.
4. Manage emotions.

To determine your level of emotional intelligence, complete Lab Assessment 7.5.

The Importance of Emotional Intelligence

Emotional intelligence is important in developing and maintaining relationships. Without emotional intelligence you would not pick up on others' feelings, or your own, that are keys to human interaction. It stands to reason that without successful human interaction, you would experience a good deal of stress. Consequently, emotional intelligence is an important component of managing stress.

Unfortunately, it appears that modern advances have negatively impacted on our ability to become emotionally intelligent. For example, lamenting the current state of technology's influence on personal interaction and, therefore, the development of emotional intelligence, Goldman states:

> Mirror neurons are one of the main classes of neurons that have been discovered in the social brain—all of these social circuits together keep things operating smoothly during interactions. But when we're online there's no channel for our social brain to get feedback. The mirror neurons have nothing to read, and so we're operating in the dark. This may create, for example, a negativity bias to e-mail, where the sender thinks the message is more positive than does the person who receives. This also means people are more likely to experience what's called "cyber-disinhibition," which

means that, say, you're having a little bit of an emotional hijack and if you were face-to-face your social circuitry might tell you "Well, it would be better to say this than that." In other words, you might be artful about it. But online it has zero feedback; that's the disinhibition. . . . So, on the downside, there also may be some emotional numbing, some deadening of empathy, and all of that means that we may be fraying social connections as more and more interactions become virtual as on Facebook and less and less face-to-face. Then there is the big experiment that is perhaps the most troubling: kids are spending more and more time during childhood online. This changes the way we have always taught social and emotional skills in life, in day-to-day interactions. If kids are spending fewer hours of time together in person and more and more hours online we might be de-skilling entire generations in essentials for a full human life.[13]

Interestingly, one way suggested by Goleman to counteract technology's influence on emotional intelligence is through meditation, which he believes is a way to enhance self-awareness.

Ways to Develop Emotional Intelligence

Emotional intelligence can be improved at any age. In fact, several programs have been developed to do that and are described on the website of the Consortium for Research on Emotional Intelligence in Organizations.[14] However, improving emotional intelligence takes a long time of concentrated effort. Goleman argues that because the neural circuits need to be modified to extend deep into the nonverbal parts of the brain, emotional intelligence training must be experiential. He uses the example of learning to ride a bicycle. Understanding what needs to be done on a cognitive level helps, but only to a limited degree. It is only by getting on a bike and riding it, falling over, and trying again repeatedly, that the skill is mastered. The same is true for most emotional learning. It usually involves a long and sometimes difficult process requiring much practice and support. One-day seminars just won't do it.

Technostress

You have a busy day planned today. You need to do research for a term paper, to study for an exam, to phone your family, to call the bank to dispute some charges on your credit card, and to meet friends after dinner. Interfering with getting all of this done are interruptions from a barrage of text messages, e-mails to which you have to respond, phone calls you have to take, and a message on your computer to download an updated version of your virus protection program and your iTunes. It's understandable that you become frustrated and stressed out—after all, who wouldn't? You have just become the victim of technostress. *Technostress* is our reaction to technology and how our lives are changing as a result. Technology lets us do more and more that we often take on too much, ending up feeling overwhelmed and stressed.[15] What with iPhones and BlackBerrys, pagers and cell phones, fax machines, and messaging and e-mail we never seem to have any *down time*. Worse yet, we too often employ more than one technological wonder at the same time, demonstrating a classical sign of stress and Type A behavior pattern called *polyphasic* behavior. Some research suggests that 85 percent of Americans feel uncomfortable with technology, and employees are interrupted at least three hours a day by technological tools.[16] Other studies found workers spending five hours a week stressed out because of technology, with one-third of workers stating technology made their blood boil more than anything else during the work day. Technology causes five hours of stress per week.[17]

Not only does technostress affect us as individuals, it also affects our relationships. Families tend to get into their techno-cocoons with one person playing computer games or Nintendo, another on the cell phone, and another glued to a high-definition television set. The result, of course, is a lack of communication among family members.

Ways to Improve Emotional Intelligence

Some experts suggest the following as a help in improving emotional intelligence:

- *Observe how you react to people.* Do you rush to judge before you know all of the facts? Do you stereotype? Look honestly at how you think and interact with other people. Try to put yourself in their place, and be more open and accepting of their perspectives and needs.

- *Look at your work environment.* Do you seek attention for your accomplishments? Humility can be a wonderful quality, and it doesn't mean that you're shy or lack self-confidence. When you practice humility, you say that you know what you did, and you can be quietly confident about it. Give others a chance to shine—put the focus on them, and don't worry too much about getting praise for yourself.

- *Do a self-evaluation.* What are your weaknesses? Are you willing to accept that you're not perfect and that you could work on some areas to make yourself a better person? Have the courage to look at yourself honestly—it can change your life.

- *Examine how you react to stressful situations.* Do you become upset every time there's a delay or something doesn't happen the way you want it to? Do you blame others or become angry at them, even when it's not their fault? The ability to stay calm and in control in difficult situations is highly valued. Keep your emotions under control when things go wrong.

- *Take responsibility for your actions.* If you hurt someone's feelings, apologize directly—don't ignore what you did or avoid the person. People are usually more willing to forgive and forget if you make an honest attempt to make things right.

- *Examine how your actions will affect others before you take those actions.* If your decision will impact others, put yourself in their place. How will they feel if you do this? Would you want that experience? If you must take the action, how can you help others deal with the effects?

Source: Mindtools.com. (2011) Emotional Intelligence: Developing Strong "People Skills." [Online] Available at: www .mindtools.com/pages/article/newCDV_59.htm. Accessed May 2012. Reproduced with permission.

So what can be done about technostress? We certainly cannot go back to the "good old days," BC—before computers. Yet, we can take control of our technological tools rather than be controlled by them. That means consciously limiting their use. Rather than checking e-mails or text messages numerous times a day, we can reserve 15 minutes in the morning, 15 minutes in the afternoon, and another 15 minutes in the evening for e-mails and text messages. When interacting with family or friends, we can purposefully refrain from answering phone calls or text messages, instead focusing on communicating with those people. When having dinner with someone and a question comes up (e.g., what year did the movie *Rocky Horror Picture Show* first come out?), we can refuse to use our iPhones to obtain immediate gratification with an answer. Consistent with the theme of this book, you are more in control of your behavior than you might think. Now, you just need to exercise that control.

Time Management

One of the tasks we are often unsuccessful at is managing our time well. There really is no reason for this, since there are effective time management techniques.[18-21] These techniques can help you with your most precious posses-sion—your time. Time spent is time gone forever. In spite of what we often profess, we cannot save time. Time moves con-tinuously and it is used—one way or another. If we waste time, there is no bank where we can withdraw time we previ-ously saved to replace the time wasted. To come to terms with our mortality is to realize that our time is limited. Given this realization and the probability that you would like to better organize your time (I've never met anyone who didn't profess that need), some techniques that can help are presented next.

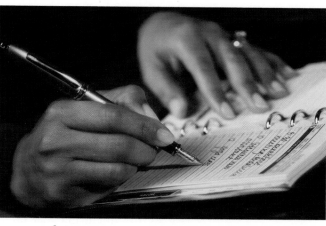

Assessing How You Spend Time

As a first step in managing time better, you might want to analyze how you spend your time now. To do this, divide your day into fifteen-minute segments. Then record what you are doing every fifteen minutes (see Table 7.1). Afterward, review this time diary and total the time spent on each activity throughout the day (see Table 7.2). For example, you might find you spent three hours watching television, one hour exercising, one hour studying, and two hours shopping. Next, evaluate that use of time. You might decide you spent too much time watching television and too little time studying. Based upon this evaluation, decide on an adjustment, but make it specific. For example, I will watch only one hour of television and will study two hours. A good way to actually make this change is to draw up a contract with yourself that includes a reward for being successful.

Using time management techniques will help you with one of life's most precious possessions—your time.

Setting Goals

The most important thing you can do to manage time is to set goals: daily, weekly, monthly, yearly, and long-range. If you don't have a clear sense of where you are headed, you will not be able to plan how to get there. Your use of time should be organized to maximize the chances of achieving your goals.

Table 7.1 Daily Record of Activity

Time (a.m.)	Activity	Time (a.m.)	Activity	Time (p.m.)	Activity	Time (p.m.)	Activity
12:00		6:00		12:00		6:00	
12:15		6:15		12:15		6:15	
12:30		6:30		12:30		6:30	
…		…		…		…	
…		…		…		…	

Activity	Total Time Spent on Activity
Talking on the telephone	2 hours
Socializing	2 hours
Studying	1 hour
Watching television	3 hours
Exercising	1 hour
Shopping	2 hours
Housework	2 hours
In class	5 hours
Sleeping	6 hours

Table 7.2
Summary of Activities (Sample)

Prioritizing

Once you have defined your goals, you need to prioritize them and your activities. Not all of your goals will be equally important. Focus on goals of major importance to you, and work on the other goals secondarily. Likewise, focus on activities most important to the achievement of your highest goals and on other activities afterward. To help with this, develop **A,B,C lists.**

A,B,C lists
A time management technique in which tasks are prioritized.

On the A list are those activities that must get done; they are so important that not to do them would be very undesirable. For example, if your term paper is due next week and today is the only day this week you can get to the library to do the research required for that paper, going to the library goes on your A list today.

On the B list are those activities you'd like to do today and that need to be done. However, if they don't get done today, it wouldn't be too terrible. For example, if you haven't spoken to a close friend and have been meaning to telephone, you might put that on your B list. Your intent is to call today, but if you don't get around to it, you can always call tomorrow or the next day.

On the C list are those activities you'd like to do if you get all the A and B list activities done. If the C list activities *never* get done, that would be just fine. For example, if a department store has a sale and you'd like to go browse, put that on your C list. If you do all of the As and Bs, then you can go browse; if not, no big loss.

In addition, you should make a list of things *not to do*. For example, if you tend to waste your time watching television, you might want to include that on your not-to-do list. In that way, you'll have a reminder not to watch television today. Other time wasters should be placed on this list as well.

Scheduling

Once you've prioritized your activities, you can then schedule them into your day. When will you go to the library? When will you grocery-shop? Don't forget to schedule some relaxation and recreation as well.

Maximizing Your Rewards

In scheduling your activities, remember what some time management experts say: We get 80 percent of our rewards from only 20 percent of our activities and, conversely, get only 20 percent of our rewards from 80 percent of the time we spend. What that tells us is that we need to make sure we identify and engage in the 20 percent of the activities that give us 80 percent of our rewards *before* we move to the other activities. Maximize your rewards by organizing your time.

Saying No

I have a friend who says, "You mean that I don't have to do everything I want to do?" What he means is that there are so many activities he would love to engage in that he overloads himself and winds up enjoying them less and feeling overburdened. Because of guilt, concern for what others might think, or a real desire to engage in an activity, we have a hard time saying no. The A,B,C lists and the scheduled activities will help identify how much time remains for other activities and will make saying no easier.

Delegating

When possible, get others to do those things that need to be done but that do not need your personal attention. Conversely, avoid taking on chores that others try to delegate to you. A word of caution: This advice does not mean that you use other people to do work you should be doing or that you do not help out others when they ask. What I am suggesting is that you be more *discriminating* about the delegation of activities. In other words: Do not hesitate to seek help when you are short on time and are overloaded, and help others only when they really need help and you have the time available.

Evaluating Tasks Once

Many of us open our mail, read through it, and set it aside. For example, I often receive a questionnaire from some graduate student doing a study on stress. My tendency is to put the questionnaire aside and fill it out later. However, that is a waste of time. If I pick it up later, I have to once again familiarize myself with the task. As much as possible, look things over only once. That means, when you first pick something up, be prepared to complete working on it *then*. And this applies to e-mails and text messages as well.

Using the Circular File

Another way of handling questionnaires is to file them—in the garbage can. How many times do we receive junk mail that is obvious from its envelope—you know, the kind addressed to "Resident"? In spite of knowing what is enclosed in that envelope and that after we read its contents we will throw it out, we still take the time to open it and read the junk inside. We would be better off bypassing the opening and reading part and going directly to the throwing-out part.

Limiting Interruptions

Throughout the day, we are likely to be interrupted from what we have planned to do. Recognizing this fact, we should actually schedule in times for interruptions. On the one hand, don't make your schedule so tight that interruptions would throw you into a tizzy. On the other hand, try to keep these interruptions to a minimum. There are several ways you can accomplish that. You can refuse to accept phone calls between certain hours. Ask your roommate or assistant to take messages and call back later. Do the same with visitors. Anyone who visits should be asked to return at a more convenient time, or you should schedule a visit with him or her for later. If you are serious about making better use of your time, you will need to adopt some of these means of limiting interruptions. Adhere to your schedule as much as you can.

Investing Time

The bottom line of time management is that you need to invest time *initially* in order to benefit by the good use of your time subsequently. Those who attend my classes or workshops often say, "I don't have the time to organize myself the way you suggest. That would put me farther in the hole." This is an interesting paradox. Those who feel they don't have time to plan the better use of their time probably need to take the time more than those who feel they do have the time. Confusing enough? Well, let me state it this way: If you are so pressed for time that you believe you don't even have sufficient time to get yourself organized, that in itself tells you that you are in need of applying time management skills. The investment in time devoted to organizing yourself will pay dividends by allowing you to achieve more of what is really important to you.

And yet, researchers inform us that in spite of making a time management plan, people tend not to follow through on it.[22] Will you be one of those people, or will you employ ways to use your time more efficiently? (See Table 7.3.)

Social Support Networking

As mentioned earlier, one of the protective factors thought to prevent stress-related illness or disease is social support. Social support is belonging, being accepted, being loved, or being needed. In different words, it is having people you can really talk to, to whom you feel close, and with whom you share your joys, stressors, problems, apprehensions, and love. Social support comes in many different forms:[23] (1) tangible support (e.g., money or the use of a car); (2) emotional support (e.g., love or caring concern); and (3) informational support (e.g., facts or advice). Social support can be provided by family members, friends, lovers, or anyone else who provides what is described above.

Table 7.3
What do College Students *Not* Spend Their Time on?

Behavior	NOT Performing Behavior
Getting vaccinated against hepatitis B	26.6%
Having dental exam and cleaning in past year	23%
Females: performing breast self-exam in past month	63%
Males: performing testicular exam in past month	64%
Using sunscreen	47%
Using a condom the last time they had sexual intercourse	41%
Participating in the recommended amount of exercise at least 3–5 days a week	24%
Doing weight training to strengthen muscles at least 3–5 days a week	55%
Getting enough sleep at least 3–5 days a week	42%
Volunteering	65%

Source: American College Health Association. *American College Health Assessment—National College Health Assessment II. Fall 2010 Reference Group Data Report.* Linthicum, MD: American College Health Association, 2011.

The manner in which social support helps manage stress is hypothesized to occur in one of two ways.[24] One hypothesis, the *direct effect theory,* views social support as a means of preventing stressors from occurring in the first place. For example, support received in the form of information and advice might prevent you from losing your job and experiencing the stress associated with that event. Another theory, the *stress buffering theory,* states that social support helps after a stressor is encountered to help prevent that stressor from resulting in negative consequences. For example, you may lose your job, but your family and friends may help you feel worthwhile nonetheless. They help you deal with and feel better about stressors.

Common sense dictates that social support can help prevent stressors from leading to negative consequences. I volunteered to conduct a monthly stress management workshop for parents residing at the Washington, D.C., Ronald McDonald House. The Ronald McDonald House is a residence for families of seriously ill children who are being treated in local hospitals and whose parents and siblings need a place to stay during the time of the treatment. Most of the families staying at the house are in the military and travel great distances—often from other countries in which they are stationed—to have their children treated. Other families are from states across the United States, far away from relatives and friends. The social support provided to families residing at the house by the staff and by other families is obviously invaluable. In fact, when we evaluated the stress management workshops I conducted there, parents stated that what they valued most was the opportunity to interact with other families experiencing a similar stressful situation. You have probably also found value in talking over your problems and stressors with friends and relatives. You may not have known it at the time, but what you were experiencing was social support.

Social support has been found to be related to several indices of health and illness. For example, in a study of women in a depressed mood, it was found that the loss of social support was related to poor quality of life.[25] African American women's psychological and physical health functioning was found to be related to the quality of their intimate relationships, as well as to how connected they felt to their neighborhood. The better the quality of the relationship and the more connected to the neighborhood, the better their health.[26] In a study of youth in an urban community, social support emerged as the strongest predictor of life satisfaction.[27]

Other studies concur with these findings. For example, social support has been found to help patients adjust to their illnesses.[28] Researchers have identified the effects of social support that result in this benefit to patients. Social support improves the immune system's effectiveness,[29] is associated with healthier neuroendocrine functioning,[30] and decreases cortisol secretion during stress.[31] Social support also increases HIV/AIDS patients' adherence to their medication regimens,[32] and helps to alleviate depressive symptoms.[33, 34] In an interesting study in Thailand, social support groups totally eliminated the previously high rate of abandonment of children with Down syndrome.[35] The rate of abandonment of these children had previously been one every other month. And, consistent with the view that when you do something for someone else, you are doing something for yourself, researchers have found that providing social support may be even more beneficial than receiving it.[36] So, go out and support others, thereby benefiting your own health.

There appears to be a difference between males and females when it comes to social support. Researchers have found that whereas males prepare to use fight-or-flight when encountering a stressor, females tend to employ the tend-and-befriend response.[37] When encountering a stressor, females are likely to "tend" their children and loved ones (to protect them) and seek the support of other females through social networks. This strategy seems to be learned at a young age. Boys report having fewer people they feel comfortable turning to for support than do girls. Boys seek the support of friends less, instead turning to exercise, watching television, and spending time on the computer as a means of coping.[38] To assess your level of social support, complete Lab 7.3 at the end of this chapter.

The development of a social support system is complex and would require a whole book to describe. Certainly, the conflict-resolution technique and the assertiveness skills discussed in this chapter contribute to improved relationships. However, one of the keys to developing social support networks is being open and caring with others. It's often easier and less threatening to stay aloof and detached from others. Fear prevents us from getting close to others. We fear that if we show love for another person, we will be rejected by that person. We fear that we will be embarrassed. We fear that we will be ridiculed. We even fear that we will find within ourselves an inability to be intimate, caring, and loving. To develop social support systems, however, requires an overcoming of these fears.

I vividly recall listening to a colleague whom I had known casually for several years give a speech upon the occasion of being awarded a professional honor. His speech was very uplifting and quite emotional. At its conclusion, my colleague was greeted with a standing ovation and hordes of well-wishers. As I was waiting to get close enough to congratulate him on the speech and the honor bestowed upon him, I noticed most women hugged him after their congratulations, whereas *all* the men shook his hand. At that time, I felt very close to my colleague. I wanted very much to grab him and hug his guts out, but fear entered my mind. What would other colleagues of mine think? What if Bob reached out with his hand, thereby rejecting my hug? Do I dare? Will I be embarrassed? Well, I rejected that

Positive healthy relationships are within your reach. The social support obtained from these relationships can help prevent illness or disease resulting from stress.

fear and, when I got close enough, hugged my colleague and told him how much I had enjoyed his speech and how deserving I believed he was of his honor. Do you know what? He hugged me harder than I hugged him! He turned out to be the "hugger" and I the "huggee"! That small incident remains with me always. If I had not taken a chance, I would have always regretted not hugging Bob. The chance taken resulted in our being closer than before. I now realize that these fleeting moments have great meaning in our lives and that they present us with opportunities that are removed only too quickly. If we don't take advantage of them when they are presented to us, we probably will never have another chance.

Why don't you take a chance? Tell someone that you love him or her. Get involved with those around you. Show people you care about them. By doing so, you will be improving your social support network. You can expect this love, involvement, and care to rebound to you, allowing you to be more effective in managing the stress in your life.

Getting Involved in Your Community

Many communities have after-school recreation or community centers. These are usually open on weekdays from when public schools let out to approximately 10 p.m. and on weekends. Children and youths of all ages attend these centers, which offer sports competition (e.g., soccer or basketball leagues), classes (e.g., arts and crafts, photography, or dance), and open recreation time (e.g., shooting pool or playing Ping-Pong). These centers provide an excellent vehicle for educating youths about conflict-resolution techniques to help prevent fights and other aggressive behavior that can cause a great deal of stress. Why not volunteer to teach a conflict-resolution class at a local community center, YMCA, Jewish community center, or other after-school program? You can really make a difference in the lives of young people in your community if you choose to.

Coping in Today's World

Have you arranged to have a satisfying life? The *Satisfaction with Life* scale[a] presented here helps you determine whether you need to improve your level of satisfaction with your life. If you do, there is still time to do that. Once completing the scale and analyzing the results, elaborate on your answers—why did you answer as you did? Then write down the things you can change to increase the satisfaction with your life. The results should be placed in your Stress Portfolio.

Satisfaction with Life Scale

Here are five statements that you may agree or disagree with. Using the 1–7 scale below, indicate your agreement with each statement.

7 = strongly agree   6 = agree   5 = slightly agree

4 = neither agree nor disagree   3 = slightly disagree

2 = disagree   1 = strongly disagree

_____ In most ways my life is close to ideal.

_____ The conditions of my life are excellent.

_____ I am satisfied with my life.

_____ So far I have gotten the important things I want in life.

_____ If I could live my life over, I would change almost nothing.

Scoring:		
	31–35	Extremely satisfied
	26–30	Satisfied
	21–25	Slightly satisfied
	20	Neutral
	15–19	Slightly dissatisfied
	10–14	Dissatisfied
	5–9	Extremely dissatisfied

[a]W. Pavot and E. Deiner, "Review of the Satisfaction with Life Scale," *Psychological Assessment* 5(1993): 164–72.

summary

- Assertiveness is expressing yourself and satisfying your own needs while not hurting others in the process. People who cannot have their needs satisfied or who perceive that their basic human rights are violated will be stressed by that situation. The use of the DESC form can help you organize a verbal assertive response. Standing straight and speaking clearly, fluently, and without hesitation can convey assertiveness nonverbally.

- Conflicts resolved to only one person's satisfaction are not effectively resolved. A three-step approach to resolve conflict is effective in satisfying both people. This approach entails active listening, identifying the points of view, and exploring alternative solutions.

- To improve communication, check out your impressions of someone's nonverbal messages, plan time to have discussions, listen better, begin disagreeing by stating a point of agreement, substitute the word "and" for the word "but," use "I" statements, and avoid "why" questions.

- Time management skills involve setting goals and prioritizing them, making schedules, saying no when that is appropriate, delegating tasks, reviewing materials only once, limiting interruptions, and assessing how time is now spent.

- Social support is belonging, being accepted, being loved, or being needed all for oneself and not for what one can do. It is having people to whom you feel close and with whom you share your joys, problems, apprehensions, and love. Social support can help protect you from the negative consequences of stress.

internet resources

Study Guides and Strategies: Time Management **www.studygs.net/timman.htm** *Describes ten applications of time management and their effects on learning.*

Assertiveness Training Web Sites **www.selfgrowth.com/assert.html** *Links to assertiveness Web sites, including numerous articles.*

Conflict Resolution Information Source **www.crinfo.org** *Resources, articles, organizations, and much more related to conflict resolution.*

Stress and Communication **www.nasdonline.org/document/212/d000012/stress-and-communication.html** *An article on stress and communication, including steps to effective conflict resolution.*

references

1. S. M. Noar, P. J. Morokoff, and C. A. Redding, "Sexual Assertiveness in Heterosexually Active Men: A Test of Three Samples," *AIDS Education and Prevention* 14(2002): 330–42.

2. R. J. Macy, P. S. Nurius, and J. Norris, "Responding in Their Best Interests: Contextualizing Women's Coping with Acquaintance Sexual Aggression." *Violence Against Women* 12(2006): 478–500.

3. M. R. Andersen and K. A. Guthrie, "Assertiveness with Physicians: Does It Predict Mammography Use?" *Women and Health* 39(2004): 1–11.

4. M. R. Andersen, J. Abullarade, and N. Urban, "Assertiveness with Physicians Is Related to Women's Perceived Roles in the Medical Encounter," *Women and Health* 42(2005): 15–33.

5. D. Buback, "Assertiveness Training to Prevent Verbal Abuse in the OR," *AORN Journal* 79(2004): 148–50, 153–58, 161–64; quiz 165–66, 169–70.

6. Valerie Manusov and April R. Trees, "Are You Kidding Me? The Role of Nonverbal Cues in the Verbal Accounting Process," *Journal of Communication* 52(2002): 640–56.

7. K. Nishiuchi, A. Tsutsumi, S. Takao, S. Mineyama, and N. Kawakami, "Effects of an Education Program for Stress Reduction on Supervisor Knowledge, Attitudes, and Behavior in the Workplace: A Randomized Controlled Trial," *Journal of Occupational Health* 49(2007): 190–98.

8. S. Mineyama, A. Tsutsumi, S. Takao, K. Nishiuchi, and N. Kawakami, "Supervisors' Attitudes and Skills for Active Listening with Regard to Working Conditions and Psychological Stress Reactions Among Subordinate Workers," *Journal of Occupational Health* 49(2007): 81–87.

9. Jerrold S. Greenberg, Clint E. Bruess, and Debra W. Haffner, *Exploring the Dimensions of Human Sexuality* (Boston: Jones and Bartlett, 2011).

10. Cary Chemiss and Daniel Goleman, "Emotional Intelligence," *Learning Matters,* 2009. Available at: www.learningmatters.com/dwn/7950/

11. Daniel Goleman, *Emotional Intelligence: Why It Can Matter More Than IQ* (New York: Bantom, 1995).

12. John D. Mayer and Peter Salovey, "What Is Emotional Intelligence?" In Peter Salovey and D. J. Sluyter. *Emotional Development and Emotional Intelligence* (New York: Basic Books, 1997).

13. Monty McKeever, "The Brain and Emotional Intelligence: An Interview with Daniel Goleman." *Trycycle*, May 18, 2011. Available at: http://danielgoleman.info/2011/05/19/the-brain-and-emotional-intelligence-an-interview-with-daniel-goleman/

14. Consortium for Research on Emotional *Intelligence* in Organizations, 2010. Available at: www.eiconsortium.org

15. Michelle M. Weil and Larry D. Rosen, *Technostress* (New York: John Wiley & Son, 1997).

16. Michelle Weil and Larry Rosen, "Technology Causes Stress at Home, Work," *Business Courier*, September 21, 1998. Available at: www.bizjournals.com/cincinnati/stories/1998/09/21/focus3.html

17. *Newslite,* May 18, 2011. Available at: http://newslite.tv/2011/05/18/technology-causes-five-hours-s.html

18. C. J. König and M. Kleinmann, "Deadline Rush: A Time Management Phenomenon and Its Mathematical Description," *Journal of Psychology* 139(2005): 33–45.

19. M. Greene, "Time Management Is Good Business," *CDS Review* 100(2007):22.

20. *Time Management: Beat Work Overload, Increase Your Effectiveness, Achieve More,* Wiltshire, England: Mind Tools, 2007. Available at www.mindtools.com/pages/main/newMN_HTE.htm

21. *Managing Your Time,* Hanover, NH: Dartmouth College, 2007. Available at www.dartmouth.edu/~acskills/success/time.html

22. König and Kleinmann, "Deadline Rush."

23. Coretta M. Jenerette, "Relationships Among Types of Social Support and QOL in Adults with Sickle Cell Disease," *Southern Online Journal of Nursing Research* 8(2008). Available at: www.snrs.org/publications/SOJNR_articles2/Vol08Num03Art04.html

24. J. C. Overholser, W. H. Norman, and I. W. Miller, "Life Stress and Support in Depressed Patients," *Behavioral Medicine,* Fall 1990, 125–31.

25. L. C. Friedman, A. E. Brown, C. Romero, M. F. Dulay, L. E. Peterson, P. Wehrma, D. J. Whisnand, L. Laufman, and J. Lomax, "Depressed Mood and Social Support as Predictors of Quality of Life in Women Receiving Home Health Care," *Quality of Life Research* 14(2005): 1925–29.

26. A. R. Black, J. L. Cook, V. M. Murry, and C. E. Cutrona, "Ties That Bind: Implications of Social Support for Rural, Partnered African American Women's Health Functioning," *Women's Health Issues* 15(2005): 216–23.

27. P. Bramston, H. Chipuer, and G. Pretty, "Conceptual Principles of Quality of Life: An Empirical Exploration," *Journal of Intellectual Disability Research* 49(2005): 728–33.

28. A. M. DeLongis, J. Capreol, S. Holtzman, T. B. O'Brien, and J. Campbell, "Social Support and Social Strain Among Husbands and Wives: A Multilevel Analysis." *Journal of Family Psychology* 18(2004): 470–79.

29. J. K. Kiecolt-Glaser, L. McGuire, T. F. Robles, and R. Glaser, "Psychoneuroimmunology and Psychosomatic Medicine: Back to the Future." *Psychosomatic Medicine* 64(2002): 15–28.

30. J. M. Turner-Cobb, S. E. Sephton, C. Koopman, J. Blake-Mortimer, and D. Spiegel, "Social Support and Salivary Cortisol in Women with Metastatic Breast Cancer," *Psychosomatic Medicine* 62(2000): 337–45.

31. Shelley E. Taylor, William T. Welch, Heejung S. Kim, and David K. Sherman, "Cultural Differences in the Impact of Social Support on Psychological and Biological Stress Responses," *Psychological Science* 18(2007): 831–37.

32. K. E. Weaver, M. M. Llabre, R. E. Dura'n, M. H. Antoni, G. Ironson, F. J. Penedo, and N. Schneiderman, "A Stress and Coping Model of Medication Adherence and Viral Load in HIV-Positive Men and Women on Highly Active Antiretroviral Therapy (HAART)." *Health Psychology* 24(2005): 385–92.

33. R. Schwarzer and B. Gutierrez-Dona, "More Spousal Support for Men Than for Women: A Comparison of Sources and Types of Support in Costa Rican Factory Workers," *Sex Roles* 52(2005): 532–33.

34. R. B. Trivedi, J. A. Blumenthal, C. O'Connor, K. Adams, A. Hinderliter, C. Dupree, K. Johnson, and A. Sherwood, "Coping Styles in Heart Failure Patients with Depressive Symptoms," *Journal of Psychosomatic Research* 67(2009): 339–46.

35. P. Wasant and C. Raichagool, "Downs Syndrome Parents' Support Group in Thailand Siriraj Hospital, Fifteen Years Experience: A Review," *Journal of the Medical Association of Thailand* 92(2009): 1256–62.

36. S. L. Brown, R. M. Neese, A. Vinokur, and D. M. Smith, "Providing Social Support May Be More Beneficial Than Receiving It: Results from a Prospective Study of Mortality," *Psychological Science* 14(2003): 320–27.

37. Shelley E. Taylor, "Tend and Befriend: Biobehavioral Bases of Affiliation under Stress," *Current Directions in Psychological Science* 15(2006): 273–77.

38. "Coping with Stress," *Washington Post Health,* September 9, 1998, 5.

LAB ASSESSMENT 7.1

How Assertive Are You?

Directions: To determine your general pattern of behavior, indicate how characteristic or descriptive each of the following statements is of you by using the code that follows. This scale was developed by Spencer Rathus.

+3 = very characteristic of me, extremely descriptive

+2 = rather characteristic of me, quite descriptive

+1 = somewhat characteristic of me, slightly descriptive

−1 = somewhat uncharacteristic of me, slightly nondescriptive

−2 = rather uncharacteristic of me, quite nondescriptive

−3 = very uncharacteristic of me, extremely nondescriptive

_____ 1. Most people seem to be more aggressive and assertive than I am.

_____ 2. I have hesitated to make or accept dates because of "shyness."

_____ 3. When the food served at a restaurant is not done to my satisfaction, I complain about it to the waiter or waitress.

_____ 4. I am careful to avoid hurting other people's feelings, even when I feel that I have been injured.

_____ 5. If a salesperson has gone to considerable trouble to show me merchandise that is not quite suitable, I have a difficult time in saying no.

_____ 6. When I am asked to do something, I insist upon knowing why.

_____ 7. There are times when I look for a good, vigorous argument.

_____ 8. I strive to get ahead as well as most people in my position.

_____ 9. To be honest, people often take advantage of me.

_____ 10. I enjoy starting conversations with new acquaintances and strangers.

_____ 11. I often don't know what to say to attractive persons of the opposite sex.

_____ 12. I will hesitate to make phone calls to business establishments and institutions.

_____ 13. I would rather apply for a job or for admission to a college by writing letters than by going through with personal interviews.

_____ 14. I find it embarrassing to return merchandise.

_____ 15. If a close and respected relative were annoying me, I would smother my feelings rather than express my annoyance.

_____ 16. I have avoided asking questions for fear of sounding stupid.

_____ 17. During an argument I am sometimes afraid that I will get so upset that I will shake all over.

_____ 18. If a famed and respected lecturer makes a statement that I think is incorrect, I will have the audience hear my point of view as well.

_____ 19. I avoid arguing over prices with clerks and salespeople.

_____ 20. When I have done something important or worthwhile, I manage to let others know about it.

_____ 21. I am open and frank about my feelings.

_____ 22. If someone has been spreading false and bad stories about me, I see him (her) as soon as possible to "have a talk" about it.

_____ 23. I often have a hard time saying no.

_____ 24. I tend to bottle up my emotions rather than make a scene.

_____ 25. I complain about poor service in a restaurant and elsewhere.

_____ 26. When I am given a compliment, I sometimes just don't know what to say.

_____ 27. If a couple near me in a theater or at a lecture were conversing rather loudly, I would ask them to be quiet or to take their conversation elsewhere.

_____ 28. Anyone attempting to push ahead of me in a line is in for a good battle.

_____ 29. I am quick to express an opinion.

_____ 30. There are times when I just can't say anything.

Reprinted from "A 30-Item Schedule for Assessing Assertive Behavior," from *Behavior Therapy* 4(1973): 398–406 with permission from Elsevier.

The Rathus Assertiveness Scale has recently been validated by

- James Quillin, Steven Besing, David Dinning, "Standardization of the Rathus Assertiveness Schedule," *Journal of Clinical Psychology* 33(2006): 418–22.
- Eiko Suzuki, Yuka Kanoya, Takeshi Katsuki, and Chifumi Sato, "Verification of Reliability and Validity of a Japanese Version of the Rathus Assertiveness Schedule," *Journal of Nursing Management* 15 (2007): 530–37.

Scoring: To score this scale, first change (reverse) the signs (+ or –) for your scores on items 1, 2, 4, 5, 9, 11, 12, 13, 14, 15, 16, 17, 19, 23, 24, 26, and 30. Now total the plus (+) items, total the minus (–) items, and subtract the minus total from the plus total to obtain your score. This score can range from –90 through 0 to +90. The higher the score (closer to +90), the more assertively you usually behave. The lower the score (closer to –90), the more nonassertive is your typical behavior. This particular scale does not measure aggressiveness.

Interpretation of Scores

High = +30 or over   Average = –29 to +29   Low = –30 or below

If you scored below –29, you could benefit from assertiveness training. Perhaps there is a workshop or course on campus that might help. Alternatively, ask your instructor for suggestions.

Source: Ford Hickson and Richard Boxford, *Assert Yourself* (London: Sigma Research, University of Portsmouth, 1999).

LAB ASSESSMENT 7.2

How Do You Resolve Conflicts?

Directions: Circle the answer that best describes how you would react to each of the following situations.

1. If a salesperson refuses to give me a refund on a purchase because I've lost the sales slip,
   a. I say, "I'm sorry—I should have been more careful," and leave without the refund.
   b. I say, "You're the only store in town that handles this brand of merchandise. I demand a refund, or I'll never shop here again."
   c. I say, "Look, if I can't have a refund, can I exchange it for something else?"

2. If I had irritated a teacher by questioning his or her theoretical position and the teacher retaliated by giving me a D on an excellent paper,
   a. I wouldn't say anything; I would realize why it happened and be quieter in my next class.
   b. I would tell the teacher he or she was dead wrong and couldn't get away with being so unfair.
   c. I would try to talk to the teacher and see what could be done about it.

3. If I worked as a TV repairperson and my boss ordered me to double-charge customers, I would
   a. go along with the boss; it's the boss's business.
   b. tell the boss that he or she is a crook and that I won't go along with this dishonesty.
   c. tell the boss that he or she can overcharge on calls but I'm charging honestly on mine.

4. If I gave up my seat on the bus to an older woman with packages, but some teenager beat her to it,
   a. I would try to find the woman another seat.
   b. I would argue with the teenager until he or she moved.
   c. I would ignore it.

5. If I had been waiting in line at the supermarket for twenty minutes and then some woman rushed in front of me, saying, "Thank you—I'm in such a hurry!"
   a. I would smile and let her in.
   b. I would say, "Look, what do you think you're doing? Wait your turn!"
   c. I would let her in if she had a good reason for being in such a hurry.

6. If a friend was to meet me on a street corner at 7:00 p.m. one night and at 8:00 p.m. he still wasn't there, I would
   a. wait another thirty minutes.
   b. be furious at his thoughtlessness and leave.
   c. try to telephone him, thinking, "Boy, he'd better have a good excuse!"

7. If my partner volunteered me for committee work with someone she (or he) knew I disliked, I would
   a. work on the committee.
   b. tell her (or him) that she (or he) had no business volunteering my time and then call and tell the committee chairperson the same.
   c. tell her (or him) that I want her (or him) to be more thoughtful in the future and then make a plausible excuse for her (or him) to give to the committee chairperson.

8. If my four-year-old son "refused" to obey an order I gave him, I would
   a. let him do what he wanted.
   b. say, "You do it—and you do it now!"
   c. say, "Maybe you'll want to do it later on."

Scoring: To score your responses for each item *except number 4,* give yourself 1 point for an *a* answer, 5 points for a *b* answer, and 3 points for a *c* answer. For item 4, give yourself 3 points for an *a,* 5 points for a *b,* and 1 point for a *c.* Add up your points. The total should fall between 8 and 40.

Your score should give you a hint regarding your usual manner of dealing with conflict. The closer you are to a score of 8, the more submissive (nonassertive) you are when involved in a conflict. The closer you are to a score of 40, the more aggressively you respond. A score near the midpoint (24) indicates you generally compromise as a means of dealing with conflict.

If your score indicates you are having problems resolving conflicts, you might consider learning a more effective way of having your needs met while still maintaining your relationships. There are several ways in which you might acquire such skills. Among these are a course or workshop on campus or in the community or, if the need is great enough, counseling through your campus's health center or privately. You might also speak with your instructor for other suggestions.

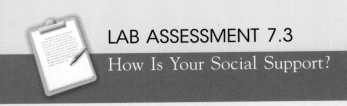

LAB ASSESSMENT 7.3

How Is Your Social Support?

Directions: To determine your social support, complete the following scale developed by Dwight Dean. For each statement, place one of the following letters in the blank space provided.

A = strongly agree
B = agree
C = uncertain
D = disagree
E = strongly disagree

_____ 1. Sometimes I feel all alone in the world.

_____ 2. I worry about the future facing today's children.

_____ 3. I don't get invited out by friends as often as I'd really like.

_____ 4. The end often justifies the means.

_____ 5. Most people today seldom feel lonely.

_____ 6. Sometimes I have the feeling other people are using me.

_____ 7. People's ideas change so much that I wonder if we'll ever have anything to depend on.

_____ 8. Real friends are as easy as ever to find.

_____ 9. It is frightening to be responsible for the development of a little child.

_____ 10. Everything is relative, and there just aren't any definite rules to live by.

_____ 11. One can always find friends, if one is friendly.

_____ 12. I often wonder what the meaning of life really is.

_____ 13. There is little or nothing I can do toward preventing a major "shooting" war.

_____ 14. The world in which we live is basically a friendly place.

_____ 15. There are so many decisions that have to be made today that sometimes I could just blow up.

_____ 16. The only thing one can be sure of today is that one can be sure of nothing.

_____ 17. There are few dependable ties between people anymore.

_____ 18. There is little chance for promotion on the job unless a person gets a break.

_____ 19. With so many religions abroad, one doesn't really know which to believe.

_____ 20. We're so regimented today that there's not much room for choice even in personal matters.

_____ 21. We are just cogs in the machinery of life.

_____ 22. People are just naturally friendly and helpful.

_____ 23. The future looks very dismal.

_____ 24. I don't get to visit friends as often as I'd like.

Source: Dwight Dean, "Alienation: Its Meaning and Measurement," *American Sociological Review* 26(1961): 753–58.

Scoring: This scale measures several factors of alienation, one of which is social isolation. High social isolation scores indicate low social support, and vice versa. The nine items making up the social isolation subscale and the scoring for those items follow:

Item	Scoring
1	A = 4, B = 3, C = 2, D = 1, E = 0
3	A = 4, B = 3, C = 2, D = 1, E = 0
5	A = 0, B = 1, C = 2, D = 3, E = 4
8	A = 0, B = 1, C = 2, D = 3, E = 4
11	A = 0, B = 1, C = 2, D = 3, E = 4
14	A = 0, B = 1, C = 2, D = 3, E = 4
17	A = 4, B = 3, C = 2, D = 1, E = 0
22	A = 0, B = 1, C = 2, D = 3, E = 4
24	A = 4, B = 3, C = 2, D = 1, E = 0

Your total score should range between 0 and 36. The higher your score, the more socially isolated you believe yourself to be. Therefore, the higher your score, the less effective you believe your social support system to be.

Social support can be an important resource to help you manage stress. Do you have people to whom you can turn to provide you with the support you need? Whom would you consult for each of the following?

1. Financial help:

   a. _____

   b. _____

   c. _____

2. Information:

   a. _____

   b. _____

   c. _____

3. Advice:

   a. _____

   b. _____

   c. _____

4. Emotional support:

   a. _____

   b. _____

   c. _____

If you find a gap in support available to you, perhaps you should start cultivating relationships so that this help is available to you if and when it is needed.

LAB ASSESSMENT 7.4

What Is Your Active Listening Style?

Directions: To determine your active listening style, for each statement below, place the letter from the scale below that best represents your listening behavior.

Scale

A = agree
B = rather agree
C = rather disagree
D = disagree

_____ 1. I talk with others personally.

_____ 2. I'm asked my advice by other people.

_____ 3. I'm the kind of person others feel it's easy to talk to.

_____ 4. I don't talk with someone else unless I have something I have to talk about.

_____ 5. I'm willing to say something to others usually.

_____ 6. I'm actually talking longer than the other person in spite of my intention to listen to him/her.

_____ 7. I begin to talk before the other person finishes talking.

_____ 8. I listen to the other person calmly while he/she is speaking.

_____ 9. I begin arguing with the other person before I know it while I'm listening to him/her.

_____ 10. While listening, I tend to talk to the other person, sticking to his/her trivial words.

_____ 11. I listen to others absentmindedly.

_____ 12. I listen to the other person, putting myself in his/her shoes.

_____ 13. I express my feelings straightforwardly.

_____ 14. I inadvertently see the other person from a critical viewpoint.

_____ 15. I listen to the other person, summarizing in my mind what he/she has said.

_____ 16. I sometimes give the other person a brief summary of what he/she has said.

_____ 17. I tend to listen to others seriously.

_____ 18. When I want to say something, I talk about it, even if I interrupt the other person.

_____ 19. I tend to hurry the other person into talking faster.

_____ 20. I can listen to the other person, even if he/she has a different opinion from mine.

_____ 21. I tend to deny the other person's opinion when it's different from mine.

_____ 22. I tend to talk in a directive and persuasive way while talking to others.

_____ 23. I tend to persist in my opinion while talking with others.

_____ 24. While listening, I get irritated from not understanding the other person's feelings.

_____ 25. I talk offensively when I'm in a bad mood.

_____ 26. When the other person is hesitating, I give him/her a chance by asking, "For example, is it like this?"

_____ 27. I listen to the other person, paying attention to his/her unexpressed feelings.

_____ 28. I listen to the other person, paying more attention to the changes of his/her feelings than to the contents of his/her talk.

_____ 29. I'm aware of my own feelings while I'm listening to others.

_____ 30. I can listen to the other person's worries, but I can't confide mine.

_____ 31. I'm pleased that I have given some advice to the other person.

Scoring: This scale is comprised of three subscales, each of which is discussed below. To score these three subscales, place the number assigned to your response alongside each statement.

Statement		Scoring
———	1	A = 3, B = 2, C = 1, D = 0
———	2	A = 3, B = 2, C = 1, D = 0
———	3	A = 3, B = 2, C = 1, D = 0
———	4	A = 3, B = 2, C = 1, D = 0
———	5	A = 3, B = 2, C = 1, D = 0
———	6	A = 0, B = 1, C = 2, D = 3
———	7	A = 0, B = 1, C = 2, D = 3
———	8	A = 3, B = 2, C = 1, D = 0
———	9	A = 0, B = 1, C = 2, D = 3
———	10	A = 0, B = 1, C = 2, D = 3
———	11	A = 3, B = 2, C = 1, D = 0
———	12	A = 3, B = 2, C = 1, D = 0
———	13	A = 3, B = 2, C = 1, D = 0
———	14	A = 0, B = 1, C = 2, D = 3
———	15	A = 3, B = 2, C = 1, D = 0

Statement		Scoring
———	16	A = 3, B = 2, C = 1, D = 0
———	17	A = 3, B = 2, C = 1, D = 0
———	18	A = 0, B = 1, C = 2, D = 3
———	19	A = 0, B = 1, C = 2, D = 3
———	20	A = 3, B = 2, C = 1, D = 0
———	21	A = 0, B = 1, C = 2, D = 3
———	22	A = 0, B = 1, C = 2, D = 3
———	23	A = 0, B = 1, C = 2, D = 3
———	24	A = 0, B = 1, C = 2, D = 3
———	25	A = 0, B = 1, C = 2, D = 3
———	26	A = 3, B = 2, C = 1, D = 0
———	27	A = 3, B = 2, C = 1, D = 0
———	28	A = 3, B = 2, C = 1, D = 0
———	29	A = 3, B = 2, C = 1, D = 0
———	30	A = 3, B = 2, C = 1, D = 0
———	31	A = 3, B = 2, C = 1, D = 0

Subscale Scores

- *Listening attitude.* Scores of 7 or higher indicate a person-centered attitude toward listening. The higher the score, the more person-centered. People with person-centered attitudes are respectful of other people's rights during communication and pay attention to what the other person is saying. To calculate your *Listening Attitude Score,* add up your scores for statements 6, 7, 9, 10, 14, 18, 19, 20, 21, 22, 23, 24, and 25.

- *Listening skill.* Scores of 6 or higher indicate good listening skills. The higher the score, the better the listening skills. People with good listening skills use active listening, reflecting back what they hear. To calculate your *Listening Skill Score,* add up your scores for statements 8, 11, 12, 15, 16, 17, 26, 27, 28, 29, and 31.

- *Conversation opportunity.* Scores of 4 or higher indicate making many opportunities to talk with colleagues and others. The higher the score, the more opportunities are made for conversation. To calculate your *Conversation Opportunity Score,* add up your scores for statements 1, 2, 3, 4, 5, 13, and 30.

If any of your subscale scores indicate you need to improve that component of your listening, re-read this chapter and/or speak to your instructor for advice. Perhaps there are books, pamphlets, or articles your instructor can recommend to improve your listening prowess. Maybe there are workshops on campus or offered in the community that can help. If you listen better, your communication with others will be more effective. In that case, you will experience less stress associated with your interactions with others.

Source: Norio Mishima, Shinya Kubota, and Shoji Nagata, "The Development of a Questionnaire to Assess the Attitude of Active Listening," *Journal of Occupational Health* 42(2000): 111–18.

Each of the following items asks you about your emotions or reactions associated with emotions. After deciding whether a statement is generally true for you, use the 5-point scale to respond to the statement. Please circle the 1 if you strongly disagree that this is like you, the 2 if you somewhat disagree that this is like you, 3 if you neither agree nor disagree that this is like you, the 4 if you somewhat agree that this is like you, and the 5 if you strongly agree that this is like you. There are no right or wrong answers. Please give the response that best describes you.

1 = strongly disagree
2 = somewhat disagree
3 = neither agree nor disagree
4 = somewhat agree
5 = strongly agree

1. I know when to speak about my personal problems to others.   1 2 3 4 5
2. When I am faced with obstacles, I remember times I faced similar obstacles and overcame them.   1 2 3 4 5
3. I expect that I will do well on most things I try.   1 2 3 4 5
4. Other people find it easy to confide in me.   1 2 3 4 5
5. I find it hard to understand the nonverbal messages of other people.   1 2 3 4 5
6. Some of the major events of my life have led me to reevaluate what is important and not important.   1 2 3 4 5
7. When my mood changes, I see new possibilities.   1 2 3 4 5
8. Emotions are one of the things that make my life worth living.   1 2 3 4 5
9. I am aware of my emotions as I experience them.   1 2 3 4 5
10. I expect good things to happen.   1 2 3 4 5
11. I like to share my emotions with others.   1 2 3 4 5
12. When I experience a positive emotion, I know how to make it last.   1 2 3 4 5
13. I arrange events others enjoy.   1 2 3 4 5
14. I seek out activities that make me happy.   1 2 3 4 5
15. I am aware of the nonverbal messages I send to others.   1 2 3 4 5
16. I present myself in a way that makes a good impression on others.   1 2 3 4 5
17. When I am in a positive mood, solving problems is easy for me.   1 2 3 4 5
18. By looking at their facial expressions, I recognize the emotions people are experiencing.   1 2 3 4 5
19. I know why my emotions change.   1 2 3 4 5
20. When I am in a positive mood, I am able to come up with new ideas.   1 2 3 4 5
21. I have control over my emotions.   1 2 3 4 5
22. I easily recognize my emotions as I experience them.   1 2 3 4 5
23. I motivate myself by imagining a good outcome to tasks I take on.   1 2 3 4 5
24. I compliment others when they have done something well.   1 2 3 4 5
25. I am aware of the nonverbal messages other people send.   1 2 3 4 5
26. When another person tells me about an important event in his or her life, I almost feel as though I experienced this event myself.   1 2 3 4 5
27. When I feel a change in emotions, I tend to come up with new ideas.   1 2 3 4 5
28. When I am faced with a challenge, I give up because I believe I will fail.   1 2 3 4 5
29. I know what other people are feeling just by looking at them.   1 2 3 4 5
30. I help other people feel better when they are down.   1 2 3 4 5

31. I use good moods to help myself keep trying in the face of obstacles.   1 2 3 4 5

32. I can tell how people are feeling by listening to the tone of their voice.   1 2 3 4 5

33. It is difficult for me to understand why people feel the way they do.   1 2 3 4 5

Scoring: Total scale scores are calculated by first reversing your scores on items 5, 28, and 33. Then sum all items scores. For example, if you scored a 5 for item 28, that 5 becomes a 1. Scores can range from 33 to 165, with higher scores indicating more characteristic emotional intelligence.

    This scale is composed of four subscales. To score each subscale, sum scores for the items comprising each subscale.

1. *Perception of emotions:* the capacity to accurately perceive emotions in the face or voice of others

    (items 5, 9, 15, 18, 19, 22, 25, 29, 32, 33).

2. *Managing emotions in the self:* the capacity of the emotions to enter into and guide the cognitive system and promote thinking

    (items 2, 3, 10, 12, 14, 21, 23, 28, 31).

3. *Social skills or managing others' emotions:* regulate and manage others' emotions so as to promote one's own and others' personal and social goals

    (items 1, 4, 11, 13, 16, 24, 26, 30).

4. *Utilizing emotions:* recognizing and accepting one's own emotions and using these emotions to achieve personal goals

    (items 6, 7, 8, 17, 20, 27).

Interpretation of Your Scores

The higher the score, the more emotional the intelligence. When U.S. college students completed the scale, the average score was approximately 125. Females scored slightly higher than males. If your score is below 125, refer to the section on ways to develop emotional intelligence in this chapter and apply some of those methods to improve your emotional intelligence.

    Subscale scores may also be analyzed to determine which component of emotional intelligence needs most improvement. To make that determination, the average subscale scores are approximately:

1. *Perception of emotions:*   38
2. *Managing emotions in the self:*   34
3. *Social skills or managing others' emotions:*   30
4. *Utilizing emotions:*   23

Source: The assessing emotions scale. Stough, C., Saklofske, D. and Parker, J. (Eds.). "The Assessment of Emotional Intelligence" with kind permission from Springer Science+Business Media B.V.

Perception Interventions

There's a story going around the sex education circuit that is used to introduce the topic of guilt about sexual behavior. It seems an elephant and an ant, in a moment of unbridled passion, spent the night making love. The next morning the ant learned that the elephant had a terminal disease and would soon die. Amazed and piqued, the ant said, "One night of passion and I spend the rest of my life digging a grave."

The ant viewed that situation as frustrating, unfair, and distressing. That needn't have been the case. The ant might have chosen to focus upon the enjoyable evening spent crawling all over the elephant's wrinkled skin (or however ants make love to elephants). Instead, the ant remembered the displeasing aspects of the situation. In short, that is what this chapter is about: perceiving life changes and other stressors as less distressing by attending to their positive aspects and deemphasizing their negative ones.

The topics discussed here relate to your inner self—your **perceptions** of events and of your own self-worth. Among these are what to focus on (selective awareness), how to perceive stressors as more humorous than threatening (humor and stress), how to reduce an inner sense of hurriedness and hostility (Type A behavior pattern), ways to feel more confident about yourself (self-esteem), the value of feeling in control of events that affect your life (locus of control), reducing unrealistic fear (anxiety), and perceiving stressors as challenging and within your control and being committed to their resolution (hardiness).

perceptions
A person's cognitive interpretation of events.

Selective Awareness

On my office door, displayed prominently in large type for every passing soul to see, was the following newspaper account:

> Bob Wieland, 44, who lost his legs in Vietnam and propels himself with his hands and no wheelchair, completed the Marine Corps Marathon at about 10:15 p.m. Sunday, 79 hours 57 minutes after he started Thursday in Arlington.

I don't know about you, but I have a hard time feeling sorry for myself whenever I think of Bob Weiland. We are all free to choose what to think and on what to focus. We can think about Bob Weiland or we can bemoan not getting that grade we wanted. Too often, though, we don't exercise this control over our thoughts but allow them to ride the seas rudderless. To complicate matters, we have been taught to be critical rather than supportive—focusing on the bad rather than the good. If you doubt the validity of this observation, consider the following:

1. When people are complimented, they often feel embarrassed. A woman being told how nice her dress is might say, "Oh, it's really quite old." The translation might be "You don't have taste enough to recognize an old *schmatta* (rag)," when the woman is really flattered but too embarrassed (due to lack of experience in being complimented) to know how to react appropriately. Or consider this exchange: You may say, "Joe, that was a very

nice thing you did." Joe answers, "Oh, it was nothing" (said with eyes looking down). Joe is really saying, "I'm too uncomfortable being told something nice. It doesn't happen very often. I'd know how to respond to criticism but have difficulty when I'm complimented."

2. When term papers are submitted to professors, too often they come back with comments directed only at improving the paper. Noticeably absent are notes underlining the good parts of the paper.

3. If you took two exams and received your grades back today, one a 43 percent and the other a 93 percent, which would you remember throughout the day—the one you passed or the one you failed?

Other examples of our inexperience in focusing on the positive can be offered, but I think the point is made. Now, what to do about it? The first step is to realize that in any situation there are both good and bad, positive and negative elements. Before I realized this, I couldn't bear to wait at airports for a plane. I defined that situation as a waste of my valuable time, unnecessary, and frustrating. Now I view the time I wait at airports as an opportunity to study people. I've learned a lot about parenting by observing a wide range of parenting styles in airport terminals. I've gotten ideas about how to coordinate my clothes by noticing well-dressed men at ticket counters. And I've become familiar with the types of literature people are interested in by noting their purchases at the gift shops located in most airports. What enjoyable and interesting places airports can be! Mind you, given the choice, I wouldn't opt for spending time at airports. The point is that I'm often not given a choice. If I want to travel by airplane (my initial choice), I must accept waiting in terminals. However, even though I may not be able to choose whether to wait at airports, I can choose how I perceive that situation. To put it physiologically, I can choose to raise my blood pressure, serum cholesterol, heart rate, and muscle tension, or I can choose not to alter these body processes. That choice is mine. Even if the situation is so bad that it couldn't possibly get any worse, I could choose to focus on the fact that things have to get better.

Some typically distressing situations are listed below. Being selectively aware of a positive aspect of each situation, write in the space provided your positive definition of that situation.

1. Waiting in a long line to purchase movie tickets. _____

    _____

2. Being stuck in bumper-to-bumper traffic. _____

    _____

3. Having to make a presentation before a group of people. _____

    _____

4. Being rejected from something because you're too old. _____

    _____

5. Having a relationship break up. _____

    _____

Right now there are situations in your life that have the potential to cause you a great deal of stress. You may not like where you live, whom you're living with, or the work you're doing. You may not feel you have enough time to yourself or for leisure-time activities. You may not like the way you look. You may be in poor health. You may be alone. Some of these stressors you may be able to change; some you will not be able to change. You now know, however, that you can become selectively aware of their positive components while deemphasizing (though not denying) their disturbing features. On a separate sheet of paper, why not list these stressors, and list the positive aspects of each on which you will choose to focus?

Why not go even further? Each time you do something that works out well, keep the memory of that with you. Tell others how proud of yourself you are. Pat yourself on the back. Take time just before bedtime (or some other convenient time of day) to recall all the good things about that day. Don't be like some of your friends who can't sleep because they still feel embarrassed about something they did that day or worried about something over which they have no control. In the words of a best seller of several years ago, "Be your own best friend." Revel in your good points and the glory of your day.

Stop to Smell the Roses

Life can be a celebration if you take the time to celebrate. It is the curse of the Great Somebody that we work long and hard to achieve some goal, bask in the glow of satisfaction only fleetingly, and proceed to work long and hard toward the next goal.

It is sad to see a person near the end of his or her life who achieved a lot but never enjoyed the achieving. In spite of acquiring money, property, fame, or doctoral degrees, he or she remains disheartened by missing out on what life is all about—living, experiencing, smelling the roses while trying not to get caught on the thorns.

What prevents us from being aware of life as we live it is often the routine of daily experience. When we experience something over and over again in the same manner, we become habituated to it. We are desensitized to that experience and interact with it out of habit, paying little attention to what we're doing. You and I do that very, very often. By way of example, I'll bet that when you travel to school or work, you take the same route each time. You probably chose this route because it was the fastest one. Other routes may be more scenic or interesting, but you chose quickness as your number-one priority. Other routes may bring you in contact with more cars and provide an opportunity to see more people, but you chose quickness as your number-one priority. Other routes may traverse rural, suburban, urban, and business areas, thereby allowing for more variety, but you chose quickness as your number-one priority.

Aside from missing out on scenery, other cars and people, and varied areas through which to travel, the sameness of whatever route we've chosen also desensitizes us to the experience. To create yet another barrier to experiencing the travel, we turn on our car radios. We travel to work or school and, before we know it, we're there. The time just flew. We lost that time and that experience by not being aware of it and not consciously smelling the roses en route. Think for a moment:

> Do you experience the getting-there or only the having-gotten-there?
>
> Have you ever consciously felt the *texture* of the steering wheel you hold so often?
>
> Do you ever listen to the *sounds* of your car and of the neighborhoods through which you travel?
>
> If you travel by public transportation, have you made an effort to talk with fellow passengers?
>
> Have you gotten off the bus or train a stop before or after your usual one to walk through different streets?

Perspective and Selective Awareness

Whenever I think of the importance of perception in general, and selective awareness in particular, I recall one day several years ago that seemed to be heading downhill in a hurry. Before noon, I had received not only a telephone call notifying me that some consulting work I was attempting to organize wasn't coming together, but also a letter stating that a grant proposal I had submitted would not be funded; and a manuscript I had submitted was rejected. As you might imagine, I was down in the dumps.

A proper perspective was soon achieved with just two phone calls. First, I received a call from a colleague at a university where I had previously taught. He told me about two former deans under whom we had worked. It seems that the married daughter of one of them awoke in the middle of the night and, not being able to sleep, arose from bed to get something in another room. Her husband, who was still sleeping when she arose, heard noises in the house, reached for his gun, and thinking her a burglar, shot his wife in the head. She subsequently died. My heart went out to Harry when I heard about his daughter's ordeal (and, consequently, his).

The second story my colleague told me during that phone call described the recent accident another dean of ours had while pruning a tree. To prune the top of the tree, he extended a ladder and proceeded to climb it. When he found part of the tree out of his reach, he leaned and stretched toward that part, tipping the ladder, falling, and landing on a tree stump. Since he was still in the hospital, I called him to offer whatever feeble support I could. When I reached him, he described the accident, his severe injuries (to this day, he experiences pain daily), and the physical therapy he would need. But he said something that I'll always remember. He told me how great the hospital staff treated him, how competent the ambulance drivers were, and how lucky he was to be alive and able to move. I called him with the intention of cheering him up, and it turned out that he cheered me up. Warren was almost killed, fearful of paralysis, and in a great deal of pain as he spoke with me, but he chose to discuss how lucky he was!

After those telephone calls, my consulting, grant proposal, and manuscript did not seem very important. I had my health, a lovely family, and a job I really enjoyed. The rest of my day would, I decided, be appreciated. I would focus on the positive.

I'm reminded of the college student who wrote her parents describing the accident she had falling out of the sixth-floor window of her dormitory. She described how she was writing with her left hand, since her right side was paralyzed. She had met a hospital orderly, however, with whom she fell in love, and they had decided to elope and marry just as soon as she recovered. Although he wasn't very educated, was of a different race and religion, and was addicted to heroin, she wrote, he had promised to make a good husband. The letter continued in this way until the closing sentence, in which the daughter stated that everything she had written so far was untrue. There was no accident, no paralysis, and no hospital orderly to marry; however, she continued, "I did fail my chemistry course and wanted you to be able to view this in its proper perspective."

How can you use this understanding to manage stress? Whenever things seem bad, remember that they can always be worse. Be thankful they aren't. Then recall all the good things in your life and be grateful for them. Developing an *attitude of gratitude* as described in the following section will also help.

An Attitude of Gratitude

As previously mentioned, I conducted stress management workshops for parents and grandparents residing at the Ronald McDonald House in Washington, D.C. I've also conducted similar workshops for Ronald McDonald House parents in Atlanta, Portland, Denver, and Houston. One of these workshops significantly impacted the way I view situations in my own life.

Parents residing at the Ronald McDonald House have children being treated at local hospitals for serious illnesses. Many have cancer or leukemia or are newborns with serious birth defects. Some have heart problems or other life-threatening illnesses. To stay at local hotels while their children are being treated would cost more than many of these families can afford. The Ronald McDonald House provides a residence for them. We like to refer to it as the "House That Love Built."

We began these stress management workshops by sharing how we came to be at the Ronald McDonald House. I shared my story and they shared theirs. At one workshop, two mothers spoke of their children's illnesses. One had a teenager who was dying of cancer in a local hospital, and the other had a newborn who was not going to live very long. As these two mothers shared their stories, all I could think of was how lucky I was to have two children who were well. I couldn't imagine how anyone—myself?—could handle the stress that these mothers were describing. "This is as bad as it gets," I thought. It was about then that *both* mothers told us that this was their second child who was dying! I thought it was as bad as it could get; then it got worse in a hurry.

In spite of the situation in which they found themselves, during these workshops the parents developed an **attitude of gratitude.** They learned to be grateful for what they had, while not denying or ignoring the reality of their children's illnesses. In every situation, there is something about which to be grateful. The mother with the teenager learned to be grateful for all the years she'd had with her son, recognizing that the mother of the newborn would never have the same time with her child. The Ronald McDonald House parents learned to be thankful for the health of their other children, for the days in which their children were feeling well and could communicate effectively, for the expertise of the hospital staff, and for the support available to them (from other family members, church or synagogue congregants, and the Ronald McDonald House staff). Too often these families focus so intently on their children's life-threatening illnesses that they are blinded to positive factors in their lives. This may be understandable, but it isn't healthy and it isn't how it has to be.

These parents told me that, because of the illness, they had conversations with their children at a very deep level, which many of us will never experience with our children. They became grateful for these conversations. They learned on whom they could rely, and they became grateful for that. They often discovered or developed a spiritual side of themselves that served them during this troubling time and long afterward.

These factors for which the Ronald McDonald House parents learned to be thankful accompanied their children's illnesses. The parents did not—could not—lose sight of the horrendous situation with which their families were confronted, but they came to realize that there were other realities in their lives, positive ones that coexisted with the reality on which they were solely focused. They learned to develop an "attitude of gratitude."

If the Ronald McDonald House parents could be grateful for aspects of their lives, the rest of us should have relatively little problem doing the same. Ever since that workshop, whenever I start feeling sorry for myself, I think of the

attitude of gratitude
Focusing on things about which to be grateful.

Optimism and Health

Being an optimist can keep you healthy. Alternatively, being a pessimist can contribute to your being unhealthy. In a large-scale study of more than 97,000 women, subjects were divided by their degree of optimism or pessimism. The more optimistic women were, the less likely it was that they developed coronary heart disease, that they died from coronary heart disease, or that they died from cancer. Furthermore, optimistic women had lower mortality for all illnesses. So start seeing the glass as half full instead of half empty. It will be good for your health, and your level of stress.

Source: H. A. Tindle, Y. F. Chang, L. H. Kuller, J. E. Manson, J. G. Robinson, M. C. Rosal, G. J. Siegle, and K. A. Matthews, "Optimism, Cynical Hostility, and Incident Coronary Heart Disease and Mortality in the Women's Health Initiative," *Circulation* 120(2009): 656–62.

Ronald McDonald House families, and it isn't long before I start feeling grateful for what I have and accepting of what I do not have. If you can learn to appreciate the positive aspects of your life, perhaps you'll consider volunteering at a Ronald McDonald House, a hospice, or a hospital near you as a way of saying thank you.

Humor and Stress

Following is the definition of an optimist. A seventy-year-old man has an affair with a young, vivacious, curvaceous, twenty-year-old woman. Before too long, she finds out she's pregnant and irately calls her lover. "You old fool! You made me pregnant!" The elderly man answers, "Who's calling, please?"

Humor is used throughout this book. It captures your interest and thereby helps you to learn more about stress than you might otherwise. In addition, humor has been shown to be an effective means of coping with stress.[1-4] It can defuse stressful situations or feelings. Research investigations have verified this conclusion. For example, Phua, Tang, and Tham found that humor prevented negative life events from resulting in mood disturbances.[5] Humor also helps in managing stress by increasing cheerfulness,[6] thereby leading to improved social support networks.[7]

Comedian Bill Cosby, whose son was murdered, advises that if you can laugh, you can survive any situation. Other famous and wise people have reminded us of the healing and beneficial effects of humor, including President Abraham Lincoln, Nazi concentration camp survivor Victor Frankl, comedian Charlie Chaplin, and author and magazine editor Norman Cousins. Although we realize the benefits of humor, it is ironic that as we get older, we laugh less. Fourteen-year-olds were found to laugh every four minutes, whereas American adults laugh only 15 times a day.[8] This is indeed unfortunate since the use of humor can help us convert a stressful situation into one with fewer unhealthy consequences.[9,10]

Humor can take several forms. It can use exaggeration/hyperbole, incongruity (two or more incompatible ideas or feelings), surprise, slapstick, sarcasm, pun, and irony.[11] Regardless of the type of humor, its effects on health have been studied for many years.[12,13]

Humor results in both physiological and psychological changes. Laughter increases muscular activity, respiratory activity, oxygen exchange, heart rate, and the production of catecholamines and endorphins. These effects are soon followed by a relaxation state in which respiration, heart rate, blood pressure, and muscle tension rebound to below normal levels.[14] Psychological effects include the relief of anxiety, stress, and tension; an outlet for hostility and anger; an escape from reality; and a means of tolerating crises, tragedy, and chronic illnesses or disabilities.[15,16]

Humor and laughter have been shown to have health benefits for the elderly[17-19] and for other populations. In fact, because humor has been shown to improve the functioning of the immune system, increase tolerance of pain, and decrease the stress response,[20,21] it has been adopted as a therapy used in hospitals. Perhaps the most famous practitioner of humor in the hospital is Patch Adams, the subject of a major feature movie starring Robin Williams. Adams discovered the benefits of dressing like a clown as a form of therapy for his patients.[22] Laughter therapy has been used with many illnesses, including cancer.[23] Bennett and colleagues[24] found that mirthful laughter correlated with increased immune

A good hearty laugh can go a long way in relieving feelings of stress.

function in cancer patients. In particular, laughter increased cancer patients' natural killer (NK) cell activity, necessary to combat the cancer. Humor and laughter have also been found useful for patients who are receiving *palliative care*—care designed to make patients comfortable rather than cure them.[25] For example, terminally ill patients who receive hospice care are receiving palliative care. Lastly, humor has even been suggested as a means of overcoming posttraumatic stress disorder and of coping with terrorism.[26] In another study,[27] patients with end-stage renal disease (kidney disease) who had a greater sense of humor increased their odds of survival by 31 percent over patients with less of a sense of humor.

Humor also can be used inappropriately and can actually cause distress. Sands states this potential of humor well: "Anyone who has seen the hurt and puzzled expression on another's face in response to an ironic remark, or remembers how he or she may have felt as an object of a joke, has witnessed humor's power to cause distress."[28] Unfortunately, Sands continues, humor's effects are not always predictable. Consequently, it is recommended that humor be used carefully to help someone else cope with stress so as not to exacerbate the situation. However, once consideration is given to the potential negative effects of humor and they are judged to be minimal, don't hesitate to use this approach when you think it would be helpful. Regarding humor-coping for yourself, look for the humorous aspects of a stressful situation or a stress-producing person and you will be better able to manage the stress involved. Complete Lab Assessment 8.1 to determine the type of humor you most frequently use.

Type A Behavior Pattern

Far from humorous are people who always seem busy, are always rushing somewhere, and never seem to slow down. We usually envision these people as business executives with perspiration-stained armpits, cigarettes dangling from their lips, and shirtsleeves rolled up, working overtime at desks piled high with papers. However, others also fit into the hurry, rush syndrome. Unfortunately, this stereotype often fits ourselves or our loved ones as well. I say "unfortunately" because a large body of research relates this behavior to the early onset of coronary heart disease.

Before proceeding, complete Lab 8.2, which is based on a scale in *Type A Behavior and Your Heart* by Meyer Friedman and Ray Rosenman.

Type A behavior pattern is "a particular complex of personality traits, including excessive competitive drive, aggressiveness, impatience, and a harrying sense of time urgency," as well as a "free-floating but well-rationalized form of hostility, and almost always a deep-seated insecurity." This behavior pattern has been found to be associated with the development of coronary heart disease. But that's putting the cart before the horse. The manner in which this association was discovered is interesting in and of itself.

Two cardiologists called in an upholsterer to reupholster the seats in their waiting room. The upholsterer inquired about the type of practice these physicians had, since he noticed that only the front edges of the chair seats were worn out. These cardiologists later realized that people who came to them with heart disease seemed to be "on edge"; they literally sat on the edges of their seats as though preparing for some action.

Meyer Friedman and Ray Rosenman, the two cardiologists, defined and named the Type A behavior pattern. They later compared patients with coronary heart disease with healthy controls (people similar in all respects except they did not have coronary heart disease) and found a significantly greater degree of Type A behavior in the patients than in the controls. These classic retrospective studies[29,30] (comparisons *after* the development of the disease) were followed by prospective studies that monitored subjects without a history of coronary heart disease, tested them for the Type A behavior pattern, and then determined (after more than 10 years) whether more Type As developed coronary heart disease than Type Bs.[31,32] Type Bs possess an opposite behavior pattern.

Type A behavior pattern
A cluster of behaviors associated with the development of coronary heart disease.

People possessing the **Type B behavior pattern** exhibit no free-floating hostility or sense of time urgency and aren't excessively competitive. As you might expect, significantly more Type As than Type Bs subsequently developed coronary heart disease.

Early research found that Type As tend to experience more job stress. Studies of nurses and teachers have verified this conclusion.[33] In addition, studies have found that Type A hospital employees were found to have significantly more health problems than did other hospital employees[34] and that young adults,[35] college teachers,[36] and nurses also suffer the effects of Type A behavior pattern.[37] Various reviews of the great body of research on the Type A behavior pattern and coronary heart disease have concluded that individuals classified as Type A more frequently suffer from coronary disease and obstruction of the coronary vessels.[38] In addition, some researchers have found that Type As who have a heart attack are more likely to have a second attack than Type Bs who have a heart attack; they also have more severe heart attacks than Type Bs.[39] However, for some as yet unexplained reason, Type As are more likely to survive a heart attack than are Type Bs.[40]

More recently, Yoshimasu and associates reported that Type A was related to an increased risk of angina pectoris (chest pain) and an acute myocardial infarction (a heart attack).[41] Furthermore, Type A subjects were more likely to be heavy smokers and use alcohol than non-Type As. Other researchers have found that Type A drivers were also more likely to experience a traffic accident than non-Type As.[42] Researchers have studied several variables in an attempt to understand these findings. In one of these studies,[43] an interesting relationship was found between Type A and recovery time from stressful events. Although Type As initially responded physiologically similarly to stressful events, it took them longer to recover to baseline levels. Fast activation–fast recovery was not associated with coronary heart disease. However, fast activation–slow recovery was. It is thought this finding is a result of greater exposure to the effects of catecholamines and cortisol.

However, as with most human behavior, Type A is more complex than simply a set of behaviors leading to a specific disease.

Part of the confusion and complexity associated with Type A appears to be related to the variables composing it. For example, researchers have identified two components of Type A behavior that appear to operate in opposing directions.[44] One of these is termed Impatience/Irritability (II), the other Achievement Striving (AS). *Impatience/Irritability* is characterized by impatience, time urgency, and irritability; *Achievement Striving* is characterized by job dedication, target setting, and hard-driving behavior. Only II is associated with physical health complaints,[45] depression,[46] job satisfaction,[47] and marital dissatisfaction.[48] It seems that AS has no relationship to these variables. Thus, researchers have suggested separating the *toxic* from the *nontoxic* components of Type A behavior to better understand its effects.[49]

Relative to the constellation of behaviors associated with Type A, it appears that hostility and anger may be the key.[50] One explanation for this association is the high catecholamine reactivity and diminished brain serotonin functions when hostility is experienced.[51] Another explanation recognizes the relationship between blood platelet aggregation/reactivity and coronary heart disease, and that during hostility, platelet reactivity increases. This has been described as "a key pathophysiological pathway in the onset of CVD (cardiovascular) events."[52] As more studies are being conducted, a further clarification of the role of the Type A behavior pattern on health will develop. For now, at least, it seems prudent to attempt to modify Type A behavior.

What can you do about your Type A behavior? First, you must realize that Type A behavior, like all other behavior, is learned. From parents who rush us to clean up or get ready for bed, teachers who expect us to complete our work in the time allotted, and bosses who require us to get a lot done, Type A behavior finds reinforcements throughout our society. In fact, it was found that Type A fathers tend to produce Type A sons.[53] Behavior that is rewarded tends to be

Hostility toward people, and even inanimate objects such as parking meters, is a characteristic of Type A behavior pattern.

repeated. The key, then, is to reward Type B behavior while ignoring or punishing Type A behavior. For example, if you rush through a traffic light as it begins to turn red in an attempt to prevent delay, that behavior should be punished. You might decide to drive clear around the block for such a Type A demonstration. But when you make it through a week without doing business over lunch or you have a week in which you engage in some form of relaxation daily, buying yourself a new article of clothing, a tennis racket, or some other reward would be in order.

One way to begin a Type A behavior modification program is to set weekly, realistic, and attainable goals and to identify rewards to be applied when these goals are achieved. Similarly, list behaviors you wish to eliminate and punishments you are prepared to apply if these behaviors are not eliminated on schedule.

Friedman and Rosenman offer some additional suggestions for decreasing Type A behavior:

1. Recognize that life is always unfinished. It's unrealistic to believe you will finish everything needing to be done without something else presenting itself to be done.

2. Listen quietly to the conversation of other people, refraining from interrupting them or in any other way attempting to speed them up.

3. Concentrate on one thing at a time.

4. Don't interfere with others doing a job you think you can do faster.

5. When confronted with a task, ask yourself
   a. Will this matter have importance five years from now?
   b. Must I do this right now? Your answers will place tasks in proper perspective.

6. Before speaking ask yourself
   a. Do I really have anything important to say?
   b. Does anyone want to hear it?
   c. Is this the time to say it?
      If the answer to any of these is no, remain quiet.

7. Tell yourself daily that no activity ever failed because someone executed it too slowly, too well.

Polyphasic behavior is doing two or more things at the same time. This often distracts from the attention each needs and deserves. It also is one component of the Type A behavior pattern.

8. Refrain from making appointments or scheduling your activities when unnecessary. Try to maintain as flexible a schedule as possible.

9. Remember that your time is precious and must be protected. When possible, pay someone else to do bothersome chores and save your time.

10. Purposely frequent restaurants, theaters, and other such places where you know there will be some waiting required. Perceive such occasions as an opportunity to get to know your companion better or, if alone, as a chance to get some "downtime" away from the books, the phone, or people seeking your time.

11. Practice eliminating polyphasic behavior (doing two or more things at the same time) by reading books that demand your entire attention and patience. A several-volume novel that is complex would work well. (Proust's *The Remembrance of Things Past* has been recommended by Friedman and Rosenman.)

12. Plan relaxing breaks from activities you know will result in tension by nature of the time or effort required to do them. Plan these breaks to occur *prior* to the feelings of tension and pressure.

13. Engage in daily practice of a recognized relaxation technique.

14. Smile at as many people as you can so as to decrease free-floating hostility.

15. Thank people for nice things they've done.

16. Remind yourself daily that, no matter how many things you've acquired, unless they've improved your mind or spirit, they are relatively worthless.

17. Consider most of your opinions as only provisionally correct, while maintaining an open mind to new ideas.

18. Seek some "aloneness" regularly.

19. Consolidate your relationships with some friends and acquaintances to make them more intimate and rewarding.

20. Spend time periodically remembering your past and the well from which you sprang.*

Self-Esteem

self-esteem
How highly one regards oneself.

Your **self-esteem**—how highly you regard yourself—affects how you behave. Self-esteem is explained shortly, but first complete Lab 8.3, checking whether the qualities described there are like or unlike yours. Then complete Lab 8.4 to assess how highly you regard your physical self—your physical self-esteem.

Why is self-esteem important? If you don't think well of yourself, you will not trust your opinions or your decisions, and you will be more apt to be influenced by others. Not "marching to the beat of your own drum" may result in your conforming to the behaviors of those with whom you frequently interact. As a matter of fact, poor self-esteem is related to drug abuse, irresponsible sexual behavior, and other "unhealthy" activities. People with high self-esteem engage in these activities to a significantly lesser extent.

We've already discussed assertiveness, success, and social support as components of stress management. Self-esteem is related to each of these. How can you assert yourself and demand your basic rights if you don't deem yourself worthy of these rights? If you hold yourself in low regard, how can you use nonverbal assertive behavior? To stand straight and steady, to speak clearly and fluently, to maintain eye contact, and to speak with assurance require a good degree of self-confidence.

*Source: From *Type A Behavior and Your Heart* by Meyer Friedman and Ray H. Rosenman, copyright © 1974 by Meyer Friedman. Used by permission of Alfred A. Knopf, a division of Random House, Inc.

Personality Types C and D and Disease

Type A behavior pattern is not the only "type" associated with illness and disease. Researchers have also identified a **Type C** and **Type D** and refer to them as personality factors.

Type C

Type C is thought to be related to the development of cancer.[54,55] Among the characteristics of Type C are:[56]

- Denial and suppression of emotions; in particular, anger, resentment, and hostility.
- Pathological niceness, a deep desire to make others happy.
- Avoidance of conflicts.
- An exaggerated need to be accepted socially.
- Extraordinarily compliant and patient.
- Poor ability to cope with stress.

Although there appears to be a correlational relationship between the possession of these traits and a diagnosis of cancer, some researchers argue that this relationship may not be cause and effect. That is, the association between Type C and cancer may result from people with these characteristics engaging in cancer-related *behaviors,* such as smoking, and not that the characteristics cause cancer themselves. In fact, the American Cancer Society states, "Many studies of cancer and personality also have failed to look at the environment or behavioral factors that might have an effect on cancer. And some studied patients only *after* they'd been diagnosed with cancer. The very knowledge of their diagnosis could affect personality."[57] In fact, in a large-scale study involving 30,000 people, researchers found no association between any personality type and the development of cancer.[58]

Type D

People possessing Type D, for depressed, are anxious, irritable, and insecure. They see the glass as half empty rather than half full. They appear tense and inhibited around other people as they go through great lengths to get others to like them.[59]

The leading researcher of Type D, Johan Denollet, identified two factors of Type D that appear related to the development of coronary heart disease: a tendency to experience negative emotions (NA) and a tendency to inhibit self-expression in social interactions (SI).[60] Denollet termed this the *NA + SI model.*[61] Study after study supports the relationship between these two factors and the subsequent development of and/or death from coronary heart disease.[62]

Type C

A personality type proposed to be associated with the development of cancer. Characterized by denial and suppression of emotions; in particular, anger, resentment, and hostility, and pathological niceness.

Type D

A personality type associated with the development of and death from coronary heart disease. Characterized by negative emotion and inhibited self-expression.

Self-esteem is learned. How people react to us; what we come to believe are acceptable societal standards of beauty, competence, and intelligence; and how our performances are judged by parents, teachers, friends, and bosses affect how we feel about ourselves. It is common sense, then, to expect our successes to improve our self-esteem and our failures to diminish it.

Lastly, how can you expect to make friends and establish intimate relationships if you don't think enough of yourself to believe that others would want to be your friend or care about you? Since you now know of the buffering effect of social support, you can imagine how poor self-esteem, resulting in a poor social support network, would be related to the development of stress-related illness and disease.

The very essence of stress management requires confidence in yourself and in your decisions to control your life effectively.

An important concept related to self-esteem is *self-efficacy*. Self-efficacy is the belief that you can be successful at doing something. In a sense, it is self-confidence. Researchers have found that self-efficacy is related to recovery from posttraumatic stress disorder,[63] academic success in college,[64] occupational stress,[65] depression,[66] life satisfaction,[67] and less stress and burnout.[68] In fact, mothers who were self-efficacious—who felt confident in their mothering role—were found to have such an effect on their children's oral health habits.[69] Their children tended to brush their teeth more often.

Because self-esteem is so important, the means of improving it deserve your serious attention. There are no magic pills to take or laser beams with which you can be zapped to improve your sense of self-worth. It has developed over a long period of time, and it will take a while for you to change it. With time, attention, effort, and energy, you can enhance your sense of self or at least feel better about those parts of you that cannot be changed.

The first thing to do is to identify that part of yourself about which you want to feel better. If it's a part of your physical self, your scores (the 3s and 4s) on Lab 8.4 will direct you to specific body parts that need work. Perhaps an exercise program can improve that part, or you need to begin a weight-control program, pay more attention to how you dress, or use makeup more effectively. After this kind of introspection, one of my students decided to have electrolysis done to remove some hair above her lips. Another student began exercises to tighten the muscles in the buttocks. What can you do to improve a part of your physical self or to feel better about parts that cannot be improved?

To identify other components of your self-esteem that you might want to improve, look for your *lowest* subscale score in Lab 8.3. This is the part of yourself that you hold in lowest regard. Next, ask yourself what you can do to perform better at work or school, in your family role, or in social settings. Perhaps you need to spend more time with your family. Maybe you need to ask your boss if you can attend a training program being offered nearby. Asking the campus librarian to help you use the library better might do the trick. Seeking honest feedback from friends about your strengths and weaknesses could help, as well as being more open with them about your thoughts, feelings, passions, and frustrations.

> Whatever you decide to do—
> *Do it now!*
> *Stick with it!*
> You really can feel better about yourself.

Locus of Control

Before reading about locus of control, complete Lab 8.5, a scale measuring locus of control, which is the perception of the amount of personal control you believe you have over events that affect your life. People with an **external locus of control** believe they have little control of such events. People with an **internal locus of control** believe they have a good deal of control of these events.

Studies indicate that "externals" are less likely to take action to control their lives, since they believe such action to be fruitless. It was found, for example, that women who had an internal locus of control perceived themselves at greater risk of developing breast cancer and were, therefore, more likely to be screened than women with an external locus of control.[70] Also, since a person with an internal locus of control thinks something can be done to affect the situation, information

external locus of control
The perception that one has little control over events that affect one's life.

internal locus of control
The perception that one has control over events that affect one's life.

is sought to be able to take appropriate action. Consequently, these people know more about their situation than do others.[71] Other studies found locus of control related to chronic fatigue syndrome,[72] sick leave from work,[73] and psychological and behavioral responses to a diagnosis of human papillomavirus.[74]

The concept of locus of control has been used to explain numerous behaviors over the years,[75,76] although it is becoming increasingly understood that you can feel in control of one part of your life (e.g., your social life) but not of another part (e.g., your academic life). If you had to guess which gambling games externals and internals prefer, what would you guess? If you guessed that externals prefer games of chance rather than skill, you were correct. Externals prefer roulette and bingo; internals prefer poker and blackjack.[77]

If you've learned anything so far from this book, I suspect it is that we are all in more control of our lives than we believe. But it is absurd to believe we are in total control of events that affect us. A colleague of mine, John Burt, coined the term **cocreator perception deficiency (CCPD)** to describe this important concept. He believes that we are all cocreators of our destiny; that some things we control, but others are beyond our control; and that too many people are deficient in this perception. According to Burt, too many people believe either that they are completely in control or that any significant control is beyond their reach, but neither is the case.

As with self-esteem, locus-of-control orientation develops over a long period of time and cannot be expected to change overnight. However, once the concept is understood, some miraculous possibilities present themselves. After a class on locus of control, one of the women came up to me and said, "You're right. I can become more in control of myself." She resolved right then and there never to smoke another cigarette (she smoked a pack a day). As she threw her half-smoked pack into the trash container on her way out, I knew she would successfully quit smoking. The last I heard, she hadn't smoked a cigarette since that day. Most of us, in contrast, need to take little steps to reacquire control of our lives and our actions. Certainly, we can exercise control over what we ingest, with whom we interact, how we spend our leisure time, and how we react to people.

One important point needs to be made explicit here: *Along with control comes responsibility.* Externals blame both their successes and their failures on things outside themselves. "Oh, I did such a good job because I work well under pressure." It's the pressure, not the person. "Oh, I didn't do too well because I didn't have enough time." It's the lack of time, not the person. Internals might say, "I did so well because of how I decided to adjust to the pressure and time constraints," or "I did poorly because I didn't work hard enough!" Internals accept responsibility for their successes and their failures.

I'm reminded of an activity in which I sometimes ask groups of people to participate. I form several teams, with team members standing at arm's length behind each other. The activity requires participants to raise their arms shoulder height, elbows straight, palms down, fingers together, and feet adjacent to one another. The first person on any team who either lowers the arms or bends the elbows disqualifies his or her entire team. The team that holds out longest is the winner. You've never seen a funnier sight! Initially, people believe the activity to be ridiculous but decide I'm such a nice fellow they'll humor me. Shortly, however, people try to convince members of other teams to drop their arms— "Your arms are *so* heavy. They hurt *so* badly. Why not drop them and relieve *all* that pain?" At the same time, they encourage their own team members to "hang in there." I've seen grown men and women endure such discomfort in this activity that, at first, I was shocked. However, discussions with the participants after this contest soon led me to believe that most of us understand and accept the responsibility accompanying freedom. Each participant was *free* to drop his or her arms at any time but instead endured physical pain because of a sense of responsibility to the rest of the team. Similarly, when we accept

cocreator perception deficiency (CCPD)

The belief that one is either the victim of circumstances or the master of circumstances, each of which is erroneous.

greater control of our lives, we also accept the consequences following the exercise of that control. We must be responsible for our behavior when we are free to choose how we behave.

Anxiety Management

Before we begin a discussion of anxiety, complete Lab 8.6. After you know how much anxiety you experience, we will explore ways to manage that anxiety.

What is this thing called anxiety? This is a difficult question to answer and one debated by experts. Charles Spielberger, the developer of the scale you completed in Lab 8.6, defines anxiety as a subjective feeling of tension, apprehension, nervousness, and worry accompanied by activation or arousal of the autonomic nervous system. For our purposes, we will define **anxiety** operationally as an unrealistic fear resulting in physiological arousal and accompanied by the behavioral signs of escape or avoidance. For you to be anxious, you must have each of the three components of our definition: You must feel fear; your heart rate, respiratory rate, blood pressure, and other physiological processes must be aroused; and you must seek to escape the stimulus making you anxious once it presents itself, or seek to avoid it in the first place. What's more, the fear you feel must be unrealistic. Those who fear heights, who find their hearts pounding when in a high place, and who immediately seek to come down are anxious. Those who fear crowds, adjust their lives to avoid crowds (have someone else shop for them, never attend a concert, and so forth), and perspire and feel faint when caught in a crowd are anxious.

Anxiety that does not diminish the quality of your life is probably not worth concern. For example, if you become anxious around snakes, avoiding the snake house when visiting the zoo or arranging never to see a snake again will probably not significantly decrease the satisfaction you derive from living. It's probably not worth the time or effort to eliminate your anxiety regarding snakes. However, if we substitute fear of flying in airplanes for fear of snakes, and add that your loved ones are scattered all over the world, your anxiety means you will not be able to see your loved ones as often as you'd like. In this instance, you'd better learn how to manage this anxiety.

Test Anxiety

One form of anxiety to which you might want to pay particular attention is test anxiety. Many students panic when they have to take tests. Before we discuss test anxiety in more detail, complete Lab 8.7.

Test anxiety has been conceptualized to consist of two major components: *worry* and *emotionality*. The worry component is concern about failing. The emotional component refers to unpleasant feelings and physiological reactions brought on by tests. If you scored high on the test anxiety scale in Lab 8.7, you might want to consult with your instructor or counselors at your campus health center.

Trait and State Anxiety

So far, we have been considering **state anxiety:** anxiety that is either temporary in nature or specific to a particular stimulus. However, a general sense of anxiety, **trait anxiety,** which is what Lab 8.6 measures, is a condition deserving serious attention. You should make a conscious effort to manage your trait anxiety if you scored high on this scale.

Panic Disorder[78]

Another type of anxiety disorder is **panic disorder.** People with panic disorder have feelings of terror that strike suddenly and repeatedly with no warning. They can't predict when an attack will occur, and many of them develop intense anxiety between episodes, worrying when and where the next one will strike.

anxiety
An unrealistic fear that manifests itself in physiological arousal and behaviors to avoid or escape the anxiety-provoking stimulus.

state anxiety
Anxiety that is either temporary in nature or specific to a particular stimulus.

trait anxiety
A general sense of anxiety not specific to a particular stimulus.

panic disorder
A condition in which feelings of terror arise from unrealistic fear, resulting in symptoms such as feeling numb, sweaty, weak, and faint.

If you are having a panic attack, most likely your heart will pound and you may feel sweaty, weak, faint, or dizzy. Your hands may tingle or feel numb, and you might feel flushed or chilled. You may have nausea, chest pain or smothering sensations, a sense of unreality, or a sense of impending doom or loss of control. You may genuinely believe you're having a heart attack or losing your mind or on the verge of death. Panic attacks can occur at any time, even during sleep. An attack generally peaks within 10 minutes, but some symptoms may last much longer.

Panic disorder affects about 6 million adult Americans[79] and is twice as common in women as in men. It most often begins during late adolescence or early adulthood, and the risk of developing panic disorder appears to be inherited. Not everyone who experiences panic attacks, however, will develop panic disorder. For example, many people have one attack but never have another.

For those who do have panic disorder, though, it's important to seek treatment. Untreated, the disorder can become very disabling. Some people's lives become so restricted that they avoid normal, everyday activities such as grocery shopping or driving. Some individuals become housebound or are able to confront a feared situation only if accompanied by a family member or some other trusted person.

Basically, people with panic disorder avoid any situation in which they would feel helpless if a panic attack were to occur. When people's lives become so restricted, as happens in about one-third of people with panic disorder, the condition is called *agoraphobia*. Early treatment of panic disorder can often prevent agoraphobia.

Panic disorder is one of the most treatable of the anxiety disorders, responding in most cases to medications or to carefully targeted cognitive-behavioral therapy. Cognitive-behavioral therapy, also called exposure therapy, involves very slowly exposing patients to the fearful situation until they become desensitized to it. Breathing and relaxation techniques can help as well.

Social Phobia (Social Anxiety Disorder)[80]

Phobias aren't just extreme fears; they are irrational fears. You may be able to ski the world's tallest mountains with ease but feel panic going above the fifth floor of an office building. **Social phobia,** also called social anxiety disorder, involves overwhelming anxiety and excessive self-consciousness in everyday social situations. It is more than just being shy. People with social phobia have a persistent, intense, and chronic fear of being watched and judged by others and being embarrassed or humiliated by their own actions. Their fear may be so severe that it interferes with work or school and other ordinary activities. Although many people with social phobia recognize that their fear of being around people may be excessive or unreasonable, they are unable to overcome it. They often worry for days or weeks in advance of a dreaded situation.

Social phobia can be limited to only one type of situation—such as a fear of speaking in formal or informal situations, or eating, drinking, or writing in front of others—or, in its most severe form, it may be so broad that a person experiences symptoms almost anytime he or she is around other people. People may even develop social physique anxiety—fear of showing their body. To assess your social physique anxiety, complete Lab 8.8. Social phobia can be very debilitating. It may even keep people from going to work or school on some days. Many people with this illness have a hard time making and keeping friends.

Physical symptoms that often accompany the intense anxiety of social phobia include blushing, profuse sweating, trembling, nausea, and difficulty talking. If you suffer from social phobia, you may be painfully embarrassed by these symptoms and feel as though all eyes are focused on you. You may be afraid of being with people other than your family.

Social phobia affects about 15 million adult Americans.[81] Women and men are equally likely to develop it. The disorder usually begins in childhood or early

Consider tests as opportunities to demonstrate how much you know about a topic. Viewed in this positive sense, exams will tend to be less anxiety-producing.

social phobia
Overwhelming fear and excessive self-consciousness in everyday situations; a chronic fear of being watched by others and not performing well. Fear of public speaking is an example.

adolescence, and there is some evidence that genetic factors are involved.[82] Social phobia can be treated successfully with psychotherapy or medications. Relaxation and breathing exercises can also help reduce symptoms.

Specific Phobias[83]

A **specific phobia** is an intense fear of something that poses little or no actual danger. Some of the most common specific phobias are centered around closed-in places, heights, escalators, tunnels, highway driving, water, flying, dogs, and injuries involving blood. Such phobias aren't just extreme fears; they are irrational fears of particular things. Although adults with phobias realize that their fears are irrational, they often find that facing or even thinking about facing the feared object or situation brings on a panic attack or severe anxiety.

Specific phobias affect an estimated 19.2 million adult Americans[84] and are twice as common in women as in men. The causes of specific phobias are not well understood, although there is some evidence that these phobias may run in families. Specific phobias usually first appear during childhood or adolescence and tend to persist into adulthood.

If the object of the fear is easy to avoid, people with specific phobias may not feel the need to seek treatment. Sometimes, though, they may make important career or personal decisions to avoid a phobic situation, and if this avoidance is carried to extreme lengths, it can be disabling. Specific phobias are highly treatable with carefully targeted psychotherapy. Relaxation and breathing exercises also can help reduce symptoms.

Coping Techniques

Unfortunately, too many people fail to cope successfully with dysfunctional anxiety and only make matters worse. You may do drugs, drink alcohol, or in some other manner alter your state of consciousness to avoid dealing with the anxiety-provoking stimulus. Obviously, these are only temporary solutions and are accompanied by unhealthy consequences. You not only keep your anxiety, but you now have a drug habit to boot. Generally speaking, anxiety has a cognitive component (thoughts) and a somatic one (bodily reactions). Techniques such as thought stopping and cognitive restructuring, both described below, have been found effective in managing the cognitive component of anxiety. Relaxation techniques such as progressive relaxation and autogenic training are effective in managing the somatic component of anxiety.

During that period of time when I was overstressed and vomiting on the sides of roads, I developed anxiety regarding speaking before large groups of people. I would decline invitations to run workshops or present speeches, would feel faint and perspire profusely when I did dare to accept such invitations, and was extremely fearful that I would either make a fool of myself or be laughed off the stage. Because my professional goals were thwarted by my anxiety, I decided I needed to do something quickly. I saw my physician, who with the best of intent, advised me there was nothing to be fearful of and prescribed Valium (a tranquilizer) for those occasions when I could anticipate anxiety. Desperate, I had the prescription filled and a week or so later took two Valium prior to a television talk show on which I was interviewed for 30 minutes. After the show, I decided I would no longer rely upon external means to control my internal fears. I embarked upon a program to manage my anxiety, employing the following techniques.

Environmental Planning

As stated previously, sometimes it is appropriate to adjust your life and environment to avoid the anxiety-provoking stimulus. For individuals anxious in crowds, living in a small town will probably be preferable to living in a large city. For those fearful of airplane crashes, living in the flight pattern or too near an airport may not be the wisest of decisions.

I employed environmental planning with subsequent television and radio shows by arriving earlier than expected and being shown around the studio. In this way, the environment became somewhat familiar to me; therefore, I experienced it as less threatening. To this day, I arrive early for public speaking appearances.

Relabeling

Remembering the selective awareness concept, you can relabel any negative experience as a positive one. All that is required is to focus upon the positive aspects rather than the negative ones. If you have test anxiety, rather than considering the test as a possibility of failure, you could consider it an opportunity to find out or to show others how much you know. Rather than conceptualizing an airplane ride as risking your life, you can relabel it as an opportunity to ride on a sea of clouds or to see your hometown from a totally new and interesting perspective. (See the section "Cognitive Restructuring" later in this chapter.)

I relabeled public speaking appearances as opportunities to relate some ideas I thought to be valid and important, to help other people improve their lives, and to test the worth of my professional activities. Previously, I viewed these occasions as chances to be ridiculed, scorned, or rejected.

Self-Talk

This technique requires some objectivity. You must ask yourself what the real risk is in the anxiety-provoking situation. Usually, the real danger is not very significant, even if the worst result should occur, and the odds of that worst result occurring are usually meager. If you study well, the odds of failing a test, for example, are usually slim, and if you do fail, so what? It's not good to fail tests, but you still will have your health. Remember the story of my two former deans! There will be other tests. If you're anxious about asking people out on dates, self-talk will help you realize what you are really afraid of: losing self-respect and feeling rejection. It will also help you understand that you probably won't be turned down for that date, but if you are, "there are plenty of fish in the sea." Even when your worst fears are realized, it's not really *that* bad.

I used self-talk to realize that people are generally polite. They won't boo or throw rotten tomatoes. If they thought me absurd, they'd probably fake listening so as not to appear rude. The worst that could realistically happen was that I wouldn't be asked back. That would mean I'd have more time for other activities. That's not all that bad.

Thought Stopping

As simple as it sounds, when you experience negative thoughts, you can shut them off. To employ thought stopping, you should learn deep muscle relaxation techniques. Then whenever you have anxious thoughts you want to eliminate, tell yourself that you will not allow these thoughts to continue, and use the relaxation technique. The pleasant sensations of relaxation will reinforce the stopping of anxious thoughts, as well as prevent these thoughts from resulting in potentially harmful physiological consequences. An alternative to stopping to do deep muscle relaxation is to substitute a more realistic thought for the negative one. I began practicing meditation to better manage my anxiety and found it to be most helpful. Any of the other deep muscle relaxation techniques might serve just as well.

An alternative approach is to wear a rubber band around your wrist and snap it whenever you have a negative thought. This might be called the "ouch technique," but it works.

Systematic Desensitization

Developed by Joseph Wolpe, **systematic desensitization** involves imagining or experiencing an anxiety-provoking scene while practicing a response incompatible

systematic desensitization
Either imagining or encountering an anxiety-provoking stimulus while practicing relaxation.

with anxiety (such as relaxation).[85] Widely used by psychotherapists, this technique was found to be nearly as effective when people used it by themselves.[86]

As part of this technique for managing anxiety, you must develop a **fear hierarchy.** The fear hierarchy is a sequence of small steps (at least 10) that leads up to the anxiety-provoking event. For example, if you fear flying in airplanes, your fear hierarchy could be as follows:

fear hierarchy
A list of small steps to move through an anxiety-provoking stimulus.

1. Deciding where to travel.
2. Telephoning the airport for a reservation.
3. Packing a suitcase for the trip.
4. Traveling to the airport.
5. Checking your luggage in at the airport.
6. Being assigned a seat at the gate.
7. Sitting in the waiting area prior to boarding.
8. Boarding the plane.
9. Being seated as the plane taxis down the runway.
10. Watching and feeling the plane leave the ground.
11. Flying above the clouds.

You can employ the desensitization procedure in a relatively safe environment by imagining yourself at an airport (**armchair desensitization**) or use it at an actual airport (*in vivo* **desensitization**). The procedure (either armchair or *in vivo*) can be summarized as follows:

armchair desensitization
A form of systematic desensitization in which the stimulus is imagined.

in vivo desensitization
A form of systematic desensitization in which the stimulus is actually encountered.

1. Learn deep muscle relaxation.
2. Develop a fear hierarchy: List a slightly feared stimulus, then a more fearsome one, and so on (include 10 to 20 steps on the fear hierarchy).
3. Relax yourself and imagine the first item on the fear hierarchy for one to five seconds. Gradually increase the time to thirty seconds in subsequent sessions.
4. After imagining the stimulus for thirty seconds, immediately switch your focus to the feeling of relaxation for thirty seconds.
5. Move down the fear hierarchy similarly. If the stimulus provokes anxiety, shut out the scene and concentrate on the feeling of relaxation.
6. If you have difficulty moving from one point on the fear hierarchy to another, add some intermediate steps. For example, on the airplane flight fear hierarchy, you may have made too big a leap between step 8 (boarding the plane) and step 9 (the plane speeding down the runway). You may need three steps between those: (a) placing your coat in the rack above your seat, (b) sitting down and fastening your seat belt, and (c) listening to the engines start.

Cognitive Restructuring

cognitive restructuring
A method of coping with anxiety that involves thinking about an anxiety-provoking event as less threatening.

Some of us tend to catastrophize events in our lives. We *have* to pass this exam! We *must* get that job! We *have* to get there on time! If we were only able to substitute *like* for *must* or *have*, we would experience less stress. And we would be perceiving situations more realistically. When we substitute a more accurate view of these events, we call that **cognitive restructuring;** that is, in our minds, we restructure or reword the description of the event and its importance to us. Cognitive restructuring enables us to see the situation more accurately, and to perceive the consequences or outcomes as less catastrophic. As a result, we experience less stress.

Cognitive restructuring has been taught to people of various ages to help them manage stressful events. For example, it has helped children who stutter to be less fearful and stressful so as to stutter less.[87] It has also helped nursing students to

Table 8.1 Anxiety Management Techniques

Technique	Description	Example
Environmental Planning	Adjusting the environment to avoid the anxiety-provoking stimulus, or to be better able to confront it.	Bringing a friend with you to the dentist.
Relabeling	Giving the anxiety-provoking stimulus a new label that will make you less anxious.	Having blood drawn may have been "labeled" a negative event when you said, "The nurse will stick a needle in my veins and may draw out too much blood or infect me." You can relabel that a positive event by stating, "I'm going to have the opportunity to find out how healthy I am and be better able to plan to stay healthy."
Self-Talk	Making statements to yourself that focus on the positive aspects of a potentially anxiety-provoking event.	You have to give a speech in front of a group of people, and you say to yourself, "I will get the chance to let everyone know how much I know about this topic."
Thought Stopping	Recognizing when you experience an anxious thought, then redirecting your attention elsewhere. Deep muscle relaxation can be used to reinforce the ability to ignore the anxious thought.	If you experience anxious thoughts about an upcoming exam, think about something else and meditate afterward.
Systematic Desensitization	Imagining or experiencing an anxiety-provoking scene stepwise (in small steps), and engaging in a relaxation exercise when able to do so.	Imagine bungee jumping by first imagining phoning for a reservation, then driving to the site, etc. and after being able to imagine that scene without experiencing anxious thoughts, doing diaphragmatic breathing.

be less fearful about their ability to help patients manage pain.[88] In addition, cognitive restructuring has been successfully used to treat panic disorder and agoraphobia,[89] to help women with breast cancer better cope with their illness,[90] to treat grief and lessen mourning in the death of a loved one,[91] and to assist older adults in managing anxiety and depression.[92]

The ABCDE Technique

Psychologist Albert Ellis theorizes that anxiety is a function of irrational beliefs. Ellis argues that we believe the following:

1. We must be thoroughly competent, adequate, and achieving.
2. We must be loved or get approval from all others almost all the time.
3. If things don't go as we wish, it is horrible and catastrophic.[93]

Ellis continues, but I think the point is made. We become afraid to fail or do something different and we develop unrealistic fears because of beliefs that, if examined, would prove to be irrational. Consequently, Ellis suggests we do just that—examine them. Ellis's method, the **ABCDE technique,** consists of examining irrational beliefs that make us anxious, changing those beliefs, and envisioning more positive consequences of our actions. The ABCDE technique involves the following steps:

A. Activating agent (identify the stressor).
B. Belief system (identify rational and irrational beliefs).
C. Consequences (mental, physical, and behavioral).
D. Dispute irrational beliefs.
E. Effect (changed consequences).[94]

The self-talk technique described earlier in the chapter is helpful in changing old thoughts (irrational beliefs) into new thoughts. For example, the fear of speaking

ABCDE technique
A method of coping with anxiety that consists of examining irrational beliefs.

After repeatedly experiencing a stressor, such as public speaking, you generally become desensitized to the anxiety associated with that event.

in front of the class might translate to "People will laugh at me and think I'm stupid." However, with self-talk—"I know many students who spoke in front of many classes and they survived"—we might interpret speaking in front of the class as a challenge rather than a threat.

Furthermore, questions such as the following can help identify irrational beliefs:

1. What facts are there (if any) to support this belief?

2. Is it a rational or an irrational belief?

Why not complete the following Managing Anxiety Formula to apply the information you've learned in this section and to better control your anxiety?

Managing Anxiety Formula

1. I experience anxiety when _____

   _____

2. Self-talk that I could use to manage this anxiety includes

   a. _____

   b. _____

   c. _____

   d. _____

   e. _____

3. Environmental planning I could do to manage this anxiety includes

   a. _____

   b. _____

   c. _____

   d. _____

   e. _____

4. If using desensitization to manage this anxiety, I would employ the following fear hierarchy:

a. _____

b. _____

c. _____

d. _____

e. _____

f. _____

g. _____

h. _____

i. _____

j. _____

5. How successful do you think the use of one or a combination of those coping techniques would be? _____ %

Resiliency

Why is it that some people who grow up in poverty or with physical or mental challenges become successful as adults, whereas others experiencing the same challenges do not? One explanation for this phenomenon is offered by resiliency theory. Resiliency theory states that people have strengths they can be taught to use to rise above adversity.[95] Rather than identify people's weaknesses or limitations, resiliency theory, instead, focuses on their strengths, and therapists work with clients to maximize the use of these strengths to cope with and overcome adversity.

Resiliency, then, is the ability to identify and make use of your strengths and assets to respond to challenges, thereby growing as an individual. These resilient characteristics are referred to as protective factors or developmental assets.[96] Researchers have found that resilient traits include happiness,[97] optimism,[98] self-determination,[99,100] creativity,[101] a sense of morality and self-control,[102] gratitude,[103] forgiveness,[104] and humility.[105] And researchers report that spirituality—that included a purpose of life, an internal locus of control, and belief in a higher power—is an important variable used by resilient people to overcome adversity.[106] These findings do not come as a surprise to those familiar with research showing that those who perceive themselves as optimistic, hopeful, and engaged in a cause have high immune system functions as measured by the number of macrophages, lymphocytes, helper T cells, natural killer cell activity, immunoglobulin A, antibodies, and interferon. Those who perceive themselves as helpless, hopeless, and depressed have a weaker immune system function.[107]

One resiliency expert states, "Chronic stressors befall people when they do not develop resilient qualities or have not grown through the disruptions in their life."[108] In other words, life's challenges, although creating disturbances, can be positive experiences when viewed as an opportunity to learn and grow from these challenges.

One way to become resilient starts with making a list of your strengths. Then when confronted by challenges, purposefully select those strengths that seem most applicable to the situation and devise means of using those strengths to overcome the challenge. When this process is complete, take time to analyze what you did, how successful it was, and how you can refine this process to increase

Resiliency

The ability to identify and make use of strengths and assets to respond to challenges, thereby growing as an individual.

the probability that you will successfully cope with future challenges. In that way you will use the experience as one that helps you grow and develop into a more resilient person.

Hardiness

Research has been directed at discovering what prevents stress from leading to illness for some people but not for others. Kobasa found three factors that differentiate the afflicted from the nonafflicted: *commitment, control,* and *challenge.*[109] Commitment is "the tendency to involve oneself in whatever one is doing, control involves the tendency to believe that and act as if one can influence the course of events, and challenge involves the related expectations that it is normal for life to change, and that changes will stimulate personal growth."[110] A key here seems to be viewing change as a challenge rather than a threat. People who have the "three Cs" are termed **hardy** and seem to be able to withstand the onslaught of stressors. They don't become ill as often from stressors. A number of studies conducted since the hardiness concept was developed have verified the buffering effects of commitment, control, and challenge on one's health.[111-113] This has been true with various populations: Army Reserve forces,[114] student teachers,[115] senior-level employees of state government agencies,[116] Israeli Army recruits,[117] and dental surgery patients.[118] One study found hardiness was even more predictive of physical and psychological health than were anxiety, job stress, hassles, social support, or Type A behavior.[119]

In addition to the prevention of illness that hardiness appears to provide, and its relationship to lower levels of blood pressure and triglycerides,[120] hardiness also affects other variables. For example, hardiness has been found related to mental health,[121] the management of chronic illness,[122] helping family caregivers from becoming depressed,[123] preventing work stress and increasing job satisfaction,[124] and preventing burnout.[125] Hardiness has also helped diminish feelings of depression in soldiers who are deployed,[126] protect police officers from the development of psychological distress and depression,[127] decrease grief symptoms among those experiencing the death of loved ones,[128] reduce stress and illness among employees,[129] and help parents prevent sleep problems in their children.[130]

The hardiness concept is being studied further. Attempts are being made to find out if people can actually be taught to become hardy, and if they can, whether they will then become less ill.

hardy
A state of mind and body that includes three factors: commitment, control, and challenge.

Are you easily angered? Do you know someone who is? Then pay attention because this hostile trait can result in cardiovascular disease and early death. Researchers from the University of Michigan measured hostility and anger in adults.[a] They interviewed these subjects and then analyzed their interaction style using the interpersonal hostility assessment technique, which emphasizes *how* participants respond rather than the content of their responses. Subjects were then asked to recall a time when they felt so angry they wanted to explode. As they did so, their systolic blood pressure, diastolic blood pressure, and heart rate were monitored. High Hostile subjects showed *greater* blood pressure responses to anger. In addition, the *duration* of time blood pressure was raised was longer in the High Hostile subjects. That translates into those with high hostility responding to a stressor, such as a situation that elicits anger, with *higher blood pressure* for a *longer period of time* than those with low hostility. Because High Hostile subjects also respond more frequently with anger, not only is their blood pressure raised, and for a longer period of time, but this occurs more frequently with them. The result is that they are subject to developing cardiovascular heart disease and the potential of dying early from that disease.

These findings are consistent with research on Type A behavior pattern, presented earlier in this chapter. In that research, hostility and anger were the variables most related to the development of coronary heart disease.

[a]B. L. Frederickson, K. E. Maynard, M. J. Helms, T. L. Haney, I. C. Siegler, and J. C. Barefoot, "Hostility Predicts Magnitude and Duration of Blood Pressure Response to Anger," *Journal of Behavioral Medicine* 23(2000): 229–43.

Summary

- Selective awareness is deciding on whether to focus on the good or on the bad in a situation or person. Focusing on the good is less stressful.

- Experiencing life as fully as possible requires conscious effort, since we become habituated to things that are repeated. Varying our experiences (such as taking different routes to school or work) can help in this process.

- Type A behavior pattern is a particular complex of personality traits, including excessive competitive drive, aggressiveness, impatience, a sense of time urgency, and a free-floating but well-rationalized form of hostility almost always accompanied by a deep-seated sense of insecurity. People exhibiting Type A behavior patterns are more prone to coronary heart disease than are Type Bs. Type Bs are less apt to contract heart disease and exhibit just the opposite behavior pattern from Type As. Hostility and holding in anger seem to be the major variables associated with ill health resulting from Type A behavior.

- Self-esteem refers to how high a regard you hold for yourself. Individuals with low self-esteem experience stress from not thinking well of themselves, not trusting their own opinions, and acting nonassertively. Self-esteem is learned and can be changed.

- Locus of control is the perception of the amount of control you believe you have over events that affect your life. An external locus of control refers to a perception of very little control (control is outside yourself). An internal locus of control refers to a perception of a great deal of control.

- Anxiety is an unrealistic fear resulting in physiological arousal and accompanied by behavioral signs of escape or avoidance. State anxiety is either temporary in nature or specific to a particular stimulus. Trait anxiety is a generalized sense of anxiousness.

- Other types of anxiety include panic disorder, social phobia, and specific phobia. Panic disorder is a condition in which feelings of terror occur as a result of unrealistic fear. Social phobia is an overwhelming fear and self-consciousness. Specific phobia is an intense fear of a specific situation that poses little or no actual danger.

- Anxiety can be managed by environmental planning, relabeling, self-talk, thought stopping, or systematic desensitization.

- Albert Ellis developed the ABCDE technique for managing anxiety. It consists of examining irrational beliefs that make us anxious, changing those beliefs, and envisioning more positive consequences of our actions.

- Resiliency is the ability to make use of strengths and assets to respond to challenges, rather than focusing on limitations and weaknesses. Resiliency theory states that life's challenges can be positive experiences when viewed as an opportunity to learn and grow from these challenges.

- Hardiness results from three factors: commitment, control, and challenge. Commitment is the tendency to involve oneself in what one is doing, control is the belief that one can influence the course of events, and challenge involves the expectation that change both is normal and will lead to personal growth. Studies have found hardiness associated with less illness, lower levels of blood pressure and triglycerides, less psychological distress, increased happiness and adjustment, and marital happiness.

internet resources

The Stress Management and Health Benefits of Laughter: The Laughing Cure **http://stress.about.com/od/stresshealth/a/laughter.htm** *An online article that describes the benefits of humor and laughter, how to use laughter to achieve these benefits, and a list of other humor and laughter resources.*

Self-Esteem and Stress Management, Ezine Articles **http://ezinearticles.com/?Self-Esteem-and-Stress-Management&id=126480** *An online article that discusses the relationship between self-esteem and stress, and how to improve self-esteem to feel less stressful.*

Stress and Aggression Reinforce Each Other at the Biological Level, Creating a Vicious Cycle, APA Online, Media Information **www.apa.org/monitor/nov04/hormones.aspx** *Presentation of the physiological and emotional effects of aggression. In particular, the relationship between aggression and the release of stress-related hormones is discussed.*

Stress Management Information **www.selfgrowth.com/stress.html** *Links to 60 articles on managing stress, as well as to stress-related websites.*

Reader's Digest: Health **www.rd.com/health/37-stress-management-tips/** *An article that lists 37 practical ways to prevent and manage stress with the specific focus on reducing anxiety.*

references

1. D. McFarlane, E. M. Duff, and E. Y. Bailey, "Coping with Occupational Stress in an Accident and Emergency Department," *Western Indian Medical Journal* 53(2004): 242–47.

2. S. Reed and P. R. Giacobbi, "The Stress and Coping Responses of Certified Graduate Athletic Training Students," *Journal of Athletic Training* 39(2004): 193–200.

3. M. Mauriello and J. T. McConatha, "Relations of Humor with Perceptions of Stress," *Psychological Reports* 101(2007): 1057–66.

4. C. M. MacDonald, "A Chuckle a Day Keeps the Doctor Away: Therapeutic Humor and Laughter," *Journal of Psychosocial Nursing and Mental Health Services* 42(2004): 18–25.

5. D. H. Phua, H. K. Tang, and K. Y. Tham, "Coping Responses of Emergency Physicians and Nurses to the 2003 Severe Acute Respiratory Syndrome Outbreak," *Academic Emergency Medicine* 12(2005): 322–28.

6. I. Papousek and G. Schulter, "Effects of a Mood-Enhancing Intervention on Subjective Well-Being and Cardiovascular Parameters," *International Journal of Behavioral Medicine* 15(2008): 293–302.

7. N. A. Kuiper and N. McHale, "Humor Styles as Mediators between Self-Evaluative Standards and Psychological Well-Being," *Journal of Psychology* 143(2009): 359–76.

8. D. S. Sobel and R. Ornstein, eds., *The Healthy Body and Healthy Mind Handbook* (New York: Patient Education Media, 1996).

9. J. R. Davidson, V. M. Payne, K. M. Connor, E. B. Foa, B. O. Rothbaum, M. A. Hertzberg, and R. H. Weisler, "Trauma, Resilience and Saliostasis: Effects of Treatment in Post-Traumatic Stress Disorder," *International Clinical Psychopharmacology* 20(2005): 43–48.

10. W. Christie and C. Moore, "The Impact of Humor on Patients with Cancer," *Clinical Journal of Oncological Nursing* 9(2005): 211–18.

11. Kundan Pandey, "Different Types of Humor," Buzzle.com, 2010. Available at: www.buzzle.com/articles/different-types-of-humor.html.

12. G. J. Boyle and J. M. Joss-Reid, "Relationship of Humor to Health: A Psychometric Investigation," *British Journal of Health Psychology* 9(2004): 51–66.

13. A. D. Ong, C. S. Bergeman, and T. L. Bisconti, "The Role of Daily Positive Emotions During Conjugal Bereavement," *The Journals of Gerontology. Series B, Psychological Sciences and Social Sciences* 59(2004): P168–76.

14. AVMA Group Health and Life Insurance Trust, "Laugh Yourself Healthy: Studies Show Humor-Health Link," *Journal of the American Veterinary Medical Association* 226(2005): 1970–71.

15. Mary Payne Bennett and Cecile A. Lengacher, "Humor and Laughter May Influence Health, I. History and Background," *Evidence-Based Complementary Alternative and Medicine* 3(2006): 61–63.

16. E. Marziali, L. McDonald, and P. Donahue, "The Role of Coping Humor in the Physical and Mental Health of Older Adults," *Aging and Mental Health* 12(2008): 713–18.

17. D. L. Mahony, W. J. Burroughs, and L. G. Lippman, "Perceived Attributes of Health-Promoting Laughter: A Cross-Generational Comparison," *Journal of Psychology* 136(2002): 171–81.

18. B. G. Celso, D. J. Ebener, and E. J. Burkhead, "Humor Coping, Health Status, and Life Satisfaction Among Older Adults Residing in Assisted Living Facilities," *Aging Mental Health* 7(2003): 438–45.

19. K. B. Colling, "Caregiver Interventions for Passive Behaviors in Dementia: Links to the NDB Model," *Aging and Mental Health* 8(2004): 117–25.

20. C. M. MacDonald, "A Chuckle a Day Keeps the Doctor Away: Therapeutic Humor and Laughter," *Journal of Psychosocial Nursing Mental Health Services* 42(2004): 18–25.

21. Paul McGhee, *Humor: The Lighter Path to Resilience and Health* (Bloomington, IN: AuthorHouse, 2010), p. 187.

22. Patch Adams, "Humour and Love: The Origination of Clown Therapy," *Postgraduate Medical Journal* 78(2002): 447–48.

23. Cancer Treatment Centers of America, *Laughter Therapy*, undated. Available at: www.cancercenter.com/complementary-alternative-medicine/laughter-therapy.cfm

24. M. P. Bennett, J. M. Zeller, L. Rosenberg, and J. McCann, "The Effect of Mirthful Laughter on Stress and Natural Killer Cell Activity," *Alternative Therapeutic Health Medicine* 9(2003): 38–45.

25. R. A. Dean and D. M. Gregory, "Humor and Laughter in Palliative Care: An Ethnographic Investigation," *Palliative and Supportive Care* 2(2004): 139–48.

26. E. A. Pasquali, "Humor: An Antidote for Terrorism," *Journal of Holistic Nursing* 21(2003): 398–414.

27. S. Svebak, B. Kristoffersen, and K. Aasarød, "Sense of Humor and Survival Among a County Cohort of Patients with End-Stage Renal Failure: A Two-Year Prospective Study," *International Journal of Psychiatry in Medicine* 36(2006): 269–81.

28. Steven Sands, "The Use of Humor in Psychotherapy," *Psychoanalytic Review* 71(1984): 458.

29. Meyer Friedman and Ray H. Rosenman, "Association of Specific Overt Behavior Pattern with Blood and Cardiovascular Findings: Blood Clotting Time, Incidence of Arcus Senilis, and Clinical Coronary Artery Disease," *Journal of the American Medical Association* 169(1959): 1286–96.

30. Meyer Friedman, A. E. Brown, and Ray H. Rosenman, "Voice Analysis Test for Detection of Behavior Pattern: Responses of Normal Men and Coronary Patients," *Journal of the American Medical Association* 208(1969): 828–36.

31. Ray H. Rosenman, Meyer Friedman, and Reuban Strauss, "A Predictive Study of Coronary Heart Disease: The Western Collaborative Group Study," *Journal of the American Medical Association* 189(1964): 15–22.

32. Ray H. Rosenman, Richard Brand, and C. David Jenkins, "Coronary Heart Disease in the Western Collaborative Group Study: Final Follow-up Experience of 8 1/2 Years," *Journal of the American Medical Association* 223(1975): 872–77.

33. G. Lavanco, "Burnout Syndrome and Type-A Behavior in Nurses and Teachers in Sicily," *Psychological Reports* 81(1997): 523–28.

34. Muhammad Jamal and Vishwanath V. Baba, "Type-A Behavior, Components, and Outcomes: A Study of Canadian Employees," *International Journal of Stress Management* 10(2003): 39–50.

35. Hans Steiner, Erika Ryst, Jessica Berkowitz, Miriam Gschwendt, and Cheryl Koopman,. "Boys' and Girls' Responses to Stress: Affect and Heart Rate During a Speech Task," *Journal of Adolescent Health,* 30 Supplement 1(2002): 14–21.

36. Muhammad Jamal and Vishwanath V. Baba, "Type-A Behavior, Job Performance and Well-Being in College Teachers," *International Journal of Stress Management* 8(2001): 231–40.

37. Sharon Glazer, Thomas A. Stetz, and Lajos Izso, Effects of Personality on Subjective Job Stress: A Cultural Analysis, *Personality and Individual Differences* 37(2004): 645–58.

38. Julia Barnard, "The Type A personality—What It Is, Associated Risks and Helpful Tips," *Ezine Articles,* 2007. Available at: http://ezinearticles.com/?The-Type-A-Personality—What-it-is,-Associated-Risks-and-Helpful-Tips&id=656093.

39. Ronald J. Burke, "Beliefs and Fears Underlying Type A Behavior: What Makes Sammy Run So Fast and Aggressively?" *Journal of Human Stress* 10(1984): 174–82.

40. David R. Ragland and Richard J. Brand, "Type A Behavior and Mortality from Coronary Heart Disease," *New England Journal of Medicine* 318(1988): 65–69.

41. Kouichi Yoshimasu and the Fukuoka Heart Study Group, "Relation of Type A Behavior Pattern and Job-Related Psychosocial Factors to Nonfatal Myocardial Infarction: A Case-Control Study of Japanese Male Workers and Women," *Psychosomatic Medicine* 63(2001): 797–804.

42. Hermann Nabi, Silla M. Consoli, Jean-François Chastang, Mireille Chiron, Sylviane Lafont, and Emmanuel Lagarde, "Type A Behavior Pattern, Risky Driving Behaviors, and Serious Road Traffic Accidents: A Prospective Study of the GAZEL Cohort," *American Journal of Epidemiology* 161(2005): 864–70.

43. Francesc Palmero, Jose Luis Diez, and Alicia Breva Asensio, "Type A Behavior Pattern Today: Relevance of the JAS-S Factor to Predict Heart Rate Reactivity," *Behavioral Medicine* 27(2001): 28–36.

44. R. L. Helmreich, J. T. Spence, and R. S. Pred, "Making It Without Losing It: Type A, Achievement Motivation, and Scientific Attainment Revisited," *Personality and Social Psychology Bulletin* 14(1988): 495–504.

45. R. S. Pred, J. T. Spence, and R. L. Helmreich, "The Development of New Scales for the Jenkins Activity Survey Measure of the Type A Construct," *Social and Behavioral Sciences Documents* 16(1986), no. 2679.

46. S. D. Bluen, J. Barling, and W. Burns, "Predicting Sales Performance, Job Satisfaction, and Depression by Using the Achievement Strivings and Impatience-Irritability Dimensions of Type A Behavior," *Journal of Applied Psychology* 75(1990): 212–16.

47. Ibid.

48. J. Barling, S. D. Bluen, and V. Moss, "Dimensions of Type A Behavior and Marital Dissatisfaction," *Journal of Psychology* 124(1990): 311–19.

49. L. Wright, "The Type A Behavior Pattern and Coronary Artery Disease," *American Psychologist* 453(1988): 2–14.

50. Pablo E. Vera-Villarroel, Ana I. Sánchez, and Juan Cachinero, "Analysis of the Relationship between the Type A Behavior Pattern and Fear of Negative Evaluation," *International Journal of Clinical and Health Psychology* 4(2004): 313–22.

51. Irene Rebollo and Dorret I. Boomsma, "Genetic and Environmental Influences on Type A Behavior Pattern: Evidence from Twins and Their Parents in the Netherlands Twin Register," *Psychosomatic Medicine* 68(2006): 437–42.

52. Daichi Shimbo, William Chaplin, Sujith Kuruvilla, Lauren Taggart Wasson, Dennis Abraham, and Matthew M. Burg, "Hostility and Platelet Reactivity in Individuals without a History of Cardiovascular Disease Events," *Psychosomatic Medicine* 71(2009): 741–47.

53. Gerdi Weidner, Gary Sexton, Joseph D. Matarazzo, Chere Pereira, and Ronald Friend, "Type A Behavior in Children, Adolescents, and Their Parents," *Developmental Psychology* 24(1988): 118–21.

54. Christine Scivicque, "Personality and Cancer: How Personality Impacts Cancer," *Suite 101.com*, October 21, 2007. Available at: http://cancer.suite101.com/artcile.cfm/personality_and_cancer

55. St. Louis Psychologists and Counseling Information and Referral, "Personality Types A, B, and C and Disease," St. Louis Psychologists and Counseling Information and Referral. Available at: www.psychtreatment.com/personality_type_and_disease.htm

56. Jean-Jacques, Dugoua, "Are You a Type C (Cancer) Personality?" *Truestar Health*, 2009. Available at: www.truestarhealth.com/members/cm_archives10ML3P1A70.html

57. American Cancer Society, "Are Some People Just Cancer-Prone?" *ACS Cancer News Center*, 2009. Available at: www.cancer.org/docroot/NWS_2_1x_Are_Some_People_Just_Cancer-Prone.asp

58. Naoki Nakaya, Yoshitaka Tsubono, Toru Hosokawa, Yoshikazu Nishino, Takayoshi Ohkubo, Atsushi Hozawa, Daisuke Shibuya, Shin Fukudo, Akira Fukao, Ichiro Tsuji, and Shigeru Hisamichi, "Personality and the Risk of Cancer," *Journal of the National Cancer Institute* 2003 95(11): 799–805.

59. Aolhealth, "Type 'D' for Distressed," Aolhealth, 2006. Available at: www.aolhealth.com/conditions/type-d-for-distressed

60. Johan Denollet, "Type D Personality: A Potential Risk Factor Refined," *Journal of Psychosomatic Research* 49(2000): 265–72.

61. Johan Denollet, "DS14: Standard Assessment of Negative Affectivity, Social Inhibition, and Type D Personality," *Psychosomatic Medicine* 67(2005): 89–97.

62. S. Pedersen and J. Denollet, "Validity of the Type D Personality Construct in Danish Post-MI Patients and Healthy Controls," *Journal of Psychosomatic Research* 57(2004): 265–72.

63. Audra K. Langley and Russell T. Jones, "Coping Efforts and Efficacy, Acculturation, and Post-Traumatic Stress Symptomatology in Adolescents Following Wildfire," *Fire Technology* 41(2005): 125–43.

64. Anna Zajacova, Scott M. Lynch, and Thomas J. Espenshade, "Self-Efficacy, Stress, and Academic Success in College," *Research in Higher Education* 46(2005): 677–706.

65. Rosa Grau, Marisa Salanova, and Jose Maria Peiro, "Moderator Effects of Self-Efficacy on Occupational Stress," *Psychology in Spain* 5(2001): 63–74.

66. Robert H. Reiman, et al., "Depressive Symptomatology Among HIV-Positive Women in the Era of HAART: A Stress and Coping Model," *American Journal of Community Psychology* 38(2006): 275–85.

67. Donna L. Coffman and Tammy D. Gilligan, "Social Support, Stress, and Self-Efficacy: Effects on Students' Satisfaction," *Journal of College Student* 4(2002–2003): 53–66.

68. Fernando D. Betoret, "Stressors, Self-Efficacy, Coping Resources, and Burnout Among Secondary School Teachers in Spain," *Educational Psychology* 26(2006): 519–39.

69. T. L. Finlayson, K. Siefert, A. I. Ismail, and W. Sohn, "Maternal Self-Efficacy and 1–5-Year-Old Children's Brushing Habits," *Community Dentistry and Oral Epidemiology* 35(2007): 272–81.

70. J. L. Rowe, G. H. Montgomery, P. R. Duberstein, and D. H. Bovbjerg, "Health Locus of Control and Perceived Risk for Breast Cancer in Healthy Women," *Behavioral Medicine* 31(2005): 33–40.

71. P. Winstead-Fry, C. G. Hernandez, G. M. Colgan, et al., "The Relationship of Rural Persons' Multidimensional Health Locus of Control to Knowledge of Cancer, Cancer Myths, and Cancer Danger Signs," *Cancer Nursing* 22(1999): 456–62.

72. E. M. van de Putte, R. H. Engelbert, W. Kuis, G. Sinnema, J. L. Kimpen, and C. S. Uiterwaal, "Chronic Fatigue Syndrome and Health Control in Adolescents and Parents," *Archives of Disease in Childhood* 90(2005): 1020–24.

73. A. Hansen, C. Edlund, and I. B. Branholm, "Significant Resources Needed for Return to Work After Sick Leave," *Work* 25(2005): 231–40.

74. J. A. Kahn, G. B. Slap, D. I. Bernstein, L. M. Kollar, A. M. Tissot, P. A. Hillard, and S. L. Rosenthal, "Psychological, Behavioral, and Interpersonal Impact of Human Papillomavirus and Pap Test Results," *Journal of Women's Health* 14(2005): 650–59.

75. A. Cabak, L. Wasilewski, A. Zdrodowska, and P. Tomaszewski, "Pain Control in Patients with Chronic Back Pain Syndrome," *Ortopedia Traumatologia Rehabilitacja* 13(2011): 361–68.

76. C. Otto, G. Bischof, H. J. Rumpf, C. Meyer, U. Hapke, and U. John, "Multiple Dimensions of Health Locus of Control in a Representative Population Sample: Ordinal Factor Analysis and Cross-Validation of an Existing Three and a New Four Factor Model," *BMC Medical Research Methodology* 11(2011): 114.

77. D. Clarke, "Motivational Differences Between Slot Machine and Lottery Players," *Psychological Reports* 96(2005): 843–48.

78. National Institute of Mental Health, *Anxiety Disorders*, 2010. www.nimh.nih.gov/Publicat/anxiety.cfm

79. National Institute of Mental Health, *Anxiety Disorders: Panic Disorder,* 2011. Available at: www.nimh.nih.gov/health/publications/anxiety-disorders/panic-disorder.shtml

80. National Institute of Mental Health, *Anxiety Disorders (Social Anxiety Disorder),* 2009. Available at: www.nimh.nih.gov/health/publications/anxiety-disorders/social-phobia-social-anxiety-disorder.shtml

81. Ibid.

82. K. S. Kendler, E. E. Walters, K. R. Truett, et al., "A Twin-Family Study of Self-Report Symptoms of Panic-Phobia and Somatization," *Behavior Genetics* 25(1995): 499–515.

83. National Institute of Mental Health, *Anxiety Disorders: Specific Phobias,* 2009. Available at: www.nimh.nih.gov/health/publications/anxiety-disorders/specific-phobias.shtml

84. Ibid.

85. Joseph Wolpe, *The Practice of Behavior Therapy,* 2nd ed. (New York: Pergamon, 1973).

86. Ronald B. Adler, *Confidence in Communication: A Guide to Assertive and Social Skills* (New York: Holt, Rinehart & Winston, 1977).

87. W. P. Murphy, J. S. Yaruss, and R. W. Quesal, "Enhancing Treatment for School-Age Children Who Stutter. I. Reducing Negative Reactions Through Desensitization and Cognitive Restructuring," *Journal of Fluency Disorders* 32(2007): 121–38.

88. R. McCaffrey, J. Zerwekh, and K. Keller, "Pain Management: Cognitive Restructuring as a Model for Teaching Nursing Students," *Nurse Educator* 30(2005): 226–30.

89. F. Galassi, S. Quercioli, D. Charismas, V. Niccolai, and E. Barciulli, "Cognitive-Behavioral Group Treatment for Panic Disorder with Agoraphobia," *Journal of Consulting and Clinical Psychology* 63(2007): 409–16.

90. J. C. Manuel, S. R. Burwell, S. L. Crawford, R. H. Lawrence, D. F. Farmer, A. Hege, K. Phillips, and N. E. Avis, "Younger Women's Perceptions of Coping with Breast Cancer," *Cancer Nursing* 30(2007): 85–94.

91. P. A. Boelen, J. de Keijser, M. A. van den Hout, and J. van den Bout, "Treatment of Complicated Grief: A Comparison Between Cognitive-Behavioral Therapy and Supportive Counseling," *Journal of Consulting and Clinical Psychology* 75(2007): 277–84.

92. C. Barrowclough, P. King, J. Colville, E. Russell, A. Burns, and N. Tarrier, "A Randomized Trial of the Effectiveness of Cognitive-Behavioral Therapy and Supportive Counseling for Anxiety Symptoms in Older Adults," *Journal of Consulting and Clinical Psychology* 69(2001): 756–62.

93. Albert Ellis and Robert Harper, *A New Guide to Rational Living* (Englewood Cliffs, NJ: Prentice Hall, 1979).

94. Albert Ellis and Catharine MacLaren, *Rational Emotive Behavior Therapy: A Therapist's Guide (Practical Therapist)* (Atascadero, CA: Impact Publishers, 2004).

95. A. D. Van Breda, *Resilience Theory: A Literature Review.* Pretoria, South Africa: South African Military Health Service, 2001. Available: www.vanbreda.org/adrian/resilience.htm

96. Glenn E. Richardson, "The Metatheory of Resilience and Resiliency," *Journal of Clinical Psychology* 58(2002): 307–21.

97. D. M. Buss, "Subjective Well-Being," *American Psychologist* 55(2000): 15–23.

98. C. Peterson, "The Future of Optimism," *American Psychologist* 55(2000): 44–55.

99. R. M. Ryan and E. Deci, "Self-Determination Theory and the Facilitation of Intrinsic Motivation, Social Development, and Well-Being," *American Psychologist* 55(2000): 68–78.

100. B. Schwartz, "Self-Determination," *American Psychologist* 55(2000): 79–88.

101. D. K. Simonton, "Creativity," *American Psychologist* 55(2000): 151–158.

102. R. F. Baumeister and J. J. Exline, "Self-Control, Morality, and Human Strength," *Journal of Social and Clinical Psychology* 19(2000): 29–42.

103. R. A. Emmons and C. A. Crumpler, "Gratitude as a Human Strength: Appraising the Evidence," *Journal of Social and Clinical Psychology* 19(2000): 59–69.

104. M. E. McCullough, "Forgiveness as a Human Strength: Theory, Measurement, and Links to Well-Being," *Journal of Social and Clinical Psychology* 19(2000): 43–55.

105. J. P. Tangney, "Humility: Theoretical Perspectives, Empirical Finding and Directions for Future Research," *Journal of Social and Clinical Psychology* 19(2000): 70–82.

106. Emily Crawford, Margaret O'Doughtery Wright, and Ann S. Masten, "Resilience and Spirituality in Youth," in Eugene C. Roehlkepartain, Pamela Ebstyne King, Linda Wagener, and Peter L. Benson, *The Handbook of Spiritual Development in Childhood and Adolescence* (Thousand Oaks, CA: Sage, 2006).

107. Richardson, "The Metatheory of Resilience and Resiliency."

108. Richardson, "The Metatheory of Resilience and Resiliency."

109. Suzanne C. Kobasa, "Stressful Life Events, Personality, and Health: An Inquiry into Hardiness," *Journal of Personality and Social Psychology* 37(1979): 1–11.

110. Salvatore R. Maddi, "Personality as a Resource in Stress Resistance: The Hardy Type" (Paper presented in the symposium on "Personality Moderators of Stressful Life Events" at the annual meeting of the American Psychological Association, Montreal, September 1980).

111. S. W. Hystad, J. Eid, and J. I. Brevik, "Effects of Psychological Hardiness, Job Demands, and Job Control on Sickness Absence: A Prospective Study," *Journal of Occupational Health Psychology* 16(2011): 265–78.

112. D. E. Stewart and T. Yuen, "A Systematic Review of Resilience in the Physically Ill," *Psychosomatics* 52(2011): 199–209.

113. I. K. Weigold and C. Robitschek, "Agentic Personality Characteristics and Coping: Their Relation to Trait Anxiety in College Students," *American Journal of Orthopsychiatry* 81(2011): 255–64.

114. P. T. Bartone, "Hardiness Protects Against War-Related Stress in Army Reserve Forces," *Consulting Psychology Journal* 51(1999): 72–83.

115. W. C. Thomson and J. C. Wendt, "Contribution of Hardiness and School Climate to Alienation Experienced by Student Teachers," *Journal of Educational Research* 88(1995): 269–74.

116. M. C. Rush, W. A. Schoel, and S. M. Barnard, "Psychological Resiliency in the Public Sector: 'Hardiness' and Pressure for Change," *Journal of Vocational Behavior* 46(1995): 17–39.

117. V. Florian, M. Mikulincer, and O. Taubman, "Does Hardiness Contribute to Mental Health During a Stressful Real-Life Situation? The Roles of Appraisal and Coping," *Journal of Personality and Social Psychology* 68(1995): 687–95.

118. I. Solcava and J. Sykora, "Relation Between Psychological Hardiness and Physiological Response," *Homeostasis in Health and Disease* 36(1995): 30–34.

119. C. F. Sharpley, J. K. Dua, R. Reynolds, and A. Acosta, "The Direct and Relative Efficacy of Cognitive Hardiness, a Behavior Pattern: Coping Behavior and Social Support as Predictors of Stress and Ill-Health," *Scandinavian Journal of Behavior Therapy* 1(1999): 15–29.

120. R. Duncko, A. Makatsori, E. Fickova, D. Selko, and D. Jezova, "Altered Coordination of the Neuroendocrine Response During Psychosocial Stress in Subjects with High Trait Anxiety," *Progress in Neuro-Psychopharmacology and Biological Psychiatry* 30(2006): 1058–66.

121. Salvatore R. Maddi, Deborah M. Khoshaba, Michele Persico, John Lu, Richard Harvey, and Felicia Bleecker, "The Personality Construct of Hardiness: II. Relationships with Comprehensive Tests of Personality and Psychopathology," *Journal of Research in Personality* 36(2002): 72–85.

122. M. V. Brooks, "Health-Related Hardiness and Chronic Illness: A Synthesis of Current Research," *Nursing Forum* 38(2003): 11–20.

123. P. C. Clark, "Effects of Individual and Family Hardiness on Caregiver Depression and Fatigue," *Research in Nursing Health* 25(2002): 37–48.

124. K. T. McCalister, C. L. Dolbier, J. A. Webster, M. W. Mallon, and M. A. Steinhardt, "Hardiness and Support at Work as Predictors of Work Stress and Job Satisfaction," *American Journal of Health Promotion* 20(2006): 183–91.

125. J. M. Otero-López, Mariño M. J. Santiago, and Bolaño C. Castro, "An Integrating Approach to the Study of Burnout in University Professors," *Psicothema* 20(2008): 766–72.

126. C. A. Dolan and A. B. Adler, "Military Hardiness as a Buffer of Psychological Health on Return from Deployment," *Military Medicine* 171(2006): 93–98.

127. M. E. Andrew, E. C. McCanlies, C. M. Burchfiel, L. E. Charles, T. A. Hartley, D. Fekedulegn, and J. M. Violanti, "Hardiness and Psychological Distress in a Cohort of Police Officers," *International Journal of Emergency Mental Health* 10(2008): 137–47.

128. L. L. Mathews and H. L. Servaty-Seib, "Hardiness and Grief in a Sample of Bereaved College Students," *Death Studies* 31(2007): 183–204.

129. C. L. Dolbier, S. E. Smith, and M. A. Steinhardt, "Relationships of Protective Factors to Stress and Symptoms of Illness," *American Journal of Health Behavior* 31(2007): 423–33.

130. N. Johnson and C. McMahon, "Preschoolers' Sleep Behaviour: Associations with Parental Hardiness, Sleep-Related Cognitions and Bedtime Interactions," *Journal of Child Psychology and Psychiatry* 49(2008): 765–73.

LAB ASSESSMENT 8.1

What Kind of Sense of Humor Do You Have?

Directions: To determine what kind of sense of humor you have, use the scale below to respond how much you agree or disagree with each statement.

1 = totally disagree

2 = mostly disagree

3 = somewhat disagree

4 = neither disagree or agree

5 = somewhat agree

6 = mostly agree

7 = totally agree

_____ 1. I usually don't laugh or joke around much with other people.*

_____ 2. If I am feeling depressed, I can usually cheer myself up with humor.

_____ 3. If someone makes a mistake, I will often tease them about it.

_____ 4. I let people laugh at me or make fun at my expense more than I should.

_____ 5. I don't have to work very hard at making other people laugh—I seem to be a naturally humorous person.

_____ 6. Even when I'm by myself, I'm often amused by the absurdities of life.

_____ 7. People are never offended or hurt by my sense of humor.*

_____ 8. I will often get carried away in putting myself down if it makes my family or friends laugh.

_____ 9. I rarely make other people laugh by telling funny stories about myself.*

_____ 10. If I am feeling upset or unhappy I usually try to think of something funny about the situation to make myself feel better.

_____ 11. When telling jokes or saying funny things, I am usually not very concerned about how other people are taking it.

_____ 12. I often try to make people like or accept me more by saying something funny about my own weaknesses, blunders, or faults.

_____ 13. I laugh and joke a lot with my closest friends.

_____ 14. My humorous outlook on life keeps me from getting overly upset or depressed about things.

_____ 15. I do not like it when people use humor as a way of criticizing or putting someone down.*

_____ 16. I don't often say funny things to put myself down.*

_____ 17. I usually don't like to tell jokes or amuse people.*

_____ 18. If I'm by myself and I'm feeling unhappy, I make an effort to think of something funny to cheer myself up.

_____ 19. Sometimes I think of something that is so funny that I can't stop myself from saying it, even if it is not appropriate for the situation.

_____ 20. I often go overboard in putting myself down when I am making jokes or trying to be funny.

_____ 21. I enjoy making people laugh.

_____ 22. If I am feeling sad or upset, I usually lose my sense of humor.*

_____ 23. I never participate in laughing at others even if all my friends are doing it.*

_____ 24. When I am with friends or family, I often seem to be the one that other people make fun of or joke about.

_____ 25. I don't often joke around with my friends.*

_____ 26. It is my experience that thinking about some amusing aspect of a situation is often a very effective way of coping with problems.

_____ 27. If I don't like someone, I often use humor or teasing to put them down.

_____ 28. If I am having problems or feeling unhappy, I often cover it up by joking around, so that even my closest friends don't know how I really feel.

_____ 29. I usually can't think of witty things to say when I'm with other people.*

_____ 30. I don't need to be with other people to feel amused—I can usually find things to laugh about even when I'm by myself.

_____ 31. Even if something is really funny to me, I will not laugh or joke about it if someone will be offended.*

_____ 32. Letting others laugh at me is my way of keeping my friends and family in good spirits.

Source: Rod A. Martin, Patricia Puhlik-Doris, Gwen Larsen, Jeanette Gray, and Kelly Weir, "Individual Differences in Uses of Humor and Their Relation to Psychological Well-Being: Development of the Humor Styles Questionnaire," *Journal of Research in Personality* 37(2003): 48–75.

Scoring: Before determining your scores on the various categories of humor, reverse the scores for each item with an asterisk (*) appearing after the statement. For example, if you answered you totally agree with item 1, instead of assigning 7 points to that statement, assign 1 point. Once you have done that, compute your scores for affiliative, self-enhancing, aggressive, and self-defeating humor by adding up the scores you assigned to each item within that subscale as below.

- *Affiliative humor:* Items 1, 5, 9, 13, 17, 21, 25, and 29   Score: _____

- *Self-enhancing humor:* Items 2, 6, 10, 14, 18, 22, 26, and 30   Score: _____

- *Aggressive humor:* Items 3, 7, 11, 15, 19, 23, 27, 31   Score: _____

- *Self-defeating humor:* Items 4, 8, 12, 16, 20, 24, 28, 32   Score: _____

Definitions of humor subscales:

- *Affiliative humor:* Humor used to enhance relationships. For example, saying funny things and telling jokes to make others feel comfortable.

- *Self-enhancing humor:* A general humorous outlook on life. For example, using jokes to cope with stress but not harming oneself or others.

- *Aggressive humor:* Humor intended to put down others. For example, using sarcasm, ridicule, or teasing.

- *Self-defeating humor:* Making self-disparaging jokes and humorous statements at one's own expense.

Interpretation of Your Scores: Means for the four Humor Styles Questionnaire scales appear below.

	Total	Males	Females
Affiliative humor	46.4	47.3	46.0
Self-enhancing humor	37.3	37.9	36.8
Aggressive humor	28.5	32.3	26.3
Self-defeating humor	25.9	27.8	24.5

Affiliative humor is related to cheerfulness, self-esteem, psychological well-being, and social intimacy. It is negatively correlated with depression, anxiety, seriousness, and bad mood. Individuals with high scores on this measure appear to be socially extraverted, cheerful, emotionally stable, and concerned for others.

Like affiliative humor, self-enhancing humor is positively related to cheerfulness, self-esteem, optimism, psychological well-being, and satisfaction with social support. It is negatively related to depression, anxiety, and bad mood.

Aggressive humor is positively related to measures of hostility and aggression. It is negatively related to seriousness. Hostility negatively affects social relationships and physical health.

Self-defeating humor is related to depression, anxiety, hostility, aggression, bad mood, and psychiatric symptoms. It is negatively related to self-esteem, psychological well-being, intimacy, and satisfaction with social supports.

So, if you want to be psychologically and physically healthy, make a conscious effort to use affiliative and self-enhancing humor, and avoid aggressive and self-defeating humor.

LAB ASSESSMENT 8.2

Are You a Type A?

Directions: Check whether the following statements are like you or unlike you.

Like Me	Unlike Me	
_____	_____	1. I explosively accentuate key words during ordinary speech.
_____	_____	2. I utter the last few words of a sentence more rapidly than the opening words.
_____	_____	3. I always move, walk, and eat rapidly.
_____	_____	4. I feel an impatience with the rate at which most events take place.
_____	_____	5. I hurry the speech of others by saying "Uh huh" or "Yes, yes," or by finishing their sentences for them.
_____	_____	6. I become enraged when a car ahead of me runs at a pace I consider too slow.
_____	_____	7. I find it anguishing to wait in line.
_____	_____	8. I find it intolerable to watch others perform tasks I know I can do faster.
_____	_____	9. I find myself hurrying my reading or attempting to obtain condensations or summaries of truly interesting and worthwhile literature.
_____	_____	10. I frequently strive to think about or do two or more things simultaneously.
_____	_____	11. I find it always difficult to refrain from talking about or bringing the theme of any conversation around to those subjects that especially interest me.
_____	_____	12. I always feel vaguely guilty when I relax or do nothing for several hours to several days.
_____	_____	13. I no longer observe the more important, interesting, or lovely objects I encounter.
_____	_____	14. I don't have any time to spare to become the things worth *being* because I am so preoccupied with getting the things worth *having*.
_____	_____	15. I attempt to schedule more and more in less and less time.
_____	_____	16. I am always rushed.
_____	_____	17. When meeting another aggressive, competitive person I feel a need to challenge that person.
_____	_____	18. In conversations, I frequently clench my fist, bang on the table, or pound one fist into the palm of another for emphasis.
_____	_____	19. I habitually clench my jaw, grind my teeth, or jerk back the corners of my mouth, exposing my teeth.
_____	_____	20. I believe that whatever success I enjoy is due in good part to my ability to get things done faster than others.
_____	_____	21. I find myself increasingly committed to translating and evaluating not only my own but also the activities of others in terms of "numbers."

Scoring

0–10 statements checked = Type B behavior pattern

0–5 statements checked = high degree of Type B behavior pattern

11–21 statements checked = Type A behavior pattern

16–21 statements checked = high degree of Type A behavior pattern

Source: From *Type A Behavior and Your Heart* by Meyer Friedman and Ray H. Rosenman, copyright © 1974 by Meyer Friedman. Used by permission of Alfred A. Knopf, a division of Random House, Inc.

LAB ASSESSMENT 8.3

How Is Your Self-Esteem?

Directions: Check whether the following statements are like you or unlike you.

Like Me	Unlike Me	
____	____	1. I'm a lot of fun to be with.
____	____	2. I always do the right thing.
____	____	3. I get upset easily at home.
____	____	4. I'm proud of my schoolwork.
____	____	5. I never worry about anything.
____	____	6. I'm easy to like.
____	____	7. I like everyone I know.
____	____	8. There are many times I'd like to leave home.
____	____	9. I like to be called on in class.
____	____	10. No one pays much attention to me at home.
____	____	11. I'm pretty sure of myself.
____	____	12. I'm not doing as well at school as I'd like to.

You have just completed sample questions from a scale used to measure self-esteem that discloses in how much esteem you hold yourself (how highly you regard yourself, your sense of self-worth). Let's score these sample items and then discuss the implications of self-esteem for stress management. Place the number 1 to the left of items 1, 4, 6, 9, and 11 of which you checked "like me." Place the number 1 to the left of items 2, 3, 5, 7, 8, 10, and 12 of which you checked "unlike me."

Some people deliberately lie on these types of inventories because they think it's clever or because they are embarrassed to respond honestly to items that evidence their low regard for themselves. Other people do not provide accurate responses because they rush through the inventory without giving each item the attention and thought necessary. In any case, this inventory contains a *lie scale* to identify the inaccurate responders. A lie scale includes items that can only be answered one way if answered accurately. A look at the items making up the lie scale will quickly elucidate the point. Items 2, 5, and 7 can only be answered one way. No one always does the right thing, never worries, or likes everyone. Add up the points you scored on the lie scale by adding the 1's you placed alongside these three items. If you didn't score at least 2, the rest of your scores are suspect; they may not be valid. Eliminating the three lie-scale items, add up the remaining 1's for your total self-esteem score.

This general self-esteem score, however, doesn't provide the kind of information needed to improve your self-esteem and thereby decrease the stress you experience. You may feel good about one part of yourself (e.g., your physical appearance) but be embarrassed about another part (e.g., your intelligence). Your general self-esteem score, however, averages these scores, and you lose this important information. To respond to this concern, the measure consists of three subscales that are specific to various components of self-esteem. The subscales and the items included within them follow:

Social self	Items 1, 6, 11
Family self	Items 3, 8, 10
School/work self	Items 4, 9, 12

To determine in how much esteem you hold yourself in social settings and interactions, add up the 1's by those three items. Do likewise to see how much regard you hold for yourself in your family interactions and in school or work settings. The closer to 3 you score, the higher is your self-esteem for that particular subscale. Remember, however, that these scores are only a rough approximation; the entire *Coopersmith Inventory* would have to be taken and scored for an accurate reading.

LAB ASSESSMENT 8.4

How Is Your Physical Self-Esteem?

Directions: How do you feel about your physical self—your physical self-esteem? In the following blanks, place the number on the scale that best represents your view of each body part listed.

1. = very satisfied
2. = OK
3. = not very satisfied
4. = very dissatisfied

_____ 1. hair		_____ 11. chest
_____ 2. face		_____ 12. eyes
_____ 3. neck		_____ 13. back
_____ 4. shoulders		_____ 14. mouth
_____ 5. hips		_____ 15. chin
_____ 6. legs		_____ 16. thighs
_____ 7. abdomen		_____ 17. arms
_____ 8. nose		_____ 18. knees
_____ 9. buttocks		_____ 19. elbows
_____ 10. hands		_____ 20. calves

Although there is no scale to evaluate your responses to this lab, the results can be quite meaningful. Lab Assessment 8.4 helps you determine which body parts are affecting how you feel about yourself—your self-esteem. Then you can either plan to improve that body part or devise a means of being more accepting of it. That may mean doing sit-ups to improve your abdomen. Or, it may mean focusing on an "attitude of gratitude" as discussed in this chapter, whereby you are purposefully grateful for the positive aspects of your body and accept that no one is perfect.

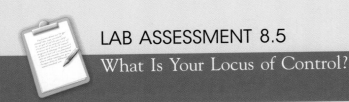

LAB ASSESSMENT 8.5

What Is Your Locus of Control?

Directions: For each numbered item, circle the answer that best describes your belief.

1. a. Grades are a function of the amount of work students do.
   b. Grades depend on the kindness of the instructor.
2. a. Promotions are earned by hard work.
   b. Promotions are a result of being in the right place at the right time.
3. a. Meeting someone to love is a matter of luck.
   b. Meeting someone to love depends on going out often so as to meet many people.
4. a. Living a long life is a function of heredity.
   b. Living a long life is a function of adopting healthy habits.
5. a. Being overweight is determined by the number of fat cells you were born with or developed early in life.
   b. Being overweight depends on what and how much food you eat.
6. a. People who exercise regularly set up their schedules to do so.
   b. Some people just don't have the time for regular exercise.
7. a. Winning at poker depends on betting correctly.
   b. Winning at poker is a matter of being lucky.
8. a. Staying married depends on working at the marriage.
   b. Marital breakup is a matter of being unlucky in choosing the wrong marriage partner.
9. a. Citizens can have some influence on their governments.
   b. There is nothing an individual can do to affect governmental function.
10. a. Being skilled at sports depends on being born well coordinated.
    b. Those skilled at sports work hard at learning those skills.
11. a. People with close friends are lucky to have met someone to be intimate with.
    b. Developing close friendships takes hard work.
12. a. Your future depends on whom you meet and on chance.
    b. Your future is up to you.
13. a. Most people are so sure of their opinions that their minds cannot be changed.
    b. A logical argument can convince most people.
14. a. People decide the direction of their lives.
    b. For the most part, we have little control over our futures.
15. a. People who don't like you just don't understand you.
    b. You can be liked by anyone you choose to like you.
16. a. You can make your life a happy one.
    b. Happiness is a matter of fate.
17. a. You evaluate feedback and make decisions based upon it.
    b. You tend to be easily influenced by others.
18. a. If voters studied nominees' records, they could elect honest politicians.
    b. Politics and politicians are corrupt by nature.
19. a. Parents, teachers, and bosses have a great deal to say about one's happiness and self-satisfaction.
    b. Whether you are happy depends on you.
20. a. Air pollution can be controlled if citizens would get angry about it.
    b. Air pollution is an inevitable result of technological progress.

Scoring: To determine your locus of control, give yourself one point for each of the following responses:

Item	Response	Item	Response
1	a	11	b
2	a	12	b
3	b	13	b
4	b	14	a
5	b	15	b
6	a	16	a
7	a	17	a
8	a	18	a
9	a	19	b
10	b	20	a

Scores above 10 indicate internality; scores below 11 indicate externality. Of course, there are degrees of each, and most people find themselves scoring near 10.

Directions: Following are a number of statements that people have used to describe themselves. Read each statement, and then circle the appropriate number to the right of the statement to indicate how you *generally* feel. There are no right or wrong answers. Do not spend too much time on any one statement, but give the answer that seems to describe how you generally feel.

	Not at All	Somewhat	Moderately So	Very Much So
1. I feel pleasant.	1	2	3	4
2. I feel nervous and restless.	1	2	3	4
3. I feel satisfied with myself.	1	2	3	4
4. I wish I could be as happy as others seem to be.	1	2	3	4
5. I worry too much over something that really doesn't matter.	1	2	3	4
6. I am happy.	1	2	3	4
7. I lack self-confidence.	1	2	3	4
8. I feel secure.	1	2	3	4
9. I am content.	1	2	3	4
10. Some unimportant thought runs through my mind and bothers me.	1	2	3	4

Scoring: You have just completed a scale that measures the degree to which you are generally anxious—trait anxiety. To score this scale, add the circled point values for items 2, 4, 5, 7, and 10. Reverse the point values for items 1, 3, 6, 8, and 9—that is, a circled 4 becomes 1 point, a circled 3 becomes 2 points, a circled 2 becomes 3 points, and a circled 1 becomes 4 points. Next, total these reversed scores and add that total to the total of the nonreversed items you previously obtained. The possible range of scores is between 10 and 40. The higher the score, the greater the trait anxiety.

Source: Modified and reproduced by special permission of the publisher, Mind Garden, Redwood City, CA 94061, from the *State-Trait Anxiety Inventory—Form Y* by Charles D. Spielberger, R. L. Gorsuch, R. Lushene, P. R. Vagg, and G. A. Jacobs. Copyright 1983 by Charles Spielberger. All rights reserved. Further reproduction is prohibited without the publisher's written consent. The complete *State-Trait Anxiety Inventory* and information about managing anxiety are available from Mind Garden, 1690 Woodside Road, #202, Redwood City, CA 94061, www.mindgarden.com.

LAB ASSESSMENT 8.7

What Is Your Level of Test Anxiety?

Directions: Read each item below to see if it reflects your experience in test taking. If it does, place a check mark on the line next to the number of the statement. Check as many as seem fitting. Be honest with yourself.

_____ 1. I wish there were some way to succeed without taking tests.

_____ 2. Getting a good score on one test does not seem to increase my confidence on other tests.

_____ 3. People (family, friends, etc.) are counting on me to do well.

_____ 4. During a test, I sometimes find myself having trains of thought that have nothing to do with the test.

_____ 5. I do not enjoy eating before or after an important test.

_____ 6. I have always dreaded courses in which the teacher has the habit of giving pop quizzes.

_____ 7. It seems to me that test sessions should not be made the formal, tense situations they are.

_____ 8. People who do well on tests generally end up in better positions in life.

_____ 9. Before or during an important exam, I find myself thinking about how much brighter some of the other test takers are.

_____ 10. Even though I don't always think about it, I am concerned about how others will view me if I do poorly.

_____ 11. Worrying about how well I will do interferes with my preparation and performance on tests.

_____ 12. Having to face an important test disturbs my sleep.

_____ 13. I cannot stand to have people walking around watching me while I take a test.

_____ 14. If exams could be done away with, I think I would actually learn more from my courses.

_____ 15. Knowing that my future depends in part on doing well on tests upsets me.

_____ 16. I know I could outscore most people if I could just get myself together.

_____ 17. People will question my ability if I do poorly.

_____ 18. I never seem to be fully prepared to take tests.

_____ 19. I cannot relax physically before a test.

_____ 20. I mentally freeze up on important tests.

_____ 21. Room noises (from lights, heating/cooling systems, other test takers) bother me.

_____ 22. I have a hollow, uneasy feeling before taking a test.

_____ 23. Tests make me wonder if I will ever reach my goals.

_____ 24. Tests do not really show how much a person knows.

_____ 25. If I score low, I am not going to tell anyone exactly what my score is.

_____ 26. I often feel the need to cram before a test.

_____ 27. My stomach becomes upset before important tests.

_____ 28. I sometimes seem to defeat myself (think negative thoughts) while working on an important test.

_____ 29. I start feeling very anxious or uneasy just before getting test results.

_____ 30. I wish I could get into a vocation that does not require tests for entrance.

_____ 31. If I do not do well on a test, I guess it will mean I am not as smart as I thought I was.

_____ 32. If my score is low, my parents will be very disappointed.

_____ 33. My anxiety about tests makes me want to avoid preparing fully, and this just makes me more anxious.

_____ 34. I often find my fingers tapping or my legs jiggling while taking a test.

_____ 35. After taking a test, I often feel I could have done better than I actually did.

_____ 36. When taking a test, my emotions interfere with my concentration.

_____ 37. The harder I work on some test items, the more confused I get.

_____ 38. Aside from what others may think of me, I am concerned about my own opinion of myself if I do poorly.

_____ 39. My muscles tense up in certain areas of my body when I take a test.

_____ 40. I do not feel confident and mentally relaxed before a test.

_____ 41. My friends will be disappointed in me if my score is low.

_____ 42. One of my problems is not knowing exactly when I am prepared for a test.

_____ 43. I often feel physically panicky when I have to take a really important test.

_____ 44. I wish teachers understood that some people are more nervous than others when taking tests, and that this could be taken into account when test answers are evaluated.

_____ 45. I would rather write a paper than take a test for a grade.

_____ 46. I am going to find out how others did before I announce my score.

_____ 47. Some people I know will be amused if I score low, and this bothers me.

_____ 48. I think I could do much better on tests if I could take them alone and/or not feel pressured by a time limit.

_____ 49. My test performance is directly connected to my future success and security.

_____ 50. During tests, I sometimes get so nervous that I forget facts I really know.

Scoring

This scale measures four _main sources_ of test anxiety and three _main expressions_ of test anxiety. If you checked more than four statements for any of these seven subscales of test anxiety variables, these sources of test anxiety may be a concern for you. Plan ways to respond to these variables more effectively. Perhaps get suggestions from your instructor or the campus counseling center.

Main Source of Test Anxiety

1. _Concerns about how others will view you if you do poorly:_
   Items 3, 10, 17, 25, 32, 41, 46, 47
2. _Concerns about your own self-image:_
   Items 2, 9, 16, 24, 31, 38, 40
3. _Concerns about your future security:_
   Items 1, 8, 15, 23, 30, 49
4. _Concerns about not being prepared for a test:_
   Items 6, 11, 18, 26, 33, 42

Main Expressions of Test Anxiety

1. _Bodily reactions:_
   Items 5, 12, 19, 27, 34, 39, 43
2. _Thought disruptions:_
   Items 4, 13, 20, 21, 28, 35, 36, 37, 48, 50
3. _General test-taking anxiety:_
   Items 7, 14, 22, 29, 44, 45

   How strong is each of these sources of test anxiety for you?

   How would you summarize your reactions to each of these sources?

   What will you do to manage any test anxiety issues raised by your responses on this scale?

Some items adapted from the Test Anxiety Inventory published by Mind Garden, Inc. www.mindgarden.com

LAB ASSESSMENT 8.8

The Measurement of Social Physique Anxiety?

Directions: Stress does not only lead to physical illness and diseases. Psychological consequences can also result, such as anxiety associated with body image. This type of anxiety is called social physique anxiety. To determine your social physique anxiety, respond to the following statements using the scale below:

1. = not at all

2. = slightly

3. = moderately

4. = very

5. = extremely characteristic

_____ 1. I am comfortable with the appearance of my physique/figure.

_____ 2. I would never worry about wearing clothes that might make me look too thin or overweight.

_____ 3. I wish I wasn't so uptight about my physique/figure.

_____ 4. There are times when I am bothered by thoughts that other people are evaluating my weight or muscular development negatively.

_____ 5. When I look in the mirror I feel good about my physique/figure.

_____ 6. Unattractive features of my physique/figure make me nervous in certain social situations.

_____ 7. In the presence of others, I feel apprehensive about my physique/figure.

_____ 8. I am comfortable with how fit my body appears to others.

_____ 9. It would make me uncomfortable to know others were evaluating my physique/figure.

_____ 10. When it comes to displaying my physique/figure to others, I am a shy person.

_____ 11. I usually feel relaxed when it is obvious that others are looking at my physique/figure.

_____ 12. When in a bathing suit, I often feel nervous about the shape of my body.

Scoring: To score this scale, first reverse the values you assigned for items 1, 2, 5, 8, and 11. In other words, if you assigned a 1 for item 11, change that 1 to a 5, and if you assigned a 4 for item 2, change that to a 2. Next, add up the points assigned to all 12 items as they now appear. The average score (mean) for college students is 37.5 for females and approximately 30.1 for males. Scores higher than these means indicate the possibility that you experience social physique anxiety.

Social physique anxiety is the degree to which you are satisfied or dissatisfied with your body. As you might expect, social physique anxiety is related to self-esteem. If you feel good about your body, you will feel good about yourself, and vice versa. Social physique anxiety is also related to insecurity and depression. Experts on social physique anxiety state that "compared to people who are low on social physique anxiety, those who are highly anxious are likely to avoid situations in which their physique is under the scrutiny of others (e.g., swimming in public), become very distressed when their physiques are on display, avoid activities that accentuate their physiques (including aerobic activities that might be beneficial to them), suffer depression related to their bodies, and attempt to improve their physiques through a variety of means, some of which may be harmful (e.g., fasting, exercising in rubber suits)" (Hart, Leary, and Rejeski, 1989, p. 96).

If you experience social physique anxiety, pay particular attention to the discussions of nutrition in Chapter 6, anxiety in the current Chapter 8, and exercise in Chapter 14. Following the guidelines in these sections should help you improve your physique/figure and lower your level of social physique anxiety. Recognizing, though, that changes in one's body and the resulting changes in social physique anxiety take time, it is also helpful to become more accepting of the body you have. Recall the discussion on "attitude of gratitude" earlier in this chapter. Be purposefully thankful for those parts of yourself you like, while working on improving those parts of your body you are committed to changing.

Adapted, with permission, from E. Hart, M.R. Leary, and W.J. Rejeski, 1989, "The Measurement of Social Physique Anxiety," _Journal of Sport and Exercise Psychology_ 11(1): 94–104.

LAB ASSESSMENT 8.9

Do You Have Irrational Beliefs?

Directions: This is an inventory about the way you believe and feel about various things. Use the following scale to state how strongly you agree or disagree with each of the numbered statements:

DS = disagree strongly

DM = disagree moderately

N = neither disagree nor agree

AM = agree moderately

AS = agree strongly

Try to avoid the neutral N response as much as possible. Select this answer *only* if you really cannot decide whether you tend to agree or disagree with a statement.

_____ 1. It is important to me that others approve of me.

_____ 2. I hate to fail at anything.

_____ 3. There is a right way to do everything.

_____ 4. I like the respect of others, but I don't have to have it.

_____ 5. I avoid things I cannot do well.

_____ 6. There is no perfect solution to anything.

_____ 7. I want everyone to like me.

_____ 8. I don't mind competing in activities where others are better than me.

_____ 9. There is seldom an easy way out of life's difficulties.

_____ 10. I can like myself even when many others don't.

_____ 11. I like to succeed at something but don't feel I have to.

_____ 12. Some problems will always be with us.

_____ 13. If others dislike me, that's their problem, not mine.

_____ 14. It is highly important to me to be successful in everything I do.

_____ 15. Every problem has a correct solution.

_____ 16. I find it hard to go against what others think.

_____ 17. I enjoy activities for their own sake, no matter how good I am at them.

_____ 18. We live in a world of chance and probability.

_____ 19. Although I like approval, it is not a real need for me.

_____ 20. It bothers me when others are better than I am at something.

_____ 21. There is seldom an ideal solution to anything.

_____ 22. I often worry about how much people approve of and accept me.

_____ 23. It upsets me to make mistakes.

_____ 24. It is better to look for a practical solution than a perfect one.

_____ 25. I have considerable concern with what people are feeling about me.

_____ 26. I often become quite annoyed over little things.

_____ 27. I feel I must handle things in the right way.

_____ 28. It is annoying but not upsetting to be criticized.

_____ 29. I'm not afraid to do things that I cannot do well.

_____ 30. There is no such thing as an ideal set of circumstances.

Source: R. G. Jones, "A Factored Measure of Ellis' Irrational Belief System, with Personality and Maladjustment Correlates," *Dissertation Abstracts,* 69(1969): 6443.

Scoring: For items 1, 2, 3, 5, 7, 14, 15, 16, 20, 22, 23, 25, 26, and 27:

DS = 1 point

DM = 2 points

N = 3 points

AM = 4 points

AS = 5 points

For items 4, 6, 8, 9, 10, 11, 12, 13, 17, 18, 19, 21, 24, 28, 29, and 30:

DS = 5 points

DM = 4 points

N = 3 points

AM = 2 points

AS = 1 point

Add up the points for each of the three subscales described below.

You have just completed a scale to measure three different types of irrational beliefs.

1. *Approval of others:* The degree to which you believe you need to have the support of everyone you know or care about. Average score: Men = 27, Women = 30.

   Items: 1, 4, 7, 10, 13, 16, 19, 22, 25, 28

2. *Self-expectations:* The degree to which you believe that you must be successful, achieving, and thoroughly competent in every task you undertake, and the degree to which you judge your worthiness as a person on the basis of your successful accomplishments. Average score: Men = 29, Women = 30.

   Items: 2, 5, 8, 11, 14, 17, 20, 23, 26, 29

3. *Perfectionism:* The degree to which you believe that every problem has a "right" or perfect solution, and the degree to which you cannot be satisfied until you find that perfect solution. Average score: Men = 29, Women = 28.

   Items: 3, 6, 9, 12, 15, 18, 21, 24, 27, 30

If you scored higher than the average, you believe these irrational beliefs to a greater extent than do most adults. Perhaps you want to step back and reevaluate these beliefs.

Spirituality and Stress

One late afternoon on a sunny April day, I drove from Phoenix, Arizona, north toward Flagstaff and arrived at Oak Creek Canyon just as the sun was setting. The canyon walls, created over many centuries, surrounded a natural river that left me breathless. All I could think was, "The wonder of it all!" Later that evening, on the ride back to Phoenix, I was accompanied by what seemed like thousands of stars in a crystal clear sky. Any of you who have been to this part of the United States knows that the stars appear so low in the night sky that they seem almost touchable. I could not drive too long—it seemed beyond my will—before I had to pull the car onto the shoulder of the roadway to get out and marvel at that sky with its twinkling ceiling.

It was impossible to be distressed that day. I was enraptured with these natural wonders and so intently focused upon them that the hassles and stressors I had experienced before I left Phoenix seemed inconsequential. Why sweat the small stuff in the face of the big stuff?

Too infrequently do we celebrate life's wonders with the attitude of gratitude that they deserve. Parents take their children for granted instead of marveling at their uniqueness and development. Students become desensitized to the beauty surrounding them on campus; to the quiet walks to the library; and to the opportunity to lie in the grass, reading Plato, Hemingway, or Poe. Professors forget to appreciate the cloistered environs in which they are honored by being allowed to devote their careers to labors of love. And creation itself often receives short shrift in a hurried society concerned with fast food, quick weight-loss diets, and electrodes that can stimulate muscular development without your even having to move. Quicker, faster, more, sooner, easier: We allow ourselves so little time to nourish the soul, to develop optimal spiritual health.

Spiritual Health

Despite all of the technological advances of recent years, 90 percent of the world's population is still involved in some form of religious or spiritual practice.[1] In fact, 45 percent of Americans used prayer for health reasons within the past year, 43 percent had prayed for their own health, and 25 percent had others pray for them.[2] Among these Americans, older people and African Americans are more likely than others to use prayer.[3,4] And it seems that when people become ill, they are even more likely to pray. For example, when cancer patients were asked if they prayed for their health, 69 percent stated they had—68 percent of whites, 81 percent of African Americans, and 73 percent of Hispanics.[5]

Spiritual health has been defined a number of ways. Some of these definitions recognize the existence of a Supreme Being, whereas others relate spirituality to one's relationships with others and one's place in this world. For example, one definition of **spiritual health** is adherence to doctrine as prescribed by a religion. The closer the adherence, the greater is the spiritual health. Another definition of spiritual health is the ability to discover and express your purpose in life; to learn how to experience love, joy, peace, and fulfillment; and to help yourself and others to achieve full potential.[6]

spiritual health
Adherence to religious doctrine; the ability to discover and express one's purpose in life; to experience love, joy, peace, and fulfillment; or to achieve and help others to achieve full potential.

Prayer can provide one with a sense of control over one's life. This man is praying at the Wailing Wall in Jerusalem.

According to leading coronary health researcher and developer of the Lifestyle Heart Trial, Dr. Dean Ornish, a lack of emotional and spiritual health is the basic cause of heart disease, because the stress that develops as a result influences the development of negative health behaviors that place the individual at risk for heart disease. Dr. Ornish's program, therefore, includes activities designed to help individuals increase their connectedness with self, others, and a higher power.[7]

The Stress Reduction clinic of Jon Kabat-Zinn also recognizes the importance of spiritual health to stress reduction and general health. Using mindfulness meditation, clinic patients are taught to live in the moment, becoming acutely aware of feelings, thoughts, and sensations. The results are decreases in chronic pain,[8] anxiety, stress, and depression.[9–12]

It has been suggested, therefore, that "it may be useful to view techniques such as meditation, imagery, and group support within a broad framework as tools for enhancing the spiritual health components of self-awareness, connectedness with others, and meaning and purpose in life rather than looking at them narrowly as superficial stress reduction techniques that simply help people 'calm down' or escape from their problems."[13]

Spiritual health may include answers to such questions as "Who am I?" "Why am I here?" and "Where am I headed?"—questions that confront you with the very fact of your existence and the meaning of your life. Answers to these questions may comfort you and alleviate stress with assurance that your life is headed in the direction you desire. Or your answers may disturb you. Perhaps you have not previously appreciated your relationship to humankind, to a Supreme Being, to nature, or to what has preceded you and what will remain when you no longer do. Should that occur, use that dissonance to make changes in your life so as to be more spiritual—take more walks in the woods, so to speak. Celebrate loved ones and natural wonders; find activities in which to make a contribution to your world and to the people who inhabit it; leave something of meaning behind; experience who you are and let others experience that as well.

Religion and Spirituality

As we will soon discuss, it is clear that religious and spiritual involvement affects health.[14–17] Yet what is not so clear are the differences and similarities between religion and spirituality.

Religion is a social entity that involves beliefs, practices, and rituals related to the sacred—sacred defined as mystical or supernatural or God, or in Eastern religious traditions, the ultimate truth or reality. Religions usually speak to life after death, and proscribe rules to guide behavior within a support group. **Spirituality** is more personal than religion in that it is something people define for themselves that is largely free of rules, regulations, and responsibilities typical of religions. Therefore, people may be spiritual but not religious. In that case, they deny a connection with any organized religion and define their spirituality in secular and individualistic terms. They consider themselves spiritual based on their view of meaning and purpose in life, connections with others (with those who came before and those who will follow) and with nature, peacefulness, and comfort with life choices.[18]

Spirituality and Health

Although both religion and spirituality have been associated with various health parameters (such as blood pressure[19]), researchers have also used religion and spirituality as interventions to improve health and alleviate stress. Some of these studies fit the traditional scientific mode, whereas others are more "exotic." In an interview pertaining to his and other researchers' studies on prayer and health, Larry Dossey describes a fascinating and controversial study he conducted.[20] A group of patients

religion
An organized entity in which people have common beliefs and engage in common practices relevant to spiritual matters.

spirituality
A person's view of life's meaning, direction, purpose, and connectedness to other things, other people, and the past and future.

with the same illness was divided into two groups. Then a group of people who described themselves as religious believers prayed for one group of patients. Patients in neither group knew whether they were the objects of the believers' prayers, and those praying had no idea for whom they were praying. The patients who were prayed for improved their health to a greater extent than did the other patients. This was a double-blind study, one of the most rigorous of research designs.

Dossey explains these findings in both spiritual and scientific terms:

> I've referred to these distant happenings as nonlocal events, because in essence they resemble the eerie, nonlocal events that physicists have demonstrated at the subatomic level between separate particles. These distant particles seem to behave as if they are united; if you change one, you change the other instantly and to the same degree. This is strongly analogous to distant, prayer-based healing, in which the separated individuals behave as if they are united. No one knows, however, if there is any real connection between the nonlocal behavior of subatomic particles and the nonlocal manifestations of intention and prayer.[21]

Dossey also points out that numerous studies have found that prayers of different religions seem to be equally effective. He lauds these findings for their validation of religious tolerance.

On the other hand, when Benson and colleagues[22] studied patients in six hospitals, they found no benefit to *intercessory prayer*—that is, others praying for patients' recovery. They divided patients into three groups: (1) 604 patients received intercessory prayer after being informed they might or might not receive a prayer; (2) 597 did not receive intercessory prayer, also after being informed they might or might not receive a prayer; and (3) 601 patients received intercessory prayer after being informed they would receive prayer. Complications occurred in 52 percent of patients in the two groups who received intercessory prayer, compared to 51 percent who did not receive prayer. In addition, complications occurred in 59 percent of patients certain of receiving intercessory prayer, compared to 52 percent of those uncertain of receiving prayer. The effects of intercessory prayer on health remain an area of controversy.

Many other, less controversial studies attest to the role of spirituality in health. For example, researchers have found spirituality or religion related to lower levels of psychological distress,[23] reduced risk of physical illness,[24] lower rates of cigarette smoking,[25] and lower mortality rates.[26] Researchers who have studied the relationship of spirituality and religion to health found them related to the adoption of healthy behaviors in general. Consequently, spiritual and religious people tend to be healthier. As one researcher stated, "a composite measure of spiritual health is more predictive of health-promoting behaviors, in general, than are isolated psychosocial variables (such as self-esteem, locus of control, connectedness, and sense of coherence)."[27]

It is not only researchers who are aware of the relationship between spirituality and health. The public also is aware. A survey found that 63 percent of Americans wanted their doctors to discuss their spiritual or religious commitment with them, but only 10 percent of doctors did so.[28] Medical schools have changed as a result of the need for physicians to discuss spirituality and religion with their patients. In 1992, very few medical schools included spirituality in their curricula. In 2000, more than half did so.[29] By 2008, two-thirds of medical schools offered some variation of spirituality-in-medicine coursework.[30]

One reason patients want to discuss spirituality with their physicians is that they have developed a *faith* in prayer to heal. In a study conducted by the Centers for Disease Control and Prevention of complementary and alternative medicine (CAM) use among American adults,[31] it was found that the most common form of CAM was praying.

Businesses also are recognizing the role of spirituality in the health and satisfaction of their employees. Some companies hire chaplains who play a role similar to that of an Army chaplain. The rationale, according to the president of Marketplace

Major Religious Traditions in the U.S.	
Among all adults... %	
Christian	**78.4**
Protestant	51.3
Evangelical churches	*26.3*
Mainline churches	*18.1*
Hist. black churches	*6.9*
Catholic	23.9
Mormon	1.7
Jehovah's Witness	0.7
Orthodox	0.6
Greek Orthodox	*<0.3*
Russian Orthodox	*<0.3*
Other	*<0.3*
Other Christian	0.3
Other Religions	**4.7**
Jewish	1.7
Reform	*0.7*
Conservative	*0.5*
Orthodox	*<0.3*
Other	*0.3*
Buddhist	0.7
Zen Buddhist	*<0.3*
Theravada Buddhist	*<0.3*
Tibetan Buddhist	*<0.3*
Other	*0.3*
Muslim*	0.6
Sunni	*0.3*
Shia	*<0.3*
Other	*<0.3*
Hindu	0.4
Other world rel.	<0.3
Other faiths	1.2
Unitarians and other liberal faiths	*0.7*
New Age	*0.4*
Native American rel.	*<0.3*
Unaffiliated	**16.1**
Atheist	1.6
Agnostic	2.4
Nothing in particular	12.1
Secular unaffiliated	*6.3*
Religious unaffiliated	*5.8*
Don't Know/Refused	**0.8**
	100

Due to rounding, figures may not add to 100 and nested figures may not add to the subtotal indicated.

*From "Muslim Americans: Middle Class and Mostly Mainstream," Pew Research Center, 2007

Source: *Pew Forum on Religion & Public Life,* "U.S. Religious Landscape Survey," 2010. Available at: http://religions .pewforum.org/reports.

Ministries, is that employees bring their spiritual issues to work with them and these issues affect their productivity.[32] In the huge Mall of America in Minneapolis, there is a 400-square-foot basement room that employees can use for a break from work. Among other things in that room are foot-washing stalls, shelves for shoes, prayer rugs, a compass to locate the direction east, and a poster displaying thirteen religions' interpretations of the Golden Rule.[33]

Spirituality and College Students

In 2003, the Higher Education Research Institute at UCLA began a seven-year study of how students' spiritual and religious qualities change during their college years.[34] The rationale for this first national longitudinal study of students' spiritual growth was that higher education should attend more to students' spiritual development since, the researchers argued, spirituality is essential to students' lives. As the researchers stated, "Assisting students' spiritual growth will help create a new generation who are more caring, more globally aware, and more committed to social justice than previous generations, while also enabling students to respond to the many stresses and tensions of our rapidly changing technological society with a greater sense of equanimity."

The study analyzed data from 14,527 students attending 136 colleges and universities nationwide. The results indicated that:[35]

- The greatest degree of spiritual growth occurs when students are actively engaged in introspective activities such as self-reflection, contemplation, and meditation.

- Charitable involvement such as community service, service-learning, helping friends with personal problems, and donating money to charity to promote spiritual growth.

- Growth in *equanimity*—the extent to which students are able to find meaning in times of hardship, feel at peace or centered, see each day as a gift, and feel good about the direction of their lives—increases students' grade point averages, leadership skills, and satisfaction with college. Equanimity also contributes to psychological well-being and the ability to get along with other races and cultures, and is best developed, the researchers state, through meditation and other self-reflection activities.

One of the purposes of the "Getting Involved in Your Community" boxes appearing in each chapter in this book is to contribute to your spiritual growth. If that occurs, you can expect to derive the accompanying benefits described above. So, don't be lazy. Actually engage in community service—by either following the suggestions in the "Getting Involved in Your Community" boxes or devising your own community service activities—and become an even better person than you were beforehand.

How Spirituality and Religion Affect Health

No one is certain about the exact mechanism that is working when spirituality affects a person's health status, but there are several theories.

Control Theory

Researchers have long known that when someone feels some degree of control over a stressor, that person's health will be less affected by the stressor than will the health of someone who perceives little or no control. There are two different approaches to increasing control: **Primary control** (similar to problem-focused coping) refers to attempts to change the situation. **Secondary control** refers to attempts to affect or control oneself. Secondary control can be more helpful in low-control situations.[36]

primary control
Attempts to change a situation; similar to problem-focused coping.

secondary control
Attempts to control oneself or one's emotional reactions; similar to emotion-focused coping.

Religion and spirituality can function as either primary control or secondary control. **Intercessory prayer** (prayers for divine intervention) is a primary control activity. Reframing a situation so as to view it as the outcome of fate or of forces of nature is a secondary control activity. Other secondary control spiritual activities that lessen emotional reactions to stress include "meditation, contemplative prayer, rituals, or scripture readings."[37] One researcher even found prayer and devotional meditations more effective than progressive relaxation or no treatment in reducing anger and anxiety.[38]

Pargament[39,40] and his colleagues categorized religious approaches to increasing control as a coping mechanism:

Self-directing: Individual perceives him- or herself as responsible for the outcome, although God or nature has provided the resources the individual needs to be successful—the "God helps those who help themselves" approach.

Collaborative: Individual works with God or with forces of nature to control the situation.

Deferring: Entire situation is turned over to God or to forces of nature, with reliance on external forces to manage or cope with the situation.

Pleading: Individual begs God or forces of nature to intervene in the situation to resolve it.

Studies have found the self-directing and collaborative approaches associated with mental health and competence, and the deferring approach associated with lower levels of self-competence.[41] However, other researchers conclude that a collaborative or deferring approach may be healthier in situations in which the individual really does have little control (e.g., when about to have surgery).[42] In this instance, secondary control is facilitated by a deferring or collaborative approach.

Social Support Theory

Others conceptualize the value of spirituality and religion in more social terms. Participation in a church, synagogue, or other spiritual group often brings one in close contact, on a very personal level, with other people of similar mind. The sense of affiliation alone may help assuage feelings of anger and anxiety, thereby positively affecting one's health. In addition, church, mosque, and synagogue affiliation or being a member of another type of spiritual group might bring into an individual's life people who can provide the various kinds of social support sometimes required to maintain health and well-being. They could provide emotional support during tough times or financial support when someone is laid off from work, or they could provide advice for overcoming temporary hardship. We know that social support is an effective means for managing stress and preventing ill effects from stressors. Therefore, it should be no surprise that religious and spiritual affiliations that provide social support can have profound effects on health.

Spirituality, Social Support, and Terrorism

Those directly involved, and those only peripherally involved, in such tragic events as those of September 11, 2001, or shootings on campuses can draw support through spiritual activities. We know that social support can take various forms, and much of this support can flow from organized spiritual activity such as attendance at religious services or from individual spiritual perspectives. For example, *emotional support* can be offered by fellow congregants or clergy. It is satisfying,

The social support obtained through organized spiritual or religious groups can take on many different forms such as financial support, emotional support, or provision of advice when it is needed.

intercessory prayer
Prayers that seek divine intervention either to prevent an occurrence or to help overcome it.

as well as important for one's physical health, to have people with whom to share feelings about stressful events. For those not inclined to participate in religious activities, sharing feelings with friends and family can serve the same purpose. Counseling services can also supply emotional support in times of need.

Sometimes emotional support is not enough, and *financial support* is required. Financial contributions made by churches, synagogues, and mosques can alleviate a significant amount of the stress people in need might otherwise experience. Again, friends and relatives can also provide financial support.

At other times, *informational support* is needed. Knowing where to go for help (e.g., social services) or what stress management techniques to use and how to use them can contribute to managing life crises. Such information is often available from clergy, teachers, family, friends, or governmental agencies.

Another type of social support that can be obtained through religious institutions or significant others is *advice support*. Sometimes being advised regarding what course of action to take can result in alleviating stress in confusing and traumatic times.

Lastly, the perception that life is meaningful, even when that meaning is elusive, can alleviate stress. Believing in an afterlife, or in a connection with those who preceded you and those who will follow, can assuage feelings of haphazardness or of feeling victimized by traumatic events. As taught in the Book of Job and reiterated in Harold Kushner's book *When Bad Things Happen to Good People,* meaning can be found even in apparently unexplainable events. It is not easy finding and accepting that lesson, but others who care for you and for whom you care can be a source of inspiration during life's challenges.

Placebo Theory

Some have argued that neither religious nor spiritual activities have any direct effect on health. Instead, they say, these health benefits are actually akin to what researchers find in other areas of study—namely, the placebo effect. When people believe something will help them, they often report that it actually does help them. It is for this reason that researchers try to conceal which research subjects are experiencing the treatment and which comprise the control group. Researchers even try to conceal this information, whenever possible, from those collecting the data as well. When both subjects and data collectors have no idea who the treatment subjects are and who the control subjects are, we call the studies **double-blind studies.** Although it is important to identify when the placebo effect is operating, it has been argued that whether it is operating or not is immaterial. As long as people either maintain health or improve it, what does it matter whether the improvement occurred because they believed a treatment would work or because the treatment actually worked? If religious and spiritual activities result in better health, for example, whether it is because of some metaphysical properties or a placebo effect may not matter to the individual at all.

Critics of this argument believe that effective treatments must be validated before time and resources are spent on replicating them. Therefore, if intercessory prayer improves health, we need to identify the particular reasons for this finding. Is it believing that prayer will work? Is it the particular nature of the prayer? Is it the result of some supernatural force? Once identified, the effective components can be applied in other treatments. With which view of the placebo effect do you most agree?

Forgiveness and Health

Take a moment and try to imagine someone who has done something so harmful to you that you cannot ever see yourself forgiving that person. Perhaps that person embarrassed you terribly, or fired you from a job you valued, or hurt a

Forgiving others is good for your own health—physical and spiritual.

member of your family. You probably feel very angry when you think of this person, and that is perfectly natural. But did you know that being so angry and unforgiving is unhealthy? It elicits a stress reaction accompanied by all the consequences of stress that we discussed earlier. In fact, studies have found that unforgiveness evokes brain activity consistent with stress, anger, and aggression,[43] stress-related hormonal secretions (in particular cortisol[44] and adrenaline[45]), an increase in blood pressure,[46] and blood chemistry consistent with a stress response.[47] Being unforgiving also negatively affects mental health[48] and renders the immune system less effective.[49] Now who would want to do that to him- or herself?

On the other hand, adopting a forgiving attitude has many health benefits. Studies have verified that forgiving results in lower levels of anxiety, depression, and stress, as well as lower blood cholesterol.[50,51] **Forgiveness** is also associated with lower self-reported illness,[52] less back pain,[53] and spiritual well-being.[54]

So, for your own mental and physical health, you should try to forgive others. However, forgiveness is not excusing, justifying, condoning, pardoning, nor forgetting a transgression.[55] Instead, it is a sincere intention not to seek revenge or avoid the transgressor (*decisional forgiveness*) and to replace negative emotions such as resentment, hate, and anger with positive emotions such as compassion, empathy, and sympathy (*emotional forgiveness*).[56] One way to become more forgiving is to recognize that you, too, have done things for which you wish to be forgiven. All of us have. Feeling gratitude for having been forgiven yourself, or wishing you were forgiven when you were not, should help you to forgive others. No one said it was easy—but it is worth striving toward, if for no other reason than it is good for your health.

In addition to wishing others to forgive us, we need to be willing to forgive ourselves. Understanding that all of us say things, do things, or wish we had done what we think we should have done but didn't, is part of the human condition that will help us forgive ourselves. That does not mean we forget the past. Rather, it means that we remember it, learn from it, but then let it go. The ability to forgive oneself is also related to improved health status (for example, higher self-esteem, less anxiety and depression, and less stress).[57,58] In fact, several studies find that forgiving oneself has the most effect on one's health.[59,60]

Lastly, sometimes we blame events in our lives on God or a Supreme Being. We may experience a life tragedy (such as the death of a child or chronic painful illness) and ascribe that to God or a Supreme Being. Consequently, we assume an unforgiving attitude toward that deity. That, too, can be unhealthy. When college students were studied, difficulty in forgiving God was associated with anxiety and depression.[61] However, researchers found the reverse to be true as well: When people forgive God, they improve their health status.[62,63]

The accompanying box entitled "Forgiving Others and Yourself" will help you get started on adopting this important spiritual and health-related concept, as will Lab Assessment 9.2, How Forgiving Are You?

forgiveness
A sincere intention not to seek revenge or avoid the transgressor (*decisional forgiveness*) and replacing negative emotions such as resentment, hate, and anger with positive emotions such as compassion, empathy, and sympathy (*emotional forgiveness*).

Volunteerism as a Spiritual and Healthy Activity

Volunteering to help others is one spiritual activity that pays big dividends, not only to those receiving the volunteer service but also to the person performing it. As Ralph Waldo Emerson once said, "It is one of the most beautiful compensations of this life that no man can sincerely try to help another without helping himself." That certainly appears to be the case with volunteerism.

Several large-scale studies of college students' community service and service-learning activities have found numerous benefits for college students. Among these

Forgiving Others and Yourself

1. List three people whom you have had trouble forgiving:

   a. _____

   b. _____

   c. _____

2. Identify three negative effects this unforgiving attitude has on you:

   a. _____

   b. _____

   c. _____

3. Choose one or more of the three people you cited above and describe what you will do to forgive them, and the date by when you will do it:

   _____

   _____

   _____

benefits are the development of a greater sense of civic responsibility (a commitment to serving the community), a higher level of academic achievement (academic self-concept, grades, degree aspirations, time devoted to academic endeavors), growth in life skills (leadership, interpersonal skills, self-confidence), increased commitment to helping others and to promoting racial understanding, and enhanced critical thinking and conflict resolution skills. In addition, benefits accrued to the colleges conducting the service activities and to the communities and agencies they served.[64,65] In a comprehensive review, the Corporation for National and Community Service reported physical and mental health benefits associated with volunteering.[66] Volunteering led to higher levels of happiness, life satisfaction, self-esteem, and sense of control over life. In addition, volunteering increased social networks that served as a buffer to stress, reduced disease risk, lowered mortality rates, and helped people cope with chronic and serious illness beyond that achieved from medical care alone.

Historically volunteerism has been associated with religious organizations. However, there is also a long history of secular volunteerism and community service in the United States and elsewhere. On many college campuses, there is an office responsible for encouraging students, faculty, and staff to participate in community service. The "Getting Involved in Your Community" box at the conclusion of each chapter in this book will get you started volunteering. Remember, by doing so you are doing something good for yourself while doing something good for someone else. What more could you ask for?

Service-Learning: A Spiritual and Academic Activity

Service-learning involves students who provide service on or off campus using the knowledge or skills they learn in class. In this way, students have the opportunity to apply what they learn in the real world, and communities receive service they might not otherwise receive.

Mitzvah Day

In Rochester, New York, 150 Jewish teenagers participate in "Mitzvah Day," one day each year that synagogues devote to community service. The variety of activities in which they participate might give you some ideas about how you can volunteer your time and benefit others while, at the same time, benefiting yourself. Here are some of the projects through which these teenagers provided service:[a]

1. Learned how to do CPR and then taught seven other people how to do it.
2. Taught a dozen people how to cook chicken soup, which was delivered to homebound individuals the following week.
3. Learned how to give manicures and hand massages so they could go to local nursing homes and provide these services to residents.
4. Learned how to dance to music from the Big Band era and then organized a Senior Ball at a nursing home during which the teenagers danced with the elders.
5. Learned how to act like a clown and perform magic tricks in preparation for putting on a show at a children's hospital.
6. Cut two inches off their hair and donated it to Locks of Love, an organization that makes wigs and provides them free of charge to children who experience hair loss from various medical treatments, illnesses, or diseases.

What service can you volunteer?

What service will you volunteer?

Marian Wright Edelman, executive director of the Children's Defense Fund, once wrote that "service is the rent we pay for living. If you see a need, don't ask, 'Why doesn't somebody do something?' Ask, 'Why don't I do something?' . . . We are not all guilty but we are all equally responsible."[b]

[a]D. Seigel, "A Cold Day in Rochester," *Tikkun* 15(2000): 61.
[b]M. W. Edelman, *The Measure of Our Success* (Boston: Beacon Press, 1992).

In each decade since 1990, the federal government has developed national health objectives intended to focus national attention and actions on improving the health of Americans. Several of these objectives for the year 2010 are directly and indirectly related to stress or other content presented in this book. Among the stress-related national health objectives are:[67]

- Increase the proportion of employees who have access to workplace programs that prevent or reduce employee stress.

- Reduce the suicide rate.

- Reduce suicide attempts by adolescents.

- Reduce the proportion of adolescents who engage in disordered eating behaviors in an attempt to control their weight.

- Reduce the proportion of persons who experience major depressive episode.

- Increase the proportion of adults with mental health disorders who receive treatment.

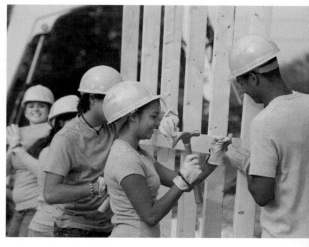

When you volunteer to help others, you inevitably help yourself. Volunteering is associated with better health and less stress.

- Increase depression screening by primary care providers.
- Increase the proportion of homeless adults with mental health problems who receive mental health services.
- Increase the proportion of adults who meet current federal physical activity guidelines for aerobic physical activity and for muscle-strengthening activity.
- Reduce the proportion of persons in the population with hypertension.
- Increase overall cardiovascular health in the U.S. population.
- Increase the proportion of Americans who have access to a food retail outlet that sells a variety of foods that are encouraged by the *Dietary Guidelines for Americans.*
- Increase the proportion of physician office visits that include counseling or education related to nutrition or weight.
- Increase the proportion of adults who are at a healthy weight and reduce the proportion of adults who are obese.

Through service-learning, you can be supportive of these stress-related national health objectives. For example, you could conduct stress management workshops for others in your community. These workshops could be offered in community centers, in schools, or in housing projects. My students have conducted stress management workshops for cancer patients, nursing home residents and staff, volunteer firefighters, and many others.

Or you could organize fitness activities for younger students attending after-school programs, or for the elderly in your community. Participants will dissipate the built-up by-products of stress and have something on which to focus other than their stressors.

You can contribute to the achievement of these stress-related national health objectives in many ways. Service-learning is one way. Through service-learning, you can make your community, and the people in it, healthier. And by doing so, you will learn more about stress and stress management. Now, how can you beat that? Perhaps your instructor will work with you to organize a service-learning activity to derive those benefits.

Closing Thoughts on Spirituality, Health, and Managing Stress

Believing that your life is not an isolated event will be one of the developmental tasks of your later years. Many years ago, psychiatrist Erik Erikson said that the main challenge facing old people is to resolve what he termed the crisis between integrity and despair.[68] When this crisis is satisfactorily resolved, you feel connected to what came before you and to what will come after you. You believe that you contributed to the chain of life and that your life has had meaning and purpose. This is spiritual health. Some people find it through a religious belief, a belief in God and life in the hereafter as a reward for good deeds in this life. Others find it in a belief that all things are connected, that what affects me also affects you and all others. These people may feel strongly about protecting the environment, volunteering to serve others, and advocating for those less fortunate than themselves.

This feeling of life having a purpose, of integrity rather than despair, can be invaluable during times of stress. It can help as an emotion-focused coping technique by allowing you to be more accepting of those things that are beyond your control, and it can provide something positive upon which to focus, thereby helping elicit a relaxation response.

Believing your life has a larger purpose can also serve as a problem-focused coping technique during stressful times. Possessing this level of spiritual health usually results in collaboration with other people in the pursuit of common goals. For some this will mean becoming a member of an organized religion—a church, synagogue, or mosque—and interacting with congregants with similar views. For others it will mean joining an organization that seeks to achieve the spiritual goals they find important. That could be joining the Sierra Club, or volunteering at a shelter for women who have experienced domestic violence, or delivering blankets to the homeless on cold winter nights. In either case, active participation in a religious group or in a secular one makes available people who can offer advice, financial support, or even shelter when that is needed during stressful times. These all serve as problem-focused coping interventions.

So, as we have seen, spiritual health not only is good for you physically and psychologically but is an important component of effective stress management. Having faith—be it in yourself, in God, or in other humans—goes a long way in helping us be soulful and happy. One author has described this another way. Gafni[69] speaks of "soul prints." Soul prints are people's unique stories, their reasons for being, their views of holy and holistic living, the unique patterns of their spirit. When people are not living their story, Gafni argues, they have **spiritual disease.** As might be expected, and as attested to by the research described earlier in this chapter, spiritual disease eventually results in physiological or psychological disease.

The lesson to be learned in all of this? Be true to yourself and to what you view as your purpose in life, contribute to enhancing the lives of others, and connect to what has come before and to what will come after. You will be healthier, happier, more fulfilled, and better able to manage stressful events. Now there's a formula for living!

spiritual disease
A condition in which people are not true to their spiritual selves and are living a "life story" that is inconsistent with their beliefs and values.

Getting Involved in Your Community

Many religious organizations—synagogues, churches, mosques—conduct educational programs of varied kinds. You can offer to teach congregants to manage stress by using prayer on which to focus when meditating. Or you can organize youth members of the congregation to provide services to others in the community, similar to the Mitzvah Day activities described in the boxed material in this chapter.

If you are not active with a religious group or are nonreligious, you can still engage in community service of a spiritual nature. For example, you can organize a group of youth who frequent an after-school community center to offer services to the community. You can start a basketball league with all team registration fees, admission fees, and any other contributions people or area businesses are willing to make donated to a shelter for the homeless in your neighborhood or town.

When you offer service to your community, you can expect to feel that your life is more meaningful and you really matter and can make a difference. This might even be used as a definition of spiritual health. Volunteer. Be healthier and more fulfilled as a result. Be a person in your community who cares, and you will make a huge contribution in helping your neighbors live less stressful lives; and you, too, will be better able to manage stress in your own life.

Many African American churches have a "church nurse" or "health ministry." These church nurses perform several functions, including comforting the family of the deceased at funeral services. Church nurses can be seen distributing tissues and water to grieving family members at these funeral services. When a parishioner becomes too excited during services—becomes "overcome with the holy spirit"—the church nurse might be seen fanning this parishioner.

Today, though, these health ministries have been transformed so that, in addition to their previous responsibilities, they may organize health fairs, conduct health screenings (e.g., blood pressure and blood glucose), and visit ill or shut-in parishioners in their homes. The health ministry may also supervise a health library so interested parishioners may have written material to consult.

Furthermore, the health ministry may arrange for health experts to speak to the congregation on health issues that are differentially distributed among African Americans: hypertension, diabetes, HIV/AIDS, and obesity.

Health ministries in African American churches combine spirituality, religiosity, and health care for the betterment of their parishioners.

summary

- Spiritual health has been defined in a number of ways. Some definitions recognize the existence of a Supreme Being; others relate spirituality to one's relationships with others and to one's place in this world. One definition of spiritual health is adherence to doctrine as prescribed by a religion. Another definition of spiritual health is the ability to discover and express your purpose in life; to learn how to experience love, joy, peace, and fulfillment; and to help yourself and others to achieve full potential. Spiritual health may include answers to such questions as "Who am I?" "Why am I here?" and "Where am I headed?" Developing one's spiritual nature can help alleviate stress by feeling connected to others, by having purpose in life, and by being better able to view hassles and stressors with proper perspective.

- Spirituality is a person's orientation toward or experiences with the transcendent existential features of life such as meaning, direction, purpose, and connectedness. Spirituality is sometimes referred to as the search for the sacred life.

- Religion is an external manifestation of spiritual experience, or an organized social entity in which individuals share some basic beliefs and practices.

- It is possible to be spiritual without being religious, or to be spiritual but antireligious. It is also possible to engage in a religious practice but to do so in a secular, spiritual manner, such as using prayer as the focus of meditation rather than as a means of praying to a Supreme Being.

- Spiritual health is related to a number of physiological conditions such as heart disease, anxiety, depression, and mortality.

- The means by which spiritual health affects other components of health has been explained by various theories: control theory, social support theory, and placebo theory. Religious approaches to increase control as a mechanism to cope include self-directing, collaboration, deferring, and pleading.

- Forgiveness is also associated with health and stress. The inability to forgive another person or a Supreme Being leads to anger, which in turn leads to ill health. For example, studies have shown an inability to forgive associated with anxiety and depression. The ability to forgive has been associated with improved mental health, lower blood cholesterol, less back pain, and spiritual well-being.

- Volunteerism, a spiritual activity, is related to a variety of benefits for the person volunteering, the people and agencies receiving the service, and the college supporting student, faculty, and staff volunteers. Volunteerism has been associated with lower mortality, better physical functioning, healthier habits, and the availability of social support. Volunteers are more sociable, are more altruistic, are in better health, have higher morale, and possess higher self-esteem.

- Believing one is connected to the past and to the future, either through a religious belief or a belief in nature and the oneness of the world, is a developmental stage related to health and the ability to manage stress.

internet resources

About Religion and Spirituality **www.about.com/religion** *Provides links that describe numerous religions' perspectives on spiritual issues.*

Faith **www.faith.com** *Provides a forum for exploring spirituality and religion without promoting any one religion or approach through articles, audio and video clips, and other resources.*

Naturalism.org **www.naturalism.org/spiritua.htm** *Discusses a naturalistic vision of oneself and the world informing spiritual experience. Takes the view that nature can generate feelings of connection and meaning that rival those offered by traditional religions, and those feelings reflect the empirical reality of our being at home in the cosmos.*

The University of Minnesota's Center for Spirituality and Healing **www.csh.umn.edu/** *The Center seeks to enrich health and well-being by providing high-quality interdisciplinary education, conducting rigorous research, and delivering innovative programs that advance integrative health and healing.*

Spirituality in Higher Education **http://spirituality.ucla.edu/** *Presents findings from a seven-year study examining the role that college plays in facilitating the development of students' spiritual qualities.*

Center for Spirituality at Work **www.cfsaw.org/about/mission.htm** *The Center's mission is to act as a bridge uniting diverse people for spiritual transformation and social justice. Building relationships and partnerships that bring together the powerless and privileged in a mutual project for social change is central to the center's activities.*

references

1. D. B. Barrett and T. M. Johnson, "World Christian Database: Atheist/Nonreligious by Country: World Christian Trends," *William Carey Library*, 2007. Available at: www.worldchristiandatabase.org/wcd

2. National Center for Complementary and Alternative Medicine, "Prayer and Spirituality in Health: Ancient Practices, Modern Science," *CAM at the NIH: Focus on Complementary and Alternative Medicine*, Winter 2005.

3. R. A. Bell, et al., "Pray for Health among U.S. Adults: The 2002 National Health Interview Survey," *Complementary Health Practice Review* 10(2005): 175–88.

4. M. S. Goldstein, et al., "The Use of Complementary and Alternative Medicine among California Adults with and Without Cancer," *Evidence Based Complementary and Alternative Medicine* 2(2005): 557–65.

5. L. E. Ross, I. J. Hall, T. L. Fairly, Y. J. Taylor, and D. L. Howard, "Prayer and Self-Reported Health among Cancer Survivors in the United States, National Health Interview Survey, 2002," *Journal of Complementary and Alternative Medicine* 14(2008): 931–38.

6. Larry S. Chapman, "Developing a Useful Perspective on Spiritual Health: Well-Being, Spiritual Potential, and the Search for Meaning," *American Journal of Health Promotion*, Winter 1987, 31–39.

7. Dean Ornish, *The Spectrum: A Scientifically Proven Program to Feel Better, Live Longer, Lose Weight, and Gain Health* (New York: Ballantine, 2008).

8. Jon Kabat-Zinn et al., "Clinical Use of Mindfulness Meditation for the Self-Regulation of Chronic Pain," *Journal of Behavioral Medicine* 8(1985): 163–90.

9. Jon Kabat-Zinn, et al., "Effectiveness of Meditation-Based Stress Reduction Program in the Treatment of Anxiety Disorders," *American Journal of Psychiatry* 149(1992): 936–43.

10. D. S. Ludwig and J. Kabat-Zinn, "Mindfulness in Medicine," *JAMA* 300(2008): 1350–52.

11. T. Meili and J. Kabat-Zinn, "The Power of the Human Heart: A Story of Trauma and Recovery and Its Implications for Rehabilitation and Healing," *Advances in Mind-Body Medicine* 20(2004): 6–16.

12. R. J. Davidson, J. Kabat-Zinn, J. Schumacher, M. Rosenkranz, D. Muller, S. F. Santorelli, F. Urbanowski, A. Harrington, K. Bonus, and J. F. Sheridan, "Alterations in Brain and Immune Function Produced by Mindfulness Meditation," *Psychosomatic Medicine* 65(2003): 564–70.

13. Steven R. Hawkes, Melisa L. Hull, Rebecca L. Thulman, and Paul M. Richins, "Review of Spiritual Health: Definition, Role, and Intervention Strategies in Health Promotion," *American Journal of Health Promotion* 9(1995): 371–78.

14. D. R. Williams and M. J. Sternthal, "Spirituality, Religion and Health: Evidence and Research Directions," *Medical Journal of Australia* 186(2007): S47–S50.

15. D. B. Bekelman, S. M. Dy, D. M. Becker, I. S. Wittstein, D. E. Hendricks, T. E. Yamashita, and S. H. Gottlieb, "Spiritual Well-Being and Depression in Patients with Heart Failure," *Journal of General Internal Medicine* 22(2007): 470–77.

16. D. P. Yoon and E. K. Lee, "The Impact of Religiousness, Spirituality, and Social Support on Psychological Well-Being Among Older Adults in Rural Areas," *Journal of Gerontological Social Work* 48(2007): 281–98.

17. K. Newlin, G. D. Melkus, D. Chyun, and V. Jefferson, "The Relationship of Spirituality and Health Outcomes in Black Women with Type 2 Diabetes," *Ethnicity and Disease* 13(2003): 61–68.

18. Harold G. Koenig, "Research on Religion, Spirituality, and Mental Health: A Review," *Canadian Journal of Psychiatry* 54(2009): 283–91.

19. J. Tartaro, L. J. Luecken, and H. E. Gunn, "Exploring Heart and Soul: Effects of Religiosity/Spirituality and Gender on Blood Pressure and Cortisol Stress Responses," *Journal of Health Psychology* 10(2005): 753–66.

20. "An Interview with Larry Dossey," *Tikkun* 15(2000): 11–16.

21. Ibid., 12.

22. Herbert Benson, et al., "Study of the Therapeutic Effects of Intercessory Prayer (STEP) in Cardiac Bypass Patients: A Multicenter Randomized Trial of Uncertainty and Certainty of Receiving Intercessory Prayer," *American Heart Journal* 151(2006): 934–42.

23. P. Wink and M. Dillon, "Religiousness, Spirituality, and Psychosocial Functioning in Late Adulthood: Findings from a Longitudinal Study," *Psychology and Aging* 18(2003): 916–24.

24. A. Etnyre, M. Rauschhuber, I. Gilliland, J. Cook, M. Mahon, D. Allwein, R. Sethness, J. Lowry, and M. E. Jones, "Cardiovascular Risk among Older Hispanic Women: A Pilot Study," *AAOHN Journal* 54(2006): 120–28.

25. R. F. Gillum, "Frequency of Attendance at Religious Services and Cigarette Smoking in American Women and Men: The Third National Health and Nutrition Examination Survey," *Preventive Medicine* 41(2005): 607–13.

26. L. H. Powell, L. Shahabi, and C. E. Thoresen, "Religion and Spirituality: Linkages to Physical Health," *The American Psychologist* 58(2003): 36–52.

27. P. J. Waite, S. R. Hawks, and J. A. Gast, "The Correlation Between Spiritual Well-Being and Health Behaviors," *American Journal of Health Promotion* 13(1999): 159–62.

28. Lydia Strohl, "Faith: The Best Medicine," *The Washingtonian*, December 2000, 63–65, 138–40.

29. Ibid.

30. Bonnie Booth, "More Schools Teaching Spirituality in Medicine," *amednews.com*, 2008. Available at: www.ama-assn .org/amednews/2008/03/10/prsc0310.htm.

31. Patricia M. Barnes, Eve Powell-Griner, Kim McFann, and Richard L. Nahin, "Complementary and Alternative Medicine Use Among Adults: United States, 2002," *Advance Data*, 343(2004): 1.

32. Dixie L. Dennis and Brent G. Dennis, "Spirituality@ Work.Health," *American Journal of Health Education,* 34(2003): 297–301.

33. S. Scott, "A Great Deal for Mall Employees," *Lexington Herald-Leader,* June 8, 2002, E3.

34. Alexander W. Astin, Helen S. Astin, and Jennifer A. Lindholm, "A National Study of Spirituality in Higher Education: Students'

Search For Meaning And Purpose," *Spirituality in Higher Education*, 2010. Available at: http://spirituality.ucla.edu/ findings/.

35. Alexander W. Astin, Helen S. Astin, and Jennifer A. Lindholm, *Cultivating the Spirit: How College Can Enhance Students' Inner Lives* (New York: Jossey-Bass, 2010).

36. E. Band and J. Weisz, "How to Feel Better When It Feels Bad: Children's Perspectives on Coping with Everyday Stress," *Developmental Psychology* 24(1988): 247–53.

37. K. I. Pargament, B. Cole, L. Vandecreek, T. Belavich, C. Brant, and L. Perez, "The Vigil: Religion and the Search for Control in the Hospital Waiting Room," *Journal of Health Psychology* 4(1999): 327–41.

38. C. Carlson, P. Bacaseta, and D. Simanton, "A Controlled Evaluation of Devotional Meditation and Progressive Relaxation," *Journal of Psychology and Theology* 16(1988): 362–68.

39. K. I. Pargament, D. S. Ensing, K. Falgout, H. Olsen, B. Reilly, K. Van Haitsma, and R. Warren, "God Helps Me: Religious Coping Efforts as Predictors of the Outcomes of Significant Negative Life Events," *American Journal of Community Psychology* 18(1990): 793–825.

40. K. I. Pargament, J. Kennel, W. Hathaway, N. Grevengoed, J. Newman, and W. Jones, "Religion and the Problem-Solving Process: Three Styles of Coping," *Journal of the Scientific Study of Religion* 27(1988): 90–104.

41. W. L. Hathaway and K. I. Pargament, "Intrinsic Religiousness, Religious Coping, and Psychological Competence: A Covariance Structure Analysis," *Journal for the Scientific Study of Religion* 29(1992): 423–41.

42. C. Bickel, J. W. Ciarrocchi, W. J. Sheers, B. K. Estadt, D. A. Powell, and K. I. Pargament, "Perceived Stress, Religious Coping Styles, and Depressive Affect," *Journal of Psychology and Christianity* 17(1998): 33–42.

43. P. Pietrini, M. Guazzelli, G. Basso, K. Jaffe, and J. Grafman, "Neural Correlates of Imaginal Aggressive Behavior Assessed by Positron Emission Tomography in Healthy Subjects," *American Journal of Psychiatry* 157(2000): 1772–81.

44. J. W. Berry and E. L. Worthington, "Forgiveness, Relationship Quality, Stress While Imagining Relationship Events, and Physical and Mental Health," *Journal of Counseling Psychology* 48(2001): 447–55.

45. R. Sapolsky, "The Physiology and Pathophysiology of Unhappiness." In E. L. Worthington, *Handbook of Forgiveness* (New York: Brunner-Routledge, 2005), 273–303.

46. C. V. O. Witvliet, T. E. Ludwig, and K. Vander Lann, "Granting Forgiveness or Harboring Grudges: Implications for Emotion, Physiology, and Health," *Psychological Science* 12(2001): 117–23.

47. K. S. Seybold, P. C. Hill, J. K. Neumann, and D. S. Chi, "Physiological and Psychological Correlates of Forgiveness," *Journal of Psychology and Christianity* 20(2001): 250–59.

48. J. W. Berry, E. L. Worthington, L. E. O'Connor, L. Parrot, and N. G. Wade, "Forgiveness, Vengeful Rumination, and Affective Traits," *Journal of Personality* 73(2005): 1–43.

49. L. Temshok and R. L. Wald, "Forgiveness and Health in Persons Living with HIV/AIDS." In E. L. Worthington, *Handbook of Forgiveness* (New York: Brunner-Routledge, 2005), 335–48.

50. J. P. Friedberg, S. Suchday, and V. S. Srinivas, "Relationship between Forgiveness and Psychological and Physiological Indices in Cardiac Patients," *International Journal of Behavioral Medicine* 16(2009): 205–11.

51. K. A. Lawler, J. W. Younger, R. L. Piferi, E. Billington, R. Jobe, K. Edmondson, and W. H. Jones, "A Change of Heart: Cardiovascular Correlates of Forgiveness in Response to Interpersonal Conflict," *Journal of Behavioral Medicine* 26(2003): 373–93.

52. K. A. Lawler, J. W. Younger, R. L. Piferi, R. Jobe, K. Edmondson, and W. H. Jones, "The Unique Effects of Forgiveness on Health: An Exploration of Pathways," *Journal of Behavioral Medicine* 28(2005): 157–67.

53. J. W. Carson, F. J. Keefe, V. Goli, A. M. Fras, T. R. Lynch, S. R. Thorp, and J. L. Buechler, "Forgiveness and Chronic Low Back Pain: A Preliminary Study Examining the Relationship of Forgiveness to Pain, Anger, and Psychological Distress," *Journal of Pain* 6(2005): 84–91.

54. E. L. Worthington, *Handbook of Forgiveness* (New York: Brunner-Routledge, 2005).

55. E. L. Worthington, C. V. Witvliet, P. Pietrini, and A. J. Miller, "Forgiveness, Health, and Well-Being: A Review of Evidence for Emotional Versus Decisional Forgiveness, Dispositional Forgivingness, and Reduced Unforgiveness," *Journal of Behavioral Medicine* 30(2007): 291–302.

56. Everett L. Worthington, Jr., Charlotte vanOyen Witvliet, Andrea J. Lerner, and Michael Scherer, "Forgiveness in Health Research and Medical Practice," *Explore* 1(2005): 169–76.

57. P. A. Mauger, J. E. Perry, T. Freeman, D. C. Grove, A. G. McBride, and K. E. McKinney, "The Measurement of Forgiveness: Preliminary Research," *Journal of Psychology and Christianity* 11(1992): 170–80.

58. K. A. Lawler, J. W. Younger, R. L. Piferi, R. L. Jobe, K. A. Edmondson, and W. H. Jones, "The Unique Effects of Forgiveness on Health: An Exploration of Pathways," *Journal of Behavioral Medicine* 28(2005): 157–67.

59. J. R. Webb and K. Brewer, "Forgiveness, Health, and Problematic Drinking Among College Students in Southern Appalachia," *Journal of Health Psychology* 15(2010): 1257–66.

60. T. Wilson, A. Milosevic, M. Carroll, K. Hart, and S. Hibbard, "Physical Health Status in Relation to Self-Forgiveness and Other-Forgiveness in Healthy College Students," *Journal of Health Psychology* 13(2008): 798–803.

61. J. Exline, A. M. Yali, and M. Lobel, "When God Disappoints: Difficulty Forgiving God and Its Role in Negative Emotion," *Journal of Health Psychology* 4(1999): 365–79.

62. J. N. Sells and T. D. Hargrove, "Forgiveness: A Review of the Theoretical and Empirical Literature," *Journal of Family Therapy* 20(1998): 21–36.

63. R. D. Enright and the Human Development Study Group, "Counseling Within the Forgiveness Triad: On Forgiving, Receiving Forgiveness, and Self-Forgiveness," *Counseling and Values* 40(1996): 107–26.

64. A. Melchior, *National Evaluation of Learn and Serve America School and Community-Based Programs* (Washington, D.C.: The Corporation for National Service, 1997).

65. A. W. Astin, L. J. Sax, and J. Avalos, "Long-Term Effects of Volunteerism During the Undergraduate Years," *Review of Higher Education* 22(1999): 187–202.

66. Corporation for National and Community Service, *Issues Brief: The Health Benefits of Volunteering: A Review of Recent Research*. Washington, DC: Corporation for National and Community Service, 2007. Available at: www.nationalservice.gov/pdf/07_0506_hbr_brief.pdf

67. Office of Disease Prevention and Health Promotion, *Healthy People 2020*. Washington, DC: U. S. Department of Health and Human Services, 2010. Available at: www.healthypeople.gov/.

68. E. Erikson, *Childhood and Society* (New York: Norton, 1963).

69. M. Gafni, "My Unique Pathology," *Tikkun* 15(2000): 8–9.

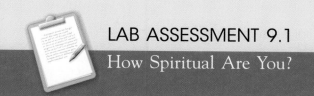

LAB ASSESSMENT 9.1

How Spiritual Are You?

Directions: In today's modern world, with the stressors encountered and the challenges faced, experts argue that spirituality can help. How spiritual are you? To find out, complete the scale below. This is an inventory that measures how spiritual—not necessarily religious—you are. Indicate your response to each statement by circling the appropriate letters using the following scale:

SA = strongly agree

A = agree

AM = agree more than disagree

DM = disagree more than agree

D = disagree

SD = strongly disagree

There is no right or wrong answer. Please respond to what you think or how you feel at this point in time.

1. I have a general sense of belonging.	SA	A	AM	DM	D	SD
2. I am able to forgive people who have done wrong to me.	SA	A	AM	DM	D	SD
3. I have the ability to rise above or go beyond a physical or psychological condition.	SA	A	AM	DM	D	SD
4. I am concerned about destruction of the environment.	SA	A	AM	DM	D	SD
5. I have experienced moments of peace in a devastating event.	SA	A	AM	DM	D	SD
6. I feel a kinship to other people.	SA	A	AM	DM	D	SD
7. I feel a connection to all of life.	SA	A	AM	DM	D	SD
8. I rely on an inner strength in hard times.	SA	A	AM	DM	D	SD
9. I enjoy being of service to others.	SA	A	AM	DM	D	SD
10. I can go to a spiritual dimension within myself for guidance.	SA	A	AM	DM	D	SD
11. I have the ability to rise above or go beyond a body change or body loss.	SA	A	AM	DM	D	SD
12. I have a sense of harmony or inner peace.	SA	A	AM	DM	D	SD
13. I have the ability for self-healing.	SA	A	AM	DM	D	SD
14. I have an inner strength.	SA	A	AM	DM	D	SD
15. The boundaries of my universe extend beyond usual ideas of what space and time are thought to be.	SA	A	AM	DM	D	SD
16. I feel good about myself.	SA	A	AM	DM	D	SD
17. I have a sense of balance in my life.	SA	A	AM	DM	D	SD
18. There is fulfillment in my life.	SA	A	AM	DM	D	SD
19. I feel a responsibility to preserve the planet.	SA	A	AM	DM	D	SD
20. The meaning I have found for my life provides a sense of peace.	SA	A	AM	DM	D	SD
21. Even when I feel discouraged, I trust that life is good.	SA	A	AM	DM	D	SD
22. My life has meaning and purpose.	SA	A	AM	DM	D	SD
23. My innerness or an inner resource helps me deal with uncertainty in my life.	SA	A	AM	DM	D	SD
24. I have discovered my own strength in time of struggle.	SA	A	AM	DM	D	SD
25. Reconciling relationships is important to me.	SA	A	AM	DM	D	SD
26. I feel a part of the community in which I live.	SA	A	AM	DM	D	SD
27. My inner strength is related to a belief in a Higher Power or Supreme Being.	SA	A	AM	DM	D	SD
28. I have goals and aims for my life.	SA	A	AM	DM	D	SD

Scoring: Write alongside each statement, the points assigned for each response:

SD = 1, D = 2, DM = 3, AM = 4, A = 5, SA = 6

This scale also has several subscales. Add up the number of points for the responses you circled for each subscale's statements to obtain a score for that subscale.

Purpose and meaning in life (searching for events or relationships that provide a sense of worth, hope, or reason for living):
Statements: 18, 20, 22, 28

Innerness or inner resources (striving for wholeness, identity, and sense of empowerment):
Statements: 8, 10, 12, 14, 16, 17, 23, 24, 27

Unifying interconnectedness (feeling of relatedness or attachment to others and with the universe):
Statements: 1, 2, 4, 6, 7, 9, 19, 25, 26

Transcendence (ability to reach or go beyond the limits of usual experience):
Statements: 3, 5, 11, 13, 15, 21

If your total scale score is over 84, you tend to be a spiritual person. The higher your score, the more spiritual you are. To interpret your subscale scores, multiply the number of items in the subscale by 3. If your subscale score is above that number, you evidence that factor. The closer to the multiple of 3 times the number of total items in that subscale, the more you evidence that factor.

Source: J. W. Howden, *Spirituality Assessment Scale* (Corsicana, TX: Judy W. Howden, 1992).

LAB ASSESSMENT 9.2

How Forgiving Are You?

Directions: In the course of our lives negative things may occur because of our own actions, the actions of others, or circumstances beyond our control. For some time after these events, we may have negative thoughts or feelings about ourselves, others, or the situation. Think about how you typically respond to such negative events. Next to each of the following items write the number (from the 7-point scale below) that best describes how you typically respond to the type of negative situation described. There are no right or wrong answers. Please be as open as possible in your answers.

1	2	3	4	5	6	7
Almost Always False of Me		More Often False of Me		More Often True of Me		Almost Always True of Me

_____ 1. Although I feel bad at first when I mess up, over time I can give myself some slack.

_____ 2. I hold grudges against myself for negative things I've done.

_____ 3. Learning from bad things that I've done helps me get over them.

_____ 4. It is really hard for me to accept myself once I've messed up.

_____ 5. With time I am understanding of myself for mistakes I've made.

_____ 6. I don't stop criticizing myself for negative things I've felt, thought, said, or done.

_____ 7. I continue to punish a person who has done something that I think is wrong.

_____ 8. With time I am understanding of others for the mistakes they've made.

_____ 9. I continue to be hard on others who have hurt me.

_____ 10. Although others have hurt me in the past, I have eventually been able to see them as good people.

_____ 11. If others mistreat me, I continue to think badly of them.

_____ 12. When someone disappoints me, I can eventually move past it.

_____ 13. When things go wrong for reasons that can't be controlled, I get stuck in negative thoughts about it.

_____ 14. With time I can be understanding of bad circumstances in my life.

_____ 15. If I am disappointed by uncontrollable circumstances in my life, I continue to think negatively about them.

_____ 16. I eventually make peace with bad situations in my life.

_____ 17. It's really hard for me to accept negative situations that aren't anybody's fault.

_____ 18. Eventually I let go of negative thoughts about bad circumstances that are beyond anyone's control.

Scoring: To calculate the scores for the Heartland Forgiveness Scale, first reverse score items 2, 4, 6, 7, 9, 11, 13, 15, and 17. Then, sum the values for the items that compose the total scale and each subscale (with appropriate items being reverse scored):

		Your Score
HFS total:	Items 1–18	_____
HFS Self subscale:	Items 1–6	_____
HFS Other subscale:	Items 7–12	_____
HFS Situation subscale:	Items 13–18	_____

Interpretation of Scores: Mean scores for the total HFS and its subscales are—

Total HFS:	92
HFS Self:	31
HFS Other:	30
HFS Situation:	31

Your **Total HFS** score indicates how forgiving you tend to be of yourself, other people, and uncontrollable situations. Higher scores indicate higher levels of forgiveness, and lower scores indicate lower levels of forgiveness.

- Scores of 18 to 54: You are usually unforgiving of yourself, others, and uncontrollable situations.

- Scores of 55 to 89: You are about as likely to forgive, as not to forgive yourself, others, and uncontrollable situations.

- Scores of 90 to 126: You are usually forgiving of yourself, others, and uncontrollable situations.

Your **Forgiveness of Self Subscale** indicates how forgiving you tend to be of yourself, with higher scores indicating higher levels of forgiveness, and lower scores indicating lower levels of forgiveness.

- Scores of 6 to 18: You are usually unforgiving of yourself.
- Scores of 19 to 29: You are about as likely to forgive yourself as you are not to forgive yourself.
- Scores of 30 to 42: You are usually forgiving of yourself.

Your **Forgiveness of Others Subscale** indicates how forgiving you tend to be of other people, with higher scores indicating higher levels of forgiveness, and lower scores indicating lower levels of forgiveness.

- Scores of 6 to 18: You are usually unforgiving of other people.
- Scores of 19 to 29: You are about as likely to forgive others as you are not to forgive others.
- Scores of 30 to 42: You are usually forgiving of other people.

Your **Forgiveness of Situations Subscale** indicates how forgiving you tend to be of negative circumstances, events, or situations that are beyond your control (such as an illness or a natural disaster). Higher scores indicate higher levels of forgiveness, and lower scores indicate lower levels of forgiveness.

- Scores of 6 to 18: You are usually unforgiving of uncontrollable situations.
- Scores of 19 to 29: You are about as likely to forgive uncontrollable situations as you are not to forgive uncontrollable situations.
- Scores of 30 to 42: You are usually forgiving of uncontrollable situations.

Source: Yamhure Thompson L., C. R. Snyder, L. Hoffmany, S. T. Michael, H. N. Rasmussen, L. S. Billings, et al., "Dispositional Forgiveness of Self, Others, and Situations," *Journal of Personality* 73(2005): 313–360.

General Applications
Relaxation Techniques

Before you begin Part 3, some instructions are necessary. Part 3 describes relaxation techniques: meditation, autogenic training, progressive relaxation, biofeedback, yoga, and others. A description of each technique, its historical development, how to do it, and its benefits are presented. Remember, these relaxation techniques are but one part of a comprehensive stress management program. Relaxation techniques relate to the level of emotional arousal on the stress model and serve as interventions between stress and illness and disease. Because you will learn how to do each technique, two additional comments need to be made.

Medical Caution

First, relaxation techniques result in changes in physiological processes. We've already seen that the relaxation response is a hypometabolic state of lowered blood pressure, heart rate, muscle tension, and serum cholesterol, with other physiological parameters being affected. Those of you using medication that is designed to affect, or that incidentally affects, a physiological parameter might be affecting that parameter too much if you engage in relaxation techniques. For example, a person with high blood pressure who is taking medication to lower the blood pressure might lower it too much if relaxation training is added to the medication. It is because of these changes in physiological processes that people who are thinking of beginning relaxation training and are under medical care or taking medication are advised to get the permission of the medical specialist supervising their care *prior* to practicing relaxation skills. In particular, those with heart conditions, epilepsy, hypertension, diabetes, and psychological problems should obtain medical permission to begin relaxation training.

Relaxation Technique Trials

Second, the opportunity to try several different relaxation techniques is designed to help you find one that you prefer and will use regularly. To structure your evaluation of these techniques so you can decide which one is best for you, use the Lab Assessment rating scale that appears at the conclusion of each chapter. Although we do not have enough research to recommend a specific relaxation technique for you, we do have guidelines when recommending relaxation techniques for your specific condition. For example, if you have a cognitive issue—such as social anxiety or low self-esteem—techniques that focus on the mind are more effective. These are termed *mind-to-muscle* relaxation techniques and include meditation and autogenic training. On the other hand, if you have a physical issue—such as tension headaches or TMJ syndrome—techniques that focus on the body are more effective. These are termed *muscle-to-mind* relaxation techniques and include progressive relaxation and yoga. The relaxation rating scale should help you determine which relaxation technique is most suited to your needs.

To use the rating scale in the lab assessments, it is best to practice each technique for at least one week (the longer, the better). Your inner environment may change from day to day (e.g., you may eat different foods at different times of the day) and your outer environment is never constant (temperature, outside noises, and quality of the air vary), so a one-day trial of one relaxation technique compared with a one-day trial of another will not allow for a valid comparison. Also, practice the technique as recommended—correct posture, frequency, time of day, type of environment—and make your practice consistent with other suggestions. After a sufficient trial period, answer each of the questions in the Lab Assessment; then sum up the point values you gave each answer. The lower the total point value is, the more that relaxation technique fits you.

10 Meditation

Meditation requires an object of focus. That can be a word (or mantra), your breathing, or a geometric shape such as the mandala shown here.

Y ou may know that some meditators wear muslin robes, burn incense, shave their hair, and believe in the Far Eastern religions. You should also know that these things are *not required* in order to benefit from meditative practice. Although wine may be a part of a Catholic religious service, not all those who drink wine embrace Catholicism. Similarly, not all those who meditate need adopt a particular religion.

What Is Meditation?

Meditation is a mind-to-muscle relaxation technique that uses an object of focus to clear the mind, thereby resulting in beneficial physiological and psychological changes. Just as physical exercise has certain psychological benefits, meditation has certain physical benefits, as we shall soon see. The purpose of meditation is to gain control over your attention so that you can choose what to focus upon rather than being subject to the unpredictable ebb and flow of environmental circumstances.

Meditation has its tradition grounded in Eastern cultures (e.g., those of India and Tibet) but has been popularized for Western cultures. The major exporter of meditation to the Western world has been the Maharishi Mahesh Yogi. The Maharishi developed a large, worldwide, and highly effective organization to teach **transcendental meditation (TM)** to a population of people experiencing more and more stress and recognizing the need for more and more of an escape. The simplicity of this technique, coupled with the effectiveness of its marketing by TM organizations, quickly led to its popularity. In a short time, in spite of an initial fee of $125 (significantly higher now), large numbers of people learned and began regular practice of TM (10,000 persons were joining the program each month during the early 1970s in the United States).

The Maharishi's background is interesting in itself. Mahest Prasod Varma (his name at birth) was born in 1918 and earned a degree in physics in 1942 from Allahabad University in India. Before he began practicing his profession, however, he met and eventually studied under a religious leader, Swami Brahmananda Saraswati. Thirteen years of religious study later, he was assigned the task of finding a simple form of meditation that everyone could readily learn. It took two years of isolated life in a Himalayan cave to develop TM, which he later spread via mass communication, advertising, and the Students International Meditation Society.

Types of Meditation

Transcendental meditation is but one form of meditative practice. Chakra yoga, Rinzai Zen, Mudra yoga, Sufism, Zen meditation, and Soto Zen are examples of other meditative systems. In Soto Zen meditation, common external objects (e.g., flowers or a peaceful landscape) are focused upon. Tibetan Buddhists use a **mandala**—a geometric figure with other geometric forms on it that has spiritual or philosophical importance—to meditate upon. Imagined sounds (thunder or a beating drum), termed **nadam,** and a silently repeated word, termed **mantra,** have also been used. Rinzai Zen meditation uses **koans** (unanswerable, illogical riddles); Zazen focuses on subjective states of consciousness; Hindu meditation employs **pranayama** (prana means "life force" and refers to breathing); and Zen practitioners have been known to focus on **anapanasati** (counting breaths from one to ten repetitively).[1] There is also a revival of the centuries-old traditional Jewish meditation. This form of meditation does not require a belief in the traditional God or membership in a synagogue. Instead, it involves focusing on repetitive prayer, receiving the light of the divine with each breath, or chanting.[2] There is even a Jewish Meditation Center in Brooklyn, New York (www.jmcbrooklyn.org).

Regardless of the type of meditation, however, one of two approaches is used: opening up of attention or focusing of attention. Opening up your attention requires a nonjudgmental attitude: You allow all external and internal stimuli to enter your awareness without trying to use these stimuli in any particular manner. As with a blotter (the inner self) and ink (the external and internal stimuli), everything is just absorbed. When the meditative method requires the focusing of attention, the object focused upon is something either repetitive (e.g., a word or phrase repeated in your mind) or something unchanging (e.g., a spot on the wall).

To understand the two basic methods of meditation, place an object in the center of your room. Try to get an object at least as high as your waist. Come on now. Your tendency will be to rush to get this chapter read rather than get the most out of it. Remember that people with the Type A behavior pattern, those most prone to coronary heart disease, rush through tasks rather than doing them well. Slow down. Get that object, and continue reading.

Now, look at that object for about five seconds. Most likely, you saw and focused upon the object while excluding the other stimuli in your field of vision. Behind the object (in your field of vision) might have been a wall, a window, a table, or maybe a poster. In spite of the presence of these other visual stimuli, you can put them in the background, ignore them, and focus your attention on one object. The object of focus is called the *figure,* and the objects in the background of your field of vision are called the *ground.* When you see and listen to a lecturer, you probably focus upon that person and his or her voice. You choose to place objects other than the lecturer in the background, as well as sounds other than the lecturer's voice. You may even be doing that now. As you read this book, you may be hearing your inner voice recite the words while placing in the background other sounds (the heating or cooling system, people and cars outside, birds chirping, or airplanes flying overhead).

Focusing-of-attention meditation is similar to focusing on the figure while excluding the ground. Opening-up-of-attention meditation blends the figure and ground together so they are one and the same.

Benefits of Meditation

Because it is so popular and can be learned quickly and easily, meditation has been one of the most researched of the relaxation techniques. The research findings evidence the physiological and psychological effects of meditation. These findings follow. However, the shortcomings of generalizing results about relaxation techniques should be recognized. For example, even though we state findings about meditation, there are many different types of meditation. Findings for different types may differ. Sometimes the level of motivation of the research subjects can affect the results obtained. The experience of the meditators has also been found to affect results (those with at least six months' experience differ from novice meditators). In spite of these limitations, though, there are some things we can say about the effects of meditation.

nadam
Imagined sounds used as the object of focus during meditation.

mantra
A word used as the object of focus during meditation.

koans
Unanswerable, illogical riddles used as the object of focus during meditation.

pranayama
A Hindu practice that involves breathing as the object of focus during meditation.

anapanasati
A Zen practice that involves counting breaths as the object of focus during meditation.

Meditation involves focusing on something that is repetitive—like this flame—or unchanging.

One can meditate to the recurring sounds of the surf coming ashore or to pleasant sounds recorded earlier and replayed at a later time. Even though the surf may be preferable for most people, noisy and crowded beaches may necessitate the use of taped music or relaxing sounds to drown out disturbing and distracting sounds. There are many innovative ways to create an environment conducive to relaxation.

Physiological Effects

The physiological effects of meditation were discovered by early research on Indian yogis and Zen masters. In 1946, Therese Brosse found that Indian yogis could control their heart rates.[3] Another study of Indian yogis found that they could slow respiration (four to six breaths per minute), decrease by 70 percent their ability to conduct an electrical current (galvanic skin response), emit predominantly alpha brain waves, and slow their heart rate to twenty-four beats fewer than normal.[4] Other early studies of yogis and Zen meditators have reported similar results.[5,6]

More recently, researchers have verified the extraordinary ability of yogis to adjust their bodies into a hypometabolic state. For example, when researchers connected electrodes to a professional yogi, they found he was able to limit his breathing to one breath per minute for an hour.[7] Other researchers verified the ability of a yoga master to feel no pain. They used magnetic resonance imaging (MRI) and magnetoencephalography (to see brain function) and found the yogi altered two parts of the brain most responsible for pain (the insula and the cingulated cortex).[8] In another study, when a yogi was connected to electrodes and his tongue was pierced, he induced a state the researchers described as similar to individuals under analgesia.[9]

Studies have verified the physiological effects of meditation.[10] Allison compared the respiration rate of a subject meditating with that subject's respiration rate while watching television and while reading a book. Respiration rate decreased most while meditating (from twelve and one-half breaths per minute to seven).[11] The decrease in respiration rate as a result of meditation is a consistent finding across research studies.[12,13]

Several researchers have found a decrease in muscle tension associated with meditation. In one study by Arambula et al., and another by Luskin et al., the decrease in muscle tension in meditators was significantly greater than that experienced by a control group of nonmeditators.[14,15]

The decrease in heart rate found by early studies on Indian yogis has also been verified in more recent studies. When meditators and nonmeditators were physiologically stimulated by viewing a film on laboratory accidents, the meditators' heart rates returned to normal sooner than the nonmeditators' heart rates.[16]

Galvanic skin response—the ability of skin to conduct an electrical current—differs between meditators and nonmeditators. The lower the conductance is, the less stress. These skin electrical conductance findings led researchers to conclude that meditators are better able to cope with stress and have more stable autonomic nervous systems.[17]

Meditation has been found to have profound effects on the brain. With the use of electroencephalograms to actually measure brain function, meditators have demonstrated the ability to "switch off irrelevant brain networks for the maintenance of focused internalized attention and inhibition of inappropriate information."[18] Electroencephalograms have also verified that meditators can change the brain waves they emit, thereby lowering their heart rates.[19]

Meditation has been demonstrated to have positive effects on blood pressure and the prevention of hypertension,[20,21] lowering baseline cortisol,[22,23] even affecting the aging process. Researchers suggest "that meditation may have salutary effects on telomere length by reducing cognitive stress and stress arousal and increasing positive states of mind and hormonal factors that may promote telomere maintenance."[24]

Much of the research discussed so far was given impetus by the work of Robert Keith Wallace. Wallace was one of the first modern researchers to study the effects of meditation scientifically. In his initial study and in his subsequent work with Herbert Benson, Wallace showed that meditation resulted in decreased oxygen consumption, heart rate, and alpha brain-wave emissions. He also demonstrated that meditation increased skin resistance, decreased blood lactate (thought to be associated with lessened anxiety) and carbon dioxide production, and increased the peripheral blood flow to arms and legs.[25,26]

There is ample evidence, therefore, that meditation results in specific physiological changes that differ from those produced by other relaxation techniques (reading, watching television, sleeping). These changes are termed the **relaxation response (trophotropic response)** and are thought to have beneficial effects upon one's health.

Psychological Effects

At this point, you realize that the mind cannot be separated from the body. Consequently, you've probably guessed that the physiological effects of meditation have psychological implications. You are right. Numerous studies have found evidence that the psychological health of meditators is better than that of nonmeditators.

For example, meditators have been found to be less anxious.[27,28] Even more significant than this, however, is the finding that anxiety can be decreased by teaching people to meditate. Schoolchildren decreased their test anxiety after 18 weeks of meditation training.[29] Several other studies have shown that people's trait and state anxiety levels decreased after they practiced meditation for varying periods of time.[30] Even students who experienced test anxiety have found meditation to relax them more.[31]

In addition to its effect of decreasing anxiety, researchers have found that meditation is related to an internal locus of control, greater self-actualization, more positive feelings after encountering a stressor, improvement in sleep behavior, decreased cigarette smoking, headache relief, and a general state of positive mental health. Even eating disorders have been found positively affected by meditation. In a study of eighteen obese women taught meditation, binge eating decreased, anxiety decreased, and a sense of control increased.[32,33]

More recently, meditation has been demonstrated to increase attention[34,35] and to be effective in treating drug addiction.[36,37] Meditation has also been found effective in improving the care of people with schizophrenia[38] and in the prevention of suicide.[39] I will now teach *you* how to meditate. In that way, you might be able to decrease your oxygen consumption and blood lactate level, change other physiological parameters, and be less anxious and more self-actualized. Are you ready?

relaxation response
The physiological state achieved when one is relaxed; also called the trophotropic response.

trophotropic response
The physiological state achieved when one is relaxed; also called the relaxation response.

How to Meditate

Although meditation was founded in Far Eastern cultures, it has significant health implications for Westerners.

Meditation is best learned in a relatively quiet, comfortable environment. However, once you become experienced, you will be able to meditate almost anywhere. As I've already mentioned, I've meditated in the passenger seat of a moving automobile in Florida, on an airplane in flight to California, in my office at the University of Maryland, and under a tree on a golf course in the Bahamas. Of course, the quiet, serene setting of the golf course was the most preferred, but the others sufficed.

Once you have located a quiet place to learn meditation, find a comfortable chair. Because sleep is a different physiological state than meditation, you will not get the benefits of meditation if you fall asleep. To help prevent yourself from falling asleep, use a straight-backed chair. This type of chair encourages you to align your spine and requires only a minimum of muscular contraction to keep you erect (though not stiff). If you can find a chair that will support your upper back and head, all the better.

Be seated in this chair with your buttocks pushed against its back, feet slightly forward of your knees, and your hands resting either on the arms of the chair or in your lap.

Let your muscles relax as best you can. Don't *try* to relax. Trying is work, not relaxation. Just assume a passive attitude in which you focus upon your breathing. Allow whatever happens to happen. If you feel relaxed, fine; if not, accept that, too.

Next, close your eyes and repeat in your mind the word "one" every time you inhale and the word "two" every time you exhale. Do not consciously alter or control your breathing; breathe regularly. Continue to do this for 20 minutes. It is recommended that you meditate twice a day for approximately 20 minutes each time.

Last, when you stop meditating, give your body a chance to become readjusted to normal routines. Open your eyes gradually, first focusing on one object in the room, then focusing upon several objects. Take several deep breaths. Then stretch while seated and, when you feel ready, stand and stretch. If you rush to leave the meditation session, you are apt to feel tired or to lose the sense of relaxation. Your blood pressure and heart rate are decreased while meditating, thus rising from the chair too quickly might make you dizzy and is not recommended.

Although you shouldn't experience any problems, if you feel uncomfortable or dizzy, or if you experience hallucinations or disturbing images, just open your eyes and stop meditating. These situations are rare but occasionally do occur. Here are several more recommendations:

1. Immediately upon rising and right before dinner tend to be good times to meditate. Do not meditate directly after a meal. After eating, the blood is pooled in the stomach area, participating in the digestive process. Since part of the relaxation response is an increased blood flow to the arms and legs, pooled blood in the abdomen is not conducive to relaxation. It is for this reason that you should meditate *before* breakfast and *before* dinner.

2. The object of meditation is to bring about a hypometabolic state. Because caffeine is a stimulant and is included in coffee, tea, cola, and some other soft drinks, and because you do not want to be stimulated but rather to relax, you should not ingest these substances before meditating. Likewise, you should avoid smoking cigarettes (which contain the stimulant nicotine) or using other stimulant drugs.

3. I'm often asked "What do I do with my head?" Well, do whatever you want to do with it. Some people prefer to keep it directly above the neck, others rest it against a high-backed chair, and still others let their chins drop onto

their chests. If you choose the last position, you may experience some discomfort in your neck or shoulder muscles for several meditation sessions. This is because these muscles may not be flexible enough; for the same reason, some of you can't touch your toes without bending your knees. With stretching, these muscles will acquire greater flexibility and will not result in any discomfort when the head hangs forward.

4. Another question I'm often asked is "How do I know when 20 minutes are up?" The answer is so simple I'm usually embarrassed to give it: look at your watch. If 20 minutes are up, stop meditating; if not, continue. Although you don't want to interrupt your meditation every couple of minutes to look at your watch, once or twice when you think the time has expired will not affect your experience. An interesting observation I have noted is that, after a while, you acquire a built-in alarm and will know when 20 minutes have gone by.

5. Whatever you do, do not set an alarm clock to go off after 20 minutes. Your body will be in a hypometabolic state, and a loud sound may startle you too much. Similarly, disconnect the telephone or take the receiver off the hook so it doesn't ring. If the phone goes off, you'll go off.

6. You will not be able to focus on your breathing to the exclusion of other thoughts for very long. You will find yourself thinking of problems, anticipated experiences, and other sundry matters. This is normal. However, when you do realize you are thinking and not focusing on your breathing, gently—without feeling as though you've done something wrong—go back to repeating the word "one" on each inhalation and the word "two" on each exhalation.

7. I'm flabbergasted by people who decide to meditate for 20 minutes and then try to rush through it. They breathe quickly, fidget around a lot, and too

Meditation Tips

- Find a quiet place.
- With your eyes closed, repeat a relaxing word (mantra) in your mind each time you exhale.
- Repeat the mantra for approximately 20 minutes, twice a day.
- Do not meditate after ingesting a stimulant (for example, caffeine or nicotine).
- Meditate before meals.
- Look at your watch or a clock to know when 20 minutes have elapsed.
- Limit distractions when learning how to meditate.
- Unplug telephones, put cell phones on vibrate or turn them off, and do not set an alarm clock.
- Let your head do whatever is comfortable.
- Do not try to "rush" through the 20 minutes.
- Assume a passive attitude. That is, do not "try" to relax.
- Allow whatever sensations are experienced to occur without evaluating or taking note of them.

often open their eyes to look at their watches in the hope that the 20 minutes have passed. During their meditations, they're planning their days and working out their problems. They'd be better off solving their problems and meditating later. Once you commit yourself to time to meditate, relax and benefit from it. Twenty minutes are twenty minutes! You can't speed it up! Relax and enjoy it. Your problems will be there to greet you later. Don't worry, they're not going anywhere. You won't lose them. The only thing you'll do, perhaps, is to perceive them as less distressing after meditating than before.

Other Types of Meditation

There are many other types of meditation. For example, *Heart Rhythm Meditation*[40] is designed to pull the richness of the universe into the person, and anchor it in the heart. This is accomplished by experiencing all emotion, simultaneously, which requires and causes expanded emotional capacity. Chanting allows attention to focus on the heart, with the rationale that turning on the heart is easier than turning off the mind.

Consciousness Meditation[41] seeks to shut down the distinction between the self and other so that the boundary between self and other dissolves. The rationale is that this boundary is an illusion. The analogy drawn is to the stars and the sky. Both are always present, although one is seen during the night and the other during the day. So it is with self and others. At the point where the personal identity dissolves, the sense of oneness with all occurs.

More mainstream than these forms of meditation is *Secular Meditation,* or the *Relaxation Response,* developed by Herbert Benson.[42] Benson proposed that neither religion nor philosophy need be a part of the meditation experience, and that a state of relaxation could be achieved following a few simple procedures. Benson instructs meditators to repeat the word "one" in his or her mind with each rhythmic breath out. Benson stated that Secular Meditation requires four requisites:

1. *A quiet environment.* Distractions interfere with the ability to focus on the object of meditation. Therefore, a quiet room or other location is required.

2. *An object of focus.* Benson suggests the word *one* as a focus, thereby precluding focusing on disturbing or stressful thoughts.

3. *A passive attitude. Trying* to make relaxation happen only interferes with it occurring. Benson instructs meditators to focus on the word *one* and accept whatever develops.

4. *A comfortable position.* Although Benson never identified a specific body position when meditating, he did state that it is important to be comfortable so relaxation can occur.

Making Time for Meditation

Meditation can be quite pleasing and can help you better manage the stress in your life—but you have to *do* it. I have known men and women who have told me they see the benefits of meditating but can't get the time or the place to meditate. Either the kids are bothering them or their roommates are inconsiderate. They say they don't have the 40 minutes a day to spare. I unsympathetically tell them that, if they don't have the time, they really need to meditate, and if they can't find a quiet place in which to spend 20 minutes, they are the ones who need to meditate the most. The time is always available, although some of us choose to use our time for activities holding a higher priority for us. If you really value your health, you'll find the time to do healthy things. The place is available, too. As I've already said,

I have left my wife, two children, and parents in my parents' apartment and sat in my car in the indoor parking garage, meditating. My health and well-being were that important to me. How important are your health and well-being to you?

If you want a more structured approach to meditation to help you get started, read *Insight Meditation*[43] by Sharon Salzberg and Joseph Goldstein. That book outlines a several-week program, taking the reader through various meditative exercises.

To assess the effects of meditation on you, complete Lab 10.1 at the end of this chapter.

Coping in Today's World

Evidence supports the view that meditation has profound effects on the brain and, consequently, awareness. Studying Buddhist monks who were long-term meditators, researchers found "electroencephalographic, high-amplitude gamma-based oscillations and phase synchrony during meditation."[a] The meaning of these changes in brain activation indicates that the brain can be trained with practice to be more coordinated, similar to training the body by physical activity. This is a change in understanding of the brain. Previously it was thought that connections in the brain were determined early in life and could not be altered. Now, brain researchers speak of *neuroplasticity,* the brain's ability to grow and develop and create new connections throughout one's life. And mental training through meditation appears to be one way to develop this capacity.

So, you can cope with today's stressors better by training your brain through regular practice of meditation.

[a]A. Lutz, L. L. Greischar, N. B. Rawlings, M. Ricard, and R. J. Davidson, "Long-Term Meditators Self-Induce High-Amplitude Gamma Synchrony During Mental Practice," *Proceedings of the National Academy of Sciences* 101 (2004): 16369–373.

summary

- Meditation is a simple mental exercise designed to gain control over your attention so you can choose what to focus upon.

- Meditation involves focusing upon either something repetitive (such as a word repeated in your mind) or something unchanging (such as a spot on the wall).

- There are different types of meditation. Some types use external objects to focus upon, others employ a geometric figure called a mandala, and others use silently repeated words or sounds.

- Meditation has been used in the treatment of muscle tension, anxiety, drug abuse, and hypertension. It lowers blood pressure, heart and respiratory rates, and the skin's electrical conductance, and it increases the blood flow to the arms and legs.

- Meditation has been found to have several beneficial psychological effects. It can help alleviate anxiety and is related to an internal locus of control, greater self-

actualization, improvement in sleep, decreased cigarette smoking, headache relief, and a general state of positive mental health.

- To learn to meditate, you need a quiet place. Sit in a straight-backed chair and in your mind repeat the word "one" when you inhale and the word "two" when you exhale with your eyes closed. These words should be repeated each time you breathe, and this should continue for 20 minutes.

- For meditation to be effective, you need to practice it regularly. It is recommended that you avoid consciously altering your breathing, forcing yourself to relax, or coming out of a meditative state too abruptly. Since digestion inhibits peripheral blood flow, it is best to meditate before eating in the morning and evening.

- Meditation's effectiveness is hindered by the administration of stimulants. Stimulants such as nicotine in cigarettes and caffeine in coffee, tea, and some soft drinks will interfere with the trophotropic (relaxation) response.

internet resources

Learning Meditation **www.learningmeditation.com/** *A website devoted to teaching how to meditate, the benefits of meditation, and offers readings and CDs to help people relax.*

The Transcendental Meditation Program **www.tm.org/** *Discusses what transcendental meditation is, its benefits, how to learn transcendental meditation, and how transcendental meditation differs from other meditation practices.*

The World Wide Online Meditation Center **www .meditationcenter.com/** *Presents a definition and uses of meditation, guidelines for getting started, shows how to engage in mindfulness meditation, describes a meditation for sending healing energy directly to an affected area, and presents several easy and effective techniques for staying in one's calm center in daily life.*

references

1. Rolf Gates and Katrina Kenison, *Meditations from the Mat: Daily Reflections on the Path of Yoga* (Peterborough, Canada: Anchor Books, 2002).

2. Jeff Roth, *Jewish Meditation Practices for Everyday Life: Awakening Your Heart, Connecting with God* (Woodstock, VT: Jewish Lights Publishing, 2009).

3. Therese Brosse, "A Psychophysiological Study of Yoga," *Main Currents in Modern Thought* 4(1946): 77–84.

4. B. K. Bagchi and M. A. Wengor, "Electrophysiological Correlates of Some Yogi Exercises." In *Electroencephalography, Clinical Neurophysiology and Epilepsy*, vol. 3 of the First International Congress of Neurological Sciences, ed. L. van Bagaert and J. Radermecker (London: Pergamon, 1959).

5. B. K. Anand, G. S. Chhina, and B. Singh, "Some Aspects of Electroencephalographic Studies in Yogis," *Electroencephalography and Clinical Neurophysiology* 13(1961): 452–56.

6. A. Kasamatsu and T. Hirai, "Studies of EEG's of Expert Zen Meditators," *Folia Psychiatrica Neurologica Japonica* 28(1966): 315.

7. M. Miyamura, K. Nishimura, K. Ishida, K. Katayama, M. Shimaoka, and S. Hiruta, "Is Man Able to Breathe Once a Minute for an Hour? The Effect of Yoga Respiration on Blood Gases," *Japanese Journal of Physiology* 52(2002): 313–16.

8. R. Kakigi, H. Nakata, K. Inui, N. Hiroe, O. Nagata, M. Honda, S. Tanaka, N. Sadato, and M. Kawakami, "Intracerebral Pain Processing in a Yoga Master Who Claims Not to Feel Pain During Meditation," *European Journal of Pain* 9(2005): 581–89.

9. E. Peper, V. E. Wilson, J. Gunkelman, M. Kawakami, M. Sata, W. Barton, and J. Johnston, "Tongue Piercing by a Yogi: QEEG Observations," *Applied Psychophysiology and Biofeedback* 31(2006): 331–38.

10. R. P. Brown and P. L. Gerbarg, "Sudarshan Kriya Yogic Breathing in the Treatment of Stress, Anxiety, and Depression: Part II—Clinical Applications and Guidelines," *Journal of Alternative and Complementary Medicine* 11(2005): 711–17.

11. J. Allison, "Respiratory Changes During Transcendental Meditation," *Lancet,* no. 7651(1970): 833–34.

12. W. E. Mehling, K. A. Hamel, M. Acree, N. Byl, and F. M. Hecht, "Randomized, Controlled Trial of Breath Therapy for Patients with Chronic Low-Back Pain," *Alternative Therapies in Health and Medicine* 11(2005): 44–52.

13. R. Vyas and N. Dikshit, "Effect of Meditation on Respiratory System, Cardiovascular System and Lipid Profile," *Indian Journal of Physiological Pharmacology* 46(2002): 487–91.

14. P. Arambula, E. Peper, M. Kawakami, and K. H. Gibney, "The Physiological Correlates of Kundalini Yoga Meditation: A Study of a Yoga Master," *Applied Psychophysiology and Biofeedback* 26(2001): 147–53.

15. F. M. Luskin, K. A. Newell, M. Griffith, M. Holmes, S. Telles, E. DiNucci, F. F. Marvasti, M. Hill, K. R. Pelletier, and W. L. Haskell, "A Review of Mind/Body Therapies in the Treatment of Musculoskeletal Disorders with Implications for the Elderly," *Alternative Therapies in Health and Medicine* 6(2000): 46–56.

16. L. I. Aftanas and S. A. Golocheikine, "Impact of Regular Meditation Practice on EEG Activity at Rest and During Evoked Negative Emotions," *International Journal of Neuroscience* 115(2005): 893–909.

17. M. J. Ott, "Mindfulness Meditation: A Path of Transformation and Healing," *Journal of Psychosocial Nursing and Mental Health Services* 42(2004): 22–29.

18. L. I. Aftanas and S. A. Golocheikine, "Non-linear Dynamic Complexity of the Human EEG During Meditation," *Neuroscience Letters* 330(2002): 143–46.

19. Y. Kubota, W. Sato, M. Toichi, T. Murai, T. Okada, A. Hayashi, and A. Sengoku, "Frontal Midline Theta Rhythm Is Correlated with Cardiac Autonomic Activities During the Performance of an Attention Demanding Meditation Procedure," *Brain Research, Cognitive Brain Research* 11(2001): 281–87.

20. S. Rosenzweig, D. K. Reibel, J. M. Greeson, J. S. Edman, S. A. Jasser, K. D. McMearty, and B. J. Goldstein, "Mindfulness-Based Stress Reduction is Associated with Improved Glycemic Control in Type 2 Diabetes Mellitus: A Pilot Study," *Alternative Therapies in Health and Medicine* 13(2007): 36–38.

21. S. I. Nidich, M. V. Rainforth, D. A. Haaga, J. Hagelin, J. W. Salerno, F. Travis, M. Tanner, C. Gaylord-King, S. Grosswald, and R. H. Schneider, "A Randomized Controlled Trial on Effects of the Transcendental Meditation Program on Blood Pressure, Psychological Distress, and Coping in Young Adults," *American Journal of Hypertension* (2009). Online ahead of print at www.nature.com/ajh/journal/vaop/ncurrent/abs/ajh2009184a.html

22. L. Witek-Janusek, K. Albuquerque, K. R. Chroniak, C. Chroniak, R. Durazo-Arvizu, and H. L. Mathews, "Effect of Mindfulness Based Stress Reduction on Immune Function, Quality of Life and Coping in Women Newly Diagnosed with Early Stage Breast Cancer," *Brain, Behavior, and Immunity* 22(2008): 969–81.

23. L. E. Carlson, M. Speca, K. D. Patel, and E. Goodey, "Mindfulness-Based Stress Reduction in Relation to Quality of Life, Mood, Symptoms of Stress, and Immune Parameters in Breast and Prostate Cancer Outpatients," *Psychosomatic Medicine* 65(2003): 571–81.

24. E. Epel, J. Daubenmier, J. T. Moskowitz, S. Folkman, and E. Blackburn, "Can Meditation Slow Rate of Cellular Aging? Cognitive Stress, Mindfulness, and Telomeres," *Annals of the New York Academy of Sciences* 1172(2009): 34–53.

25. Robert Keith Wallace, "Physiological Effects of Transcendental Meditation," *Science* 167(1970): 1751–54.

26. Robert Keith Wallace and Herbert Benson, "The Physiology of Meditation," *Scientific American* 226(1972): 84–90.

27. Tony Toneatto and Linda Nguyen, "Does Mindfulness Meditation Improve Anxiety and Mood Symptoms? A Review of the Controlled Research," *The Canadian Journal of Psychiatry* 52(2007): 260–66.

28. A. Finucane and S. W. Mercer, "An Exploratory Mixed Methods Study of the Acceptability and Effectiveness of Mindfulness-based Cognitive Therapy for Patients with Active Depression and Anxiety in Primary Care," *BMC Psychiatry* 6(2006): 14.

29. O. Mason and I. Hargreaves, "A Qualitative Study of Mindfulness-based Cognitive Therapy for Depression," *British Journal of Medical Psychology* 74(2001): 197–212.

30. M. M. Delmonte, "Meditation and Anxiety Reduction: A Literature Review," *Clinical Psychology Review* 5(2002): 91–102.

31. G. Paul, B. Elam, and S. J. Verhulst, "A Longitudinal Study of Students' Perceptions of Using Deep Breathing Meditation to Reduce Testing Stresses," *Teaching and Learning in Medicine* 19(2007): 287–92.

32. J. L. Kristeller and C. B. Hallett, "An Exploratory Study of a Meditation-based Intervention for Binge Eating Disorder," *Journal of Health Psychology* 4(July 1999): 357–63.

33. Ruth A. Baer, Sarah Fischer, and Debra B. Huss, "Mindfulness-Based Cognitive Therapy Applied to Binge Eating: A Case Study." *Cognitive and Behavioral Practice* 12(2005): 351–58.

34. L. I. Aftanas and S. A. Golocheikine, "Human Anterior and Frontal Midline Theta and Lower Alpha Reflect Emotionally Positive State and Internalized Attention: High-Resolution EEG Investigation of Meditation," *Neuroscience Letters* 310(2001): 57–60.

35. J. D. Creswell, B. M. Way, N. I. Eisenberger, and M. D. Lieberman, "Neural Correlates of Dispositional Mindfulness During Affect Labeling," *Psychosomatic Medicine* 69(2007): 560–65.

36. K. Hoppes, "The Application of Mindfulness-based Cognitive Interventions in the Treatment of Co-occurring Addictive and Mood Disorders," *CNS Spectrums* 11(2006): 829–51.

37. M. Yücel and D. I. Lubman, "Neurocognitive and Neuroimaging Evidence of Behavioural Dysregulation in Human Drug Addiction: Implications for Diagnosis, Treatment and Prevention," *Drug and Alcohol Review* 26(2007): 33–39.

38. D. M. Ziedonis, D. Smelson, R. N. Rosenthal, S. L. Batki, A. I. Green, R. J. Henry, I. Montoya, J. Parks, and R. D. Weiss, "Improving the Care of Individuals with Schizophrenia and Substance Use Disorders: Consensus Recommendations," *Journal of Psychiatric Practice* 11(2005): 315–39.

39. J. M. Williams, D. S. Duggan, C. Crane, and M. J. Fennell, "Mindfulness-based Cognitive Therapy for Prevention of Recurrence of Suicidal Behavior," *Journal of Clinical Psychology* 62(2006): 201–10.

40. Institute of Applied Meditation, *What Are the Types of Meditation?* 2007. Available at www.appliedmeditation.org/ Heart_Rhythm_Practice/meditation_types_of.shtml

41. Buddhistplace.ca, Relocation of Consciousness via Meditation, 2007. Available at http://buddhistplace.ca/consciousness-meditation.php

42. Herbert Benson, *The Relaxation Response* (New York: Avon, 1975).

43. Sharon Salzberg and Joseph Goldstein, *Insight Meditation: A Step-by-Step Course on How to Meditate* (Gilroy, CA: Sounds True, 2002).

LAB ASSESSMENT 10.1

Is Meditation for You?

Directions: Practice meditation as suggested and regularly. After at least a one-week trial period, rate each statement, using the following scale:

1 = very untrue

2 = somewhat untrue

3 = not sure

4 = somewhat true

5 = very true

_____ 1. It felt good.

_____ 2. It was easy to fit into my schedule.

_____ 3. It made me feel relaxed.

_____ 4. I handled my daily chores better than I usually do.

_____ 5. It was an easy technique to learn.

_____ 6. I was able to close out my surroundings while practicing this technique.

_____ 7. I did not feel tired after practicing this relaxation technique.

_____ 8. My fingers and toes felt warmer directly after trying this relaxation technique.

_____ 9. Any stress symptoms I had (headache, tense muscles, anxiety) before doing this relaxation technique disappeared by the time I was done.

_____ 10. Each time I concluded this technique, my pulse rate was much lower than when I began.

Now sum up the values you responded with for a total score. Save this score and compare it with scores for other relaxation techniques you try. The higher the score is, the more appropriate a particular relaxation skill is for you.

Describe any recurring thoughts you experienced during meditation:

_____

_____

_____

Describe any difficulties you experienced during meditation:

_____

_____

_____

Autogenic Training, Imagery, and Progressive Relaxation

You're at a magic show and, before you realize what you've done, you've volunteered to be hypnotized on stage. The hypnotist asks you to follow the pendulum-like movement of her chained watch as she slowly and softly mutters, "You're getting tired. Your eyelids are becoming heavy and are difficult to keep open. Your body feels weighted down—very full and heavy. You are relaxed, totally relaxed. You will now listen to my voice and obey its instructions." After several more sentences, you are willing to crow like a rooster, look at your watch on cue, or even stand up when a certain word is spoken. How is it that people can be made to do embarrassing things and be laughed at by other people? Whatever the reason, hypnosis can be a powerful tool if used appropriately. People who have had difficulty giving up cigarettes or other drugs, flying on airplanes, or losing weight have been helped by hypnosis.

An interesting aspect of hypnosis is that we can hypnotize ourselves. Autohypnosis is the basis of the relaxation technique to which the first part of this chapter is devoted—autogenic training.

Autogenic Training

Around 1900, Oskar Vogt (a brain physiologist) noted that some patients were able to place themselves in a hypnotic state. Vogt called this condition **autohypnosis.** These patients reported less fatigue, less tension, and fewer psychosomatic disorders (e.g., headaches) than other patients. German psychiatrist Johannes Schultz had used hypnosis with his patients. In 1932, he developed **autogenic training,** using the observations of Vogt as its basis. Schultz had found that patients he hypnotized developed two physical sensations: general body warmth and heaviness in the limbs and torso. Schultz's autogenic training consisted of a series of exercises designed to bring about these two physical sensations and, thereby, an autohypnotic state. The generalized warmth was a function of the dilation of blood vessels, resulting in increased blood flow. The sensation of heaviness was caused by muscles relaxing. Because both vasodilation and muscle relaxation are components of the relaxation response, autogenic training exercises have been employed as a relaxation technique designed to help people better manage the stresses in their lives.

Schultz described autogenic training as a technique to treat neurotic patients and those with psychosomatic illness.[1] However, its use quickly expanded to healthy people who wanted to regulate their own psychological and physiological processes. Part of the reason that autogenic training became a well-known relaxation technique was its description in several sources by Schultz's student Wolfgang Luthe.[2-4] The details of how to do autogenic training as described by Schultz and Luthe appear in a later section of this chapter. For now, we will only mention the need for a passive attitude toward autogenic training exercises. Trying to relax gets in the way of relaxing. You just have to do the exercises and let what happens happen.

We should also note that, although autogenic training and meditation both lead to the relaxation response, they get there by different means. Meditation uses the mind to relax the body. Autogenic training uses the bodily sensations of heaviness and warmth to first relax the body and then expand this relaxed state to the mind

autohypnosis
Being able to place oneself in a hypnotic state.

autogenic training
A relaxation technique that involves imagining one's limbs to be heavy, warm, and tingling.

by the use of imagery. This distinction will become more clear to you after the description of autogenic training exercises and your practice of them.

Those to whom I have taught meditation and autogenic training report interesting and contradictory reactions. Some prefer meditation, because it requires very little learning, can be done almost anywhere, and allows the mind to be relatively unoccupied. Meditation only requires the mind to focus upon something repetitive, such as a mantra, or something unchanging, such as a spot on the wall. Others find meditation boring and prefer autogenic training's switches of focus from one part of the body to another and its use of imagery to relax the mind. Whichever works for you is the relaxation technique you should employ. Use the rating scale in Lab 11.1 at the end of this chapter to help you evaluate the benefits you derive from your practice of autogenic training.

To summarize, autogenic training is a relaxation technique that uses exercises to bring about the sensations of body warmth and heaviness in the limbs and torso and then uses relaxing images to expand physical relaxation to the mind.

Benefits of Autogenic Training

Autogenic means "self-generating." That means you do the procedure to yourself. It also refers to the self-healing nature of autogenics. As you will now see, autogenic training has been shown to have physiological as well as psychological benefits. Although there is some question as to whether any valid means are available for prescribing a particular relaxation technique for particular people, there is some indication that those who have an internal locus of control find autogenics more effective than do those with an external locus of control.[5]

Physiological Effects

The physiological effects of autogenic training are similar to those of other relaxation techniques that elicit the trophotropic response. Heart rate, respiratory rate, muscle tension, and serum-cholesterol level all decrease. Alpha brain waves and blood flow to the arms and legs increase. Autogenics has been used to improve the immune function in people with cancer[6] and to improve the quality of life of people with multiple sclerosis.[7] In addition, those suffering from headaches have experienced relief through autogenics.[8-10] Autogenics has even been used to help people with drug abuse.[11]

Other studies have also documented the benefits of autogenics for a range of physiological and psychological conditions. Autogenics has been employed to help women alleviate menstrual discomfort.[12] When autogenic training was provided to students with scoliosis, and their teachers were instructed in decreasing emotional distress in these students, fewer needed braces for their condition.[13] And, when researchers provided autogenic training for students experiencing dyspnea (labored breathing), they concluded that autogenics helped these students breathe better.[14] The researchers conceptualized dyspnea as a symptom that provided patients with a way of expressing their reactions to perceived or anticipated stress. Thus, they suggested, stress reduction interventions (autogenic training) could prove extremely helpful in resolving this symptom. Even more recently, autogenic training has been found to help people with insomnia get to sleep,[15] treat substance abuse,[16] relieve pain,[17] and decrease tics associated with Tourette syndrome.[18]

Psychological Effects

In one dramatic demonstration of the psychological effects of autogenics, a subject was able to withstand for a minute and a half the pain of a third-degree burn brought about by a lighted cigarette placed on the back of the hand.[19] I don't suggest you attempt such a feat; still, it makes us marvel once again about the influence our minds exert over our bodies. In any case, autogenics can aid those with chronic illnesses that result in pain (e.g., arthritis) to tolerate that pain better.[20]

Autogenics has also been effective in treating people of all ages who experience anxiety. These have included postwar Kosovo high school students,[21] patients undergoing coronary angioplasty,[22] and those wishing to employ self-help treatments for anxiety.[23] In addition, autogenic training has been found to reduce anxiety and depression, decrease tiredness, and help people increase their resistance to stress.[24,25] For example, a woman who couldn't wear dentures without gagging was taught to control the gagging by learning autogenics.[26] Another woman who couldn't drive an automobile because of a previous accident and the associated anxiety was helped with autogenics.[27] Even pregnant women were found to experience less pain and less anxiety during childbirth when employing autogenics.[28] Migraine sufferers have found relief with autogenics,[29] as have people with multiple sclerosis[30] and women with chest pain.[31] When autogenics was learned and practiced, patients with Meniere's disease experienced less vertigo (dizziness) and insomnia,[32] and even athletes have improved athletic performance and prevented injury by employing autogenic training to control anxiety associated with competition.[33] Furthermore, firefighters experiencing post-traumatic stress disorder have been able to control their cardiac activity and deal better with related psychological issues through the use of autogenic training.[34]

How to Do Autogenic Training

Before describing autogenic training exercises, we should note that people with psychological problems who employ autogenics to alleviate these problems should do so in clinical situations with trained clinicians (e.g., a clinical psychologist or psychiatrist). When autogenics is used in this manner, it may take anywhere from two months to one year before a person becomes proficient.

Although the six initial stages of autogenic training and the second phase (autogenic meditation) are described below, the autogenic training practice that you will experience is a modified version of the standard procedures. Since the purpose of autogenics described here is relaxation rather than therapy, this modified version (easier to learn and found effective for teaching the relaxation response) will suffice.

Prerequisites

Schultz and Luthe cite several factors essential to successful autogenic training:

1. High motivation and cooperation.
2. A reasonable degree of self-direction and self-control.
3. Maintenance of particular body posture conducive to success (see "Body Position," below).
4. Reduction of external stimuli to a minimum and mental focusing on the process to the exclusion of the external environment.
5. Concentrated attention on the bodily sensations.

Body Position

There are three basic positions for doing autogenics: one reclining and two seated. In the reclining position (see Figure 11.1), you lie on your back, feet slightly apart, toes pointing away from the body. Cushion any part of the body that feels uncomfortable. Use blankets or pillows for cushioning, but be careful not to misalign the body (e.g., by using pillows under the head that make the chin almost touch the

Figure 11.1

The reclining position. Relaxation can be enhanced even more when barefoot and wearing loose-fitting clothing.

Figure 11.2

The first seated position.

Figure 11.3

The second seated position.

chest). Your arms should lie alongside your body but not touch it, with a slight bend at the elbows and the palms facing upward.

The seated positions (see Figures 11.2 and 11.3) have two advantages: You can do them almost anywhere, and they are less apt to result in sleep. On the other hand, they don't allow as much total muscle relaxation as the reclining position. The best chair to use is a straight-backed one that will provide support for your head and align it with your torso. Your buttocks should be against the back of the chair, and the seat of the chair should be long enough to support your thighs. Your arms, hands, and fingers may relax on the arms of the chair or be supported in your lap.

The second seated position uses a stool or a low-backed chair, upon which you sit without support for your back. Sit at the forward part of the chair with your arms supported on your thighs, hands and fingers dangling loosely. The head hangs loosely, with the chin near the chest. Your feet should be placed at shoulder width, slightly forward of your knees.

Whichever position you choose, make sure your body is relaxed and that it is supported by as little muscular contraction as possible.

Six Initial Stages of Autogenic Training

Here are the six initial stages of autogenic training that precede the use of imagery:

1. Focus on sensations of heaviness throughout the arms and legs (beginning with the dominant arm or leg).
2. Focus on sensations of warmth throughout the arms and legs (beginning with the dominant arm or leg).
3. Focus on sensations of warmth and heaviness in the area of the heart.
4. Focus on slow, calm breathing.
5. Focus on sensations of warmth in the abdomen.
6. Focus on sensations of coolness in the forehead.

These stages are sequential; you need to master the skills of each stage before practicing the next. Sample instructions for each of these stages appear below. Repeat each statement three times.

Stage 1: Heaviness
> My right arm is heavy …
> My left arm is heavy …
> Both of my arms are very heavy.
> My right leg is heavy …
> My left leg is heavy …
> Both of my legs are very heavy.
> My arms and legs are very heavy.

Stage 2: Warmth
> My right arm is warm …
> My left arm is warm …
> Both of my arms are very warm.
> My right leg is warm …
> My left leg is warm …
> Both of my legs are very warm.
> My arms and legs are very warm.

Stage 3: Heart
> My heartbeat is calm and regular. (Repeat four or five times.)

Stage 4: Respiration
> My breathing is calm and relaxed …
> It breathes me. (Repeat four or five times.)

Stage 5: Abdomen
     My abdomen is warm. (Repeat four or five times.)
Stage 6: Forehead
     My forehead is cool. (Repeat four or five times.)

With experience in autogenics, it should take you only a few minutes to feel heaviness and warmth in your limbs, a relaxed and calm heart and respiratory rate, warmth in your abdomen, and coolness in your forehead. Remember, though, that it usually takes several months or more of regular practice to get to that point. Regular practice means 10 to 40 minutes per day. However, don't be too anxious to master autogenics, since trying too hard will interfere with learning the skills. Proceed at your own pace, moving to the next stage only after you have mastered the previous stage.

An Autogenic Training Experience

The six initial stages and the phases of autogenic meditation take a good deal of time to work through. A set of instructions follows that will take you through a modified autogenic training experience. Note that each of the six initial stages is presented at one sitting and that visualization is also a part of this exercise. For relaxation purposes, my students and others for whom I have conducted relaxation training report these instructions to be effective.

This exercise should be practiced at least once daily but preferably twice: once upon waking and once just before dinner. You can either memorize the phrases, ask someone to read them to you, or recite them into a tape recorder. In any case, these phrases should be presented calmly, softly, and with sufficient pause between them for you to be able to bring about the sensations to which each phrase refers.

Now, assuming that you are ready and haven't just eaten or ingested a stimulant, are located in a relatively quiet, comfortable environment, and have approximately 30 minutes for relaxation, position yourself in one of the three autogenic positions previously described. Repeat the following phrases:

I am calm.

It is quiet.

I am relaxed.

My right arm (if right-handed) is heavy. (Repeat four or five times.)

My right arm is warm. (Repeat four or five times.)

My right arm is tingly.

My right arm is heavy and warm.

My right arm is weighted down and feels warm.

My left arm is heavy. (Repeat four or five times.)

My left arm is warm. (Repeat four or five times.)

My left arm is tingly.

My left arm is heavy and warm.

My left arm is weighted down and warm.

Both my arms are heavy and warm. (Repeat four or five times.)

(Repeat the phrases above for the legs, beginning with the dominant leg.)

My heart is beating calmly.

I am relaxed.

My heart is calm and relaxed. (Repeat four or five times.)

My breathing is regular.

My breathing is calm.

My breathing is calm and relaxed. (Repeat four or five times.)

It breathes me. (Repeat four or five times.)

My abdomen is warm. (Repeat four or five times.)

I feel warmth throughout my abdomen. (Repeat four or five times.)

My forehead is cool. (Repeat four or five times.)

I am calm.

I am relaxed.

I am quiet.

Now think of a relaxing scene.

(Refer to the scene you identified earlier in this chapter as relaxing for you.)

Imagine yourself there.

See this scene clearly.

Experience it.

Be one with it.

Hear the sounds.

See the colors.

This scene relaxes you.

You are calm.

You are quiet.

You are at peace.

Your mind is quiet.

Your whole body is quiet, heavy, warm, and relaxed.

Your thoughts are of your quiet, heavy, warm body and of your scene.

Tell yourself you feel quiet, you feel relaxed, you feel calm.

Now prepare to leave your scene.

Count backward from five.

With each number, you will be more alert.

With each number, you will be closer to opening your eyes.

Five.

You are leaving your scene.

You wave goodbye.

Four.

You are back in this room.

You are seated (or reclined).

You know where you are.

Three.

Prepare to open your eyes.

Think of what you will see when you open your eyes.

Two.

Open your eyes.

Focus upon one object in the room.

Take a deep breath.

One.

Focus on objects about the room.

Take several deep breaths.

When you feel ready, stretch your arms and legs.

Now stand and stretch.

Take several more deep breaths.

Now proceed with your regular activities, knowing that you are refreshed and revitalized.

To assess the effects of autogenics for you complete Lab 11.1.

Imagery

Part of autogenic training employs images of relaxing scenes to translate body relaxation into mind relaxation. Some people visualize a sunny day spent on a sailboat on a quiet lake. Others find it relaxing to imagine birds flying gently through the air, the ocean surf reaching the shore, or a cozy, carpeted room warmed by a fire. What image do you find relaxing? The following questions will help you to identify your own relaxing image.

1. What is the temperature at the scene? _____

2. Who is there? _____

3. What colors are present in your scene? _____

   _____

4. What sounds are present in your scene? _____

   _____

5. What movement is occurring? _____

   _____

6. How are you feeling? _____

   _____

Sometimes called **autogenic meditation,** visualization of relaxing images begins by rotating your eyeballs inward and upward as if you are attempting to look at your own forehead. The next step involves practicing visualizing one color in your whole field of vision—any color you choose. Next, visualize colors making pictures. When that is accomplished, practice visualizing one object against a dark background. This object should be seen clearly, be immobile, and be viewed for a long duration (practice sessions may run from 40 to 60 minutes).

The next phase of autogenic meditation instructs you to visualize abstract ideas (such as freedom). This phase usually runs from two to six weeks. After this training period, you may then practice focusing upon feeling states while visualizing yourself in various situations. For example, you may focus upon your feelings as you imagine yourself floating on a cloud.

The next phase involves the visualization of other people, first neutral people (e.g., a storekeeper you know), then family or friends. It is hoped that such visualization will result in insight into relationships you have with these people. In particular, relationships with people with whom you are in conflict are thought to be improved by autogenic meditation insights.

Although you would do best to develop your own image of relaxation (different people find different things relaxing), an example of relaxing imagery appears in the "Imagery Exercise" box. In any relaxing imagery, there should be a very vivid scene. Use as many of your senses as you can to make the image as real as possible. You should smell the smells, hear the sounds, see the colors, feel the sensations, and even taste the tastes present. Images can be of clouds, valleys, a willow tree, a field of wildflowers, a cool forest, a log cabin, a clear stream, a sloping hill, or just about any other scene that would relax you. I have chosen a sunny beach as the image to use as an example. Others might choose an image of a rainbow, or parts of the immune system attacking invaders or cancer cells, or performing

autogenic meditation
Visualization of relaxing images used during autogenic training.

Imagining a relaxing scene—for example, a beach, lake, or park—can be very calming on the mind, especially if the image is very vivid. What scene would relax you?

An Imagery Exercise

You are driving to the beach with your car window rolled down and no radio on in your car. The wind is blowing through your hair, and the sun is beating down on your thighs through the car window. You can see people walking with beach chairs and blankets, clad in bathing suits and carrying food in picnic baskets and coolers. You park your car, and as you are walking to the beach, you hear the surf rolling onto the shore and can smell the salt in the air. You find a quiet spot of beach away from other people and spread your blanket out there. Being tired from the drive, you are relieved to allow your muscles to relax as you apply sunblock and lie on the blanket, with your feet extending beyond, onto the sand.

As you relax, you can taste the salt in the air. Droplets of ocean seem to fall on you as you hear the pounding of the surf and hear it ever so gently rolling back to sea. Everything seems light and yellow and tan and blue. The sun's bright yellow on the sand's relaxing tan contrasted with the ocean's vivid blue seems just the right combination of serenity. You decide to close your eyes and take in all the sensations through other senses.

The sun seems to move over your body. First your arms warm up from the intensity of the sun's rays. You can feel the heat pass through them, and the feeling is one of relaxation. Next your legs become caressed by the sun as they, too, become warm. The sun moves to warm your chest now and your whole chest area becomes heated and relaxed. But it doesn't stop there. The sun moves to your abdomen, bringing its relaxing warmth there. And, as though you've willed it, the sun next moves to your forehead, bringing warmth and relaxation there. Your whole body now feels warm and relaxed. Your muscles are relaxed, and your body feels as though it's sinking into the sand. Your body feels warm and heavy. Your body tingles from the sun's warmth.

You hear the sea gulls as you relax. They are flying over the ocean. They are free and light and peaceful. As they fly out to sea, they are carrying your problems and worries with them. You are relieved of your problems and worries and relaxed. You think of nothing but your body's heaviness and warmth and tingling sensation. You are totally relaxed.

You have relaxed all day like this, and now the sun is setting. As you feel the sun leaving, you slowly open your eyes, feeling wonderfully relaxed and content. You have no worries; you have no cares. You look at the sea gulls, which have left your problems and worries out at sea, and you thank them. Feeling alert, you stand and stretch, feeling the still warm—yet cooling—sand between your toes, and you feel terrific. You feel so good that you know the car ride home will be pleasant. You welcome the time to be alone, in your car, at peace, without problems or cares. You fold your blanket and leave your piece of beach, taking with you your relaxation and contentment. You say goodbye to your beach as you walk from it, knowing you can return anytime you desire.

well on an exam. The point is to select an image that you will find relaxing. Remember, imagery has been shown to be extremely effective in eliciting either the stress or the relaxation response,[35,36] so use it to your advantage.

Physiological Effects

In addition to its usefulness in managing stress, imagery has been demonstrated to have physiological benefits. When children and adolescents with chronic headaches were taught imagery, 88 percent reported a decrease in the frequency of their headaches, and 26 percent said they were headache-free after learning how to use imagery.[37] Chronic pain sufferers in general,[38] as well as children in hospices experiencing pain,[39] have had their pain decrease when learning to use imagery. Imagery has even helped women with osteoporosis experience less pain and to improve their self-rated quality of life.[40]

Psychological Effects

Imagery has also been found to have beneficial psychological effects. For example, when sexual assault survivors with posttraumatic stress disorder (PTSD) and chronic nightmares learned imagery, they slept better and experienced a decrease in PTSD severity.[41] Imagery has also been found to help both older adults with mild or moderate depression[42] and breast cancer patients to decrease their anxiety and depression.[43] Even problem gamblers were able to decrease their urge to gamble by the use of imagery.[44] Lastly, imagery can be used to alleviate anxiety about an event so you can perform better. For example, athletes have employed imagery to picture themselves competing effectively, thereby decreasing physiological arousal that might interfere with their performance. I have written a book to help athletes do just this.[45]

Progressive Relaxation

I'll never forget my first lesson in downhill skiing. Having been selected the most valuable player on my college basketball team and having found success at some local tennis tournaments, I considered myself an accomplished athlete. An accomplished skier I was not and never became.

The area where I learned to ski (rather, attempted to learn to ski) had three slopes: beginner, intermediate, and advanced. My first lesson, this first day ever on a pair of skis, consisted of one hour of falling, learning how to rise (no easy task in snow with long, thin objects protruding fore and aft from my feet), and snowplowing. Believing my entry on the Olympic team as a downhill slalom racer assured after this lesson, I immediately attacked the intermediate course. With ineffective snowplowing to avoid some skiers and a loud "Watch out!" that worked even better to avoid a crash with most of the others, I managed to get to the bottom of the slope without even getting snow on my ski outfit. As I waited for the lift to return me to the top so I could break the downhill speed record, I was awed by the grace and ease with which the more accomplished skiers appeared to be floating downhill. Effortlessly, it seemed, they moved left, then right, then tucked, then stopped smoothly at the bottom.

I never learned to ski well. In fact, the very next (and last) time I was silly enough to find myself at the top of a series of ski slopes and recklessly let my fragile body begin sliding downward, I found that my snowplowing was good enough to get me about one-third down a zigzagging slope, though I wound up a little farther and farther behind at each successive curve. The one-third point was where I attempted to save my body from the oncoming woods by turning to the left, only to learn that it was too late and my skills were too few. Using my brains as the only way out, I sat down and skidded just short of a threatening blue spruce. Recalling something about wisdom being the better part of valor, I removed my skis, smacked the snow off my derrière, and marched downhill to spend the rest of the day in what was for me a more natural habitat—the fireplace-warmed lodge.

Bracing

I relate this embarrassing story because what I really want to discuss is the grace and effortlessness I observed in the good skiers. The reason they appeared this way is that they were using proper *form*. Some of you have probably had lessons in tennis, golf, or another sport, during which you were taught the proper form. Proper form means moving the body to accomplish the task most effectively—with the least amount of energy. Proper form allows you to be effective and efficient. What has always been interesting to me is that too much muscular contraction can often interfere with using proper form. The approach of Tim Gallwey in teaching tennis is to prevent the mind from scaring the body into tensing so much that proper form is impossible.[46] For example, Gallwey instructs players to try to read the writing on the ball as it comes toward them rather than worry about having to hit a backhand return.

Doing things effectively and efficiently is important for our daily routines as well. Too often, we use too much muscular contraction, with the consequences being backache, headache, pains in the neck or shoulders, and other illnesses. Unnecessary muscular contraction occurs when your shoulders are raised, your hands are holding something too tightly, your forearm muscles are tensed, or your abdominal muscles are sort of squeezing you in. These are all signs of bracing: the muscles contracted, the body ready for some action it seldom takes. As McGuigan states, "The person who falls victim to stressors reflexively reacts to them, often emotionally. If such muscular reactions are prolonged, as they often are, they can eventually lead to the malfunction of some system of the body. Such chronic overtension may lead to a variety of psychosomatic (somatoform) and psychiatric disorders."[47]

The next time you drive an automobile, notice how tightly you grasp the steering wheel. With the power steering of most modern cars, the steering wheel need only be held gently. To do otherwise is to brace.

The next time you take notes during a lecture, notice how tightly you hold the pen or pencil. If you hold too tightly or press down too hard, you are bracing.

The next time you visit a dentist, notice how you cling to the arms of the chair. The chair will probably not move, so your grip on it is unnecessary. You are bracing.

On numerous occasions, we use muscular contraction inefficiently, and the result is poor health. However, we can learn to use our muscles in a more healthy manner through a relaxation technique called progressive relaxation.

What Is Progressive Relaxation?

Progressive relaxation is a technique used to induce nerve-muscle relaxation. Developed by Edmund Jacobson and described in his book *Progressive Relaxation*, this technique was originally designed for hospital patients who appeared tense.[48] Jacobson, a physician, observed that tense patients, as evidenced by such small muscle movement as frowning or wrinkling the forehead, did not recuperate quickly or well. Seeking to intervene in this residual muscle tension syndrome, Jacobson taught his patients a series of exercises that first required them to contract a muscle group, then relax it, moving (or progressing) from one muscle group to another. The purpose of first contracting the muscle is to teach people to recognize more readily what muscle tension feels like.[49] At first glance this appears unnecessary, but remember our discussion of bracing. The purpose of the relaxation phase is to become familiar enough with this sensation so that it can be voluntarily induced. The idea, then, is to sense more readily when we are muscularly tense and, on those occasions, to be able to relax those muscles. "One who has acquired the ability to momentarily relax in the face of a stressor creates the opportunity to rationally select the most appropriate mode of responding. That is, rather than reflexively reacting, one can pause and consider the nature of the threat, weigh the consequences of various possible reactions, and then engage in the most effective one."[50]

Sometimes termed **neuromuscular relaxation** (because the nerves control muscular contraction) or **Jacobsonian relaxation** (named after its developer), progressive relaxation starts with one muscle group, adds another when the first is relaxed, and progresses through the body until total body relaxation occurs. It starts with the distal muscle groups (the feet and legs) and moves to the proximal muscle groups (the head and trunk) afterward. Like autogenic training, progressive relaxation relaxes the mind by first relaxing the body. However, unlike autogenic training and meditation, progressive relaxation does not produce a hypnotic state. Like

progressive relaxation
A relaxation technique involving contracting and relaxing muscle groups throughout the body; also called neuromuscular relaxation or Jacobsonian relaxation.

neuromuscular relaxation
A relaxation technique involving contracting and relaxing muscle groups throughout the body; also called progressive relaxation or Jacobsonian relaxation.

Jacobsonian relaxation
A relaxation technique involving contracting and relaxing muscle groups throughout the body; also called progressive relaxation or neuromuscular relaxation.

the other relaxation techniques presented in this book, progressive relaxation should be practiced regularly, and you should expect to become more proficient as you gain experience with the technique.

Benefits of Progressive Relaxation

This relaxation technique has proved effective in helping people relax and does not require any special equipment. Although it takes several years of practice as originally described by Jacobson, benefits can result in several weeks of three daily practice sessions of just five minutes each.[51] Nevertheless, progressive relaxation has been shown to have both physiological and psychological benefits.

Physiological Effects

In describing Jacobson's research on the effects of progressive relaxation, Brown states that learned relaxation of skeletal muscles can be generalized to smooth muscles, causing relaxation of the gastrointestinal and cardiovascular systems.[52] Other researchers have found progressive relaxation effective in treating headaches,[53] backaches,[54] side effects of cancer,[55-58] insomnia,[59,60] pain,[61,62] and high blood pressure (although meditation is even more effective).[63,64] When diabetics were trained in stress management techniques that included progressive relaxation, 32 percent had lower than their baseline levels of HbA1c, a marker for blood glucose, compared to only 12 percent of control subjects at 12 months after the program.[65] It appears that conditions resulting from bracing or ineffective muscular tension can be alleviated, or at least their symptoms diminished, with regular practice of progressive relaxation—even writer's cramp.

Psychological Effects

Progressive relaxation has been demonstrated to have wide-ranging effects upon psychological well-being, as well as upon behavioral change. For example, both depression[66] and anxiety[67,68] were lessened in people trained in progressive relaxation. Even insomniacs were helped to sleep by using this relaxation technique.[69] Alcoholism,[70] and even batting slumps[71] were aided by regular practice of progressive relaxation. When baseball players were taught progressive relaxation, they were better able to perform (bat) under stress than their teammates who did not practice relaxation techniques. They had higher batting averages. This should not be surprising, since we know that stress (up at the plate or before an audience) can interfere with performance. In an interesting study, Rausch and colleagues[72] taught university students how to do progressive relaxation. Then she had them watch graphic slides of trauma and its aftermath while measuring their anxiety. The students taught progressive relaxation elicited a greater reduction in anxiety than those taught meditation or than the control group. Dialysis patients also decreased their trait and state anxiety through progressive relaxation.[73] Even patients with heart failure reduced their psychological distress by employing progressive relaxation.[74] And college students improved their academic performance after employing progressive relaxation.[75] Now, how can you beat that? Lastly, Italian peacekeepers in Afghanistan, who understandably experience a great deal of stress, used progressive relaxation to effectively manage anxiety, depression, and posttraumatic stress disorder symptoms.[76] In the stress management classes I teach, several students have been performers (a singer and a violinist come to mind) who reported performing better when using stress management techniques.

How To Do Progressive Relaxation

As with the other relaxation techniques, learning progressive relaxation necessitates several prerequisites, as well as learning the appropriate body position for performing the exercises.

Muscle tension can often be easily seen. Obviously, this drill instructor is not having a calm discussion with this sailor. His muscle tension is visible in his facial expression and body language.

Cues Identifying Tension

First of all, it is helpful to recognize that you are tense. You may have aches in your shoulders, back, neck, or head. Your body may feel stiff. You may sense that you are generally holding yourself too tightly or rigidly. You may have difficulty sitting comfortably, or your hands may tremble.

As you become more experienced with regular practice of progressive relaxation, you will more readily recognize these signs of tension and be better prepared to relax them away. In addition, regular practice will help prevent these signs of tension from occurring in the first place.

Look for these signs of tension and use them as cues to doing progressive relaxation. A good idea is to check for these cues just prior to meals so you can relax them away before eating. As we've discussed earlier, food in your stomach results in the blood flow increasing to that area of your body. This makes it more difficult to bring about relaxation, since the relaxation response includes increasing the blood flow to the arms and legs.

Prerequisites

When learning progressive relaxation, seek a relatively quiet, distraction-free environment. That means any telephones must be removed from the room or the receiver removed from the cradle and muffled with a towel. The lights should be dimmed and the threat of cats, dogs, kids, or roommates disturbing you eliminated. If after making adjustments in your environment, the noise is still impeding your learning, you might try headphones or cotton in your ears to block out the noise. Make sure you remove or loosen any tight clothing or jewelry and that the room is warm. It is difficult to relax in a cold environment, because the blood doesn't readily travel to cold extremities. Removing your shoes is also advisable.

Finally, approach the exercises knowing that any discomfort can quickly be eliminated by just stopping the exercise. Learning is designed to proceed slowly, so don't expect to be proficient at progressive relaxation after only a few sessions. Don't contract a muscle that is strained, pained, or cramped. There's always another day. Lastly, if you have high blood pressure, try a different relaxation technique since contractions can raise systolic blood pressure.

Body Position

To do progressive relaxation, stretch out on the floor (see Figure 11.4). The idea is to have your body supported by the floor rather than by your muscles. Lying on your back, let your arms and legs go. You can rest your hands on your abdomen or at your sides, and your legs and feet will most likely rotate outward. Just relax. You can support your neck with a pillow (small enough to fit behind your neck between your shoulders and where your head is resting on the floor); you may also find that a pillow placed under your knees feels comfortable. If not, re-arrange your body so that you are comfortable. After you have more experience with progressive relaxation, you will be able to relax particular muscle groups when seated or even when standing in line (for example, those muscles in the neck) (see Figure 11.5). However, it is best to learn these exercises while reclined.

Figure 11.4

Reclining position for progressive relaxation exercise. Relaxation can be enhanced even more when barefoot and wearing loose-fitting clothing.

Figure 11.5

Muscle tension and relaxation exercises.

(a) Tightening the calf muscles by pointing the toes.

(b) Raising the shoulders in a shoulder stretch.

(c) Tightening facial muscles.

(d) Stretching the neck muscles.

After you become proficient, you can eliminate the contraction phase and focus totally on relaxation. It may take several weeks or months of regular practice, though, to develop the "muscle sense" that the contraction phase teaches. Because this phase teaches you to recognize muscle tension, it is important not to rush to eliminate it. But, as you will soon find out, it is the relaxation phase that is most pleasant and has the most health-related benefits. If you are having difficulty with progressive relaxation, you can even work with a partner.

Exercises

Stress management experts have developed several variations of muscle relaxation exercises. For example, Forman and Myers suggest contracting a muscle group by pushing against an immovable object.[77] They recommend pushing down with the fingertips on a desktop, for instance. Their reasoning is that this resistance technique requires more muscular contractions, which in turn increases the ability to recognize the difference between the contracted and relaxed states. Smith, in contrast, recommends eleven isometric squeeze exercises: hand squeeze, arm squeeze, arm and side squeeze, back squeeze, shoulder squeeze, back and neck squeeze, face squeeze, front of neck squeeze, stomach and chest squeeze, leg squeeze, and foot squeeze.[78] (After all those squeezes, you're probably entitled to squeeze someone you love.) Smith argues that, too often, students of progressive relaxation are taught to stretch the muscles too quickly during the contraction phase. He believes isometric contractions will be experienced as more pleasurable, thereby being more effective in teaching relaxation.

The exercises that follow are simple enough to learn yet powerful enough to be used for the control of stress and tension. Try them several times a day for at least a week. Then complete the rating scale in Lab Assessment 11.3 to evaluate progressive relaxation's benefits to you, compared with the other relaxation techniques you have tried.

The following instructions, which were developed by Jenny Steinmetz, can be read to you, memorized, or recited into a tape recorder. Follow each instruction carefully and completely. Don't skip any part of the body (unless injured) and don't skip any exercises. Also, make sure that you spend twice as much time relaxing a muscle as you do tensing that muscle. We begin with the hips, thighs, and calves.

Relaxation of the hips, thighs, and calves (four or five minutes):
Let go of all tensions and relax.
Now flex your buttocks and thighs.
Flex your thighs by pressing down your heels as hard as you can.
Relax and notice the difference.
Straighten your knees and flex your thigh muscles again.
Hold the tension.
Relax your hips and thighs …
Allow the relaxation to proceed on its own.
Press your feet and toes downward, away from your face, so that your calf muscles become tense.
Study that tension.
Relax your feet and calves.
This time, bend your feet toward your face so that you feel tension along your shins.
Bring your toes right up.
Relax again … keep relaxing for a while …
Now let yourself relax further all over …
Relax your feet, ankles, calves and shins, knees, thighs, buttocks, and hips …
Feel the heaviness of your lower body as you relax still further.
Now spread the relaxation to your stomach, waist, and lower back.
Let go more and more deeply …
Make sure no tension has crept into your throat.
Relax your neck and your jaws and all your facial muscles.
Keep relaxing your whole body like that for a while …
Let yourself relax.
Now you can become twice as relaxed as you are merely by taking in a really deep breath and slowly exhaling, with your eyes closed, so that you

become less aware of objects and movements around you, and thus prevent any surface tensions from developing.

Breathe in deeply and feel yourself becoming heavier.

Take in a long, deep breath and exhale very slowly …

Feel how heavy and relaxed you have become.

In a state of perfect relaxation, you should feel unwilling to move a single muscle in your body.

Think about the effort that would be required to raise your right arm.

As you think about that, see if you can notice any tensions that might have crept into your shoulders and arm.

Now you decide not to lift the arm, but to continue relaxing …

Observe the relief and the disappearance of the tension.

Just carry on, relaxing like that … continue relaxing …

When you wish to get up, count backward from four to one.

You should now feel fine and refreshed, wide awake and calm.

Relaxation of the chest, stomach, and lower back (four or five minutes):

Relax your entire body to the best of your ability.

Feel that comfortable heaviness that accompanies relaxation.

Breathe easily and freely in and out …

Notice how the relaxation increases as you exhale …

As you breathe out, just feel that relaxation.

Now breathe right in and fill your lungs.

Inhale deeply and hold your breath.

Study the tension.

Now exhale, let the walls of your chest grow loose, and push the air out automatically.

Continue relaxing, and breathe freely and gently …

Feel the relaxation, and enjoy it.

With the rest of your body as relaxed as possible, fill your lungs again.

Breathe in deeply, and hold it again.

Now breathe out, and appreciate the relief, just breathe normally …

Continue relaxing your chest, and let the relaxation spread to your back, shoulders, neck, and arms …

Merely let go, and enjoy the relaxation.

Now let's pay attention to your abdominal muscles, your stomach area.

Tighten your stomach muscles; make your abdomen hard.

Notice the tension.

And relax, let the muscles loosen, and notice the contrast.

Once more, press and tighten your stomach muscles.

Hold the tension and study it.

And relax; notice the general well-being that comes with relaxing your stomach.

Now draw your stomach in.

Pull the muscles right in and feel the tension this way.

Now relax again … let your stomach out …

Continue breathing normally and easily, and feel the gentle massaging action all over your chest and stomach.

Now pull your stomach in again, and hold the tension.

Once more pull in, and feel the tension.

Now relax your stomach fully …

Let the tension dissolve as the relaxation grows deeper.

Each time you breathe out, notice the rhythmic relaxation both in your lungs and in your stomach …

Notice how your chest and your stomach relax more and more …

Let go of all contractions anywhere in your body.

Now direct your attention to your lower back.

Arch up your back, make your lower back quite hollow, and feel the tension along your spine.

Now settle down comfortably again, relaxing the lower back.

Just arch your back up, and feel the tension as you do so.

Keep the rest of your body as relaxed as possible.

Localize the tension throughout your lower back area.

Relax once more, relaxing further and further …

Relax your lower back, relax your upper back, spread the relaxation to your stomach, chest, shoulders, arms, and facial area …

These parts relax further and further and further and even deeper.

Relaxation of the face, neck, shoulders, and upper back (four or five minutes):

Let all your muscles go loose and heavy.

Just settle back quietly and comfortably.

Wrinkle up your forehead now, wrinkle it tighter.

And now stop wrinkling up your forehead.

Relax and smooth it out …

Picture the entire forehead and scalp becoming smoother, as the relaxation increases.

Now frown and crease your brows, and study the tension.

Let go of the tension again …

Smooth out the forehead once more.

Now close your eyes.

Keep your eyes closed, gently, comfortably, and notice the relaxation.

Now clench your jaws, push your teeth together.

Study the tension throughout the jaws.

Relax your jaws now …

Let your lips part slightly …

Appreciate the relaxation.

Now press your tongue hard against the roof of your mouth.

Look for the tension.

All right, let your tongue return to a comfortable and relaxed position.

Now purse your lips; press your lips together tighter and tighter.

Relax the lips …

Notice the contrast between tension and relaxation …

Feel the relaxation all over your face, all over your forehead, and scalp, eyes, jaws, lips, tongue, and throat …

The relaxation progresses further and further.

Now attend to your neck muscles.

Press your head back as far as it can go, and feel the tension in the neck.

Roll it to the right, and feel the tension shift …

Now roll it to the left.

Straighten your head, and bring it forward.

Press your chin against your chest.

Let your head return to a comfortable position, and study the relaxation …

Let the relaxation develop.

Shrug your shoulders right up.

Hold the tension.

Drop your shoulders and feel the relaxation …

Neck and shoulders relaxed.

Shrug your shoulders again, and move them around.

Bring your shoulders up and forward and back.

Feel the tension in your shoulders and in your upper back.

Drop your shoulders once more and relax …

Let the relaxation spread deep into the shoulders right into your back muscles.

Relax your neck and throat, and your jaws and other facial areas, as the pure relaxation takes over and grows deeper … deeper … even deeper.

Relaxation of the arms (four or five minutes):

Settle back as comfortably as you can and let yourself relax to the best of your ability.

Now, as you relax, clench your right fist.

Clench it tighter and tighter, and study the tension as you do so.

Keep it clenched, and feel the tension in your right fist, hand, and forearm. Now relax …

Let the fingers of your right hand become loose …

Observe the contrast in your feelings.

Now, let yourself go and allow yourself to become more relaxed all over.

Once more, clench your right fist really tight.

Hold it, and notice the tension again.

Now, let go, relax, let your fingers straighten out …

Notice the difference once more.

Now repeat that with your left fist.

Clench your left fist while the rest of your body relaxes.

Clench that fist tighter, and feel the tension.

And now relax … again, enjoy the contrast.

Repeat that once more, clench the left fist, tight and tense.

Now do the opposite of tension—relax and feel the difference …

Continue relaxing like that for a while.

Clench both fists tighter and tighter, both fists tense, forearms tense.

Study the sensations … and relax …

Straighten out your fingers and feel that relaxation …

Continue relaxing your hands and forearms more and more.

Now bend your elbows, and tense your biceps.

Tense them harder, and study the tension feeling.

All right, straighten out your arms …

Let them relax, and feel the difference again …

Let the relaxation develop.

Once more, tense your biceps.

Hold the tension, and observe it carefully.

Straighten the arms, and relax …

Relax to the best of your ability …

Each time pay close attention to your feelings when you tense up and when you relax.

Now straighten your arms; straighten them so that you feel the most tension in the triceps muscles along the back of your arms.

Stretch your arms, and feel the tension.

And now relax …

Get your arms back into a comfortable position …

Let the relaxation proceed on its own …

The arms should feel comfortably heavy as you allow them to relax.

Straighten the arms once more so that you feel the tension in the triceps muscles. Feel that tension … and relax.

Now let's concentrate on pure relaxation in the arms without any tension …

Get your arms comfortable and let them relax further and further …

Continue relaxing your arms even further …

Even when your arms seem fully relaxed, allow yourself to go that extra bit further …

Allow yourself to achieve deeper and deeper levels of relaxation.[*]

*Source: Jenny Steinmetz, *Managing Stress Before It Manages You* (Palo Alto, CA: Bull Publishing 1980), 20–27.

Other Short Exercises

There may be occasions when you choose not to devote as much time to relaxation as the exercises just presented require. In those instances, you can still practice a modified, simplified, and quick version of progressive relaxation. For example, you may be working at your desk and notice that your shoulder muscles are tense. To relax them, you can tense them further—raising your shoulders as high as you can get them—and then let them relax. Focus on the sensations of your relaxed shoulder muscles, paying particular attention to any warm and tingly sensations.

Another quick exercise you can do involves your abdominal muscles. Make these muscles tense by keeping your abdominal area flat but tight. Notice how you breathe with these muscles tensed—with the expansion of your chest muscles alone. Be aware of the sensations of breathing this way. Now relax your abdominal muscles and let your abdominal area stick out. Breathe by the expansion and contraction of your abdominal area rather than your chest. To help breathe this way, place the palm of your hand on your abdomen. Let your hand rise and fall as your abdomen rises when you inhale and falls when you exhale. Notice how relaxed you feel breathing in this manner.

You can improvise your own quick, modified version of progressive relaxation by identifying any particular muscle group that feels tense and then tensing it further. Next, relax that muscle group and focus upon the feelings of relaxation. After approximately five minutes of such an exercise, you can begin to feel less tense and more relaxed—and better able to proceed with the rest of your day. You might even do such exercises on schedule each day, considering that five minutes as a "vacation period" in which you leave your daily cares to travel to a more relaxed state.

To assess the effects of progressive relaxation on you, complete Lab Assessment 11.3.

Getting Involved in Your Community

At a conference I attended a while ago, a 71-year-old woman who was a participant in the Foster Grandparent Program rose to describe her volunteer experience. She was a "cuddler" for "crack babies" at Johns Hopkins University Hospital. I will never forget the smile on her face as she described how the babies stopped crying and calmed down when she held them. The audience was moved to applause.

You, too, can have an impact on the well-being of those in your community. For example, you might offer to teach autogenic training, imagery, or progressive relaxation to teenage, unmarried mothers at a local high school. These women experience a great deal of stress as a result of being a student while caring for a child. The respite that these relaxation techniques could offer them would be most welcomed. Or you might teach autogenics, imagery, or progressive relaxation to a support group of working mothers, a group that also experiences a great deal of stress.

Will you give some of your time and stress-related knowledge to make the lives of your community's neighbors better?

Coping in Today's World

Complementary and alternative medicine (CAM) continues to be of interest to the American public and is now accessed with greater frequency than ever before. Among CAM therapies are several that employ relaxation techniques to improve health. To protect the American public from spending their money on ineffective CAM therapies, or employing CAM therapies rather than proven traditional medical interventions when these traditional interventions are more effective, the federal government established the National Center for Complementary and Alternative Medicine (NCCAM). NCCAM, a unit of the National Institutes of Health, funds research to test the safety and effectiveness of CAM therapies. A brief summary of research findings pertaining to select CAM therapies is presented here.[a]

- Acupuncture has been found to be effective in the short-term alleviation of chronic low back pain and to help relieve pain in the knee from osteoarthritis.

- Massage therapy can help people feel better if accompanied by physical therapy and instruction regarding proper posture. Massage therapy has also been shown to have beneficial effects on the immunological system, such as reducing levels of substance P (a protein associated with pain).

- Mind-body therapies, such as meditation, have been shown to "improve postsurgical outcomes and reduce mortality rates from coronary heart disease by using techniques to reduce anger, hostility and stress," and have been shown to

be "effective in treating incontinence, chronic low-back pain, headaches, insomnia, and nausea, vomiting, pain and functional problems caused by chemotherapy."[b]

- Using magnetic resonance imagery (MRI), meditation has been found to increase left brain activity, which is associated with positive emotional feelings. It also activates parts of the brain that enhance attention and control of the nervous system.

- Biofeedback has been shown to be effective in treating more than 100 medical conditions, among which are migraine headache, arthritis, and fibromyalgia. This benefit is achieved by patients learning to control their heart rates, muscle tension, rate and pattern of breathing, blood pressure, and skin temperature.

- Cognitive behavioral therapy—a form of psychotherapy in which patients explore the meaning they attach to their surroundings and events in their lives and the influence that meaning has on their behavior—helps relieve stress. Consequently, cognitive behavioral therapy is effective as an adjunct treatment for coronary heart disease and chronic pain.

[a]National Center for Complementary and Alternative Medicine. *Mind-Body Medicine: An Overview*, 2007. Available at http://nccam.nih.gov/health/backgrounds/mindbody.htm
[b]J. W. Payne, "What Really Works? Forget Hearsay. Here's How Science Sizes up Some Therapies." *Washington Post*, July 12, 2005, HE01.

summary

- Autogenic training is a relaxation technique that consists of a series of exercises designed to bring about body warmth and heaviness in the limbs and torso. In addition, relaxing images are employed to expand physical relaxation to the mind.

- Autogenic training results in the trophotropic (relaxation) response. *Autogenic* means "self-generating" and refers to the fact that the response is self-induced.

- Autogenics has been used in the treatment of Raynaud's disease, migraine headaches, insomnia, hypertension, bronchial asthma, constipation, writer's cramp, indigestion, ulcers, hemorrhoids, tuberculosis, diabetes, and lower back pain.

- Prerequisites for doing autogenics include high motivation, a measure of self-direction, maintenance of the recommended body position, blocking out the external environment, focusing inward, and giving up ego boundaries.

- Autogenic training can be done while you are lying down or in a seated position. Cushion parts of your body that feel uncomfortable, and let your body relax.

- The six initial stages of autogenic training involve focusing on heaviness in the limbs, warmth in the limbs, heaviness and warmth in the area of the heart, regular breathing, sensations of warmth in the abdomen, and sensations of coolness in the forehead.

- Sometimes called autogenic meditation, visualization of relaxing images begins by rotating the eyeballs inward and upward. The next step involves choosing one color to visualize and then numerous colors. Next follows visualization of abstract images and then of people.

- People often use more muscular contraction than necessary. This can lead to backache, headache, and pains in the shoulders and neck.

- Muscular tension that prepares the body for action that is never taken is termed bracing. Raising your shoulders throughout the day is an example of bracing.

- Progressive relaxation is a technique used to induce nerve-muscle relaxation. It involves contraction of a muscle group and then relaxation of it, progressing from one muscle group to another throughout the body.

- The contraction phase of progressive relaxation is designed to help people better recognize when they are bracing. The relaxation phase is designed to help people recognize and bring on a relaxed state when they choose.

- Progressive relaxation has been used to treat tension headaches, migraine headaches, backaches, and other conditions. It has also been used to treat psychological conditions, such as poor self-concept, depression, anxiety, and insomnia.

- When learning progressive relaxation, seek a distraction-free environment and lie on your back. Proceed slowly and carefully, stopping if you experience muscle cramping or pain.

- It may take several weeks or months of regular practice of progressive relaxation before you develop the "muscle sense" that the contracting phase teaches, but the relaxation will benefit you much sooner.

internet resources

Guided Imagery **www.guidedimageryinc.com** *Stress and the benefits of imagery are examined. Includes information about how to obtain guided imagery audiotapes.*

Stress Management Associates **www.stresscontrol.com** *A program designed to facilitate education and training in relaxation and stress management.*

Short-Term Therapy for Long-Term Living **www.autogenictraining.org/**

Defines autogenic training, discusses how it relates to stress and illness, how autogenic training works, its benefits, and lists autogenic training courses available.

Stress Education Center **www.dstress.com** *This website guides the reader through a relaxation exercise and also includes information about how to obtain additional resources (tapes and books) for coping with stress.*

references

1. Johannes Schultz, *Das Autogene Training* (Stuttgart: Georg-Thieme Verlag, 1953).

2. Wolfgang Luthe, ed., *Autogenic Therapy*, 6 vols. (New York: Grune and Stratton, 1969).

3. Wolfgang Luthe, "Method, Research and Application of Autogenic Training," *American Journal of Clinical Hypnosis* 5(1962): 17–23.

4. Johannes Schultz and Wolfgang Luthe, *Autogenic Training: A Psychophysiologic Approach to Psychotherapy* (New York: Grune and Stratton, 1959).

5. P. M. Lehrer, "Varieties of Relaxation Methods and Their Unique Effects," *International Journal of Stress Management* 3(1996): 1–15.

6. M. Hidderley and M. Holt, "A Pilot Randomized Trial Assessing the Effects of Autogenic Training in Early Stage Cancer Patients in Relation to Psychological Status and Immune System Responses," *European Journal of Oncology Nursing: The Official Journal of European Oncology Nursing Society* 8(2004): 61–65.

7. G. Sutherland, M. B. Andersen, and T. Morris, "Relaxation and Health-Related Quality of Life in Multiple Sclerosis: The Example of Autogenic Training," *Journal of Behavioral Medicine* 28(2005): 249–56.

8. T. Zsombok, G. Juhász, X. Gonda, J. Vitrai, and G. Bagdy, "Effect of Autogenic Training with Cognitive and Symbol Therapy on the Treatment of Patients with Primary Headache," *Psychiatria Hungarica* 20(2005): 25–34.

9. T. Zsombok, G. Juhász, A. Budavari, J. Vitrai, and G. Bagdy, "Effect of Autogenic Training on Drug Consumption in Patients with Primary Headache: An 8-Month Follow-Up Study," *Headache* 43(2003): 251–57.

10. G. Juhász, T. Zsombok, X. Gonda, N. Nagyne, E. Modosne, and G. Bagdy, "Effects of Autogenic Training on Nitroglycerin-Induced Headaches," *Headache* 47(2007): 371–83.

11. G. Potter, "Intensive Therapy: Utilizing Hypnosis in the Treatment of Substance Abuse Disorders," *American Journal of Clinical Hypnosis* 47(2004): 21–28.

12. E. B. Blanchard and M. Kim, "The Effect of the Definition of Menstrually-Related Headache on the Response to Biofeedback Treatment," *Applied Psychophysiology and Biofeedback* 30(2005): 53–63.

13. S. Matsunaga, K. Hayashi, T. Naruo, S. Nozoe, and S. Komiya, "Psychologic Management of Brace Therapy for Patients with Idiopathic Scoliosis," *Spine* 30(2005): 547–50.

14. R. D. Anbar, "Stressors Associated with Dyspnea in Childhood: Patients' Insights and a Case Report," *American Journal of Clinical Hypnosis* 47(2004): 93–101.

15. A. Bowden, A. Lorenc, and N. Robinson, "Autogenic Training as a Behavioural Approach To Insomnia: A Prospective Cohort Study," *Primary Health Care Research and Development* 26(2011): 1–11.

16. B. Pikó, E. Kovács, and P. Kriston, "The Significance of the Relationship Between External/Internal Locus of Control and Adolescent Substance Use in Behavioral Medicine," *Orvosi Hetilap* 152(2011): 331–37.

17. M. P. Jensen, D. M. Ehde, K. J. Gertz, B. L. Stoelb, T. M. Dillworth, A. T. Hirsh, I. R. Molton, G. H. Kraft, "Effects of Self-Hypnosis Training and Cognitive Restructuring on Daily Pain Intensity and Catastrophizing in Individuals with Multiple Sclerosis and Chronic Pain," *International Journal of Clinical and Experimental Hypnosis* 59(2011): 45–63.

18. J. E. Lazarus and S. K. Klein, "Nonpharmacological Treatment of Tics in Tourette Syndrome Adding Videotape Training to Self-Hypnosis," *Journal of Developmental and Behavioral Pediatrics* 31(2010): 498–504.

19. B. Gorton, "Autogenic Training," *American Journal of Clinical Hypnosis* 2(1959): 31–41.

20. F. Stetter and S. Kupper, "Autogenic Training: A Meta-Analysis of Clinical Outcome Studies," *Applied Psychophysiology and Biofeedback* 27(2002): 45–98.

21. J. S. Gordon, J. K. Staples, A. Blyta, and M. Bytyqi, "Treatment of Posttraumatic Stress Disorder in Postwar Kosovo High School Students Using Mind-Body Skills Groups: A Pilot Study," *Journal of Traumatic Stress* 17(2004): 143–47.

22. N. Kanji, A. R. White, and E. Ernst, "Autogenic Training Reduces Anxiety After Coronary Angioplasty: A Randomized Clinical Trial," *American Heart Journal* 147(2004): E10.

23. A. F. Jorm, H. Christensen, K. M. Griffiths, R. A. Parslow, B. Rodgers, and K. A. Blewitt, "Effectiveness of Complementary and Self-Help Treatments for Anxiety Disorders," *Medical Journal of Australia* 181(2004): S29–S46.

24. N. Kanji, A. White, and E. Ernst, "Autogenic Training to Reduce Anxiety in Nursing Students: Randomized Controlled Trial," *Journal of Advanced Nursing* 53(2006): 729–35.

25. B. R. Jojić and L. M. Leposavić, "Autogenic Training as a Therapy for Adjustment Disorder in Adults," *Srpski arhiv za celokupno lekarstvo* 133(2005): 505–09.

26. Jack A. Gerschman, et al., "Hypnosis in the Control of Gagging," *Australian Journal of Clinical and Experimental Hypnosis* 9(1981): 53–59.

27. Jon D. Boller and Raymond P. Flom, "Behavioral Treatment of Persistent Posttraumatic Startle Response," *Journal of Behavior Therapy and Experimental Psychiatry* 12(1981): 321–24.

28. C. A. Smith, C. T. Collins, A. M. Cyna, and C. A. Crowther, "Complementary and Alternative Therapies for Pain Management in Labour," *Cochrane Database Systematic Reviews (Online)* 4(October 18, 2006). CD003521.

29. E. H. Kang, J. E. Park, C. S. Chung, and B. H. Yu, "Effect of Biofeedback-Assisted Autogenic Training on Headache Activity and Mood States in Korean Female Migraine Patients," *Journal of Korean Medical Science* 24(2009): 936–40.

30. M. P. Jensen, J. Barber, J. M. Romano, I. R. Molton, K. A. Raichle, T. L. Osborne, J. M. Engel, B. L. Stoelb, G. H. Kraft, and D. R. Patterson, "A Comparison of Self-Hypnosis Versus Progressive Muscle Relaxation in Patients with Multiple Sclerosis and Chronic Pain," *International Journal of Clinical and Experimental Hypnosis* 57(2009): 198–221.

31. E. A. Asbury, N. Kanji, E. Ernst, M. Barbir, and P. Collins, "Autogenic Training to Manage Symptomology in Women with Chest Pain and Normal Coronary Arteries," *Menopause* 16(2009): 60–65.

32. F. Goto, K. Nakai, T. Kunihiro, and K. Ogawa, "Case Report: A Case of Intractable Meniere's Disease Treated with Autogenic Training," *Biopsychosocial Medicine* 2(2008): 3.

33. Y. E. Noh, T. Morris, and M. B. Andersen, "Psychological Intervention Programs for Reduction of Injury in Ballet Dancers," *Research in Sports Medicine* 15(2007): 13–32.

34. S. Mitani, M. Fujita, S. Sakamoto, and T. Shirakawa, "Effect of Autogenic Training on Cardiac Autonomic Nervous Activity in High-Risk Fire Service Workers for Posttraumatic Stress Disorder," *Journal of Psychosomatic Research* 60(2006): 439–44.

35. T. S. Newmark and D. F. Bogacki, "The Use of Relaxation, Hypnosis, and Imagery in Sport Psychiatry," *Clinics in Sports Medicine* 24(2005): 973–77.

36. G. Elkins, M. H. Rajab, and J. Marcus, "Complementary and Alternative Medicine Use by Psychiatric Inpatients," *Psychological Reports* 96(2005): 163–66.

37. Daniel P. Kohen and Robert Zajac, "Self-Hypnosis Training for Children and Adolescents," *Journal of Pediatrics* 150(2007): 635–39.

38. W. A. Lewandowski, "Patterning of Pain and Power with Guided Imagery," *Nursing Science Quarterly* 17(2004): 233–41.

39. C. Russell and S. Smart, "Guided Imagery and Distraction Therapy in Paediatric Hospice Care," *Paediatric Nursing* 19(2007): 24–25.

40. C. L. Baird and L. P. Sands, "Effect of Guided Imagery with Relaxation on Health-Related Quality of Life in Older Women with Osteoarthritis," *Research in Nursing and Health* 29(2006): 442–51.

41. B. Krakow, M. Hollifield, R. Schrader, M. Koss, D. Tandberg, J. Lauriello, L. McBride, T. D. Warner, D. Cheng, T. Edmond, and R. Kellner, "A Controlled Study of Imagery Rehearsal for Chronic Nightmares in Sexual Assault Survivors with PTSD: A Preliminary Report," *Journal of Traumatic Stress* 13(2000): 589–609.

42. R. McCaffrey, "The Effect of Healing Gardens and Art Therapy on Older Adults with Mild to Moderate Depression," *Holistic Nursing Practice* 21(2007): 79–84.

43. L. Freeman and L. Dirks, "Mind-Body Imagery Practice among Alaska Breast Cancer Patients: A Case Study," *Alaska Medicine* 48(2006): 74–84.

44. M. G. Kushner, K. Abrams, C. Donahue, P. Thuras, R. Frost, and S. W. Kim, "Urge to Gamble in Problem Gamblers Exposed to a Casino Environment," *Journal of Gambling Studies* 23(2007): 121–32.

45. Jerrold S. Greenberg and George B. Dintiman, *Managing Athletic Performance Stress: Getting the Mind Out of the Way* (Kill Devil Hills, NC: National Association of Speed and Explosion, 2009).

46. W. Timothy Gallwey, *The Inner Game of Tennis* (New York: Random House, 1997).

47. F. J. McGuigan, "Stress Management Through Progressive Relaxation," *International Journal of Stress Management* 1(1994): 205–14.

48. Edmund Jacobson, *Progressive Relaxation* (Chicago: University of Chicago Press, 1938).

49. James H. Humphrey, *Childhood Stress in Contemporary Society* (New York: The Haworth Press, 2004), 132–33.

50. McGuigan, "Stress Management," 205–14.

51. M. Matsumoto and J. C. Smith, "Progressive Muscle Relaxation, Breathing Exercises, and ABC Relaxation Theory," *Journal of Clinical Psychology* 57(2001): 1551–57.

52. Barbara B. Brown, *Stress and the Art of Biofeedback* (New York: Harper & Row, 1977), 45.

53. T. Devineni and E. B. Blanchard, "A Randomized Controlled Trial of an Internet-based Treatment for Chronic Headache," *Behaviour Research and Therapy* 43(2005): 277–92.

54. R. W. Ostelo, M. W. van Tulder, J. W. Vlaeyen, S. J. Linton, S. J. Morley, and W. J. Assendelft, "Behavioural Treatment for Chronic Low-Back Pain," *Cochrane Database of Systematic Reviews* 1(2005): CD002014.

55. H. J. Yoo, S. H. Ahn, S. B. Kim, W. K. Kim, and O. S. Han, "Efficacy of Progressive Muscle Relaxation Training and Guided Imagery in Reducing Chemotherapy Side Effects in Patients with Breast Cancer and in Improving Their Quality of Life," *Supportive Care in Cancer* 13(2005): 826–33.

56. A. Molassiotis, H. P. Yung, B. M. Yam, F. Y. Chan, and T. S. Mok, "The Effectiveness of Progressive Muscle Relaxation Training in Managing Chemotherapy-Induced Nausea and Vomiting in Chinese Breast Cancer Patients: A Randomized Controlled Trial," *Supportive Care in Cancer* 10(2002): 237–46.

57. E. Campos de Carvalho, F. T. Martins, and C. B. dos Santos, "A Pilot Study of a Relaxation Technique for Management of Nausea and Vomiting in Patients Receiving Cancer Chemotherapy," *Cancer Nursing* 30(2007): 163–67.

58. C. Figueroa-Moseley, P. Jean-Pierre, J. A. Roscoe, J. L. Ryan, S. Kohli, O. G. Palesh, E. P. Ryan, J. Carroll, and G. R. Morrow, "Behavioral Interventions in Treating Anticipatory Nausea and Vomiting," *Journal of the National Comprehensive Cancer Network* 5(2007): 44–50.

59. W. F. Waters, M. J. Hurry, P. G. Binks, C. E. Carney, L. E. Lajos, K. H. Fuller, B. Betz, J. Johnson, T. Anderson, and J. M. Tucci, "Behavioral and Hypnotic Treatments for Insomnia Subtypes," *Behavioral Sleep Medicine* 1(2003): 81–101.

60. A. D. Krystal, "Treating the Health, Quality of Life, and Functional Impairments in Insomnia," *Journal of Clinical Sleep Medicine* 3(2007): 63–72.

61. C. L. Baird and L. Sands, "A Pilot Study of the Effectiveness of Guided Imagery with Progressive Muscle Relaxation to Reduce Chronic Pain and Mobility Difficulties of Osteoarthritis," *Pain Management Nursing* 5(2004): 97–104.

62. K. L. Kwekkeboom and E. Gretarsdottir, "Systematic Review of Relaxation Interventions for Pain," *Journal of Nursing Scholarship* 38(2006): 269–77.

63. R. H. Schneider, C. N. Alexander, F. Staggers, D. W. Orme-Johnson, M. Rainforth, J. W. Salerno, W. Sheppard, A. Castillo-Richmond, V. A. Barnes, and S. I. Nidich, "A Randomized Controlled Trial of Stress Reduction in African Americans Treated for Hypertension for Over One Year," *American Journal of Hypertension* 18(2005): 88–98.

64. M. Schwickert, J. Langhorst, A. Paul, A. Michalsen, and G. J. Dobos, "Stress Management in the Treatment of Essential Arterial Hypertension," *MMW Fortschritte der Medizin* 148(2006): 40–42.

65. Richard S. Surwit, Miranda A. L. van Tilburg, Nancy Zucker, Cynthia C. McCaskill, Priti Parekh, Mark N. Feinglos, Christopher L. Edwards, Paula Williams, and James D. Lane, "Stress Management Improves Long-Term Glycemic Control in Type 2 Diabetes," *Diabetes Care* 25(2002): 30–34.

66. L. A. Pawlow, P. M. O'Neil, and R. J. Malcolm, "Night Eating Syndrome: Effects of Brief Relaxation Training on Stress, Mood, Hunger, and Eating Patterns," *International Journal of Obesity and Related Metabolic Disorders* 27(2003): 970–78.

67. D. H. Powell, "Behavioral Treatment of Debilitating Test Anxiety Among Medical Students," *Journal of Clinical Psychology* 60(2004): 853–65.

68. Y. L. Cheung, A. Molassiotis, and A. M. Chang, "The Effect of Progressive Muscle Relaxation Training on Anxiety and Quality of Life After Stoma Surgery in Colorectal Cancer Patients," *Psychooncology* 12(2003): 254–66.

69. K. Morgan, S. Dixon, N. Mathers, J. Thompson, and M. Tomeny, "Psychological Treatment for Insomnia in the Regulation of Long-Term Hypnotic Drug Use," *Health Technology Assessment* 8(2004): iii–iv, 1–68.

70. A. P. Greeff and W. S. Conradie, "Use of Progressive Relaxation Training for Chronic Alcoholics with Insomnia," *Psychological Reports* 82(1998): 407–12.

71. Kenneth J. Kukla, "The Effects of Progressive Relaxation Training upon Athletic Performance During Stress," *Dissertation Abstracts International* 37(1977): 6392.

72. Sarah M. Rausch, Sandra E. Gramling, and Stephen M. Auerbach, "Effects of a Single Session of Large-Group Meditation and Progressive Muscle Relaxation Training on Stress Reduction, Reactivity, and Recovery," *International Journal of Stress Management* 13(2006): 273–90.

73. Y. K. Yildirim and C. Fadiloglu, "The Effect of Progressive Muscle Relaxation Training on Anxiety Levels and Quality of Life in Dialysis Patients," *EDTNA/ERCA Journal* 32(2006): 86–88.

74. D. S. Yu, D. T. Lee, and J. Woo, "Effects of Relaxation Therapy on Psychologic Distress and Symptom Status in Older Chinese Patients with Heart Failure," *Journal of Psychosomatic Research* 62(2007): 427–37.

75. H. M. De Vos, and D. A. Louw, "The Effect of Hypnotic Training Programs on the Academic Performance of Students," *American Journal of Clinical Hypnosis* 49(2006): 101–12.

76. M. Di Nicola, L. Occhiolini, L. Di Nicola, P. Vellante, R. Di Mascio, M. Guizzardi, V. Colagrande, and E. Ballone, "Stress Management and Factors Related to the Deployment of Italian Peacekeepers in Afghanistan," *Military Medicine* 172(2007): 140–43.

77. Jeffrey W. Forman and Dave Myers, *The Personal Stress Reduction Program* (Englewood Cliffs, NJ: Prentice Hall, 1987), 72.

78. Jonathan C. Smith, *Relaxation Dynamics: Nine World Approaches to Self-Relaxation* (Champaign, IL: Research Press, 1985), 65.

LAB ASSESSMENT 11.1

Is Autogenic Training for You?

Directions: Practice autogenic training as suggested and regularly. After at least a one-week trial period, rate each statement, using the following scale.

1 = very untrue
2 = somewhat untrue
3 = not sure
4 = somewhat true
5 = very true

_____ 1. It felt good.

_____ 2. It was easy to fit into my schedule.

_____ 3. It made me feel relaxed.

_____ 4. I handled my daily chores better than I usually do.

_____ 5. It was an easy technique to learn.

_____ 6. I was able to close out my surroundings while practicing this technique.

_____ 7. I did not feel tired after practicing this relaxation technique.

_____ 8. My fingers and toes felt warmer directly after trying this relaxation technique.

_____ 9. Any stress symptoms I had (headache, tense muscles, anxiety) before doing this relaxation technique disappeared by the time I was done.

_____ 10. Each time I concluded this technique, my pulse rate was much lower than when I began.

Now sum up the values you responded with for a total score. Save this score and compare it with scores for other relaxation techniques you try. The higher the score is, the more appropriate a particular relaxation skill is for you.

Describe any recurring thoughts you experienced during autogenic training:

_____

_____

_____

Describe any difficulties you experienced during autogenic training:

_____

_____

_____

LAB ASSESSMENT 11.2

Is Imagery for You?

Directions: Practice imagery as suggested and regularly. After at least a one-week trial period, rate each statement, using the following scale.

1 = very untrue

2 = somewhat untrue

3 = not sure

4 = somewhat true

5 = very true

_____ 1. It felt good.

_____ 2. It was easy to fit into my schedule.

_____ 3. It made me feel relaxed.

_____ 4. I handled my daily chores better than I usually do.

_____ 5. It was an easy technique to learn.

_____ 6. I was able to close out my surroundings while practicing this technique.

_____ 7. I did not feel tired after practicing this relaxation technique.

_____ 8. My fingers and toes felt warmer directly after trying this relaxation technique.

_____ 9. Any stress symptoms I had (headache, tense muscles, anxiety) before doing this relaxation technique disappeared by the time I was done.

_____ 10. Each time I concluded this technique, my pulse rate was much lower than when I began.

Now sum up the values you responded with for a total score. Save this score and compare it with scores for other relaxation techniques you try. The higher the score is, the more appropriate a particular relaxation skill is for you.

Describe any recurring thoughts you experienced during the imagery exercise:

_____

_____

_____

Describe any difficulties you experienced during the imagery exercise:

_____

_____

_____

LAB ASSESSMENT 11.3

Is Progressive Relaxation for You?

Directions: Practice progressive relaxation as suggested and regularly. After at least a one-week trial period, rate each statement, using the following scale.

1 = very untrue

2 = somewhat untrue

3 = not sure

4 = somewhat true

5 = very true

_____ 1. It felt good.

_____ 2. It was easy to fit into my schedule.

_____ 3. It made me feel relaxed.

_____ 4. I handled my daily chores better than I usually do.

_____ 5. It was an easy technique to learn.

_____ 6. I was able to close out my surroundings while practicing this technique.

_____ 7. I did not feel tired after practicing this relaxation technique.

_____ 8. My fingers and toes felt warmer directly after trying this relaxation technique.

_____ 9. Any stress symptoms I had (headache, tense muscles, anxiety) before doing this relaxation technique disappeared by the time I was done.

_____ 10. Each time I concluded this technique, my pulse rate was much lower than when I began.

Now sum up the values you responded with for a total score. Save this score and compare it with scores for other relaxation techniques you try. The higher the score is, the more appropriate a particular relaxation skill is for you.

Describe any recurring thoughts you experienced during progressive relaxation:

_____

_____

_____

Describe any difficulties you experienced during progressive relaxation:

_____

_____

_____

Other Relaxation Techniques

My friend and colleague, Dr. Jack Osman, goes around the country offering his lecture, "Fat Is Where It's At." A good speaker, creative, and well informed, Jack is always looking for new ways to have his audience appreciate that the charts listing how much you should weigh for your sex and height (and sometimes body build) are invalid. We were sitting in my office one day when Jack described his latest motivational device, soon to be tested on an unsuspecting audience. "I'm going to purchase old bathroom scales from junkyards. They'll probably cost a dollar apiece. Then I'll get a sledgehammer. The first thing I'm going to do after I'm introduced to the audience is use that sledgehammer to whack the hell out of a scale. I'll hit that sucker until it begs for mercy."

Being the gentleman that he is (really), Jack cares about those he educates. He wants them to know that weight charts consider not body fat but, rather, total weight. A well-developed weight lifter, for instance, may weigh more than the weight chart advises but not be "overfat."

Your body's weight can be conveyed to you by a scale, or your degree of fat can be determined by a skin caliper. The scale and caliper give you feedback about your body. If you use a heart monitor when you work out, you are also using biofeedback equipment.

Biofeedback

Biofeedback has been defined as the use of "electronic instruments or other techniques to monitor and change subconscious activities, many of which are regulated by the autonomic nervous system."[1] That's just a fancy way of saying biofeedback is receiving information about what is occurring in your body at a particular time and then helping you to control that occurrence. A biofeedback instrument is just a tool used to obtain a measure about the part of your body in which you are interested. Consequently, a basal body thermometer is a biofeedback instrument—albeit slow and not as accurate as more sophisticated equipment—since it gives you information about a parameter of the body (its core temperature).

To better understand the concept of biofeedback and biofeedback instrumentation, tape a basal body thermometer to your middle finger, making sure the sensitive bulb of the thermometer is against the skin of your finger. In a short period of time (five minutes), the thermometer will stabilize at a reading, indicating the temperature at the surface of that finger. Record that temperature here:

_____ °F

Your task now is to increase the temperature at the surface of that finger by increasing the peripheral blood flow. As you should recall, either meditation or autogenic training will result in more blood flow to the arms and legs (and fingers and toes). Therefore, use either of these relaxation techniques for 10 or 15 minutes to accomplish your task and then record the temperature of the surface of your finger here:

_____ °F

biofeedback
The use of electronic instruments or other techniques to monitor and change subconscious activities, many of which are regulated by the autonomic nervous system.

Biofeedback, however, is also a process. It has been determined, and more than adequately validated, that once people are fed back information about their body processes, they can be taught to control these processes.

Biofeedback really involves three phases:

1. *Measuring* the physiological parameter (The sensitive mercury in the bulb of the thermometer senses temperature.)

2. *Converting* this measurement to some understandable form (The mercury in the thermometer rises in a tube calibrated by degrees Fahrenheit, allowing the temperature of the finger to be determined visually.)

3. *Feeding back* this information to the person who is learning to control his or her body processes

Before this system could be developed, however, researchers had to demonstrate that body processes previously believed to be involuntary could, in fact, be brought under voluntary control. The early research in biofeedback was directed toward demonstrating this fact. It was shown, for instance, that subjects could change their heart rate,[2-4] the electrical conductance of their skin (galvanic skin response),[5-7] the dilation of their blood vessels,[8] and the brain waves they emitted.[9,10] Numerous other physiological parameters can also be controlled by biofeedback training: muscle tension, blood pressure, penile erection, and secretion of hydrochloric acid in the stomach, to name a few. Although it still has not been determined *how* people control their physiology, that they can is no longer questioned.

Benefits of Biofeedback

Biofeedback has many benefits, not the least of which is the demonstration (objectively and physiologically) that we have much greater control of ourselves than most of us realize. If we can demonstrate through measurable means that we can control blood pressure and brain waves, shouldn't we be able to control cigarette smoking and exercise behavior? If we can increase or decrease heart rate or the amount of stomach acid we secrete, how difficult could it be to conquer stage fright or an alcohol problem? Biofeedback demonstrates to us that our behavior, as well as our physiology, is pretty much our own doing. That being the case, we must accept responsibility for our behavioral choices.

In addition, biofeedback has specific physiological and psychological benefits. These benefits are presented next.

Physiological Effects

As we shall soon see, biofeedback has been used to improve the physical health of many people. However, an interesting point is made by Elmer Green and his associates:

> In actuality, there is no such thing as training in brain wave control, there is training only in the elicitation of certain subjective states. . . . What are detected and manipulated (in some as yet unknown way) are subjective feelings, focus of attention, and thought processes.[11]

Once again, the relationship between mind and body is demonstrated. Changes in subjective states result in changes in physiology during biofeedback practice.

In any case, **electromyographic (EMG) biofeedback** alone, which focuses upon muscle tension, has been effective in treating the following conditions:

asthma	ulcers
hypertension	muscle spasms
bruxism	nerve-muscle injuries (stroke, paralysis)
hyperkinesia	spasmodic torticollis
spasticity	tinnitus
cerebral palsy	migraine headache

electromyographic (EMG) biofeedback

Biofeedback that measures muscle contraction.

dystonias	tension headache
dysphonia	colitis

More specifically, researchers have found EMG biofeedback effective in health conditions that require muscle control such as posture,[12] leg muscle control,[13-16] temporomandibular joint (TMJ) pain,[17] defecatory disorders (e.g., chronic constipation),[18,19] urinary incontinence,[20,21] asthma,[22] epilepsy,[23] and even for attention deficit/hyperactivity disorder (ADHD).[24,25]

Scoliosis—an S-shaped curvature of the spine—is also being remedied through biofeedback. To correct this curvature of the spine, many patients wear a body brace, which may be uncomfortable and psychologically disturbing. Because this condition occurs most often in adolescent girls, a body brace can be particularly bothersome during this developmental period. Neal Miller and Barry Dworkin developed an alternative to the typical body brace.[26] This harness is made of a nylon fiber, which makes it lightweight and less cumbersome than other braces. Its supports run both vertically and horizontally. A sensor determines when the wearer is not standing straight, and a tone then sounds. Such innovative uses of biofeedback are the wave of the future.

Thermal biofeedback (temperature) has been effective in treating conditions related to blood flow. As such, thermal biofeedback has been used to treat complications from diabetes,[27,28] recurrent headache,[29] Raynaud's disease (restricted blood flow to the fingers and toes),[30] and high blood pressure.[31] Additionally, thermal biofeedback has been used with patients with palmarhyperhidrosis (a fancy name for sweating of the palms).[32]

thermal biofeedback
Biofeedback that measures temperature.

However, researchers found contradictory results regarding some of these benefits and uses of biofeedback. For example, Kaushik et al.,[33] Powers and Andrasik,[34] and Biondi[35] found that biofeedback helped subjects in their studies reduce the pain of headache. Yet, other researchers found it ineffective for headaches. For example, when Szekely studied the use of biofeedback to treat headaches resulting from menstrual pain, she did not find it to be an effective treatment;[36] and a review of research concluded there was contradictory evidence for the effectiveness of biofeedback for treating menstrual pain.[37]

Psychological Effects

Biofeedback has been used to help people improve their psychological health and make changes in their health-related behavior. Phobias, anxiety, stage fright, insomnia, alcoholism, drug abuse, depression, and hyperactivity in children have been successfully treated with biofeedback. Tension headaches, sexual dysfunction, substance abuse, and even stuttering have responded to biofeedback as well.[38-40]

In addition, biofeedback has been shown to be effective in treating anxiety[41] and burnout,[42] obsessive-compulsive disorder[43] enhancing health locus of control,[44] regulation of mental state,[45] psychogenic cough,[46] phobia,[47] depression,[48] and post traumatic stress disorder.[49]

How to Relax Using Biofeedback

Biofeedback equipment is not designed to be used during the routine stressful moments we all experience daily. Rather, it is a training device. Biofeedback is used to train people to gain greater control of their physiological processes. You can't walk around all day long attached to some biofeedback apparatus or "hook up" whenever you are stressed. The equipment is used to teach you the sensations of relaxation and its physiological correlates: decreased muscle tension, heart rate, respiratory rate, blood pressure, and so forth. The hope is that, once you are able to control more of your physiological responses to stressors, you will not react to stress dysfunctionally.

Since you cannot remain connected to biofeedback equipment forever, another relaxation technique is usually taught to you and used in conjunction with

Biofeedback instrumentation comes in various forms and measures various physiological parameters. Included is (a) a galvanic skin response (electrical conductivity) instrument with accompanying kit. To make biofeedback training more interesting, and to encourage the bodily changes desired, different displays are offered. Two of these displays are depicted in (b) and (c).

(a)

(b)

(c)

biofeedback for purposes of stress management. Autogenic training, meditation, and progressive relaxation have all been employed in this manner. In one respect, the biofeedback equipment just objectively verifies that the other relaxation technique has been learned. Of course, it also may facilitate such learning by serving as a reinforcer and quickly identifying what is and what is not working.

An example of how I used biofeedback with one of my students will illustrate this last point. After teaching several different types of relaxation techniques to my students and providing them with sufficient time for practice of these techniques, I found one of my students frustrated. It seems he felt that none of the techniques helped him to relax. He said he really didn't remember relaxing much during his 50-odd years of life. When we worked with the biofeedback equipment, however, it was a different story. With electromyographic biofeedback, this student was able to demonstrate a remarkably low frontalis (forehead) muscle tension. Since the frontalis muscle is believed to be a mirror to general body relaxation, I was glad to see this student finally achieve a deep state of relaxation. Afterward, we spoke, and he told me that, for some reason, whenever he imagined a tunnel with black walls with purple blotches on them, the equipment reported he was at a very low level of muscular tension. He had never seen that tunnel before, nor could he associate it with any symbolic meaning. However, the vision of it relaxed him. The biofeedback training, then, served this student well, because it helped him to identify an image that he could recall whenever he chose to, enabling him to relax.

How to Arrange for Biofeedback Training

In spite of the limited availability of biofeedback equipment, its high cost, and the frequent need to also learn another relaxation technique, you can still do biofeedback training if you're cagey enough. Seek out the psychology, counseling, health education, or similar department on a college campus, and you'll often find biofeedback equipment. Next, make yourself available to faculty and graduate students who need subjects for their biofeedback research. Perhaps there's even a course that employs biofeedback as a component. If so, enroll in it.

In addition to universities, many hospitals have biofeedback equipment. Perhaps you can qualify for third-party payment (health insurance) for biofeedback training. Perhaps the hospital personnel are also conducting biofeedback research and need subjects.

Diaphragmatic Breathing

When you are distressed, your breathing becomes rapid and shallow, and it stems from your chest. There are several different ways that people breathe. When you expand the upper third of the chest, you are doing *upper costal breathing* (named after the intercostal muscles that connect the ribs). Most people breathe by expanding the middle third of their chest (approximately at the sixth rib down). This is known as *thoracic breathing* or *middle costal breathing*. However, the more relaxing and healthier form of breathing is to expand the belly, lower costal breathing. This is called **diaphragmatic breathing,** because you expand the diaphragm when you breathe this way. Sometimes we make a deep sigh to relieve stress by inhaling a large amount of air and exhaling it slowly. This we call *very deep breathing,* and it is quite effective as an immediate response to stress.

diaphragmatic breathing
Deep breathing that expands the belly rather than just the chest.

To help people practice breathing diaphragmatically, Krucoff and Krucoff recommend the following (see Figure 12.1):[50]

1. Lie on your back and place a book on your belly. Make the book rise with your breathing.
2. Sit with your right hand on your abdomen and your left hand on your chest and make your right hand rise as you breathe.
3. Use a second hand on a clock and inhale for five seconds and exhale for five seconds.
4. Repeat a mantra and breathe in synchrony as you say it in your mind. Zen master Thich Nhat Hanh suggests repeating, "Breathing in I calm myself, breathing out I smile."

Let's practice diaphragmatic breathing. Lie on your back, with the palms of your hands placed on your lower stomach area. As you breathe, expand your chest area while keeping your stomach flat. Become aware that this is thoracic breathing and learn to recognize it as such. Next, expand your abdomen so that your stomach rises and falls with each breath while your chest size remains relatively constant (it will expand some). Recognize this type of breathing as diaphragmatic breathing. Practice it at various times of the day (when seated doing school work, for instance).

Figure 12.1

Diaphragmatic Breathing

King Kong wasn't concerned with holding in his abdomen and showing a "six pack." Doesn't he look relaxed as he breathes diaphragmatically?

Diaphragmatic breathing is basic to all forms of relaxation. It is difficult being relaxed if you are breathing thoracically. In addition, diaphragmatic breathing may be helpful in treating migraine, Raynaud's disease, hypertension, asthma, and anxiety.

Many other breathing exercises can help you relax. Consistent with what we discussed earlier about relaxation techniques, these breathing exercises require you to focus on something other than events that have the potential to elicit a stress response. In this case, you focus on your breathing. When doing the two exercises described next, be sure *not* to try to control the rate of your breathing. Instead, regulate the *phases* of your breathing: inhalation and exhalation. Inhale deeply and slowly, and exhale completely and slowly.

- *Color breathing:* While seated comfortably, imagine the ground below you is filled with an energizing red color. Slowly inhale and visualize drawing in this red color through your feet, legs, and upward throughout your body. Then slowly exhale the red color out of your body, imagining the space around you turning completely red. Try this exercise with other colors as well. Some colors may be more relaxing for you than others.
- *Nasal switching:* Whether or not you realize it, you typically breathe through one nostril at a time, switching nostrils periodically. Paying attention to which nostril you are using and practicing switching from one nostril to the other will help you focus away from stressors you encounter. Breathe through one nostril for a series of breaths, and then focus on breathing through the other nostril for the same number of breaths.

Body Scanning

body scanning
A relaxation technique that searches for relaxed body parts and transports that sensation to less relaxed areas.

Even when you are tense, there is some part of your body that feels relaxed. **Body scanning** requires you to search for that part and, identifying it, spread that sensation to the more tense parts of yourself. For example, if you pay attention to your bodily sensations, you may find that your calf muscles feel particularly relaxed. You would then focus upon the feelings in your calf muscles, becoming aware of the sensations experienced there. Then you would attempt to transfer these sensations to other parts of your body that are more tense—for example, your shoulder muscles. The relaxed sensation can be imagined to be a warm ball that travels to various bodily locations, warming and relaxing them.

Body Scan Relaxation Exercise

To begin a body scan, find a comfortable spot either in a chair or lie down. You can engage in this exercise with a partner. If you do, take turns reading this exercise to each other in a very slow and low voice, taking adequate pauses for your partner to finish cycles of breathing.

1. Close your eyes. Begin with five complete breath cycles. Inhale deeply into your belly while you count to four . . . and exhale completely counting from four back down to one. Breathe. Again inhaling deeply into the belly . . . and exhaling completely. (Pause until five full breaths have been completed.)

2. Next focus on your forehead. Notice how it feels. Are your muscles tightened? Is your brow furrowed? Become aware of any tension you are holding in your forehead. With your next exhalation, let any tension go and feel your forehead relax. (Pause for two breaths)

3. Move to the area around your eyes. Notice how your eyes feel. Are they tired, are you squinting, do you perceive fatigue in the muscles around your eyes? With the next three complete breath cycles, release the outer corners of your eyes with the exhale.

4. Continue to breathe slowly, pulling air into your nose and down deep into your belly and then letting go of tension with your exhalation. Release.

5. Come down to your mouth and jaw. Observe any anxiety or stress that you are holding in the muscles around your mouth and the bones of your jaw. With your next exhalation, let your lower jawbone drop down and your mouth open slightly. Release the tension completely in your mouth and jawbone. Inhale and then exhale releasing the tension. (Pause for one breath, wait until the mouth is open slightly.)

6. Become aware of the juncture between your neck and shoulders. Concentrate on bringing your inhalation deep into your belly and with the exhalation releasing your shoulders so they float down toward your feet. Feel the weight of your collarbone drop several inches with your exhalation. Breathe in and feel your neck lengthening as you leave your shoulders down in the relaxed position. Exhale and feel your shoulders drop lower and lower.

7. Shift your attention to your elbows, wrists, and fingers. Can you perceive any tension or clenching in these joints and the muscles that support them? (Read slowly.) Just take notice of this as you feel your upper arm, lower arm, the palms of your hands, your thumb and fingers. Use your inhalation to pull fresh cleansing air deep into your body's center and, with the exhalation, release the tension in your arms and hands. Feel your arms get heavy as they let go and sink to the floor.

8. Sense the floor beneath you. Give your complete weight to the floor and let it support your whole being. Continue your slow inhalations and exhalations as you let your body sink down into the floor . . . lower (pause) and lower (pause.) Exhale completely and discharge all of the stress and tension that has built up in the muscles of your back. Let the ground support you now.

9. Internally scan your upper and lower legs for signs that you are contracting your muscles unnecessarily. Inhale and hold this awareness about your lower body. Exhale slowly and completely. With your next inhalation let go of all the worry and stress that you have stored in your lower body. Exhale and let your legs feel heavy against the floor. Let your feet drop away at your ankle joint.

10. Breathe. Release. Revisit your forehead, eyes, mouth, and jawbone. If any tension has slipped back into these areas, just use your deep slow exhalations to erase it and let go again. Feel your neck long and your shoulders down, the floor rising up to support your back and pelvis, legs and feet. Feel your connection to the Earth and let gravity support you. Breathe.[51]

Once your body is relaxed, perform an inventory to identify any parts that are still tense. Then focus on the relaxed parts trying to transfer that sense of relaxation to the tense part.

Massage and Acupressure

Many cultures developed forms of massage. Traditional Chinese and Indian medical care have over the centuries viewed massage as an important component of treatment. In the eighteenth century, Per Hendrik Ling developed what we today know as Swedish massage. In the past 20 to 30 years, Swedish massage has been embraced by therapists for physiological, psychological, and spiritual health.

Several techniques that originally derived from European massage have been developed in recent years. One of these is **reflexology.** In reflexology, areas of the foot are believed to correspond to organs or structures of the body. Damage to these body parts is manifested in a "reflex zone" of the foot. Treatment then consists of massaging this zone.

Another technique associated with massage is **aromatherapy.** In aromatherapy, oils derived from plants are mixed with massage oil. This lubricant has a pleasing smell and, some claim, has medicinal qualities such as the ability to heal wounds, fight infection, assist in circulation of blood, and aid in digestion. Proponents of aromatherapy state that the beneficial effects are a result of the pharmacological properties of the plant material being absorbed into the bloodstream through the skin and by the breathing in of the aromas.

Massage has a way of relaxing the muscles of a tense body. Various forms of massage exist, but acupressure massage (**shiatsu**)—pressing down on points of the body where knots or bands of muscle tension frequently occur—appears to be one of the more popular forms. Although any object can be used to employ pressure, most often the hands are used for massaging. To use acupressure correctly, you can obtain a chart of acupressure points at *TensionRelief info* at www.tensionrelief.info/charts.html.

Massage, as opposed to acupressure, involves warming a massage lotion (such as vitamin E or body lotion) and employing one of several techniques: caressing, gliding, or kneading. Never press directly on the vertebrae, just on their sides, and never apply hard pressure on the neck or lower back region.

The different techniques used during massage include[52]

1. *Effleurage*—gentle stroking along the length of a muscle.
2. *Petrissage*—gentle pressure applied across the width of a muscle.
3. *Friction*—vigorous pressure by circular motions of the thumb or fingertips.
4. *Kneading*—squeezing across the width of a muscle.
5. *Hacking*—light slaps or karate chops.

The American Massage Therapy Association[53] cites research highlighting the benefits of massage. These include decreasing feelings of fatigue[54] and pain[55] in cancer patients, alleviating back pain,[56] decreasing pain from arthritis of the knee,[57] boosting immune system functioning,[58] decreasing carpal tunnel symptoms,[59] lowering blood pressure,[60] reducing the frequency of headaches,[61] and easing alcohol withdrawal symptoms.[62]

Yoga and Stretching

Yoga comes from a root word that has many meanings: to bind, join, attach, and yoke; to direct and concentrate one's attention; or communion with God. Actually, yoga should more accurately be called "yogas" since there are so many types: Prana Yoga, Brahma Yoga, Kriya Yoga, Kundalini Yoga, Raja Yoga, Tantra Yoga, and the most widely known in the Western world, Hatha Yoga (involving stretching exercises). It is no wonder, therefore, that yoga is proposed to serve many different functions: from cleansing the body, to activating the nervous system, to improving one's intelligence or

reflexology
A massage technique that massages a "reflex zone" in the foot in which damage to body parts is thought to be manifested.

aromatherapy
The use of plant material added to massage oil thought to have pharmacological qualities that improve health.

massage
A relaxation technique that involves manipulating points in the body that are muscularly tense.

shiatsu
Acupressure massage.

yoga
A set of Hindu relaxation techniques.

Yoga can relax the mind and the body, especially when one focuses on the position being sought. In that way, concentration is on the yoga position rather than on the stressors of the day.

sex life. Researchers have found yoga to have beneficial physiological and psychological effects. For example, when asthmatics were taught yoga, they were found to breathe more comfortably and to judge their quality of life to have improved.[63] Diabetics were able to lower their blood glucose levels, use less medication, and increase their number of insulin receptors.[64] Older men and women—65 to 85 years of age—taught yoga improved their flexibility and reported feeling more energetic and less fatigued.[65] Further, lymphoma patients were able to sleep better by engaging in yoga.[66] They required less sleep medication, slept longer, and got to sleep faster. Psychological benefits of yoga include improvement in anxiety and depression disorders.[67, 68] This finding can be explained by the research of Streeter and colleagues,[69] who found an increase in brain gamma-aminobutyric acid (GABA) in yoga participants. Lower amounts of GABA are associated with anxiety and depression. Lastly, yoga has been found to contribute to a reduction in symptoms in moderately ill schizophrenia patients.[70] The stretching involved in yoga can be quite relaxing, and the prescribed yoga positions (called **asanas**) encourage this benefit. However, be careful not to stretch in a way that is uncomfortable—remember, you're trying to relax—or in a way in which you will injure yourself. And be sure to maintain relaxed breathing, proper balance, and good form. Although space here does not allow a complete description of the yogic stretching positions, some simple postures (asanas) are presented in Figures 12.2–12.9. There are many other sources you can consult if you wish to learn more about Hatha Yoga.[71, 72]

When engaging in yoga, regulated breathing techniques are used. These are called **pranayamas.** Numerous studies have documented the relationship between deep slow breathing and the activation of the parasympathetic nervous system.[73, 74] As a result, significant decreases in respiration rate, oxygen consumption, and carbon dioxide elimination occur.[75] There are several ways to regulate breathing during yoga. One of these employs a time ratio of 1-4-2: inhale for one second, hold the breath for four seconds, and exhale for two seconds. Another breathing technique involves alternating between nostrils. To practice alternate-nostril breathing, begin by sitting comfortably for a few minutes breathing normally. Then follow these instructions:[76]

1. *Left nostril:* Place the thumb of the right hand on the right nostril. Press the side of the nostril gently with the thumb to close the opening. Exhale slowly through the left nostril. When the exhale is complete, there may be a natural pause. When ready, inhale slowly through the left nostril.

2. *Switch:* Gently pinch both nostrils closed.

3. *Right nostril:* Release the thumb and exhale slowly through the right nostril. When the exhale is complete, there may be a natural pause. When ready, inhale slowly through the right nostril.

asanas
Body positions used during the practice of yoga.

Pranayamas
Regulated breathing techniques used in yoga.

Figure 12.2
Cat Pose

Place your hands directly beneath your shoulders, your back horizontal and flat, and look down. As you breathe out, perform the following movements: (1) press downward so your shoulders are lifted, (2) pull your abdominal muscles back toward your spine, and (3) contract your buttocks. That should bring you into the Cat Tilt.

Figure 12.3
Warrior Pose

To get into the Warrior Pose, perform the following movements: (1) place your feet approximately four feet apart with your left foot 90 degrees to the left, (2) bend your left knee, (3) raise your arms so they are parallel to the floor, and (4) turn your head to the left. Maintain this position for 30 seconds to one minute.

Figure 12.4
Easy Pose

To get into the Easy Pose, perform the following movements: (1) sit on the floor or a mat, (2) cross your legs, (3) place your feet beneath your knees, (4) hold onto your knees, and (5) keep your head and body straight. If you choose to, you can meditate in this position.

Figure 12.5
Half Spinal Twist

To get into the Half Spinal Twist, perform the following movements: (1) kneel and sit on your feet, (2) lean to your right, (3) lift your left leg over your right leg and place the foot of the left leg to the outside of your right knee, (4) bring the right heel inward toward your buttocks while keeping your spine erect, and (5) stretch your arms straight out to the left at shoulder height and twist them around toward the left. Repeat this sequence so that you twist to the right.

Figure 12.6
Leg Reclining Lunge

To get into the Leg Reclining Lunge, perform the following movements: (1) lie on the floor or a mat, (2) bring your right knee close to your chest, (3) hold the sole of your right foot with both hands, (4) pull the knee to the side of your chest so the right heel is directly over your right knee, and (5) while keeping your back straight, pull downward with your hands attempting to touch the right knee to the floor. Maintain this position for 30 seconds to one minute, and then switch sides.

Figure 12.7
Crane Pose

To get into the Crane Pose, perform the following movements: (1) place your hands on the ground, (2) lift your heels, (3) shift your weight to your hands, and (4) lift your feet off the ground while balancing on your hands. Maintain this position for 30 seconds to one minute, or as long as you can.

Figure 12.8
Cobra Pose

To get into the Cobra Pose, perform the following movements: (1) lie on your abdomen on the ground or a mat, (2) place your hands flat on the mat under your armpits, (3) push up on your arms raising your chest and abdomen off the mat, and (4) tilt your head and chin upward.

Figure 12.9
Corpse Pose

To get into the Corpse Pose, perform the following movements: (1) lie on your back with your legs spread out, (2) relax your arms to the sides of your body with the palms facing upward, (3) stretch your body by imagining someone is pulling your legs, arms, and head away from your torso, and (4) breathe diaphragmatically from your abdomen, concentrating on your breath and your body. Maintain this position for several minutes.

4. *Switch:* Gently pinch both nostrils closed, then release the left nostril and exhale.

5. Repeat the cycle for about five to ten minutes.

Repetitive Prayer

Cardiologist Herbert Benson, author of *The Relaxation Response*[77] and other books[78,79] and stress researcher, wondered if prayer—in particular, repetitive prayer—would have the same relaxation-inducing effect as meditation. Benson's initial interest in prayer stemmed from his frustration with people giving up meditation. He thought that if they meditated on prayer, they might be more apt to stay with their relaxation program. Benson did find that repetitive prayer—such as "Hail Mary, full of grace" for Catholics, "Shalom" for Jews, and "Our Father who art in heaven"—did evoke the relaxation response.[80] Benson called this finding the "faith factor." Interestingly, a small group of runners and walkers took off (no pun intended) on Benson's idea and jogged or walked in cadence with the prayer they repeated. They called this exercise "aerobic prayers." If prayer or religion is an important part of your life, perhaps you might want to try to relax by repeating a prayer or a phrase from a prayer with which you are familiar.

Repetitive prayer can be relaxing as it focuses attention away from stressors.

There are several different ways to perform repetitive prayer for relaxation. Cooper[81] suggests sitting in a comfortable chair with your eyes closed and concentrate on breathing regularly. As you exhale, for ten to twenty minutes repeat silently a word or phrase that conforms to your beliefs. For example, you might choose "The Lord is my shepherd" from the Twenty-third Psalm. Then engage in a second, similar session at some point later in the day.

Dain[82] offers still another way to use repetitive prayer divided into three steps.

Step 1: *Quieting the mind.* In a quiet environment, say to yourself, "You now relax and let go. You now relax and let God. You now relax and let go all tension, stress, and strain. You are now relaxing in mind and body." Then declare in a more personal way, "I now relax and let go. I now relax and let go all tension, stress, and strain. I am now relaxing in mind and body. Yes, I relax and let go." Focus on the feeling of the physical strain or muscle tension you may be experiencing. Gently instruct your body to let go, to relax.

Step 2: *Breathing.* Drop your head to your chest and as you exhale, let go of the feelings of any strain you feel in your chest or abdominal area. Imagine that constriction leaving you through those external breaths.

Step 3: *The peaceful state.* Say "peace" to your mind and body. Saying the words, "peace, be still" will help to rid you of any unwanted thoughts or emotions that remain in your mind that have not yet been released. Recite: "I feel the peace of God. I rest in his peace. Peace, sweet peace".

Quieting Reflex

Psychologist Charles Stroebel developed a relaxation technique designed to elicit relaxation quickly. Stroebel says that, with practice, the **Quieting Reflex (QR)**[83] can relax you in merely six seconds. In fact, Elizabeth Stroebel, Charles's wife, tested a variation of the Quieting Reflex—the Kiddie QR—with young children and found it effective in helping them relax as well.[84] The Quieting Reflex has been shown to be effective for stress headaches, migraine headaches, sleep problems, stress and high blood pressure, and for people who frequently have the fight or

Quieting Reflex (QR)
A six-step relaxation technique that results in relaxation in seconds.

flight response, also including those who suffer from various anxiety disorders.[85] To practice the QR,

1. Think about something that makes you afraid or anxious.
2. Smile inside. This breaks up the anxious facial muscle tension.
3. Tell yourself, "I can keep a calm body and an alert mind."
4. Inhale a quiet, easy breath.
5. Let your jaw go loose as you exhale; keep your upper and lower teeth slightly apart.
6. Imagine heaviness and warmth moving throughout your body—from head to toes.

As difficult as it may be to imagine, these six steps can be done in merely six seconds—that is, with practice.

Instant Calming Sequence

Instant Calming Sequence (ICS)
A relaxation technique that elicits relaxation quickly in a five-step approach.

Author and developer of the Health and Fitness Excellence program, Robert Cooper, teaches a relaxation technique that he says takes just seconds to elicit the relaxation response. The **Instant Calming Sequence (ICS)**[86] is based on Cooper's belief that the most effective way to manage stressful situations is to recognize the first signs of stress and immediately begin to respond. ICS's five steps are

Step 1: *Uninterrupted breathing.* In the face of the stressor, keep breathing smoothly, deeply, and evenly.

Step 2: *Positive face.* Flash a slight smile as soon as you recognize you are being stressed.

Step 3: *Balanced posture.* Keep your chest high, head up, neck long, chin in, and in other ways balanced. Imagine being lifted from a hook at the top of your head.

Step 4: *Wave of relaxation.* Send a "wave of relaxation" to those parts of your body that appear tense.

Step 5: *Mental control.* Acknowledge the reality of the situation. Cooper suggests saying, "What's happening is real, and I'm finding the best possible solution right now."

Mindfulness

mindfulness
Focusing attention on the present moment to relax.

Mindfulness is focusing your attention on the present moment. It is paying attention to each moment, living in the here-and-now. Instead of the *what-ifs* and *if-onlys,* the focus is on the *what-is.* Its opposite, mindlessness, is going through life ignoring the present moment because of attention directed toward the goal rather than the experience. Mindlessness occurs when you drive to school or work and describe yourself as being on automatic pilot. All of a sudden, you are at your destination without having really experienced the trip. How sad it is that some people reach the end of their lives without ever having truly experienced the trip along the way.

Mindfulness dates all the way back to Eastern and Western traditions of religion, philosophy, and psychology. It recognizes existentialist philosophy, such as that of Albert Camus, which argues that *who we are* is more important than *what we do.* When patients have been taught to have this focus, mindfulness has been found effective in treating pain associated with fibromyalgia,[87] improving cancer patients' psychosocial adjustment to their disease,[88] and helping with depression and anxiety,[89] insomnia,[90] and irritable bowel syndrome.[91] In fact, studies using magnetic resonance imaging (MRI) reveal that mindfulness-based stress reduction results in changes in the gray matter of the brain that is associated with learning and memory, regulation of emotions, and perception.[92] Because stress is often caused by a preoccupation with the past (guilt, shame, regret) or with the future (fear of upcoming events), mindfulness is an excellent way to help manage stress.[93]

In fact, mindfulness has had some miraculous effects on people undergoing an enormous amount of stress. For example, organ transplant patients used mindfulness and were then able to sleep better; the quality and duration of their sleep improved.[94] They also experienced less anxiety and depression. Bone marrow transplant recipients also benefited from employing mindfulness.[95] They experienced fewer emotional and psychological problems. And after an extensive review of studies on the effects of mindfulness practiced by cancer patients, it was concluded they experienced improvements in mood, sleep, and stress reduction.[96] More specifically, when breast and prostate cancer patients enrolled in an 8-week mindfulness program the result was improvement in their quality of life, symptoms of stress, and quality of sleep.[97] Even smokers were able to abstain from smoking and decrease stressful feelings more effectively when taught mindfulness.[98] Given what we know about stress, it is not surprising that brain and immune system function have also been found to improve for a group of research subjects using mindfulness, versus for a control group.[99]

Psychological benefits are derived from the practice of mindfulness as well. When a group of college students participated in a one-month mindfulness program, they reported feeling more relaxed and experiencing a more positive mood.[100] Another group of research subjects volunteered for an 8-week mindfulness program and experienced reductions in negative psychological symptoms, an increase in a specific sense of control over their lives, and increased spirituality.[101] Lastly, after being horrifically attacked while jogging in Central Park in New York City, Trisha Meili employed mindfulness to restore her emotional and physical functioning. She presented her experience with mindfulness as a copresenter with Dr. Jon Kabat-Zinn, the leading mindfulness researcher, at a conference in Boston in May 2003, concluding that mindfulness can play a significant role in recovery from devastating injury.[102]

Mindfulness can be developed in a number of ways. One is to focus on your breathing, called mindful breathing.[103] In this way, the mind is quieted and attention is drawn to the here-and-now. Another way to develop mindfulness is presented in the box entitled "The Mindfulness Process." Still other mindfulness activities include:

Mindful eating

Focus on what you are eating. Eliminate all distractions, such as reading a newspaper or watching television while eating. Eat slowly and deliberately, paying full attention to each piece of food, its look, its smell, how the food is cut, and the texture and taste of the food. Become totally absorbed only by your eating.

Mindful listening

Focus on the sounds around you. Perhaps you hear the sound of your computer, cars traveling by, the television or radio in an adjourning room, or the sound of birds outside. Be absorbed with these sounds.

Mindful walking

Direct your complete attention to the act of walking. Concentrate on how the ground feels under your feet, how you are breathing, and what is happening around you, such as the presence of objects or other people. More mindfulness exercises appear in the book *The Complete Idiot's Guide to Mindfulness.*[104] or at the Guided Meditation Site.[105]

Music and Relaxation

Sound can have a relaxing effect with the result of other physiological and psychological benefits. Imagine closing your eyes and listening to the surf roll up to a beach, or birds chirping in the woods, or the wind rustling through the leaves. We call that "white noise" since it can wipe out more disturbing sounds. White noise is often used in conjunction with the practice of a relaxation technique as a way of drowning out distracting sounds.

Another form of sound that can be relaxing is soothing music. My guess is that you probably already use music as a means of relaxation. However, remember that music can stimulate as well as relax, depending on the type of music and the level of the sound and beat. When the music listened to is soothing, it can reduce blood pressure,[106] diminish feelings of depression,[107] decrease anxiety,[108] and even enhance spirituality.[109] An interesting study even found that when music was played in a neonatal intensive care unit, premature infants had increased oxygen saturation levels, increased weight, and shorter hospital stays.[110] Obviously, music has the potential to produce many beneficial effects, not the least of which is to facilitate relaxation.

How does this relaxation occur just by listening to music? With the use of MRIs and other technology, brain imaging studies[111–113] have found that music has profound effects on the brain. In particular, the basal ganglia and the motor areas of the brain's cortex are affected. In addition, slow tempo music synchronizes brain waves, thereby resulting in a lower respiratory rate, a slower heart rate, lower blood pressure, less muscle tension, and enhanced effectiveness of the immune system.[114] At least one researcher even believes that music is so powerful that listening to it can "change brain functioning to the same extent as medication, in many instances."[115]

So go ahead, listen to music to relax. Just make sure it has a slow tempo and is not too loud. If it is too upbeat, you may be stimulating yourself, instead of relaxing. And, if it is too loud, you may do damage to your hearing—and that certainly would not be relaxing.

Tai Chi

Tai Chi is an exercise and relaxation technique that originated in China about 300 years ago. It was conceived as a form of martial arts using the Taoist philosophy of Yin and Yang (opposite forces) and breathing techniques.[116] Tai Chi (also known as taiji or taijiquan) uses slow, smooth, dancelike movements along with meditation and control of breathing. The person engaging in Tai Chi tries to integrate the mind and body through respiration, and mental and visual concentration, thereby eliciting a relaxation response.

Five basic principles guide the practice of Tai Chi:[117]

1. *Relaxation*—the conservation of energy by using just the required amount to perform the movements
2. *Separating Yin and Yang*—employing opposing forces such as speed and stillness, force versus relaxation
3. *Turning the Waist*—development of a flexible waist
4. *Keeping an Erect Back*—to maintain balance and relaxation, the body must remain perpendicular to the ground
5. *Total Body Movement*—rather than moving limb by limb, the body moves as one, all the time consistent with the preceding four principles

There have not been a lot of empirical studies of the effects of Tai Chi. However, to engage in Tai Chi requires a great deal of focus and, as we have stated elsewhere in this book, such a focus takes one's mind away from stressors, daily hassles, and worries. As a result, it is no surprise that practitioners report that Tai Chi elicits a relaxation response. Studies have found Tai Chi helps one respond to chronic arthritis by increasing muscular strength and balance.[118,119] As

Tai Chi
An exercise and relaxation technique developed in China that involves focused, slow, rhythmic movement.

Music can be relaxing if it is not too loud or too fast in tempo.

Tai Chi requires slow, balanced movements and focused breathing. The result is a relaxed state.

a result, practitioners of Tai Chi are less likely to fall and injure themselves.[120] Diabetes patients also benefit from Tai Chi. Researchers found that engaging in Tai Chi for as little as eight weeks in one study[121] and twelve weeks in another[122] resulted in lower blood glucose levels and increased nerve conduction (poor nerve conduction is one of the effects of diabetes). Other benefits of engaging in Tai Chi are decreased blood pressure and total serum cholesterol.[123] And there are even psychosocial benefits: lower trait and state anxiety, increased self-efficacy, greater perceived social support, and less stress.[124, 125] If you are interested in pursuing Tai Chi, a first stop might be checking out the website of the American Tai Chi and Qigong Association: www.americantaichi.org.

Pets and Stress

Many stress management techniques have one thing in common: a focus on something that will take a person's mind off daily worries and stressors. Often that focus is on a word or object, such as with meditation. Sometimes it is on internal feelings, such as with autogenics and progressive relaxation. At other times it is on an activity, such as with Tai Chi or yoga. Similarly, focusing on pets can alleviate stress, for several reasons. Pets allow us to focus on their care and away from our own concerns. They provide social support in the form of companionship, and they can provide entertainment.

Numerous research studies support the beneficial health effects and, in particular, stress-related benefits of pets.[126] For example, women were asked to perform a stress task in the laboratory and then, two weeks later, at home.

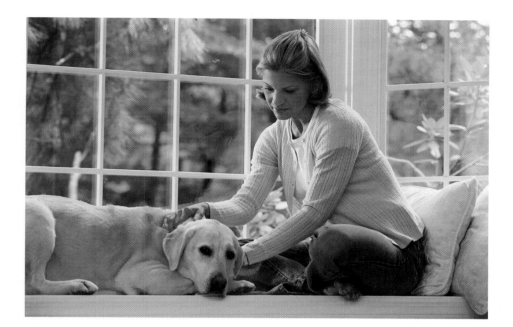

Having a pet has been shown to help manage stress. Even just petting a dog has been found to lower blood pressure—for the owner and the dog.

Getting Involved in Your Community

Just think of all of the people in your community who are "stressed out." There are people with various life-threatening illnesses, people living in conditions of poverty, and people whose loneliness is almost too much for them to bear. Sometimes these people band together to form groups from which they derive support. As such, there are groups of people living with cancer who call themselves cancer survivors, there are groups of single parents who seek advice and emotional support from other single parents, and there are counseling groups organized into group therapy sessions to support the growth and development of its members. Knowing your community (either off-campus or on-campus), you can probably identify individuals and/or groups that experience a significant amount of stress.

Wouldn't it be wonderful if you could somehow help these individuals or group members feel just a little bit better, a little less "stressed out"? Well, you can. You may not be able to alleviate the condition about which they experience stress, but you certainly can help them find moments of respite in spite of the turmoil of their daily existence. Now that you have studied various relaxation techniques, you can volunteer to teach members of your community how to relax. Then, when they feel particularly stressful, they can take a few moments to imagine themselves in a different place in a different time—through the use of imagery, for instance.

In fact, one might argue that to have this knowledge and to merely stand by, observing the stressful situations in which your neighbors find themselves without sharing this knowledge is downright negligent. It certainly is uncaring. We are all busy, but some of us can make a difference—albeit a small one—in other people's lives, and if we can, we probably owe it to our community to take the time and energy to do so.

While at home, the women were divided into three groups. Each group performed the task under different conditions. One group performed it with a friend present, one with a dog present, and the third with neither present. The group with a dog showed less physiological reactivity than did the other two groups.[127,128] In a similar experiment, women were given mental arithmetic and cold pressor stress tests. Pet owners among the women had lower heart rates and lower blood pressure levels even before the stress tests. During the test, the lowest physiological reactivity and the quickest recovery time occurred among pet owners. Furthermore, their reactivity and recovery time were less when the pet was present.[129]

It is not only women who benefit from pets. It is well known that petting a dog, for instance, lowers the blood pressure of both the pet owner and the dog.[130] One study found that elders who were not pet owners deteriorated more quickly in their ability to perform daily tasks than did pet owners.[131] When hospitalized, elderly pet owners stayed in the hospital an average of eight days, and elderly individuals who were not pet owners stayed in the hospital for thirteen days.

In an interesting study,[132] researchers wanted to determine the effect of dogs in decreasing physiological arousal and behavioral distress among children experiencing a routine physical examination. Children three to six years of age were given two physical exams—one without a dog present, the other with a dog. The children's blood pressure and heart rates were lower when the dog was present. In addition, the children with the dog present manifested less behavioral distress.

Pets have been used to help people cope with particular conditions. For example, when pets were used with patients with spinal cord injuries, the patients experienced less stress and an increase in their self-esteem, and they were better able to express their feelings.[133] Pet therapy also has been used successfully with people experiencing posttraumatic stress disorder.[134]

Organizations that study and support pet ownership cite research showing that pets can[135]

- Reduce blood pressure and levels of stress hormones.
- Improve chances of survival after a life-threatening illness.
- Reduce health care costs by preventing illness and promoting recovery.
- Provide companionship and improve social interaction.
- Promote social responses from withdrawn people.
- Reduce aggressive behavior by those prone to violence.
- Enrich the lives of older people and those who are lonely and depressed.

The Mayo Clinic reports that living with and caring for a pet[136]

- *Helps people recover from heart attacks.* Researchers have found that people who own dogs are more likely than those who are not dog owners to be alive one year after a heart attack.
- *Protects the heart and blood vessels.* Pet owners tend to have lower heart rates and lower blood pressure levels. Furthermore, pet owners physiologically react less to stressful events and recover from them faster than do people who are not pet owners.
- *Helps manage blood pressure.* Blood pressure levels decrease when a person owns a pet, even if the person is taking medication for hypertension.
- *Improves mood and well-being.* Elderly pet owners are less likely to experience depression, are better able to tolerate living alone, and are more active than elders who do not have a pet. People with AIDS who own a pet

report feeling less depressed. Pets also reduce loneliness among nursing home residents.

It is for these reasons that clinical psychologists and stress management experts often prescribe interacting with a pet as a way of coping with life's stressors. Recognizing the value of pets, hospitals have developed pet programs with dogs trained to behave in acceptable ways in that setting. Nursing homes have adopted pet programs for elders, as have organizations that treat people with various disabilities.

If you are experiencing undue stress, perhaps you might consider having a pet as a means to help you cope with that stress. Pets can be obtained from your local ASPCA and many other outlets in your community. If you think this is a good idea but are not inclined to have a dog or a cat, perhaps tropical fish would do the trick?

Coping in Today's World

They seemingly come at us from every angle, from every direction, from all areas of our lives, regardless of our age. I am speaking of *stressors.* If it isn't the cell phone ringing, the e-mail and text messages, or the PDAs designed so we can always "be in touch," it is the surveillance cameras recording our every move on the street or when driving past traffic lights. Some workers, such as telephone operators, have their work performance constantly monitored and their lunch hour timed to the minute. Depending on our past experiences, there may be databases that include our fingerprints, face recognition, DNA, or retinal images.

Add to this volatile stressor mix the fact that road rage seems to be increasing; people and politicians appear to have lost any semblance of civility; and our cherished athletes too often "lose it" and, in fits of anger, violently attack one another.

And then, there are *boomerang kids* or *adultolescents.* These are adult children who move back home with their parents to save money or delay their financial and/or emotional independence. That creates what has been termed the *sandwich generation.* These are adults who are sandwiched between caring for their adult children while also caring for their own aged parents. This sense of responsibility to loved ones both younger and older can be extremely stressful. Where do those who have reluctantly joined the sandwich generation find the time to care for themselves or to maintain positive relationships with their own partners?

Even schoolchildren are not immune to modern-day stressors. Large numbers feel pressured to do well in school. In the United States, approximately 30 percent of 15-year-olds and 23 percent of 13-year-olds feel very pressured by their schoolwork, and approximately one-third of 15-year-old students feel their teachers expect too much of them.[a]

There are physical strains as well. Schoolchildren lug heavy backpacks, while adults sit hunched over computers and work desks at angles that only exacerbate the typical stressors and strains associated with aging.

Given these modern-day stressors, the need to engage in effective relaxation techniques—regularly—is vital. The specific technique chosen is unimportant, as long as it results in a relaxation response. My friend Paul has tanks of tropical fish. He has red ones, green ones, yellow ones—of all sizes and shapes. When Paul comes home from work, he sits by those fish tanks and watches the fish swim back and forth, up and down. He watches those fish so intently that he is almost in the tank swimming with them. When he is that interested in what the fish are doing, he cannot be thinking of the stressors and hassles he experienced that day. This is an effective relaxation technique for Paul. It matters little if this technique appears in professional journals or not. It works for Paul, and therefore he ought to continue employing this technique of managing his stress. What ways of managing stress work for you? That is, how can you elicit a relaxation response? Of course, there are many methods of relaxation described in this book. Still, there are others that are also effective. Seek these out and make them a part of your daily stress management routine.

[a]D. Smith, "Stressed at School," *Washington Post,* September 9, 2000, A14.

summary

- Biofeedback is the use of instrumentation to receive information about occurrences within the body. People fed back such information can learn to control these body processes.

- Biofeedback involves three phases: measuring the physiological parameter, converting this measurement to some understandable form, and feeding back this information to the person learning to control his or her body processes.

- Biofeedback has been used to help people control their heart rates, skin's electrical conductance, blood vessels' dilation, and brain waves. Biofeedback has also been used to control muscle tension, blood pressure, penile erection, and secretion of hydrochloric acid.

- Electromyographic biofeedback has been used to treat asthma, hypertension, ulcers, muscle spasms, migraine and tension headaches, colitis, cerebral palsy, and other conditions.

- Thermal biofeedback has been used to treat Raynaud's disease, migraine headaches, and hypertension.

- When used for relaxation purposes, biofeedback is often employed in conjunction with another relaxation technique. Oftentimes, autogenics or meditation is used during biofeedback training.

- There are many types of relaxation techniques other than meditation, autogenic training, progressive relaxation, and the use of biofeedback instrumentation. Among these are diaphragmatic breathing, body scanning, massage and acupressure, yoga and stretching, repetitive prayer, Quieting Reflex, the Instant Calming Sequence, mindfulness, music, Tai Chi, and pet ownership.

internet resources

Holistic-Online **www.holistic-online.com/stress/stress_home.htm** *Addresses general information about stress and coping strategies. Examines the numerous relaxation techniques in brief, including massage, meditation, acupuncture, biofeedback, yoga, and reiki.*

The Biofeedback Webzine **www.webideas.com/biofeedback** *News, meetings, and research, including a searchable database for biofeedback-related topics.*

American Yoga Association **www.americanyogaassociation.org** *A description of yoga, its history, synopses of books and tapes, as well as an online yoga lesson.*

Yoga Journal Magazine **www.yogajournal.com** *A magazine about the practice and philosophy of yoga.*

Stress Management and Relaxation Central **www.futurehealth.org/stresscn.htm** *Provides information and tools for managing stress, including relaxation and hypnosis tapes and books, articles and biofeedback instruments, and computer products.*

references

1. Rod R. Seeley, Trent D. Stephens, and Philip Tate, *Anatomy and Physiology,* 8th ed. (New York: McGraw-Hill, 2008), 580.

2. D. W. Shearn, "Operant Conditioning of Heart Rate," *Science* 137(1962): 530–31.

3. T. W. Frazier, "Avoidance Conditioning of Heart Rate in Humans," *Psychophysiology* 3(1966): 188–202.

4. Neal E. Miller, "Learning of Visceral and Glandular Response," *Science* 163(1969): 434–45.

5. H. D. Kimmell and F. A. Hill, "Operant Conditioning of the GSR," *Psychological Reports* 7(1960): 555–62.

6. H. D. Kimmel, "Instrumental Conditioning of Autonomically Mediated Behavior," *Psychological Bulletin* 67(1967): 337–45.

7. W. A. Greene, "Operant Conditioning of the GSR Using Partial Reinforcement," *Psychological Reports* 19(1976): 571–78.

8. L. V. DiCara and Neal E. Miller, "Instrumental Learning of Vasomotor Responses by Rats: Learning to Respond Differentially in the Two Ears," *Science* 159(1968): 1485.

9. Joseph Kamiya, "Conscious Control of Brain Waves," *Psychology Today* 1(1968): 57–60.

10. Barbara B. Brown, "Recognition Aspects of Consciousness Through Association with EEG Alpha Activity Represented by a Light Signal," *Psychophysiology* 6(1970): 442–52.

11. Elmer E. Green, A. M. Green, and E. D. Walters, "Voluntary Control of Internal States: Psychological and Physiological," *Journal of Transpersonal Psychology* 2(1970): 1–26.

12. J. S. Oh, H. S. Cynn, J. H. Won, O. Y. Kwon, and C. H. Yi, "Effects of Performing an Abdominal Drawing-In Maneuver During Prone Hip Extension Exercises on Hip and Back Extensor Muscle Activity and Amount of Anterior Pelvic Tilt,"

Journal of Orthopaedic and Sports Physical Therapy 37(2007): 320–24.

13. J. Jonsdottir, D. Cattaneo, A. Regola, A. Crippa, M. Recalcati, M. Rabuffetti, M. Ferrarin, and A. Casiraghi, "Concepts of Motor Learning Applied to a Rehabilitation Protocol Using Biofeedback to Improve Gait in a Chronic Stroke Patient: An A-B System Study with Multiple Gait Analyses," *Neurorehabilitaion and Neural Repair* 21(2007): 190–94.

14. F. Massaad, T. M. Lejeune, and C. Detrembleur, "Reducing the Energy Cost of Hemiparetic Gait Using Center of Mass Feedback: A Pilot Study," *Neurorehabilitation and Neural Repair* 24(2010): 338–47.

15. S. Ferrante, E. Ambrosini, P. Ravelli, E. Guanziroli, F. Molteni, G. Ferrigno, and A. Pedrocchi, "A Biofeedback Cycling Training to Improve Locomotion: A Case Series Study Based on Gait Pattern Classification of 153 Chronic Stroke Patients," *Journal of Neuroengineering and Rehabilitation* 8(2011): 47.

16. R. Stanton, L. Ada, C. M. Dean, and E. Preston, "Biofeedback Improves Activities of the Lower Limb After Stroke: A Systematic Review," *Journal of Physiotherapy* 57(2011): 145–55.

17. A. Crider, A. G. Glaros, and R. N. Gevirtz, "Efficacy of Biofeedback-based Treatments for Temporomandibular Disorders," *Applied Psychophysiology and Biofeedback* 30(2005): 333–45.

18. A. E. Bharucha, "Constipation," Best Practice and Research, *Clinical Gastroenterology* 21(2007): 709–31.

19. H. J. Mason, E. Serrano-Ikkos, and M. A. Kamm, "Psychological State and Quality of Life in Patients Having Behavioral Treatment (Biofeedback) for Intractable Constipation," *American Journal of Gastroenterology* 97(2002): 3154–59.

20. A.Y. Zhang, G. J. Strauss, and L. A. Siminoff, "Effects of Combined Pelvic Floor Muscle Exercise and a Support Group on Urinary Incontinence and Quality of Life of Postprostatectomy Patients," *Oncology Nursing Forum* 34(2007): 47–53.

21. T. I. Klausner, "The Best Kept Secret: Pelvic Floor Muscle Therapy for Urinary Incontinence," *Advance for Nurse Practitioners* 13(2005): 43–46, 48.

22. K. A. Long, L. J. Ewing, S. Cohen, D. Skoner, D. Gentile, J. Koehrsen, C. Howe, A. L. Thompson, R. K. Rosen, M. Ganley, and A. L. Marsland, "Preliminary Evidence for the Feasibility of a Stress Management Intervention for 7- to 12-Year-Olds with Asthma," *Journal of Asthma* 48(2011): 162–70.

23. R. D. Sheth, C. E. Stafstrom, and D. Hsu, "Nonpharmacological Treatment Options for Epilepsy," *Seminars in Pediatric Neurology* 12(2005): 106–13.

24. P. N. Friel, "EEG Biofeedback in the Treatment of Attention Deficit Hyperactivity Disorder," *Alternative Medicine Review* 12(2007): 146–51.

25. V. J. Monastra, S. Lynn, M. Linden, J. F. Lubar, J. Gruzelier, and T. J. LaVaque, "Electroencephalographic Biofeedback in the Treatment of Attention-Deficit/ Hyperactivity Disorder," *Applied Psychophysiology and Biofeedback* 30(2005): 95–114.

26. Neal E. Miller, "RX: Biofeedback," *Psychology Today,* February 1985, 54–59.

27. R. A. McGinnis, A. McGrady, S. A. Cox, and K. A. Grower-Dowling, "Biofeedback-assisted Relaxation in Type 2 Diabetes," *Diabetes Care* 28(2005): 2145–149.

28. B. I. Rice, "Clinical Benefits of Training Patients to Voluntarily Increase Peripheral Blood Flow: The Warmfeet Intervention," *The Diabetes Educator* 33(2007): 442, 444–45, 447–48, 454.

29. F. Andrasik, "What Does the Evidence Show? Efficacy of Behavioural Treatments for Recurrent Headaches in Adults," *Neurological Sciences* 28(2007): S70–S77.

30. M. K. Karavidas, P. S Tsai, C. Yucha, A. McGrady, and P. M. Lehrer, "Thermal Biofeedback for Primary Raynaud's Phenomenon: A Review of the Literature," *Applied Psychophysiology and Biofeedback* 31(2006): 203–16.

31. W. Linden and J. V. Moseley, "The Efficacy of Behavioral Treatments for Hypertension," *Applied Psychophysiology and Biofeedback* 31(2006): 51–63.

32. M. Hashmonai, D. Kopelman, and A. Assalia, "The Treatment of Primary Palmar Hyperhidrosis: A Review," *Surgery Today* 30(2000): 211–18.

33. R. Kaushik, R. M. Kaushik, S. K. Mahajan, and V. Rajesh, "Biofeedback Assisted Diaphragmatic Breathing and Systematic Relaxation Versus Propranolol in Long Term Prophylaxis of Migraine," *Complementary Therapies in Medicine* 13(2005): 165–74.

34. S. W. Powers and F. Andrasik, "Biobehavioral Treatment, Disability, and Psychological Effects of Pediatric Headache," *Pediatric Annals* 34(2005): 461–65.

35. D. M. Biondi, "Physical.Treatments for Headache: A Structured Review," *Headache* 45(2005): 738–46.

36. Barbara Szekely, "Nonpharmacological Treatment of Menstrual Headache: Relaxation-Biofeedback Behavior Therapy and Person-Centered Insight Therapy," *Headache* 26(1986): 86–92.

37. M. L. Proctor, P. A. Murphy, H. M. Pattison, J. Suckling, and C. M. Farquha, "Behavioural Interventions for Primary and Secondary Dysmenorrhoea," *Cochrane Database of Systematic Reviews* (Online) (July 18, 2007): CD002248.

38. W. C. Scott, D. Kaiser, S. Othmer, and S. I. Sideroff, "Effects of an EEG Biofeedback Protocol on a Mixed Substance Abusing Population," *American Journal of Drug and Alcohol Abuse* 31(2005): 455–69.

39. G. Dorey, M. J. Speakman, R. C. Feneley, A. Swinkels, and C. D. Dunn, "Pelvic Floor Exercises for Erectile Dysfunction," *BJU International* 96(2005): 595–97.

40. J. T. Seo, J. H. Choe, W. S. Lee, and K. H. Kim, "Efficacy of Functional Electrical Stimulation-Biofeedback with Sexual Cognitive-Behavioral Therapy as Treatment of Vaginismus," *Urology* 66(2005): 77–81.

41. I. Marc, N. Toureche, E. Ernst, E. D. Hodnett, C. Blanchet, S. Dodin, and M. M. Njoya, "Mind-Body Interventions During Pregnancy for Preventing or Treating Women's Anxiety," *Cochrane Database of Systematic Reviews* (Online) (July 6, 2011): CD007559.

42. J. L. Balk, S. C. Chung, R. Beigi, and M. Brooks, "Brief Relaxation Training Program for Hospital Employees," *Hospital Topics* 87(2009): 8–13.

43. A. Lazarov, R. Dar, Y. Oded, and N. Liberman, "Are Obsessive-Compulsive Tendencies Related to Reliance on External Proxies for Internal States? Evidence from Biofeedback-Aided Relaxation Studies," *Behaviour Research and Therapy* 48(2010): 516–23.

44. W. W. Chen, "Enhancement of Health Locus of Control Through Biofeedback," *Perceptual Motor Skills* 80(1995): 466.

45. Philip Bate, "The Role of Biofeedback in Treating ADD and Other Mental Symptoms," *International Guide to the World of Alternative Health.* 2010. Available at: www.alternativementalhealth.com/articles/biofeedback.htm

46. B. Reigel, et al., "Psychogenic Cough Treated with Biofeedback and Psychotherapy: A Review and Case Report," *American Journal of Physical Medicine and Rehabilitation* 74(1995): 155–58.

47. P. J. Nada, "Heart Rate Variability in the Assessment and Biofeedback Training of Common Mental Health Problems in Children," *Medicinski Arhiv* 63(2009): 244–48.

48. S. W. Choi, S. E. Chi, S. Y. Chung, J. W. Kim, C. Y. Ahn, and H. T. Kim, "Is Alpha Wave Neurofeedback Effective with Randomized Clinical Trials in Depression? A Pilot Study," *Neuropsychobiology* 63(2011): 43–51.

49. G. Tan, T. K. Dao, L. Farmer, R. J. Sutherland, and R. Gevirtz, "Heart Rate Variability (HRV) and Posttraumatic Stress Disorder (PTSD): A Pilot Study," *Applied Psychophysiology and Biofeedback* 36(2011): 27–35.

50. Carol Krucoff and Mitchell Krucoff, *Healing Moves: How to Cure, Relieve, and Prevent Common Ailments with Exercise* (New York: Harmony Books, 2000).

51. Triangle Acupuncture Clinic, "Body Scan Relaxation Exercise." Undated. Available at: http://triangleacupunctureclinic.com/docs/fertility/body_scan_relaxation_exercise.pdf.

52. Andrew Vickers and Catherine Zollman, "ABC of Complementary Medicine: Massage Therapies," *British Medical Journal* 319(1999): 1254–57.

53. American Massage Therapy Association, *2009 Massage Therapy Industry Fact Sheet.* 2009. Available at: www.amtamassage.org/news/MTIndustryFactSheet.html#9

54. J. Currin and E. A. Meister, "A Hospital-Based Intervention Using Massage to Reduce Distress among Oncology Patients," *Cancer Nursing* 31(2008): 214–21.

55. American College of Physicians, "Massage Therapy May Have Immediate Positive Effect on Pain and Mood for Advanced Cancer Patients," *Science Daily.* September 16, 2008. Available at: www.sciencedaily.com/releases/2008/09/080915174534.htm

56. M. Preyde, "Effectiveness of Massage Therapy for Subacute Low Back Pain: A Randomized Controlled Trial," *Journal of Soft Tissue Manipulation* 8(2003): 4–10.

57. A. I. Perlman, A. Sabina, A. L. Williams, V. Y. Njike, and D. L. Katz, "Massage Therapy for Osteoarthritis of the Knee," *Archives of Internal Medicine* 166(2006): 2533–38.

58. D. Zeitlin, S. E. Keller, S. C. Shiflett, S. J. Schleifer, and J. A. Bartlett, "Immunological Effects of Massage Therapy During Academic Stress," *Psychosomatic Medicine* 62(2000): 83–87.

59. T. Field, Miguel Diego, Christy Cullen, Kristin Hartshorn, Alan Gruskin, Maria Hernandez-Reif, and William Sunshine, "Carpal Tunnel Syndrome Symptoms Are Lessened Following Massage," *Journal of Bodywork and Movement Therapies* 8(2004): 9–14.

60. M. Hernandez-Reif, T. Field, J. Krasnegor, H. Theakston, Z. Hossain, and I. Burman, "High Blood Pressure and Associated Symptoms Were Reduced by Massage Therapy," *Journal of Bodywork and Movement Therapies* 4(2000): 31–38.

61. C. Quinn, C. Chandler, and A. Moraska, "Massage Therapy and Frequency of Chronic Tension Headaches," *American Journal of Public Health* 92(2002): 1657–61.

62. M. Reader, R. Young, and J. P. Connor, "Massage Therapy Improves the Management of Alcohol Withdrawal Syndrome," *Journal of Alternative and Complementary Medicine* 11(2005): 311–13.

63. R. Manocha, G. B. Marks, P. Kenchington, D. Peters, and C. M. Salome, "Sahaja Yoga in the Management of Moderate to Severe Asthma: A Randomised Controlled Trial," *Thorax* (2002): 110–15.

64. B. K. Sahay, "Role of Yoga in Diabetes," *Journal of the Association of Physicians in India* 55(2007): 121–26.

65. B. S. Oken, D. Zajdel, S. Kishiyama, K. Flegal, C. Dehen, M. Haas, D. F. Kraemer, J. Lawrence, and J. Leyva, "Randomized, Controlled, Six-Month Trial of Yoga in Healthy Seniors: Effects on Cognition and Quality of Life," *Alternative Therapies in Health and Medicine* 12(2006): 40–47.

66. L. Cohen, C. Warneke, R. T. Fouladi, M. A. Rodriguez, and A. Chaoul-Reich, "Psychological Adjustment and Sleep Quality in a Randomized Trial of the Effects of a Tibetan Yoga Intervention in Patients with Lymphoma," *Cancer* 100(2004): 2253–260.

67. C. Smith, H. Hancock, J. Blake-Mortimer, and K. Eckert, "A Randomised Comparative Trial of Yoga and Relaxation to Reduce Stress and Anxiety," *Complementary Therapies in Medicine* 15(2007): 77–83.

68. A. Michalsen, P. Grossman, A. Acil, J. Langhorst, R. Lüdtke, T. Esch, G. B. Stefano, and G. J. Dobos, "Rapid Stress Reduction and Anxiolysis Among Distressed Women as a Consequence of a Three-Month Intensive Yoga Program," *Medical Science Monitor* 11(2005): CR555–CR561.

69. C. C. Streeter, J. E. Jensen, R. M. Perlmutter, H. J. Cabral, H. Tian, D. B. Terhune, D. A. Ciraulo, and P. F. Renshaw, "Yoga Asana Sessions Increase Brain GABA Levels: A Pilot Study," *Journal of Alternative and Complementary Medicine* 13(2007): 419–26.

70. G. Duraiswamy, J. Thirthalli, H. R. Nagendra, and B. N. Gangadhar, "Yoga Therapy as an Add-On Treatment in the Management of Patients with Schizophrenia—A Randomized Controlled Trial," *Acta Psychiatrica Scandinavika* 116(2007): 226–32.

71. Ulrica Norberg, *Hatha Yoga: The Body's Path to Balance, Focus, and Strength* (New York: Skyhorse Publishing, 2008).

72. Leslie Kaminoff, Sharon Ellis, and Amy Matthews, *Yoga Anatomy* (Champaign, IL: Human Kinetics, 2007).

73. D. Driscoll and G. DiCicco, "The Effects of Metronome Breathing on the Variability of Autonomic Activity Measurements," *Journal of Manipulative and Physiological Therapeutics* 23(2007): 610–14.

74. R. M. Kaushik, R. Kaushik, S. K. Mahajan, and V. Rajesh, "Effects of Mental Relaxation and Slow Breathing in Essential Hypertension," *Complementary Therapies in Medicine* 14(2006): 120–26.

75. R. Viyas and N. Dikshit, "Effect of Meditation on Respiratory System, Cardiovascular System and Lipid Profile," *Indian Journal of Physiology and Pharmacology* 46(2002): 487–91.

76. Adam Burke, "The Role of Breath in Yoga Traditions: Alternate Nostril Breathing," *Biofeedback* 36(2008): 67–69.

77. Herbert Benson and Miriam Z. Klipper, *The Relaxation Response* (New York: William Morrow, 2000).

78. Herbert Benson and William Proctor, *Beyond the Relaxation Response* (East Rutherford, NJ: Berkley Publishing Group, 1985).

79. Herbert Benson and Marg Stark, *Timeless Healing: The Power and Biology of Belief* (New York: Simon & Schuster, 1996).

80. Stephen Kiesling and T. George Harris, "The Prayer War," *Psychology Today*, October 1989, 65–66.

81. Kenneth H. Cooper, *Can Stress Heal?* (Nashville, TN: Thomas Nelson, 1997).

82. Victoria Dain, "Prayer and Relaxation," *Abundant Horizons*. 2011. Available at: www.abundanthorizons.com/peace/prayer-of-relaxation/.

83. Charles F. Stroebel, *QR: The Quieting Reflex* (New York: Berkley Books, 1983).

84. Sandy Rovner, "Learning Ways to Beat Stress," *Washington Post Health*, September 22, 1987, 16.

85. "Deep Breathing Exercises for Stress Relief," *Stress Management*: 2011. Available at: www.stress-management-for-peak-performance.com/deep-breathing-exercises.html.

86. Bobbie Hasslebring, "Health and Fitness According to Robert Cooper," *Medical Selfcare*, September/October 1989, 52–56, 69–70.

87. S. Schmidt, P. Grossman, B. Schwarzer, S. Jena, J. Naumann, and H. Walach, "Treating Fibromyalgia with Mindfulness-Based Stress Reduction: Results from a 3-Armed Randomized Controlled Trial," *Pain* 152(2011): 361–69.

88. D. Ledesma and H. Kumano, "Mindfulness-Based Stress Reduction and Cancer: A Meta-Analysis." *Psycho-Oncology* 18(2009): 571–79.

89. A. Chiesa and A. Serretti, "Mindfulness Based Cognitive Therapy for Psychiatric Disorders: A Systematic Review and Meta-Analysis," *Psychiatry Research* 187(2011): 441–53.

90. S. N. Garland, L. E. Carlson, M. C. Antle, C. Samuels, and T. Campbell, "I-CAN SLEEP: Rationale and Design of a Non-Inferiority RCT of Mindfulness-Based Stress Reduction and Cognitive Behavioral Therapy for the Treatment of Insomnia in Cancer Survivors," *Contemporary Clinical Trials* 32(2011): 747–54.

91. D. J. Kearney, K. McDermott, M. Martinez, and T. L. Simpson, "Association of Participation in a Mindfulness Programme with Bowel Symptoms, Gastrointestinal Symptom-Specific Anxiety and Quality of Life," *Alimentary Pharmacology and Therapeutics* 34(2011): 363–73.

92. Britta Holzol, James Carmody, Mark Vangel, Christina Congleton, Sita M. Yerramsetti, Tim Grade, and Sara W. Lazar, "Mindfulness Practice Leads to Increases in Regional Gray Matter Density," *Psychiatry Research: Neuroimaging* 191(2011): 36–43.

93. A. Chiesa and A. Serretti, "Mindfulness-Based Stress Reduction for Stress Management in Healthy People: A Review and Meta-Analysis," *Journal of Alternative and Complementary Medicine* 15(2009): 593–600.

94. M. J. Kreitzer, C. R. Gross, X. Ye, V. Russas, and C. Treesak, "Longitudinal Impact of Mindfulness Meditation on Illness Burden in Solid-Organ Transplant Recipients," *Progress in Transplantation* 15(2005): 166–72.

95. S. Horton-Deutsch, P. O'Haver Day, R. Haight, and M. Babin-Nelson, "Enhancing Mental Health Services to Bone Marrow Transplant Recipients Through a Mindfulness-based Therapeutic Intervention," *Complementary Therapies in Clinical Practice* 13(2007): 110–15.

96. J. E. Smith, J. Richardson, C. Hoffman, and K. Pilkington, "Mindfulness-based Stress Reduction as Supportive Therapy in Cancer Care: Systematic Review," *Journal of Advanced Nursing* 52(2005): 315–27.

97. L. E. Carlson, M. Speca, K. D. Patel, and E. Goodey, "Mindfulness-based Stress Reduction in Relation to Quality of Life, Mood, Symptoms of Stress and Levels of Cortisol, Dehydroepiandrosterone Sulfate (DHEAS) and Melatonin in Breast and Prostate Cancer Outpatients," *Psychoneuroendocrinology* 29(2004): 448–74.

98. J. M. Davis, M. F. Fleming, K. A. Bonus, and T. B. Baker, "A Pilot Study on Mindfulness Based Stress Reduction for Smokers," *BMC Complementary and Alternative Medicine* 7(2007): 2.

99. R. J. Davidson, J. Kabat-Zinn, J. Schumacher, M. Rosenkranz, D. Muller, S. F. Santorelli, F. Urbanowski, A. Harrington, K. Bonus, and J. F. Sheridan, "Alterations in Brain and Immune Function Produced by Mindfulness Meditation," *Psychosomatic Medicine* 65(2003): 564–70.

100. S. Jain, S. L. Shapiro, S. Swanick, S. C. Roesch, P. J. Mills, I. Bell, and G. E. Schwartz, "A Randomized Controlled Trial of Mindfulness Meditation Versus Relaxation Training: Effects on Distress, Positive States of Mind, Rumination, and Distraction," *Annals of Behavioral Medicine* 33(2007): 11–21.

101. J. A. Astin, "Stress Reduction Through Mindfulness Meditation. Effects on Psychological Symptomatology, Sense of Control, and Spiritual Experiences," *Psychotherapy and Psychosomatics* 66(1997): 97–106.

102. T. Meili and J. Kabat-Zinn, "The Power of the Human Heart: A Story of Trauma and Recovery and Its Implications for Rehabilitation and Healing," *Advances in Mind-Body Medicine* 20(2004): 6–16.

103. Eric P. Trunnell and Jerry F. Braza, "Mindfulness in the Workplace," *Journal of Health Education* 26(1995): 285–91.

104. Anne Ihnen and Carolyn Flynn, *The Complete Idiot's Guide to Mindfulness* (Exton, PA: Alpha, 2008).

105. Christopher Lloyd Clarke, "Mindfulness Activities," *The Guided Meditation Site*. Undated. Available at: www.the-guided-meditation-site.com/mindfulness-activities.html

106. American Cancer Society, "Music Therapy," *Making Treatment Decisions*. 2009. Available at: www.cancer.org/docroot/ETO/content/ETO_5_3X_Music_Therapy.asp

107. F. Moradipanah, E. Mohammadi, and A. Z. Mohammadil, "Effect of Music on Anxiety, Stress, and Depression Levels in Patients Undergoing Coronary Angiography," *East Mediterranean Health Journal* 15(2009): 639–47.

108. M. Yang, L. Li, H. Zhu, I. M. Alexander, S. Liu, W. Zhou, and X. Ren, "Music Therapy to Relieve Anxiety in Pregnant Women on Bedrest: A Randomized, Controlled Trial," *MCN: American Journal of Maternal and Child Nursing* 34(2009): 316–23.

109. Michael J. Lowis and Jenny Hughes, "A Comparison of the Effects of Sacred and Secular Music on Elderly People," *Journal of Psychology* 131(1997): 45–55.

110. Charles Marwick, "Music Hath Charms for Care of Preemies," *Journal of the American Medical Association* 283(2000): 468.

111. Joyce L. Chen, Virginia B. Penhune, and Robert J. Zatorrea, "The Role of Auditory and Premotor Cortex in Sensorimotor Transformations," *Annals of the New York Academy of Sciences* 1169(2009): 15–34.

112. Jessica A. Grahn, "The Role of the Basal Ganglia in Beat Perception: Neuroimaging and Neuropsychological Investigations," *Annals of the New York Academy of Sciences* 1169(2009): 35–45.

113. Joel S. Snyder, Edward W. Large, and Virginia Penhune, "Rhythms of the Brain: Basic Science and Clinical Perspectives," *Annals of the New York Academy of Sciences* 1169(2009): 13–14.

114. Elizabeth Scott, "Music and Your Body: How Music Affects Us and Why Music Therapy Promotes Health," *About.com*, 2009. Available at: http://stress.about.com/od/tensiontamers/a/music_therapy.htm

115. Emily Saarman, "Symposium Looks at Therapeutic Benefits of Musical Rhythm," *Stanford News Service*. 2006. Available at: www.stanford.edu/dept/news/pr/2006/pr-brainwave-053106.html

116. National Center for Complementary and Alternative Medicine, *Tai Chi for Health Purposes* (Washington, DC: National Center for Complementary and Alternative Medicine, 2007).

117. Erica S. Sandlund and Torsten Norlander, "The Effects of Tai Chi Chuan Relaxation and Exercise on Stress Responses and Well-Being: An Overview of Research," *International Journal of Stress Management* 7(2000): 140–41.

118. R. E. Taylor-Piliae, W. L. Haskell, C. M. Waters, and E. S. Froelicher, "Change in Perceived Psychosocial Status Following a 12-Week Tai Chi Exercise Programme," *Journal of Advanced Nursing* 54(2006): 313–29.

119. R. E. Taylor-Piliae, W. L. Haskell, N. A. Stotts, and E. S. Froelicher, "Improvement in Balance, Strength, and Flexibility after 12 Weeks of Tai Chi Exercise in Ethnic Chinese Adults with Cardiovascular Disease Risk Factors," *Alternative Therapies in Health and Medicine* 12(2006): 50–58.

120. J. H. Choi, J. S. Moon, and R. Song, "Effects of Sun-Style Tai Chi Exercise on Physical Fitness and Fall Prevention in Fall-Prone Older Adults," *Journal of Advanced Nursing* 51(2005): 150–57.

121. J. H. Wang, "Effects of Tai Chi Exercise on Patients with Type 2 Diabetes," *Medicine and Sport Science* 52(2008): 230–38.

122. J. W. Hung, C. W. Liou, P. W. Wang, S. H. Yeh, L. W. Lin, S. K. Lo, and F. M. Tsai, "Effect of 12-Week Tai Chi Chuan Exercise on Peripheral Nerve Modulation in Patients with Type 2 Diabetes Mellitus," *Journal of Rehabilitation Medicine* 41(2009): 924–29.

123. J. C. Tsai, W. H. Wang, P. Chan, L. J. Lin, C. H. Wang, B. Tomlinson, M. H. Hsieh, H. Y. Yang, and J. C. Liu, "The Beneficial Effects of Tai Chi Chuan on Blood Pressure and Lipid Profile and Anxiety Status in a Randomized Controlled Trial," *Journal of Alternative and Complementary Medicine* 9(2003): 747–54.

124. Taylor-Piliae et al., "Change in Perceived Psychosocial Status."

125. Tsai, et al., "Beneficial Effects of Tai Chi Chuan."

126. Stephen D. Shappell, "Health Benefits of Pets," *HealthCenterOnline*, 2004. www.healthcenteronline.com/Health_Benefits_of_Pets.html

127. Karen Allen, Jim Blascovich, Joe Tomaka, and Robert M. Kelsey, "Presence of Human Friend and Pet Dogs as Moderators of Autonomic Responses to Stress in Women," *Journal of Personality and Social Psychology* 61(1991): 582–89.

128. K. Allen, B. E. Shykoff, and J. L. Izzo, Jr., "Pet Ownership, but Not ACE Inhibitor Therapy, Blunts Home Blood Pressure Responses to Mental Stress," *Hypertension* 38(2001): 15–20.

129. Karen Allen, Jim Blascovich, and Wendy B. Mendes, "Cardiovascular Reactivity and the Presence of Pets, Friends, and Spouses: The Truth About Cats and Dogs," *Psychosomatic Medicine* 64(2002): 727–39.

130. Christine R. McLaughlin, "Furry Friends Can Aid Your Health," *Discovery Health Channel,* 2004, www.health.discovery.com/centers/aging/powerofpets/powerofpets_print.html

131. Parminder Raina, D. Waltner-Toews, B. Bonnett, C. Woodward, and T. J. Abernathy, "Influence of Companion Animals on the Physical and Psychological Health of Older People: An Analysis of a One-Year Longitudinal Study," *American Geriatric Society* 47(1999): 323–29.

132. S. L. Nagengast, M. M. Baun, M Megel, and J. M. Leibowitz, "The Effects of the Presence of a Companion Animal on Physiological Arousal and Behavioral Distress in Children During a Physical Examination," *Journal of Pediatric Nursing* 12(1997): 323–30.

133. C. M. Counsell, J. Abram, and M. Gilbert, "Animal Assisted Therapy and the Individual with Spinal Cord Injury," *SCI Nursing* 14(1997): 52–55.

134. Joan Froling, "Service Dog Tasks for Psychiatric Disabilities: Service Dog Tasks for Panic Disorder, PTSD, and Depression," *International Association of Assistance Dog Partners (IAADP)*. 2009. Available at: www.iaadp.org/psd_tasks.html.

135. Dafoni Carlisle, "A Pet for Life," *Pets & Health*, 2004. www.hda-online.org.uk/hdt/0802/pets.html

136. Mayo Foundation for Medical Education and Research, *The Health Benefits of Caring for a Pet,* 2006. www.mayoclinic.com

LAB ASSESSMENT 12.1

How Do You Cause Stress, and What Will You Do About It?

When I conduct stress management workshops or teach stress management classes, the participants already know what causes them stress. They want to learn instead how to manage that stress and how to prevent stress from making them ill. One assumption is that stress comes at them from others: The professor expects too much work in too short a period of time; the parent expects chores to be done immediately; the boss demands the work be done as the boss prescribes and in the time frame the boss expects. It seems that everyone is "emitting" stress with the exception of the participant. Seldom is thought given as to how participants cause others stress. This lab is devoted to that consideration. If we all caused others less stress, there would be less need to use relaxation techniques to manage stress. That is not to say that relaxation techniques would no longer be useful, just that the urgency to use them would diminish. With that result, relaxation techniques would be employed in a more relaxed fashion and might be expected to be more effective.

List three people about whom you care. One should be a family member, one a friend, and the other anyone else you wish to list:

1. Family member: _____

2. Friend: _____

3. Anyone else: _____

For each person listed, cite three ways in which you cause that person stress:

1. Family member:

    a. _____

    b. _____

    c. _____

2. Friend:

    a. _____

    b. _____

    c. _____

3. Anyone else:

    a. _____

    b. _____

    c. _____

Now, list three ways in which you can cause that person less stress:

1. Family member:

    a. _____

    b. _____

    c. _____

2. Friend:

    a. _____

    b. _____

    c. _____

3. Anyone else:

    a. _____

    b. _____

    c. _____

Choose one way you can cause less stress for each person listed. Commit yourself to doing that by writing a contract and having someone sign it as a witness. Then at some specified date, report back to the witness regarding what you did and how it worked out. If we each caused others less stress, wouldn't this be a better world?

LAB ASSESSMENT 12.2

Pets: Stress Busters in Spite of It All?

My son's dog has a degenerative condition that will diminish the quality of, and shorten, the dog's life. As you might imagine, my son is quite stressed out about that. That led me to wonder if pets cause more stress than the stress-busting benefits ascribed to them. What do you think? If you have or have had a pet, answer the questions below with that pet in mind. If you have never had a pet, you probably know someone who has. In that case, answer the questions relative to that person and his or her pet.

What are the stressful aspects of having a pet?

1. _____

2. _____

3. _____

4. _____

5. _____

What are the stress-related beneficial aspects of having a pet?

1. _____

2. _____

3. _____

4. _____

5. _____

Do the beneficial aspects outweigh the stressful aspects? Why did you answer as you did?

_____

_____

_____

If you had it to do all over again, would you, or the person you are thinking about, have another pet? Why do you think that is so?

_____

_____

_____

What can you conclude about pets and stress?

_____

_____

_____

part 4

General Applications

Physiological Arousal and Behavior Change Interventions

13 Physiological Arousal Interventions

My father was admitted to the hospital on a sunny day in September, just days before his 69th birthday. He had experienced a few small strokes and several minor heart attacks that resulted in his being scheduled for coronary bypass surgery the next morning. My mother, brothers, and I left him at about 8 p.m., promising to return before the time of his surgery—8 a.m. When we arrived the next day, bright and early at 7:00 a.m., my father was not behaving as usual. It did not take long before we realized he had suffered a stroke in the middle of the night. Obviously, surgery was postponed with the intent of having my father recover sufficiently to be a candidate for the bypass.

It took three weeks in the hospital before the surgeons determined surgery could be performed. I will never forget the presurgery conference, at which all the things that could go wrong, given that my father was a high-risk patient, were discussed. Yet the surgery went well. Dad was alert afterward and we were all optimistic. Unfortunately, that mood lasted only a few short days before my father suffered another, more serious stroke that left him uncommunicative and unable to care for himself. We did not even know if he understood us. My father's death provided a relief from his prolonged ordeal and was neither unexpected nor unwelcomed when it occurred a couple of weeks later.

The stress I experienced from the time of my father's admission to the hospital through his strokes and subsequent death was greater than I had ever known. All my stress management strategies were called into action. Of those coping techniques, I found exercise particularly effective.

When emotions build up, we seek physical outlets. It feels good to "let it all out" so we slam doors, punch walls, and scream loudly, throwing our whole bodies into it. Now that you are familiar with the stress response and recognize that the body has been physically prepared to do something physical (fight-or-flight), you can appreciate the value of using your body in some active way.

In attempting to do this, some people behave in unacceptable or dysfunctional ways. I have a friend who punched a wall, only to find it surprisingly softer than his knuckles. The repair of his swollen hand occurred several weeks prior to the repair of the hole in the wall. Other people beat up their spouses or children when distressed or wind up fighting with anyone in sight. However, there are socially acceptable ways of using the stress products in a manner that will make you feel better without violating anyone else's rights.

Let me tell you about Dick. Dick and I played tennis together, and Dick never won. Our talents were not dissimilar, but Dick seemed invariably to hit the ball harder than necessary and, consequently, could not control it as I did. One day I suggested to him that he hit easier but try to control the ball better. You know, it's not how hard you hit it but where it goes. Dick's response taught me an important lesson. He said that the ball represented his boss, his wife, or anyone else he was upset with at the moment. No way was he going to hit that "sucker" easier! I was concerned about winning; Dick was concerned about his health. I was frustrated when I hit a poor shot; as long as Dick got "good wood" on that ball, he was satisfied. Dick used physical exercise to alleviate stressful feelings and the buildup of stress products.

That is what this chapter is about—how to use exercise to manage stress. In particular, exercise is presented as a means of *using* the stress products—increased heart and respiratory rates, blood fats, muscle tension, and so forth—so they are not able to affect your health negatively. In addition, exercise can redirect your attention from stressors to the exercise. Since exercise results in physiological arousal and involves purposeful behavioral decisions, it is discussed in this part of the book.

Exercise and Health

Aerobic and Anaerobic Exercise

There are two basic types of exercise, aerobic and anaerobic. **Aerobic exercises** are usually of relatively long duration, use large muscle groups, and do not require more oxygen than you can take in. **Anaerobic exercises** are of shorter duration, done "all out," and for which oxygen inhaled is insufficient for the intensity of the activity. Aerobic exercises include jogging, bicycling, long-distance swimming, walking, and rope jumping. Anaerobic exercises include sprinting and short swimming races. Aerobic exercise is the kind that builds up cardiovascular endurance; however, both aerobic and anaerobic exercises are effective for managing stress and using stress products. Either form of exercise helps you use your body physically—which is what the fight-or-flight response prepares you for—as well as focuses your attention away from stressors you would otherwise be thinking about.

aerobic exercise
Exercise of relatively long duration, using large muscle groups, that does not require more oxygen than can be inhaled.

anaerobic exercise
Exercise of short duration that requires more oxygen than can be inhaled.

Physical Health

When people speak of health, most often they are referring to physical health. Physical health is the status of your body and its parts. Aerobic exercise does the following:

1. Improves the functioning of the lungs and circulatory system so that transportation of food and oxygen to cells is facilitated.

2. Provides the lungs with greater elasticity to breathe in more air by expanding more.

3. Delays the degenerative changes of aging.

4. Increases the production of red blood cells in the bone marrow, resulting in a greater ability to transport oxygen to the parts of the body where it is needed.

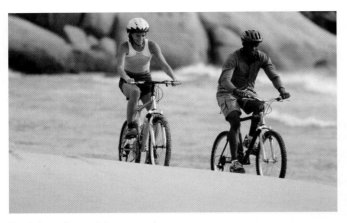
Physical exercise can help manage stress by using built-up stress by-products.

5. Helps to maintain normal blood pressure in normotensives and lower blood pressure in hypertensives.

6. Results in a quicker recovery time from strenuous activity.

7. Strengthens the heart muscle the way other muscles are strengthened—by exercising it.

8. Results in a lower pulse rate, indicating that the heart is working more efficiently.

9. Burns calories, thereby helping to prevent hypertension, heart disease, diabetes, and other conditions related to excess body fat.

10. Accelerates the speed and efficiency with which food is absorbed.

11. Tones muscle to improve strength and create a more visually appealing physique.

12. Increases endurance.

13. Improves posture.

14. Decreases low-density lipoproteins (associated with heart disease) and serum cholesterol.

15. Raises high-density lipoproteins (protective against heart disease).

physical fitness
Ability to do one's work and have energy remaining for recreational activities. Consists of muscular strength, muscular endurance, cardiorespiratory endurance, flexibility, body composition, and agility.

Most of us know that regular exercise can improve our physical fitness, but many of us do not know what that term actually means. **Physical fitness,** the ability to do one's work and have energy remaining for recreational activities, is comprised of several components:[1]

1. *Muscular strength:* the absolute maximum force that a muscle can generate, the most that can be lifted in one lift.

2. *Muscular endurance:* the ability to do continuous muscular work, the amount of work that can be done over time.

3. *Cardiorespiratory endurance:* the ability of the circulatory system (heart, lungs, and blood vessels) to supply oxygen to the muscles and remove waste products of muscular contraction.

4. *Flexibility:* the ability to move the joints of the body through their fullest range of motion.

5. *Body composition:* the proportion of lean body mass (bones and muscles) to the percentage of body fat.

6. *Agility:* the ability to move with quickness, speed, and balance.

Physical fitness, however, does not develop from just any physical activity. Certain activities are better than others. Figure 13.1 depicts the benefits of several sports and exercises, and Table 13.1 gives the energy required by various activities (the amount of calories used). Your attention is directed not only to the total physical fitness rating for each of these sports, but to the individual fitness component scores. If you have a particular need, certain sports will be better than others. For example, if you need to lose weight, you'd be advised to jog (it gives you a score of 21). If you want to develop cardiovascular fitness, you need to expend approximately 300 calories per exercise session, three times a week, or approximately 1,000 calories per week. Therefore, the activities using more calories per hour are better for you. But if flexibility is your concern, you'd be better off doing calisthenics or playing handball or squash (they give you scores of 19 and 16, respectively).

If you exercise, you will be more aware of bodily sensations. For example, you will more readily recognize muscle tension. Further, an exercised body will improve

A rating of 21 indicates maximum benefit. Ratings were made on the basis of regular (minimum of four times per week), vigorous (duration of 30 minutes to one hour per session) participation in each activity.

	Jogging	Bicycling	Swimming	Skating (ice or roller)	Handball/Squash	Skiing—cross country	Skiing—downhill	Basketball	Tennis	Calisthenics	Walking	Golf*	Softball	Bowling
Physical Fitness														
Cardiorespiratory endurance (stamina)	21	19	21	18	19	19	16	19	16	10	13	8	6	5
Muscular endurance	20	18	20	17	18	19	18	17	16	13	14	8	8	5
Muscular strength	17	16	14	15	15	15	15	15	14	16	11	9	7	5
Flexibility	9	9	15	13	16	14	14	13	14	19	7	8	9	7
Balance	17	18	12	20	17	16	21	16	16	15	8	8	7	6
General Well-being														
Weight control	21	20	15	17	19	17	15	19	16	12	13	6	7	5
Muscle definition	14	15	14	14	11	12	14	13	13	18	11	6	5	5
Digestion	13	12	13	11	13	12	9	10	12	11	11	7	8	7
Sleep	16	15	16	15	12	15	12	12	11	12	14	6	7	6
Total	148	142	140	140	140	139	134	134	128	126	102	66	64	51

*Ratings for golf are based on the fact that many Americans use a golf cart and/or caddy. If you walk the links, the physical fitness value moves up appreciably.

Figure 13.1

Physical fitness scorecard for selected sports and exercise.

your physical self-esteem. In these ways, exercise will help you to be less stressed. In addition, exercising will allow you to focus on something other than your daily problems, as well as use the products of stress such as increased blood glucose, heart rate, and muscle tension.

Psychological Health

The benefits of exercise for psychological health include the following:

1. Having more self-esteem due to feeling fit and feeling good about your body.

2. Being more positively perceived by others, since a more attractive physical appearance leads other people to consider you more poised, sensitive, kind, sincere, and more socially and occupationally successful.

3. Feeling more alert and able.

4. Being a better worker, since healthy men and women miss fewer days of work, have less illness, are involved in fewer accidents, and have a better attitude toward work.[2]

5. Decreasing feelings of depression and anxiety.[3–5]

6. Being better able to manage stress, with a resulting decrease in stress-related behaviors.[6,7]

Table 13.1

Table 13.1

Energy expenditure chart by a 150-pound person in various activities

	Energy Costs Cals/Hour
A. Sedentary Activities	
Lying down or sleeping	90
Sitting quietly	84
Sitting and writing, card playing, etc.	114
B. Moderate Activities	**(150–350)**
Bicycling (5 mph)	174
Canoeing (2.5 mph)	174
Dancing (Ballroom)	210
Golf (twosome, carrying clubs)	324
Horseback riding (sitting to trot)	246
Light housework, cleaning, etc.	246
Swimming (crawl, 20 yd per min)	288
Tennis (recreational doubles)	312
Volleyball (recreational)	264
Walking (2 mph)	198
C. Vigorous Activities	**More than 350**
Aerobic dancing	546
Basketball (recreational)	450
Bicycling (13 mph)	612
Circuit weight training	756
Cross-country skiing	690
Football (touch, vigorous)	498
Ice skating (9 mph)	384
Racquetball	588
Roller skating (9 mph)	384
Jogging (10-min mile, 6 mph)	654
Scrubbing floors	440
Swimming (crawl, 45 yd per min)	522
Tennis (recreational singles)	450

Source: President's Council on Physical Fitness and Sports, *Exercise and Weight Control* (Washington, D.C.: President's Council on Physical Fitness and Sports, 2007). www.fitness.gov/exerciseweight.pdf

In addition to all of these benefits, exercise can be fun. That is reason enough to engage in it.

It should be pointed out that exercise can also result in unhealthy outcomes, if performed incorrectly (see Figure 13.2). For example, exercise done in a rubberized sweat suit has the potential to dehydrate you and may even precipitate heat stroke or a heart attack. Exercising while wearing inappropriate clothing (e.g., dressing too warmly in the summer and too lightly in the winter) can also lead to physical consequences. In addition, your attitude when exercising is important. For example, if you associate your self-esteem with winning a sports event (such as a tennis match or basketball game) and instead you lose, you may feel less adequate and less confident. Furthermore, should you be injured while exercising, you might develop a sense of vulnerability that far exceeds reality. In all of these examples, exercise resulted in negative outcomes. And yet, it was not

Being Paid to Exercise

More than a few companies are realizing the tremendous benefits exercise can have for their employees and, more important to them, on their bottom line. As a result, companies are paying employees to work out. Quaker Oats found that, by paying employees up to $600 a year, they could save $2.8 million a year. The Providence General Medical Center in Everett, Washington, which paid employees between $250 and $325, saved almost $2.2 million a year. Other companies may not pay employees to exercise but choose, instead, to encourage them to engage in healthy activities by providing fitness facilities on-site or by contributing to membership fees their workers pay to join health clubs.

When employees exercise regularly, they are sick less frequently; therefore, their days being absent from work decrease, they use their health insurance less frequently, resulting in a decrease in the company's health insurance premiums, and they are more alert, which translates into better decisions and greater productivity.

Source: Carol Krucoff, "Cash for Working Out: Exercise Pays Off at Companies with Financial Incentive Programs," *Washington Post,* November 4, 1997, 24.

the exercise that was the culprit; rather, it was the exerciser who did not approach the activity in an appropriate manner. As stated frequently in this book, you are in control of many aspects of your life, and that includes the manner in which you approach exercise. It is in your power to make it a positive experience or organize it so it has unhealthy consequences.

One reason for the psychological benefits of exercise is the release of chemical substances by the body during exercise. One of these types of substances is a brain neurotransmitter called **endorphins.** Endorphins act as opiates might act—that is, they decrease pain and produce feelings of well-being. The much discussed and researched "runners' high"—a feeling of peace and euphoria reported by long-distance runners—is suspected of being a result of endorphin secretions by the brain.[8,9] Evidence for endorphins' effects can be found in studies that use naloxone—a substance that blocks the effects of opiates—to interfere with these euphoric feelings.[10]

Endorphins are not the only chemicals the body secretes during exercise. Dopamine is also produced. Dopamine is thought to be an antidepressant as well as an activator of erotic and sexual feelings. In addition, when you are about to exercise, the hormones epinephrine and norepinephrine are released. These substances prepare your body for the physical activity that will soon follow. Levels of these hormones remain elevated until you cease exercising. At that point, signals from the parasympathetic nervous system stop epinephrine and norepinephrine secretions, and a calming sensation occurs. Physically fit people return to their usual resting state sooner than individuals who are less fit. Those who are extremely well conditioned rebound below their resting heart rate and catecholamine levels. This *parasympathetic rebound* is one of the reasons why exercise is so helpful as a stress management tool. There is plenty of evidence of a physiological basis for the psychological and stress-reducing benefits of exercise.

endorphins
Brain neurotransmitters that decrease pain and produce feelings of well-being.

Figure 13.2
RICE

If exercise results in a minor injury, applying the RICE formula is recommended:

Rest:	Do not use the injured part of your body until it is healed.
Ice:	Place ice on the injured part for about 10 minutes at a time.
Compress:	Wrap the injured part in a bandage to diminish swelling.
Elevate:	Keep the injured body part raised to increase blood flow to the area.

Can Physical Fitness and Exercise Make You Smarter?

Several research findings indicate that physical fitness and exercise can increase cognitive functioning. The evidence for this conclusion is severalfold: Moderate- to high-intensity exercise has been shown to result in large increases of cerebral blood flow, supplying glucose and oxygen to enhance brain functioning.[11] Exercise results in increases of norepinephrine,[12] serotonin,[13] and endorphins.[14] Research in mice has shown that increases in norepinephrine are associated with an increase in memory. It is suspected that exercise may lead to changes in the brain itself or in the brain environment, leading to enhanced cognitive functioning. In a meta-analysis of studies pertaining to exercise and cognitive functioning, Etnier and colleagues[15] concluded that "exercise that is administered as a chronic treatment to produce fitness gains, or exercise that has been adopted by an individual for a sufficiently long period of time to produce fitness gains, may be a useful intervention for enhancing cognitive abilities."

So, if you want to get smart, exercise![16]

In addition, the U.S. Department of Health and Human Services reports the following benefits for adults of exercise:[17]

- Lower risk of early death.
- Lower risk of coronary heart disease.
- Lower risk of stroke.
- Lower risk of high blood pressure.
- Lower risk of adverse blood lipid profile.
- Lower risk of type 2 diabetes.
- Lower risk of colon and breast cancer.
- Prevention of weight gain.
- Weight loss, particularly when combined with reduced calorie intake.
- Improved cardiorespiratory and muscular fitness.
- Prevention of falls.
- Reduced depression.

The Healthy Way to Exercise

Have you ever seen someone jogging on a hot summer day wearing a rubberized sweat suit? Any time you overdress for exercise you are endangering your health. Your body needs to cool itself, and the evaporation of perspiration is its primary method. If you interfere with this cooling process, you can overtax your heart or court heatstroke or heat exhaustion. The result could even be death.

Sounds ridiculous, doesn't it? You think you're doing something *for* your health and instead you're doing something *against* it. People don't flirt with rubberized sweat suits because they want to see how far they can tempt the gods. They are probably just trying to lose a little more weight and think the more they perspire, the more weight they will lose. They don't know that the fluid lost through perspiration will be replenished by

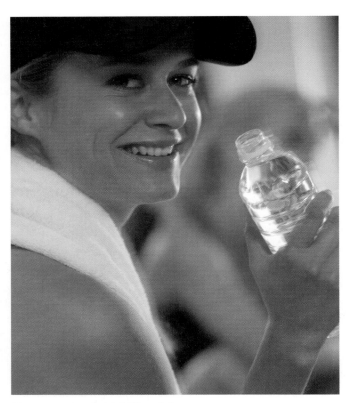
It is necessary to replenish fluid loss during and after exercise.

Figure 13.3

Physical Activity Readiness
Questionnaire - PAR-Q
(revised 2002)

PAR-Q & YOU

(A Questionnaire for People Aged 15 to 69)

Regular physical activity is fun and healthy, and increasingly more people are starting to become more active every day. Being more active is very safe for most people. However, some people should check with their doctor before they start becoming much more physically active.

If you are planning to become much more physically active than you are now, start by answering the seven questions in the box below. If you are between the ages of 15 and 69, the PAR-Q will tell you if you should check with your doctor before you start. If you are over 69 years of age, and you are not used to being very active, check with your doctor.

Common sense is your best guide when you answer these questions. Please read the questions carefully and answer each one honestly: check YES or NO.

YES	NO		
☐	☐	1.	Has your doctor ever said that you have a heart condition <u>and</u> that you should only do physical activity recommended by a doctor?
☐	☐	2.	Do you feel pain in your chest when you do physical activity?
☐	☐	3.	In the past month, have you had chest pain when you were not doing physical activity?
☐	☐	4.	Do you lose your balance because of dizziness or do you ever lose consciousness?
☐	☐	5.	Do you have a bone or joint problem (for example, back, knee or hip) that could be made worse by a change in your physical activity?
☐	☐	6.	Is your doctor currently prescribing drugs (for example, water pills) for your blood pressure or heart condition?
☐	☐	7.	Do you know of <u>any other reason</u> why you should not do physical activity?

If you answered

YES to one or more questions

Talk with your doctor by phone or in person BEFORE you start becoming much more physically active or BEFORE you have a fitness appraisal. Tell your doctor about the PAR-Q and which questions you answered YES.

- You may be able to do any activity you want — as long as you start slowly and build up gradually. Or, you may need to restrict your activities to those which are safe for you. Talk with your doctor about the kinds of activities you wish to participate in and follow his/her advice.
- Find out which community programs are safe and helpful for you.

NO to all questions

If you answered NO honestly to <u>all</u> PAR-Q questions, you can be reasonably sure that you can:
- start becoming much more physically active — begin slowly and build up gradually. This is the safest and easiest way to go.
- take part in a fitness appraisal — this is an excellent way to determine your basic fitness so that you can plan the best way for you to live actively. It is also highly recommended that you have your blood pressure evaluated. If your reading is over 144/94, talk with your doctor before you start becoming much more physically active.

→ **DELAY BECOMING MUCH MORE ACTIVE:**
- if you are not feeling well because of a temporary illness such as a cold or a fever — wait until you feel better; or
- if you are or may be pregnant — talk to your doctor before you start becoming more active.

PLEASE NOTE: If your health changes so that you then answer YES to any of the above questions, tell your fitness or health professional. Ask whether you should change your physical activity plan.

<u>Informed Use of the PAR-Q</u>: The Canadian Society for Exercise Physiology, Health Canada, and their agents assume no liability for persons who undertake physical activity, and if in doubt after completing this questionnaire, consult your doctor prior to physical activity.

No changes permitted. You are encouraged to photocopy the PAR-Q but only if you use the entire form.

Source: *Physical Activity Readiness Questionnaire (PAR-Q)* © 2002. Reprinted with permission from the Canadian Society for Exercise Physiology, www.csep.ca/.

---

drinking water and by urinating less. They don't know of the dangers they are inviting. The problem is a lack of knowledge.

This section describes how to exercise in a healthy manner. Among the topics discussed are what to do before exercise, which exercises are appropriate, and how fatigued you should get, as well as a word about competition. In addition, a sample exercise program will be offered. All of this is designed to aid you in making exercise an effective stress management technique.

One way to decide whether you are ready to exercise is to answer the questions on the *Physical Activity Readiness Questionnaire (PAR-Q)*. The PAR-Q is presented in Figure 13.3. If you answer yes to one or more questions in Figure 13.3, call your personal physician or health care provider before increasing your physical activity. On the basis of personal characteristics and medical history, people's readiness for

Everyone can benefit from exercise and alleviate stress by doing so, in spite of barriers such as lack of time, low level of fitness, and physical challenges.

target heart rate range
The low and the high heart rate during exercise to strive toward.

exercise is determined, as well as the intensity of exercise in which they ought to engage. Those individuals who are apparently healthy, and who are not aware of any condition or symptom that would affect exercising, can safely engage in exercise of moderate intensity without a medical examination or exercise test. Anyone not in the apparently healthy category should obtain an exercise test, medical examination, medical supervision while exercising, or a combination of all three.

Principles of Exercise

Intensity, Frequency, and Duration

Intensity refers to how HARD you exercise. *Frequency* is how OFTEN you exercise. And *duration* pertains to how LONG you exercise. You need not be a marathoner to derive the benefits of physical activity. In fact, research summarized in the Surgeon General's report on physical activity and health[18] concludes that moderate physical activity for 30 to 45 minutes per day provides numerous health benefits. "Moderate exercise" means such activities as gardening, brisk walking, bicycling, and working around the house. It should be obvious to you after having already read the first half of this book that, for stress management, exercise of any kind can be effective. Physical activity requires a focus of attention on the activity itself; thus, you cannot be thinking about your stressors and hassles. This is a form of selective awareness.

Of course, more strenuous exercise can result in even greater benefits. For strenuous exercise to have a beneficial cardiovascular effect, it should be done with the heart rate raised to 60 to 80 percent of its maximum. Compute your maximal heart rate and your **target heart rate (THR) range,** by completing the box. A good rule to follow is to take your pulse—every 5 minutes if you are just

Computing Your Target Heart Rate Range

1. Determine your resting heart rate (RHR) by taking your pulse (see Chapter 1 page 12).

   _____ (RHR)

2. Use the following formula to compute your target heart rate range.

   220 − _____ − _____ X .60 + _____ = _____
        (Your age) (RHR)   (RHR)   (Lower end of THR)

   220 − _____ − _____ X .80 + _____ = _____
        (Your age) (RHR)   (RHR)   (Upper end of THR)

You should be exercising so your heart rate is between your low and high target heart rate, your *target heart rate range*—sometimes referred to as your *exercise benefit zone* (EBZ). If you are more interested in losing weight, exercising closer to your lower target heart rate is recommended. If you seek cardiorespiratory benefits, exercising closer to the higher target heart rate should be the goal.

beginning to exercise and every 15 minutes if you are more experienced—during exercise to determine if you are not working hard enough or if you are working too hard. The pulse rate should be taken for 10 seconds and multiplied by 6 to get its 1-minute rate (see Chapter 1 for instructions on how to do this).

For a training effect to occur, you should exercise 20 to 30 minutes three or four days each week. Because cardiorespiratory endurance decreases after 48 hours, you should make sure to exercise at least every other day. You might want to schedule your exercise as you do other events in your life. In this way, you might view it as a commitment and be more apt to do the exercise, rather than assuming you'll exercise when you have the time and finding yourself continually postponing it.

Assessing Your Cardiorespiratory Fitness

Many exercise programs focus on cardiorespiratory endurance. The publicity surrounding the benefits of exercise for the nation's leading killer (heart disease) is probably responsible for the emphasis on improving the functioning of the heart, circulatory system, and lungs. If you were to concentrate on only one component of fitness, this would be the best one to choose. Exercises that overload the oxygen transport system (aerobic exercise) lead to an increase in cardiorespiratory endurance and often an increase in strength for selected large muscle groups.[19]

One way to assess your cardiorespiratory fitness is to take the *Rockport Fitness Walking Test.* After a 5- to 10-minute warm-up that includes stretching and slow walking, walk one mile (on an oval track is fine) as quickly as possible. Record your starting and finishing time, and then compute the time it took to walk the mile. Table 13.2 provides an interpretation of your cardiorespiratory fitness.

Starting an Exercise Program

Assuming you have determined you're a candidate for exercise, how do you begin? *Slowly!* If you have been sedentary, a good way to start is by walking. Walking can be quite enjoyable when you notice the surroundings—the foliage, the sounds, the

Table 13.2 Fitness Classification for 1-Mile Walk Test

Fitness Category	Age (years)			
	13–19	20–29	30–39	40+
	Men			
Very poor	>17:30	>18:00	>19:00	>21:30
Poor	16:01–17:30	16:31–18:00	17:31–19:00	18:31–21:30
Average	14:01–16:00	14:31–16:30	15:31–17:30	16:01–18:30
Good	12:30–14:00	13:00–14:30	13:30–15:30	14:00–16:00
Excellent	<12:30	<13:00	<13:30	<14:00
	Women			
Very poor	>18:00	>18:30	>19:30	>20:00
Poor	16:31–18:00	17:01–18:30	18:01–19:30	19:01–20:00
Average	14:31–16:30	15:01–17:00	16:01–18:00	18:00–19:00
Good	13:00–14:30	13:30–15:00	14:00–16:00	14:30–17:59
Excellent	<13:00	<13:30	<14:00	<14:30

2020 National Health Objectives Related to Physical Fitness

1. *Reduce the proportion of adults who engage in no leisure-time physical activity.*
2. *Increase the proportion of adults who meet current federal physical activity guidelines for aerobic physical activity and for muscle-strengthening activity.*
3. *Increase the proportion of adolescents who meet current federal physical activity guidelines for aerobic physical activity and for muscle-strengthening activity.*
4. *Increase the proportion of the nation's public and private schools that require daily physical education for all students.*
5. *Increase the proportion of adolescents who participate in daily school physical education.*
6. *Increase regularly scheduled elementary-school recess in the United States.*
7. *Increase the proportion of school districts that require or recommend elementary-school recess for an appropriate period of time.*
8. *Increase the proportion of children and adolescents who do not exceed recommended limits for screen time.*
9. *Increase the number of States with licensing regulations for physical activity provided in child care.*
10. *Increase the proportion of the nation's public and private schools that provide access to their physical activity spaces and facilities for all persons outside of normal school hours (that is, before and after the school day, on weekends, and during summer and other vacations).*
11. *Increase the proportion of physician office visits that include counseling or education related to physical activity.*
12. *Increase the proportion of employed adults who have access to and participate in employer-based exercise facilities and exercise programs.*
13. *Increase the proportion of trips made by walking.*
14. *Increase the proportion of trips made by bicycling.*
15. *Increase legislative policies for the built environment that enhance access to and availability of physical activity opportunities.*

buildings, the people, the sky, the colors. If you walk briskly, it can also be good exercise. After years of trying, I finally convinced my father to get off the bus one stop sooner on the way home from work and walk the rest of the way. He told me he never felt better. His body felt limber, he had a sense of accomplishment, and he felt less stressed.

Swimming and bicycle riding are other good ways to begin exercise programs if done moderately. If your body's like mine, you probably don't qualify to play the role of Tarzan anyhow, so take it easy. Since your body is supported by water when swimming and by the seat when biking, if you start slowly, these are excellent beginning activities. Swimming and biking can also be done more strenuously when you get in better shape.

Another good strategy for getting started is to exercise with a friend. It is easier to exercise regularly if you and a friend schedule it into your weekly routine. Then, when you feel like blowing off the exercise that day, you won't because you have an obligation to your friend. Besides, it is enjoyable spending time with friends and this alone might encourage you to start an exercise program. You and your friend could also monitor your progress together. Whether your goal is to lose weight, to become more cardiovascularly fit, or to feel less stressed, you can keep a record of where you are relative to those goals at the beginning of your exercise program and as the weeks go by.

How to Exercise

You should remember several points when exercising. First, keep in mind that exercise *trains,* too much exercise *strains.* I never cease being amazed at friends of mine who jog long distances but are always complaining about a knee that hurts, an Achilles tendon that is tender, or the presence of shinsplints. They approach running as a religion rather than as exercise for leisure and health. Do you exercise at a pace and with a frequency that makes it healthy and fun rather than harmful? Have a fun run, not strain and pain.

Do's and Don'ts

Warm-Up and Cool-Down

Research has indicated that beginning exercise too abruptly can cause cardiac rhythm problems.[20] Since these problems have the potential to result in heart attacks (even in an otherwise healthy heart), a 10- or 15-minute warm-up is recommended before any strenuous exercise. The warm-up will also help to stretch the muscles and will decrease the chance of muscle strains during the exercise itself.

After exercising vigorously, there is the possibility of too much blood pooling in the veins. This can lead to fainting. Though this possibility is somewhat remote, you should take a 5- or 10-minute cool-down period after strenuous exercise. Walking and stretching exercises serve as a good cool-down.

Clothing

Light-colored clothing that reflects the sun's rays is cooler in the summer, and dark clothes are warmer in the winter. When the weather is very cold, it's better to wear several layers of light clothing than one or two heavy layers. The extra layers help trap heat, and it's easy to shed one of them if you become too warm.

You should wear something on your head when it's cold, or when it's hot and sunny. Wool watch caps or ski caps are recommended for winter wear, and some form of tennis or sailor's hat that provides shade and can be soaked in water is good for summer.

If you dress properly, you can exercise in almost any weather, but it's advisable not to exercise outdoors when it's extremely hot and humid. On such days, plan to exercise early in the morning or in the evening.

Fluids

Drink plenty of water before and after exercising. The American College of Sports Medicine recommends drinking 14 to 22 oz. of water two hours before exercise, 6 to 12 oz. during exercise, and after exercise 16 to 24 oz. for every pound of body weight lost.[21]

Equipment

Use appropriate equipment. Poor-fitting sneakers or a tennis racket with too large a grip can lead to injury and more stress rather than less.

Know Your Body

Become aware of how your body usually feels so you can recognize when it doesn't feel right. The following may be signs of overtraining and may indicate that you should cut down on your exercise:

1. Unusual soreness in muscles and joints.
2. Unusual heaviness in arms and legs.
3. Inability to relax.
4. Persistent tiredness.
5. Unusual loss of appetite.
6. Unusual loss of weight.
7. Constipation or diarrhea.
8. Repeated injury.

Competition and Enjoyment

When I first started long-distance running, I was very competitive. Each time I went out, I tried to beat my best personal record. My wristwatch was as important a piece of equipment as my running shorts and shoes. Pretty soon I stopped enjoying running. It became a thing I had to do. Running became discouraging, because there was a day I ran so well that subsequent runs could never be as fast. I started developing aches in my legs and stiffness in my knees.

It was at that point that I decided to make a change. From that day on, I have never worn a wristwatch while jogging and have never had anyone else time me. I run at a pace that affords me a training effect and is comfortable. If someone attempts to pass me or if I am about to pass someone else, I'll try to carry on a brief conversation: "Nice day for a run, isn't it? How far are you going? Do you like those running shoes?" I now pay attention to the color of the trees (what a great time of year autumn is for running), hear the sound of my running shoes crunching the snow (what a great time of year winter is for running), notice the budding of flowers (what a great time of year spring is for running), and actually enjoy the feel of the sun on my body (what a great time of year summer is for running). Get the picture? For me, jogging has now become an enjoyable and stress-reducing technique rather than a pain and a stressor.

Competition, either with others or just with ourselves, often changes a recreational activity into one that does not recreate. Now, competition can be positive. It often takes competition for us to realize our potential. For example, you'll never know how good your return of service is in tennis unless your opponent hits a good serve for you to return. Too often, though, competition means we are comparing ourselves with others or with an idealized self. When we come off second best (or even worse), we often do not enjoy the activity, or we develop a diminished sense of self-worth, or both. Further, we plug our satisfaction into an end result rather than enjoying the experience regardless of the outcome. All of this can add to stress reactivity rather than help to manage stress.

If you can use competition in a healthy manner to actualize your potential, more power to you. Continue what you're doing. However, if you're like my friend Don, who one day—after missing a return of serve—flung his tennis racket over a fence and several trees into a creek and then had the nerve to ask if I would help him get it before it floated too far downstream, you'd be advised to approach sports and exercise differently. Realize you're not a professional athlete and that sports and exercise should be fun. Do your best, try hard, but enjoy the effort in spite of how it turns out. Use sports and exercise to manage stress, not create it.

Choosing an Exercise Program

There are many different types of exercise programs. In this section, several exercise possibilities are described and addresses provided where you can get information about others. Also consult the sources listed in the "References" section at the chapter's conclusion for still more information about options for exercise.

Swimming

It may surprise you to know that as long ago as January 1980 there were almost 2 million in-ground swimming pools in the United States and another 2 million above the ground. Obviously, swimming is a viable exercise for many of us. Swimming can provide benefits similar to other exercises but has one decided advantage: it diminishes the chances of athletic injury; when you are submerged up to the neck, the water supports 90 percent of your weight.[22] Therefore, your feet and legs need only support 10 percent of your body weight and will not be injured as easily as during weight-bearing exercises (e.g., basketball).

Many people use lap swimming to keep fit and to manage stress. Others do not have access to pools large enough to swim laps but can still use the water to obtain adequate exercise. These people can participate in aqua dynamics. **Aqua dynamics** is a program of structured exercises conducted in limited water areas involving standing water drills (e.g., alternate toe touching, side-straddle hopping, toe bouncing, and jogging in place); poolside standing drills (such as stretching out the arms, pressing the back flat against the wall, and raising the knees to the chest); gutter-holding drills (such as knees to chest; hop-twisting; front, back, and side flutter kicking; bobbing; and treading water). If you have your own pool and feel it is too small for lap swimming, you might want to write to the President's Council on Physical Fitness and Sports, Washington, D.C. 20201, for the *Aqua Dynamics* booklet.

Rope Jumping

Rope jumping is another excellent exercise. When I was 13, my friend Steven and I both fell head over heels in love with 12-year-old, blonde, adorable, vivacious Jill. I'm talking about the heart-pounding, palm-perspiring, any-spare-time-spent-with-her love. Steven and I would do anything for Jill. We even spent hours playing *Who Stole the Cookie from the Cookie Jar?* while our friends played baseball or basketball. That was the summer I learned to jump rope, the whole time made frantic by the thought that this was a "sissy" activity. If my other friends had seen me, I would have died.

Well, I'm no longer crippled by that thought because I have since learned that the gender you were born with need not stop you from engaging in an enjoyable activity. I have also learned that rope jumping is an excellent way to develop cardiorespiratory endurance, strength, agility, coordination, and a sense of wellness. Fortunately, many other people have learned a similar lesson, and rope jumping has become very popular. Here are some pointers for jumping rope:

1. Determine the best length for your rope by standing on the center of the rope. The handles should then reach to each armpit.

2. When jumping, keep your upper arms close to your body, with your elbows almost touching your sides. Have your forearms out at right angles, and turn the rope by making small circles with your hands and wrists. Keep your feet, ankles, and knees together.

---

aqua dynamics
A program consisting of structured exercises conducted in limited water areas.

3. Relax. Don't tense up. Enjoy yourself.

4. Keep your body erect, with your head and eyes up.

5. Start slowly.

6. Land on the balls of your feet, bending your knees slightly.

7. Maintain a steady rhythm.

8. Jump just one or two inches from the floor.

9. Try jumping to music. Maintain the rhythm of the music.

10. When you get good, improvise. Create new stunts. Have fun.

The American Heart Association recommends rope jumping stunts. If interested, write to receive a brochure describing these stunts.

Bicycling

Biking can take place outside on the road or inside on a stationary bicycle. Either road or stationary biking can use the built-up stress products and help you develop physical fitness if done regularly and at the proper intensity. To bike on the road, you need a bicycle with gears; they vary greatly in cost. If you shop around or buy a secondhand bicycle, you can probably get a good ten-speed for half the cost of a new one. You will also need a helmet, gloves with padded palms, and pant clips or special clothing. Of course, many people bike with less sophisticated equipment and still get the benefits of the exercise.

Another alternative is to bike and never go anywhere; this is especially appealing on a snowy day. For this you need a stationary bicycle. While riding a stationary bicycle, you need to pay attention to adjusting it correctly. In particular, you should make sure the handlebars and the seat are where they should be. The seat needs to be adjusted so that your knee is just slightly bent when the pedal is in its lowest position (a 5 to 10 degree of knee bend). The handlebars need to be set so you are relaxed and leaning slightly forward.

Walking

Walking is an excellent lead-in to other, more vigorous physical fitness activities, but usually it is not a sufficient stimulus for young people to raise their heart rates high enough for a training effect. However, for the deconditioned, overweight, or elderly person who is beginning an exercise program, walking is recommended, or for younger people, if they increase the pace sufficiently to reach their target heart rate. If you take up walking, use the following rule to gauge your readiness to progress to other, more vigorous forms of fitness activities: Depending on your age and gender, once you reach the Average fitness category in Table 13.2, you are ready.

Of course, we are referring to natural-gait walking. Race walking or speed walking is another story altogether. These forms of exercise are an excellent means of using the built-up stress by-products, as well as a means to develop an increased level of physical fitness. In race walking, the lead foot must be on the ground when your trailing leg pushes off, and you must keep your knee straight as your body passes over that leg. What is surprising to many people is that a race walker burns about the same number of calories as does a jogger. For example, whereas a jogger will burn off 493 calories per hour, a race walker at the same pace will burn off 457 calories per hour.[23] To perform race walking correctly, remember the following guidelines:

1. Keep your back straight and walk tall.

2. Point your feet straight and plant them at a 40-degree angle to the ground.

3. As you pull forward with one leg, push straight back with the other leg until the toe of that leg is off the ground.

4. Stretch your hips forward rather than from side to side.

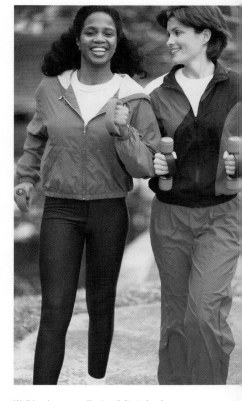

Walking is an excellent activity to begin an exercise program, especially if you have not engaged in physical activity regularly. Some walkers increase the intensity of walking by carrying dumbbells. Walking can also provide social support when the walk is shared with others.

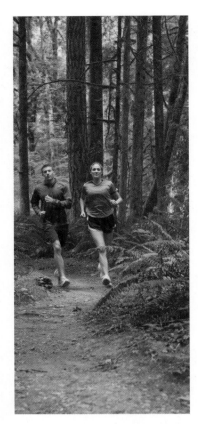

Jogging is an excellent activity to combine the physical benefits of exercise with the psychological benefits of relaxation. Running in a pleasing environment, enjoying the sounds of nature, and focusing on one's bodily sensations can also be a meaningful spiritual experience.

If you are interested in learning more about walking or have decided to participate in this activity, there are a couple of organizations you may want to contact. The Walkablock Club of America, walk@walkablock.com, (925) 373-4816, and the Rockport Walking Institute, P.O. Box 480, Marlboro, MA 01752, can provide advice and encouragement for your walking program.

Jogging

Running is such a good form of exercise because it requires a minimum of equipment (the only expense is a good pair of running shoes), it can be done almost anywhere, anytime, and it does not require a special skill.

In most sports, we are taught to run for speed and power. In running for fitness, the objectives are different and so is the form. Here are some suggestions (see Figure 13.4) to help you develop a comfortable, economical running style:

1. Run in an upright position, avoiding excessive forward lean. Keep your back as straight as you comfortably can and keep your head up. Don't look at your feet.
2. Carry your arms slightly away from the body, with elbows bent so that forearms are roughly parallel to the ground. Occasionally, shake and relax your arms to prevent tightness in your shoulders.
3. Land on the heel of the foot and rock forward to drive off the ball of the foot. If this proves difficult, try a more flat-footed style. Running only on the balls of your feet will tire you quickly and make your legs sore.
4. Keep your stride relatively short. Don't force your pace by reaching for extra distance.
5. Breathe deeply, with your mouth open.

The American Podiatry Association recommends the following running program:[24]

1–6 Weeks

Warm up with walking and stretching movement.

Jog 55 yards; walk 55 yards (four times).

Jog 110 yards; walk 110 yards (four times).

Jog 55 yards; walk 55 yards (four times).

Pace: 110 yards in about 45 seconds.

6–12 Weeks

Increase jogging and reduce walking.

Pace: 110 yards in 30 to 37 seconds.

12–24 Weeks

Jog a 9-minute mile. (However, since you need to work out aerobically for 20 to 30 minutes to gain cardiorespiratory endurance, you should add other exercise as well.)

30+ Weeks

On the second workout each week, add variety—continuous jogging or running and walking alternately at a slow, varying pace for distances up to 2 miles.

Stretching

Stretching is an excellent stress reduction technique. There are two basic types of stretching.

Active stretching is where you hold a position by muscular contraction, for example, bringing your leg up high and then holding it there. Active stretching increases flexibility and strengthens the active muscles. Active stretches are usually quite difficult to hold for more than 10 seconds and rarely should be held longer than 15 seconds. Many of the positions found in various forms of yoga are active stretches.

Figure 13.4

Running correctly.

Keep head and jaw relaxed.

Run upright; don't slouch

Move arms up and back, not across the body.

Avoid twisting the torso.

Keep your hands relaxed.

Align hips with head and shoulders.

Arms should form a 90° angle at your elbows.

Increase leg lift and stride length to take pressure off the knees.

Lift knees to lengthen your stride.

Land on your heel. Then roll off the front of your foot for a better push-off.

Static stretching involves holding a position in a relaxed fashion without muscular contraction, that is, making no contribution to the range of motion. For example, bending at the waist and reaching for your toes. In this instance, gravity aids the stretch. Static stretches should be held for at least 30 seconds, working up to 1 minute. Static stretching is preferable to active stretching, although neither is related to injury prevention. A better method of stretching before exercising is *dynamic stretching*. Dynamic stretching consists of functional-based exercises that use sport-specific movements to prepare the body for movement.[25] The stretches gradually increase the reach and speed of movement of a body part. Dynamic stretching differs from *ballistic stretching* in that it involves stretching the legs and arms in a controlled, gentle manner that reaches the limits of the range of motion. Ballistic stretches, by contrast, involve trying to force a part of the body beyond its range of motion. One expert's recommendation is to "perform dynamic stretches before a workout and static stretches

Figure 13.5   Dynamic Stretches

(a) The hurdlers knee raise

(b) Heel up quad stretch

(c) Leg swings

(d) Walking tip toe

(e) Forward leg swing

(f) Side leg swing

(g) Forward lunge and torso twist

after a workout. Studies have shown that static stretching before a workout deactivates muscles and makes them weaker."[26] Illustrations of several dynamic stretches are shown in Figure 13.5. A word of caution: Never stretch a muscle that has not been warmed up. To do so courts injury, since the muscle may tear or strain. Also, don't bounce or strain into the stretch.

Table 13.3 American College of Sports Medicine's Guidelines on Quantity and Quality of Exercise

Cardiorespiratory exercise	• Adults should get at least 150 minutes of moderate-intensity exercise per week. • Exercise recommendations can be met through 30–60 minutes of moderate-intensity exercise (five days per week) or 20–60 minutes of vigorous-intensity exercise (three days per week). • One continuous session and multiple shorter sessions (of at least 10 minutes) are both acceptable to accumulate desired amount of daily exercise. • Gradual progression of exercise time, frequency, and intensity is recommended for best adherence and least injury risk. • People unable to meet these minimums can still benefit from some activity.
Resistance exercise	• Adults should train each major muscle group two or three days each week using a variety of exercises and equipment. • Very light or light intensity is best for older persons or previously sedentary adults starting exercise. • Two to four sets of each exercise will help adults improve strength and power. • For each exercise, 8–12 repetitions improve strength and power, 10–15 repetitions improve strength in middle-age and older persons starting exercise, and 15–20 repetitions improve muscular endurance. • Adults should wait at least 48 hours between resistance training sessions.
Flexibility exercise	• Adults should do flexibility exercises at least two or three days each week to improve range of motion. • Each stretch should be held for 10–30 seconds to the point of tightness or slight discomfort. • Repeat each stretch two to four times, accumulating 60 seconds per stretch. • Static, dynamic, ballistic, and PNF stretches are all effective. • Flexibility exercise is most effective when the muscle is warm. Try light aerobic activity or a hot bath to warm the muscles before stretching.
Neuromotor exercise	• Neuromotor exercise (sometimes called "functional fitness training") is recommended for two or three days per week. • Exercises should involve motor skills (balance, agility, coordination, and gait), proprioceptive exercise training and multifaceted activities (Tai Chi and yoga) to improve physical function and prevent falls in older adults. • 20–30 minutes per day is appropriate for neuromotor exercise.

Source: Garber, Carol Ewing, Blissmer, Bryan, Deschenes, Michael R., Franklin, Barry A., Lamonte, Michael J., Lee, I-Min, Nieman, David C., and Swain, David P. Quantity and Quality of Exercise for Developing and Maintaining Cardiorespiratory, Musculoskeletal, and Neuromotor Fitness in Apparently Healthy Adults: Guidance for Prescribing Exercise. *Medicine and Science in Sports and Exercise* 43(2011): 1334–1359.

Weight Training

Weight training has become more and more popular. People are beginning to realize that aerobic fitness is only one piece of the physical fitness equation. Muscular strength and endurance are also important. Weight training also has benefits for managing stress. Not only can weight training use built-up stress by-products, but the increased self-confidence and self-esteem from feeling that your body is attractive can help you manage stressors more effectively. If you are interested in pursuing a weight-training program, a good start might be to enroll in a weight-training course at your college or one offered through a YMCA, Jewish community center, or local recreation center. Reading about the proper way to weight train or working with a trainer can also help Exercise Guideline you prevent injury.

Exercise Guidelines

The American College of Sports Medicine (ACSM) publishes guidelines regarding the recommended quantity and quality of exercise for adults.[27] These guidelines are based on current scientific evidence on physical activity, which informs the recommendations on aerobic exercise, strength training, and flexibility. ACSM's overall recommendation is for most adults to engage in at least 150 minutes of moderate-intensity exercise each week. The ACSM guidelines appear in Table 13.3. The Centers for Disease Control and Prevention (CDC) also recommends how to exercise healthfully. These recommendations appear in Table 13.4.

Exercise and the Elderly

Exercise is not only for the young. People of all ages can benefit from it. Among the benefits of exercise for the elderly is the slowing of declines in aerobic capacity, in cardiovascular fitness, in flexibility, and in muscle mass that inevitably occur with aging.[28] In addition, exercise decreases blood pressure, produces favorable changes in

Table 13.4 Adding Physical Activity to Your Life

There are a lot of ways to get the physical activity you need. If you're thinking, "How can I meet the guidelines each week?", don't worry. You'll be surprised by the variety of activities you have to choose from. To meet the guidelines for aerobic activity, basically anything counts, as long as it's done at a moderate or vigorous-intensity for at least 10 minutes at a time. If you're not sure where to start, here are some examples.

Moderate Aerobic Activity Routines

	Monday	Tuesday	Wednesday	Thursday	Friday	Saturday	Sunday	Physical Activity TOTAL
Example 1	30 minutes of brisk walking	30 minutes of brisk walking	Resistance band exercises	30 minutes of brisk walking	30 minutes of brisk walking	Resistance band exercises	30 minutes of brisk walking	**150 minutes moderate-intensity aerobic activity AND 2 days muscle strengthening**
Example 2	30 minutes of brisk walking	60 minutes of playing softball	30 minutes of brisk walking	30 minutes of mowing the lawn		Heavy gardening	Heavy gardening	**150 minutes moderate-intensity aerobic activity AND 2 days muscle strengthening**

Vigorous Aerobic Activity Routines

	Monday	Tuesday	Wednesday	Thursday	Friday	Saturday	Sunday	Physical Activity TOTAL
Example 3	25 minutes of jogging	Weight lifting	25 minutes of jogging	Weight lifting	25 minutes of jogging			**75 minutes vigorous-intensity aerobic activity AND 2 days muscle strengthening**
Example 4	25 minutes of swimming laps		25 minutes of running	Weight training	25 minutes of singles tennis	Weight training		**75 minutes vigorous-intensity aerobic activity AND 2 days muscle strengthening**

Mix of Moderate and Vigorous Aerobic Activity Routines

	Monday	Tuesday	Wednesday	Thursday	Friday	Saturday	Sunday	Physical Activity TOTAL
Example 5	30 minutes of water aerobics	30 minutes of jogging	30 minutes of brisk walking / Yoga		30 minutes of brisk walking	Yoga		**90 minutes moderate-intensity aerobic activity AND 30 minutes vigorous-intensity aerobic activity AND 2 days muscle strengthening**
Example 6	45 minutes of doubles tennis		Rock climbing		30 minutes of vigorous hiking / Weight lifting		45 minutes of doubles tennis	**90 minutes moderate-intensity aerobic activity AND 30 minutes vigorous-intensity aerobic activity AND 2 days muscle strengthening**

Source: Centers for Disease Control and Prevention. *Adding Physical Activity to Your Life.* (Atlanta, GA: Centers for Disease Control and Prevention, 2009). Available at: www.cdc.gov/physicalactivity/downloads/pa_examples.pdf.

blood lipids, helps prevent osteoporosis, improves glucose tolerance, increases bone density thereby decreasing the chances of a bone break, and helps maintain strength, endurance, and flexibility in the arms and legs. These physiological benefits foster continued independence in performing activities of daily living (such as dressing, bathing, and shopping). Even older adults who are not interested in pursuing sports often find it easier to carry groceries, climb stairs, or play with children if they maintain muscular strength.[29] In addition, it will be easier for them to maintain balance, thereby lessening their susceptibility to falling.

Furthermore, regular exercise can enhance wellness and social health when engaged in with other people. It can also contribute to spiritual health when it occurs outdoors and when attention is paid to nature and the surroundings. And, of course, exercise uses the built-up by-products of stress. Consequently, the negative consequences of stress can be reduced if seniors engage in physical activity on a regular basis.

Seniors are advised to participate in moderately intense physical activity 30 minutes a day at least three to five times a week. Climbing stairs, walking, doing yard work, gardening, cycling, and doing heavy housework all qualify. Yet the majority of Americans do not exercise regularly. One of the U.S. government's Healthy People 2010 objectives was to increase the percentage of Americans exercising regularly to 30 percent. In 2008, 34 percent of older adults engaged in the recommended amount of exercise. The 2020 national objective is for 37 percent of older adults to meet this target.[30]

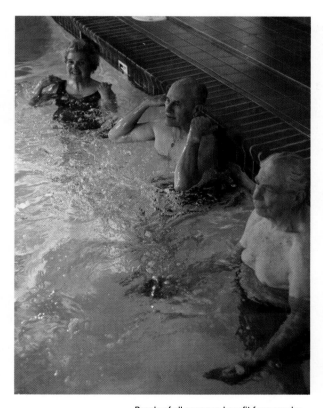

Exercise—Keeping It Going

Among other benefits, physical fitness has been shown to decrease the risk of coronary heart disease by 62 percent,[31] decrease the risk of breast cancer in women by 14 percent,[32] and decrease the risk of stroke by one-third.[33] Exercise can also help you manage stress by using the products of stress: muscle tension, serum cholesterol, and increased heart and respiratory rate.

This chapter has provided you with the information you need to begin an exercise program. You can do it. You can exercise regularly and improve your physical and psychological health. You can use those stress products before they result in illness or disease. You are in control of your exercise behavior, and you can exercise (no pun intended) that control.

People of all ages can benefit from regular exercise, physically and psychologically.

Figure 13.6

The Physical Activity Pyramid.

As with the Food Guide Pyramid, the Physical Activity Pyramid promotes a balanced diet of physical activity. Follow this guide and you will be physically healthier than you would have been otherwise.

Source: © Board of Regents of the University System of Georgia by Georgia State University (1999).

Do Sparingly
Play computer games, Watch TV, Use labor saving devices like escalators

Recreational Activities
2–3 days/week
Golf, Bowling, Baseball, Soccer, Hiking, In-line Skating, Dancing, Canoeing, Yoga, Martial Arts

Aerobic Exercise
3–5 days/week
Running, Cycling, Cross Country Skiing, In-line Skating, Stair Stepping

Flexibility Exercise
3–5 days/week
Static stretching of major muscle groups. Hold each pose 10–30 seconds

Strength Exercise
2–3 days/week
8–10 exercises
1 set of 8–12 reps Bicep curl, Tricep Press, Squats, Lunges, Push-ups

Take the stairs
Garden
Wash and wax your car
Rake leaves
Mow the lawn

Physical Activity
Most Days of the Week
Accumulate 30+ minutes

Walk to do your errands
Walk the dog
Clean your house
Play with your kids

Coping in Today's World

Fitness activities can have a significant effect on physical health, mental and emotional health, and spiritual health. Witness Rabbi Hirscel Jaffe. Rabbi Jaffe used marathon running as a means of fighting the cancer he experienced. When he recovered, he decided to share his good fortune and began helping others overcome diversity.

Rabbi Jaffe began counseling cancer patients, became a co-editor of *Gates of Healing* (a book distributed to hospital patients), wrote a highly acclaimed book called *Why Me, Why Anyone?* and developed a videotape entitled *Hanging on to Hope.* In 1988, he received the American Cancer Society's Award of Courage from President Ronald Reagan.

With his physical self healed, Rabbi Jaffe decided he needed to express his spirituality. He visited American hostages in Iran in 1980, and in 1992 he led a unity march in Newburgh, New York to protest the appearance of the Ku Klux Klan in his town. More than 3,000 people participated in that march.

Those who knew him best called him the "Running Rabbi"—both for his marathon participation and his tireless efforts on behalf of others. Rabbi Jaffe demonstrates how physical activity can improve physical, mental, and emotional health and provide expression of one's spirituality. What better way of coping with stress can one devise?

summary

- Aerobic exercise is of relatively long duration, uses large muscle groups, builds cardiovascular fitness, and does not require more oxygen than you can take in. Anaerobic exercise is of short duration and high intensity and requires more oxygen than you can take in.

- Exercise improves the functioning of the lungs and circulatory system, delays the degenerative changes of aging, increases the blood's ability to transport oxygen to body parts, strengthens the heart muscle, burns calories, and lowers serum cholesterol.

- Physical fitness consists of several components: muscular strength, muscular endurance, cardiorespiratory endurance, flexibility, body composition, and agility.

- The psychological benefits of exercise include improving self-esteem, being perceived more positively by others, feeling more alert, having a better attitude toward work, decreasing feelings of depression and anxiety, and being better able to manage stress.

- Endorphins are released by the brain during exercise and produce a euphoric, relaxed state.

- The American College of Sports Medicine has developed recommendations regarding the need for testing prior to commencing an exercise program. ACSM guidelines state that if you are apparently healthy—no signs or symptoms of cardiorespiratory disease—then you can start a moderate exercise program without the need for exercise testing or a medical examination. If signs or symptoms have occurred, you are advised to obtain a medical examination or be supervised during exercise, depending on the degree of the symptoms.

- The intensity, frequency, and duration of exercise are important considerations if cardiorespiratory endurance is the goal.

- When exercising, do warm-up and cool-down routines, wear clothing appropriate to the weather, drink plenty of fluids, use properly fitted equipment, and recognize when your body is telling you you're overdoing it.

- An exercise program can consist of a number of activities such as swimming, rope jumping, bicycling, walking, jogging, step aerobics, water aerobics, stretching, and weight training.

- There are many organizations from which you can obtain more information about specific physical fitness activities or a particular sport.

internet resources

Mayo Clinic: Fitness Basics **www.mayoclinic.com/health/ fitness/MY00396** *Information presented about fitness including stretching and flexibility, aerobic exercise, strength training, and sports nutrition.*

The President's Council on Physical Fitness and Sports: Resources **www.fitness.gov/resources_health.htm** *Lists organizations related to physical fitness from which an array of information can be obtained. Also included are a listing of federal agencies, physical activity fact sheets, and state resources.*

American College of Sports Medicine **www.acsm.org/** *Provides guidelines for engaging in exercise and position statements regarding healthy ways to stay fit. Funds research and provides information on injury prevention, weightlessness and space physiology, exercise and aging, exercise and cardiovascular disease risk factors, and exercise and heart rate response.*

Heart Information Network **www.heartinfo.org** *Provides guidelines about heart conditions, diet, and more.*

references

1. Jerrold S. Greenberg, George B. Dintiman, and Barbee Myers Oakes, *Physical Fitness and Wellness,* 3rd ed. (Champaign, IL: Human Kinetics, 2004), 6.

2. President's Council on Physical Fitness and Sports, *Building a Healthier Company* (Washington, D.C.: President's Council on Physical Fitness and Sports, n.d.).

3. Deborah Brauser, "Regular Physical Activity Significantly Reduces Depression Risk," *Medscape Medical News.* 2010. Available at: www.medscape.com/viewarticle/732021.

4. E. W. Martinsen, "Physical Activity and Depression: Clinical Experience," *Acta Psychiatrica Scandanavica.* 2007. Available at: onlinelibrary.wiley.com/doi/10.1111/j.1600-0447.1994.tb05797.x/abstract.

5. Mayo Clinic Staff, "Depression and Anxiety: Exercise Eases Symptoms," *Depression: Major Depression.* 2009. Available at: www.mayoclinic.com/health/depression-and-exercise/MH00043.

6. J. J. Daubenmier, G. Weidner, M. D. Sumner, N. Mendell, T. Merritt-Worden, J. Studley, and D. Ornish, "The Contribution

of Changes in Diet, Exercise, and Stress Management to Changes in Coronary Risk in Women and Men in the Multisite Cardiac Lifestyle Intervention Program," *Annals of Behavioral Medicine* 33(2007): 57–68.

7. S. Haugland, B. Wold, and T. Torsheim, "Relieving the Pressure? The Role of Physical Activity in the Relationship Between School-Related Stress and Adolescent Health Complaints," *Research Quarterly for Exercise and Sport* 74(2003): 127–35.

8. Bradley Hack, "Exercise Valuable for Mental Health," *Fit Society Page: A Quarterly Publication of the American College of Sports Medicine*, 2007. Available at www.acsm.org/AM/ Template.cfm? Section=Search&section=20033&template=/CM/ContentDisplay.cfm&ContentFileID=28

9. L. Carrasco, C. Villaverde, and C. M. Oltras, "Endorphin Responses to Stress Induced by Competitive Swimming Event," *Sports Medicine and Physical Fitness* 47(2007): 239–45.

10. S. A. Shankarappa, E. S. Piedras-Rentería, and E. B. Stubbs, Jr. "Forced-Exercise Delays Neuropathic Pain in Experimental Diabetes: Effects on Voltage-Activated Calcium Channels," *Journal of Neurochemistry* 118(2011): 224–36.

11. M. C. Chang, S. H. Ahn, Y. W. Cho, S. M. Son, Y. H. Kwon, M. Y. Lee, W. M. Byun, and S. H. Jang, "The Comparison of Cortical Activation Patterns by Active Exercise, Proprioceptive Input, and Touch Stimulation in the Human Brain: A Functional MRI Study," *NeuroRehabilitation* 25(2009): 87–92.

12. N. Miyai, M. Arita, I. Morioka, S. Takeda, and K. Miyashita, "Ambulatory Blood Pressure, Sympathetic Activity, and Left Ventricular Structure and Function in Middle-Aged Normotensive Men with Exaggerated Blood Pressure Response to Exercise," *Medical Science Monitor* 11(2005): CR478–CR484.

13. H. Marin and M. A. Menza, "The Management of Fatigue in Depressed Patients," *Essential Psychopharmacology* 6(2005): 185–92.

14. E. E. Cohen, R. Ejsmond-Frey, N. Knight, and R. I. Dunbar, "Rowers' High: Behavioural Synchrony Is Correlated with Elevated Pain Thresholds," *Biology Letters* 6(2010): 106–8.

15. J. L. Etnier, W. Salazar, D. M. Landers, S. J. Pertruzello, M. Han, and P. Nowell, "The Influence of Physical Fitness and Exercise upon Cognitive Functioning: A Meta-Analysis," *Journal of Sport and Exercise Psychology* 19(1997): 249–77.

16. C. W. Cotman and C. Engesser, "Exercise Enhances and Protects Brain Function," *Exercise and Sports Sciences Reviews,* 30(2002): 75–79.

17. U.S. Department of Health and Human Services, *2008 Physical Activity Guidelines for Americans* (Washington, DC: U.S. Department of Health and Human Services, 2009).

18. U.S. Public Health Service, *Physical Activity and Health: A Report of the Surgeon General* (Washington, D.C.: U.S. Department of Health and Human Services, 1996).

19. Greenberg, Dintiman, and Oakes, *Physical Fitness and Wellness.*

20. S. Pasupathy, K. M. Naseem, and S. Homer-Vanniasinkam, "Effects of Warm-Up on Exercise Capacity, Platelet Activation and Platelet-Leucocyte Aggregation in Patients with Claudication," *British Journal of Surgery* 92(2005): 50–55.

21. American College of Sports Medicine, "Nutrition and Athletic Performance," *Medicine and Science in Sports and Exercise* 32 (2000): 2130–45.

22. "Water Aerobics: A Great Way to Improve Cardiovascular Fitness," *Aerobic-Exercises.com.* 2009. Available at: www.aerobics-exercises.com/water_aerobics.php

23. NutriStrategy, *Calories Burned During Exercise.* 2007. Available at: www.nutristrategy.com/activitylist4.htm

24. American Podiatry Association, *Jogging Advice from Your Podiatrist* (Washington, D.C.: American Podiatry Association, n.d.).

25. Douglas Mann and Margaret Jones, "Guidelines to the Implementation of a Dynamic Stretching Routine," *Strength and Conditioning Journal* 21(1999): 53–55.

26. Srdjan Popovic, "Static Stretching vs. Dynamic Stretching," *Bloom to Fit.* 2010. Available at: www.bloomtofit.com/static-stretching-vs-dynamic-stretching.

27. Carol Ewing Garber, Bryan Blissmer, Michael R. Deschenes, Barry A. Franklin, Michael J. Lamonte, I-Min Lee, David C. Nieman, and David P. Swain, "Quantity and Quality of Exercise for Developing and Maintaining Cardiorespiratory, Musculoskeletal, and Neuromotor Fitness in Apparently Healthy Adults: Guidance for Prescribing Exercise," *Medicine and Science in Sports and Exercise* 43(2011): 1334–59.

28. Greenberg, Dintiman, and Oakes, *Physical Fitness and Wellness.*

29. "Strength Training Among Adults Aged > 65 Years—United States, 2001," *Morbidity and Mortality Weekly Report* 53(2004): 25–28.

30. U.S. Department of Health and Human Services, *Healthy People 2020* (Washington, DC: U.S Department of Health and Human Services, 2011). Available at: www.healthypeople.gov/2020/default.aspx.

31. S. Yu, J. W. G. Yarnell, P. M. Sweetnam, and L. Murray, "What Level of Physical Activity Protects Against Premature Cardiovascular Death? The Caerphilly Study," *Heart* 89(2003): 502–6.

32. Anne McTiernan, Charles Kooperberg, Emily White, Sara Wilcox, Ralph Coates, Lucile L. Adams-Campbell, Nancy Woods, and Judith Ockene, "Recreational Physical Activity and the Risk of Breast Cancer in Postmenopausal Women: The Women's Health Initiative Study," *Journal of the American Medical Association* 290(2003): 1331–36.

33. Sudhir Kurl, Jan A. Laukkanen, Rainer Rauramaa, Timo A. Lakka, Juhani Sivenius, and Jukka T. Salonen, "Cardiorespiratory Fitness and the Risk of Stroke in Men," *Archives of Internal Medicine* 163(2003): 1682–88.

LAB ASSESSMENT 13.1

Can You Overcome Roadblocks to Exercise?

All of us know we should be exercising. It is good for our bodies and our minds, and it is one of the most effective stress management strategies. Yet, too many Americans live sedentary lives—not because they don't want to exercise or don't believe the claims regarding the benefits of exercise. Rather, there are barriers/roadblocks to their exercising that are so strong, and for which they do not have effective strategies to overcome, that these roadblocks interfere with them doing what they know they should do. This lab is designed to help you identify and plan to overcome roadblocks that interfere with you engaging in regular exercise and, thereby, be better at managing the stress you experience.

Directions: Two examples of commonly experienced roadblocks to exercising appear here, with strategies to bypass these roadblocks. List the roadblocks specific to you and the strategies you can use to bypass those roadblocks.

Roadblock	Strategy
You may have a lot to do with little time to get it done. Term papers are due, midterm or final exams are approaching, you are invited to a party, you are expected to attend a dinner celebrating your sister's birthday, your team is scheduled for an intramural game, and your professor is holding a study session.	When lumped together, responsibilities often appear overwhelming. In this case, use the *divide and conquer* strategy. Buy a large calendar and schedule the activities of the semester by writing on the calendar when you will perform them. Do not forget to include nonacademic activities as well as those related to school. You will soon realize you have plenty of time. You simply need to be organized. That realization will go a long way in relieving unnecessary stress.
Exercise just isn't fun anymore, and you no longer look forward to your workout sessions. Even if you do get into the workout, you are not motivated to put forth much effort.	You may be experiencing some of the emotional and physical effects of overtraining or exercising too often. To renew your interest, try one or more of the following: • Change aerobic activities every other day as a cross-training technique. If you are jogging daily, substitute cycling or lap swimming two or three times weekly. • Change the time you exercise. Try early mornings, noon, or just before bedtime to see if your mood improves. • Vary the level of difficulty (intensity) of your workouts. Work out hard and easy on alternate days. • Exercise with friends and make it a social occasion as well as a workout.

Roadblock	Strategy
1. _____ _____ _____ _____	1. _____ _____ _____ _____
2. _____ _____ _____ _____ _____	2. _____ _____ _____ _____ _____

Now you need to actually implement that strategy so you are more likely to engage in regular exercise and, as a result, better manage the stress you experience.

LAB ASSESSMENT 13.2

Can You Differentiate Between Exercise Myths and Facts?

Directions: For each of the statements below, place an F in the space provided if you think the statement is a FACT, and an M if you think the statement is a MYTH.

_____ 1. The most important component of overall health is physical health.

_____ 2. Being physically fit makes you healthier, but you probably won't feel any different about yourself.

_____ 3. The more you exercise, the more benefits you will achieve.

_____ 4. "No pain, no gain" means that you must train until it hurts to reap the benefits.

_____ 5. You are more likely to stick with an exercise program if you maintain the same exercise program each workout.

_____ 6. Stretching activities are excellent warm-ups for an exercise program.

_____ 7. Weight training decreases flexibility.

_____ 8. Exercise is stressful because of the toll it takes physically.

All of the statements above are myths. An explanation follows:

1. Health consists of more than just physical health. It includes social, emotional, mental, and spiritual health as well. Who is to say which component of health is more important than another for any individual?

2. If you become physically fit, you will feel better about yourself and your self-esteem will improve. You will develop more confidence, feel less depressed, and experience a sense of more control in your life. The benefits of exercise go well beyond the healthy changes that occur within your body.

3. Too little exercise and the benefits are limited. On the other hand, too much exercise can place you at risk of overuse injuries. Sprains, strains, and fatigue can result when exercising too intensely or too frequently. Instead, there is an optimal level of exercise that will provide the benefits sought while minimizing the risk of injury or illness.

4. Exercise should be difficult, but it should not hurt. If you experience anything other than discomfort, you are exercising too intensely or too often. Cut back before you become injured.

5. Many people find their motivation tends to decrease when engaging in the same exercise routine for weeks or months. Cross-training is a way to put the pizzazz back in your workout. Switching activities once or twice a week may provide the variety you need to stay motivated over the long haul.

6. You should never stretch cold muscles. That can subject you to risk of injury or muscle soreness. Instead, begin an exercise session with a routine that involves large muscle groups, such as walking or jogging, for at least five minutes or until perspiring. After that, you can stretch to complete the warm-up.

7. When you perform weight training exercises correctly through the full range of motion, flexibility actually improves.

8. Exercise is an excellent way of managing stress. It uses up the body's stress by-products—muscle tension, increased heart rate and blood pressure, serum cholesterol—that have prepared the body to do something physical, fight-or-flight.

Strategies for Decreasing Stressful Behaviors

Why can't I get to the gym regularly? Why did I drink too much at the party last Saturday night? Why can't I learn to relax? How many times do we say we wish we had or had not done something? Some of the activities or actions that we *take* or *fail to take* are stressful to us. For example, we say to ourselves we are going to go out and meet new people, but somehow we never get around to doing it; we are going to change our diet but do not stick to the new diet. We worry about our inability to change our behavior. We feel less in control of ourselves. Consequently, our self-esteem may decline. In sum, we may experience a fight-or-flight response when we cannot behave as we would like to. The focus of this chapter is to present a number of behaviors that are stressful to you, either because you want to give them up and cannot or because you want to adopt them but have been unable to. It also describes methods that will help you make changes in these behaviors. With greater control of your behaviors, you will be better at managing stress.

Health and Lifestyle Behaviors

In this chapter, two types of behaviors are discussed: health behaviors and lifestyle behaviors. Health behaviors are considered a subclass of lifestyle behaviors and are differentiated for emphasis. **Health behaviors** are defined as activities undertaken by people who believe themselves to be healthy for the purpose of preventing disease or detecting it in an asymptomatic stage.[1] Examples of health behaviors are limiting sugar and salt in your diet, avoiding smoking cigarettes, using a seat belt, engaging in physical exercise, limiting your use of alcoholic beverages, and practicing relaxation techniques. **Lifestyle behaviors** encompass the whole host of activities in which people engage. Examples of lifestyle behaviors include everyday activities such as doing chores, going to school or work, and enjoying leisure times. Examples of other, less common lifestyle behaviors are asking someone for assistance, writing a letter to a friend, listening intently to a speaker, and meeting new people.

health behaviors
Activities that are taken by people who believe themselves to be healthy and that are designed to maintain health, a subclass of lifestyle behaviors.

lifestyle behaviors
All of the activities in which people engage.

Health-Behavior Assessment

Before you can go about changing your health-related behaviors, you need to first identify which behaviors need changing. Lab Assessment 14.1, at the end of this chapter, will help you assess how well you are doing at staying healthy and identify areas that need improvement. Lab 14.1 is adapted from the *National College Health Assessment* and the Office of Disease Prevention and Health Promotion of the Public Health Service, U.S. Department of Health and Human Services.

Selected Lifestyle Behaviors

Lab Assessment 14.2 presents a list of lifestyle activities that some people find stressful. The purpose of Lab 14.2 is to help you identify lifestyle behaviors that you would like to adopt. Feel free to choose other lifestyle activities that are not on this selected list that you would like to adopt. It is important to identify these behaviors, because your inability to engage in these activities worries you and causes you distress.

Later in this chapter, we present techniques that you can use to change your behavior, thereby better managing stress in your life. However, before we look at strategies to change lifestyle and health behaviors, there are a few more sets of factors that need to be considered. The first is barriers to action.

Barriers to Action

Good intentions are abundant. Yes, I plan to contact you. Yes, I plan to stop smoking, lose weight, save money, or get involved. But somehow I never have the time. It is too hot to jog today. I will start running tomorrow. I am embarrassed to speak in front of a group of people. I will do it another time. I really want to develop hobbies, but I have so many other obligations. Excuses, excuses.

It would be more fruitful to consider these "excuses" **barriers**—that is, barriers that we perceive as preventing us from engaging in a number of activities. To the person whose spouse brings home a high-calorie dessert, the lack of family support is a barrier to maintaining weight. A series of rainy days is a barrier to the novice jogger. A heavy work or school schedule is a barrier to getting involved in worthwhile causes. The lack of availability of low-salt foods is a barrier to reducing one's intake of salt. In other words, to help you understand ways to change health and lifestyle behaviors, it is useful to identify the barriers in the way of adopting the behaviors you want to adopt. Lab Assessment 14.3 lists a number of possible factors—barriers—that may have kept you from engaging in these activities.

barriers
Reasons given or situations that interfere with someone engaging in behaviors that he or she wishes to engage in.

Locus of Control

Another aspect of health and lifestyle behavior change concerns the issue of personal control. (Refer to our discussion of locus of control in Chapter 8.) Although **locus of control** can be a generalized perception of the control you have over events that affect your life, it can also be specific to parts of your life. For example, you may believe you can control your social life and events that affect it—for example, going out and meeting people—but you may believe that your health is a matter of chance or luck: "It's whom you're born to, not what you do." The locus of control for health is the focus of this section.

locus of control
The perception of the amount of control one has over events that affect one's life.

Some people feel that it's their physician's responsibility to keep them well: "That's what I'm paying her for." However, a growing number of people feel that they actually do have control over their health and other life outcomes: "Yes, I can prevent illness from stress." "Yes, I can maintain a desired weight."

You should now have completed several Lab Assessments. These assessments should assist you in determining the following:

1. What health behaviors you need to change to reduce your risk of illness and injury.

2. Which lifestyle changes you are *distressed* about and would like to change.

3. What barriers are preventing you from carrying out these changes in health and lifestyle activities.

4. Your perceptions of control over your health.

Now we are ready to examine ways of making changes in your health and lifestyle behaviors.

Methods for Decreasing Stressful Behaviors

One day, after having to loosen my belt still another notch, I decided I'd had enough. I was going to lose weight, and I was going to start immediately. I knew it would be difficult but it would be less expensive than having to buy a whole new wardrobe. So I developed a plan that included writing a contract to change my eating behavior. In that contract, it stated I would refrain from eating while doing something else, like watching television. The plan also included my wife, whose job it was to encourage me along the way and to sign the contract as a witness.

I also used a smaller plate. The smaller portions filled up the plate, and I did not feel that I was depriving myself. In addition, I increased the portions of the lower-calorie foods, such as salads and vegetables, and decreased the portions of the higher-calorie foods, such as meats and certain starches. If I snacked during the day, it was a piece of low-calorie fruit. If I was able to successfully follow the rules that I set down in my contract, I would reward myself by purchasing a CD at the end of the week.

The preceding account describes a diet plan that includes a number of psychological and behavioral techniques that can be used to change and modify health and lifestyle behaviors. In this section, we will examine some frequently used methods of decreasing stressful behaviors:

1. Self-monitoring
2. Tailoring
3. Material reinforcement
4. Social reinforcement
5. Social support
6. Self-contracting
7. Contracting with a significant other
8. Shaping
9. Reminders
10. Self-help groups
11. Professional help

Some of these techniques overlap and have procedures in common. However, they are listed separately in order to give emphasis to different aspects of the techniques.

Self-Monitoring

One aspect common to many of these methods involves the monitoring of behavior. **Self-monitoring** is a process of observing and recording your own behavior.[2] Suppose you are a person who tends to be late to meetings and appointments. You have good intentions, but somehow you are not able to make it on time. You may not realize how often you are late or how late you are to appointments and meetings. Self-monitoring is a method to increase your awareness of your behavior. Every time you have an appointment or a meeting, note whether you arrived on time. If you are late, note how many minutes (or hours?!) you were late. This will help you avoid being late by making you aware of just how much of a problem this behavior is. In addition, self-monitoring will provide a benchmark to compare your behavior at the start of your behavioral change program with the change you have actually made. In this manner, your progress becomes, in itself, reinforcing.

self-monitoring
The process of observing and recording behavior.

Tailoring

Programs that are adapted to the specific routines, lifestyles, abilities, and unique circumstances of an individual are said to be tailored to that individual.[3,4] Let's say you find yourself under a lot of pressure and are having difficulty relaxing. You decide that you will begin a relaxation program. Someone suggests that you awake a half hour earlier and do your relaxation exercises in the morning. You awake the following Monday a half hour earlier and do your relaxation exercises. You feel tired Monday evening but continue on Tuesday, Wednesday, and Thursday

tailoring

Making a behavior change program specific to the life of the individual.

mornings. You feel tired on these evenings as well and oversleep on Friday morning. The following week you oversleep on Thursday and Friday mornings and feel discouraged. What you need is **tailoring.**

Since you are not a "morning person," it would make sense to do your relaxation exercises after school or work. The program should be adapted to your particular schedule. It should be tailored to your unique characteristics and circumstances. Programs that are tailored to the specific characteristics of a person tend to be more effective. For example, if Sunday evening is a quiet time in your weekly schedule, then that would be a good time to call those people whom you have been meaning to call.

Before you initiate a behavior change program, examine your schedule and lifestyle. When is the best time to do your chores? What time must you leave in order to be on time for your appointments and meetings? When should you exercise? When is the best time to engage in relaxation?

If you consistently brush your teeth twice a day (e.g., early morning and late at night), relaxation techniques could be practiced at that time. In other words, relaxation techniques would be *paired* with teeth-brushing behavior. If you do not consistently brush your teeth twice a day, then relaxation techniques could be embedded into another part of your schedule (e.g., after work or before dinner). Tailoring offers you a way to maximize your success in a behavior change program by allowing you to fit the change into your particular circumstances.

Material Reinforcement

material reinforcement

Rewarding a behavior with a tangible object.

An important component in programs to increase healthy behavior is reinforcement, or reward. If you remember, I stayed with my diet all week and therefore rewarded myself with a CD. The CD is, of course, **material reinforcement.** You could reward yourself (self-reward) or you could be rewarded by another. If I refrain from smoking for a week, I could buy myself a book or magazine. Or I could be in a smoking-cessation program in which I receive five dollars a week for not smoking. Other examples of material reinforcement include bonuses, commissions, clothes, tickets for a show or concert, antiques, or any other items of value. Both material and social reinforcement increase the probability of the behavior being repeated. A point to note: What is reinforcing for Jack may not be reinforcing for Jill. If a person does not like to attend folk concerts, then tickets to a folk concert are *not* a reinforcer. A reinforcer is something of value to a particular individual. Money is a powerful and useful reinforcer, because it can be exchanged for a countless number of objects that are rewarding and valued.

Social Reinforcement

social reinforcement

Rewarding a behavior with social approval by someone else.

Reinforcement may also take the form of social reinforcement. Another person (a friend, roommate, spouse, or coworker) can be a source of encouragement and can assist you in overcoming various hurdles. Also, this person can be a source of social reinforcement. The significant other can tell you that you are doing a good job and give you praise. Acknowledgment, praise, a pat on the back, and even a smile are forms of **social reinforcement.** Research supports the observation that social reinforcement increases the frequency of the behavior that it follows.[5]

Imagine you are trying to stop smoking. You go a full day without smoking and your roommate says, "That's great." That statement from your roommate is an example of social reinforcement. Or suppose you are at work and you take on a new assignment. The assignment turns out well, and your boss pats you on the back. You feel good about the completed assignment and take on another new assignment. In our interactions with other people, we sometimes tell others they are doing a good job. These forms of social reinforcement are useful methods of encouraging people to continue what they are doing.

However, a word of caution should be added. What you are doing is for yourself. Therefore, do not expect a pat on the back every time you do a good job or a good deed. Your own sense of satisfaction may be all you need to continue the behavior. If you engage in regular practice of a relaxation technique, for instance, the sensation obtained and the knowledge that you are doing something that is healthy may be enough to encourage you to continue this behavior.

Social Support

A concept related to social reinforcement is social support. Social support, as noted earlier in this book, can reduce stress directly. It also can reduce stress indirectly. If you are having a difficult time trying to stay on a diet, emotional support from a trusted friend can relieve some of your stress by providing expressions of empathy, love, trust, and caring[6] to improve your coping ability and reduce stress. Informational support, another type of social support, can also help. For example, advice, suggestions, and information on how to stay on a diet can improve coping ability and relieve stress.

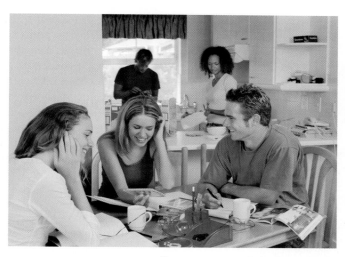

There are many ways to develop a network of social support on a college campus. You can join a campus group or organize study time with your classmates.

Self-Contracting

Once you have established a base rate for a particular behavior (e.g., I am late two out of three times), then you can create a set of rules for changing that behavior and set up a contract.[7,8] A contract takes the form of an "if-then" rule. For example, *if* I am on time to a meeting, *then* I will watch TV tonight. "Being on time to a meeting" is the behavior of interest, and "watching TV tonight" is the reward or consequence of the behavior. In addition, if I am *not* on time to a meeting today, then I will *not* watch TV tonight. I did not exhibit the desired behavior; therefore, I do not reap the reward. **Self-contracting** means that you administer your own rewards. As part of this procedure, then, you must list things that you would consider rewarding. Obviously, different things are rewarding for different people.

self-contracting
Making a contract with oneself to change a behavior.

Contracting with a Significant Other

Contracting with another person may be even more successful than self-contracting. Contracting with significant others makes the contract a *public* commitment. A **significant other** may be a spouse, a partner, a roommate, a friend, or a relative. The significant other does not necessarily have to live under the same roof. A significant other is a person who has meaning to you, in whom you can confide, and to whom you can be made accountable.

For example, you decide that you want to initiate an exercise program. You plan to jog vigorously for 20 minutes at a time, three times a week: Monday, Wednesday, and Friday. If you successfully carry out this exercise program, you will buy yourself a DVD on Saturday. You write up a contract specifying what activity (jogging for 20 minutes), how frequently (three times a week: Monday, Wednesday, and Friday), and what reward (a DVD) you will receive if you successfully complete the activity. Because you are contracting with a significant other, you show your spouse or close friend your contract. You discuss the contract with your significant other, actually sign the contract in his or her presence (making a public behavioral commitment), and may have the significant other sign the contract (a witness) as well. In general, contracting has been found to be a useful technique in a variety of health and lifestyle situations.[9] A sample contract appears in Chapter 5.

significant other
Another person who is important to an individual.

cold turkey
Stopping a behavior all at once.

Shaping

It is difficult to go **cold turkey**—stopping the undesired behavior all at once. Therefore, programs have been established to "shape" desired behaviors. **Shaping**

shaping
Changing a behavior a little bit at a time.

is the process of introducing components of a program sequentially as the individual learns and performs prior steps in the sequence. A series of short-term goals are selected that get closer and closer to the ultimate goal.[10] The steps are graded in order of difficulty. For example, if you want to reduce your caloric intake by 1,000 calories a day, you may begin by reducing your dinner by 250 calories. Once you have successfully completed this part of the program, you may then reduce your lunch by 250 calories a day. If you want to start an exercise program, you can begin by exercising once a week for 20 minutes. Once you are able to carry out this task, you could increase your program to twice a week for 30 minutes, then three times a week for 30 minutes. Shaping has been widely used in a variety of behavioral programs.

Reminders

reminder system
A means of reminding oneself to perform a particular behavior.

If you intended to save money this pay period but forgot, why not place a note on each payday on your kitchen calendar? Set up a **reminder system.** Then place a check mark on the calendar *after* you put money into your savings each pay period. A calendar that you look at each day is an ideal place to put reminder messages: Write Joe on Friday; exercise on Monday at 4:30 p.m.; call Mom on Saturday. The bathroom mirror or your refrigerator are other good places for reminders. In some cases, you could ask a significant other to remind you (as long as it does not lead to arguments or antagonisms).

Self-Help Groups

Many people with alcohol problems have found successful solutions to their problems with self-help groups such as Alcoholics Anonymous. Other self-help groups include Gamblers Anonymous, Weight Watchers, Overeaters Anonymous, self-help drug programs, self-help psychiatric groups, self-help divorce groups, and self-help groups for battered and abused spouses and children. The self-help movement has generated numerous groups to assist people with common problems. You may be able to locate a self-help group where you live that deals with your particular concern.

Professional Help

If a self-help group is not available, then professional help is an alternative. Physicians, nurses, psychiatrists, psychologists, therapists, social workers, counselors,

Getting Involved In Your Community

Do you know people who have trouble controlling their alcohol drinking behavior? Or who want to improve their grades but never seem to study enough? Or who intend to set aside time to exercise or practice a relaxation technique but never get around to it? Or who want to lose weight but continue to eat foods high in calories? Perhaps the person you know with these problems is a roommate, a friend, or a relative. The inability to control these behaviors can be extremely stressful for many people.

You can help your roommate, friend, or relative by teaching them the effective behavior management techniques you learned in this chapter, and by serving as a witness to a contract they sign regarding a change in behavior. In other words, you can help people important to you—those in your "immediate community"—to be less stressed by helping them to be more in control of their lives—in this case, their behaviors.

Techniques for Controlling Stressful Behaviors

There are many ways to manage behaviors so desired behaviors are adopted and undesirable ones are refrained from performing. Following are some of the techniques to control behavior that have been shown to be effective.

Self-Monitoring
Observing and recording behavior to determine which behavior needs changing and the influences on that behavior.

Tailoring
Adapting behaviors to routines, lifestyles, abilities, and circumstances to make it more likely that that behavior can fit a person's situation.

Material Reinforcement
Providing a tangible reward when a desired behavior is performed.

Social Reinforcement
Having another person provide a reward, such as encouragement or praise, when a desired behavior is performed.

Social Support
Having another person provide support to encourage adoption of a desired behavior. Social support can be emotional, informational, or financial.

Self-Contracting
Writing a contract that specifies the desired behavior and rewards that will be provided to oneself when that behavior is performed.

Contracting with Significant Other
Writing a contract that specifies the desired behavior and rewards that will be provided by a close relative or friend when that behavior is performed.

Shaping
Introducing components of a desired behavior sequentially and providing a reward when each component is performed successfully.

Reminders
Leaving reminders, such as notes on refrigerators or calendars, to perform the desired behavior.

Self-Help Groups
Joining a group with similar interest in performing a behavior, which will encourage the adoption of a desired behavior.

and health educators are available in almost every community and can assist you in health and lifestyle behavior changes.

Application of Behavior Change Techniques

To better understand the variety of techniques used to modify the stressful behaviors described in this chapter and to integrate the material presented, an illustrative example follows.

Example: Exercise

Exercise can be considered a health behavior and a lifestyle behavior. We have included it among the health behaviors because of its importance to health in such areas as cardiovascular health and weight control.

Let's say that you completed the health-behavior questionnaire (Lab 14.1), and exercise/fitness was one of the behaviors you were distressed about not engaging in regularly. You decide to change that behavior. You turn to the barriers-to-action questionnaire (Lab 14.3). The greatest barriers to exercise are time, inconvenience, and fatigue. Now you are ready to turn to the "Methods" section to decrease stressful behaviors. The first thing that you need to know is how often you exercise. If you do not exercise at all, then you already know the answer. If you exercise occasionally, then you need to *self-monitor* your exercise behavior. Observe and record the duration, frequency, and intensity of your exercise.

The next step is to write a *contract*. For example, you can state, "I will vigorously jog 20 minutes from 6:00–6:20 p.m. on Monday, Wednesday, and Friday." The contract can be either a *self-contract* or a *contract with a significant other*. Contracts with significant others are more effective because they make you accountable to another person. Therefore, let's assume that you show the contract to your spouse, partner, roommate, or close friend and he or she witnesses and signs it.

To overcome the three barriers of time, inconvenience, and fatigue, you need to *tailor* your exercise schedule to your unique circumstances. Three 20-minute periods a week is only one hour a week. Given your time constraints, can you spare one hour a week? After or before work, you can set aside time to engage in your thrice-weekly exercise activity.

To increase the probability that you will succeed in your exercise program, *social* or *material reinforcement* should follow your exercise. Your spouse, partner, roommate, or close friend could tell you how well you are doing, and at the end of the week, you could treat yourself to a CD, book, movie, or other reward.

If you have difficulty initiating and maintaining a thrice-weekly exercise schedule, then *shaping* might help. Start with one day a week. Once that has been successfully maintained, increase your exercise to twice a week. After that has been established, initiate a thrice-weekly program.

To maintain the program over time, use *reminders*. A note on your calendar, by your bed, on your dresser, or even taped to the bathroom mirror could be used to remind you that today is exercise day. You could also use another person to remind you that today is exercise day. If all else fails, you might ask *self-help* and *professional help groups* for assistance.

This example includes all the methods of decreasing stressful behaviors: self-monitoring, self-contracting, contracting with a significant other, tailoring, social reinforcement, material reinforcement, shaping, reminders, self-help groups, and professional groups.

Behavior Change Theories and Stress

Theories can help *explain* behavior or help in *changing* behavior. These two purposes of theory are interrelated: If we can explain why a behavior is adopted or not adopted, we can intervene and control or change that behavior. There are many theories you can employ to take charge of your stress-related behavior. A good source to consult if you want to learn about these theories of health behavior is *Health Behavior and Health Education,* edited by Karen Glanz and her colleagues (see note 1 at the end of this chapter). Several theories are presented here as examples of how behavior change theories can be helpful in coping with stress.

Stages of Change Theory

James Prochaska and his colleagues theorize that people are at different points in motivation, or readiness, to change a behavior.[11] For example, some of your classmates probably exercise regularly. Others may know the reasons they should exercise but have never gotten around to doing it. Still others of your classmates have actually made a plan to incorporate exercise into their routine but have never implemented that plan or, at least, not for long. Stages of Change theory recognizes that people are at different stages in terms of their readiness to change their health behavior.

- *Precontemplation.* One is unaware of the problem or the need to change. Consequently, no action to change is even contemplated. For example, if you don't know the benefits of relaxation techniques, you are not likely to be thinking about engaging in them.
- *Contemplation.* One is thinking about changing a behavior but has not taken any action to do so. For example, you know that exercise is a good way to manage stress and are thinking about starting an exercise program, but not soon.
- *Decision/determination.* One actually starts planning to change the behavior. For example, you start researching stress management programs offered in your area and write to obtain their fees and schedules.
- *Action.* One implements a stress management program. For example, you start jogging every other day, and meditate daily.
- *Maintenance.* One continues the changed behavior over time. For example, you exercise at a health club throughout the year, and you continue to engage in a relaxation technique each day.

Stages of Change theory has been applied with various populations and related to numerous health issues. For example, it has been used with cigarette smoking in adolescents in Bulgaria[12] and Korea,[13] adults in Germany[14] and Appalachia,[15] and hospitalized African Americans.[16] The theory has also been used to train health promoters working with Mexican American diabetes patients.[17] The result was a significant reduction in unhealthy blood factors related to diabetes and lower low-density lipoprotein cholesterol and blood pressure. In working with other diabetes patients, researchers used Stages of Change theory to increase physical activity levels, reduce weight gain, and achieve other beneficial changes in risk factors for diabetes and cardiovascular disease.[18] Still other researchers applied the theory to sleep apnea (pauses in breathing while sleeping)[19] posttraumatic stress disorder,[20] and use of contraceptives.[21]

Recognizing the stage of change at which you are located will help you strategize to take charge of your stress-related behavior. If you are at the precontemplation level, you might need to begin by reading about the benefits of managing stress to motivate you to move toward engaging in stress management activities regularly. If you are at the contemplation stage, you might realize that you value stress management techniques and know that you need to start planning to engage in those activities. Perhaps the first step is to speak with someone who is knowledgeable about stress management, such as your instructor. If you are ready for the action stage, you will need to make concrete plans to exercise regularly, engage in a relaxation technique daily, change your perception of events (see the discussion on developing an attitude of gratitude in Chapter 8), and try other stress management techniques. Write down the steps you will take and the dates by which you will take them. Again, your instructor might be a good resource to help you develop your plan. If you are at the action stage, keep a journal to monitor changes in your pulse rate, days in which you experience perceived stress, days in which you exercise and engage in a relaxation technique, and other stress-related variables. In that way, you will be reinforcing the continuation of your healthy coping behavior. Lastly, if you have been coping with stress effectively and are at the maintenance stage of change, you could schedule your exercise and relaxation times—for example, in your date book—or place reminders to engage in these and other stress-related activities on your refrigerator.

An Example of Stages of Change Theory in Use

Cindy has no idea she should be practicing a method of relaxation to manage stress. She never heard of such a thing. She is at the *precontemplation* stage. Her friend Tonya, though, took a stress management course last semester and learned how to manage stress. Concerned about her friend, she shares with Cindy what she learned. Now knowing the reasons she should incorporate a relaxation technique into her daily routine, Cindy finds herself in *contemplation*. She is thinking about meditating. Knowing Stages of Change theory, she seeks encouragement from her family. She also asks Tonya to help her devise a plan to meditate daily, and they do that. Cindy is now at the *decision/determination* stage. At this stage, she decides to meditate at 10 a.m. when her roommate is in class and the room is quiet. Her goal is to meditate at least three days the first week and, afterward, five days a week. She implements her plan (*action* stage) and after a week evaluates how she is doing. Cindy realizes that meditating at 10 a.m. does not work since there is a lot of noise from other residents in her dorm. She changes that to 2 p.m. She also learns she needs more encouragement and social support, so she suggests Tonya and she keep a journal describing their experiences while meditating to share with each other. Soon Cindy is meditating daily, but her schedule is changing and she sometimes forgets to make the time to engage in this relaxation technique. Employing Stages of Change theory, however, she writes herself reminders to meditate and leaves them on her bathroom mirror. This helps her avoid relapsing into not meditating. She is now in the *maintenance* stage.

Health Belief Model

Health Belief model

A way of conceptualizing how people make decisions regarding their health behavior. Constructs include perceptions of *susceptibility* to and *severity* of illness or disease, *benefits* of the behavior and *barriers* to performing it, *cues* to encourage, and *confidence* in being able to perform the behavior.

Another way of conceptualizing health behavior decisions is the **Health Belief model.** You have a final examination and you are trying to decide whether to study for it or, instead, party with your friends. If you do not study for the exam, you will likely fail the course. If that meant you would flunk out of school, you probably would study to avoid that serious consequence. However, if you are a graduating senior, you have a 3.98 grade point average, and this course is not needed to graduate, you still might not study, even though you recognize the likely outcome is that you will fail the course. In this case, the consequence is not considered serious enough to encourage studying.

This example presents two of the constructs of the Health Belief model, *perceived susceptibility* and *perceived severity*. Other constructs include *perceived benefits* of the behavior with *perception of barriers* to engaging in the behavior, *cues* to encourage the behavior, and *confidence* in your ability to perform the behavior successfully (see Table 14.1).

Table 14.1
Health Belief Model Constructs

Perceived Susceptibility:	One's opinion of the likelihood of getting the condition, illness, or disease if the recommended health behavior is not adopted
Perceived Severity:	One's opinion of the seriousness or severity of the condition, illness, or disease likely to be acquired if the recommended health behavior is not adopted
Perceived Benefits:	One's opinion of how effective the recommended health behavior is in reducing the risk or seriousness of the condition, illness, or disease
Perceived Barriers:	One's opinion of the *costs* associated with taking the recommended action (for example, financial, time, energy, or psychological costs)
Cues to Action:	Strategies to activate and encourage recommended health behaviors
Self-Efficacy:	Confidence in one's ability to perform the recommended health behaviors effectively

Source: National Cancer Institute, *Theory at a Glance: A Guide for Health Promotion Practice,* NIH publication no. 97-3896 (Washington, D.C.: Department of Health and Human Services, 1997).

Example of Health Belief Model in Use

Ginny loves to ride her bike. She rides to school, to the market, and for exercise at least three days a week. Although her friend Sasha encourages her to wear a helmet when biking, Ginny hates the feeling of tightness around her chin and thinks she looks *uncool* biking with a helmet. Should she wear a helmet or not? Ginny decides to make this decision systematically using the Health Belief model that she learned about in her health course.

Ginny decides to find out how *susceptible* she is to a *serious* condition if she bikes without a helmet. She researches the number of bicycle accidents and finds them to occur frequently. Furthermore, she learns that head trauma that can result in paralysis or even death is one of those accidents (*perceived severity*). Reading on, Ginny learns that bicycle helmets are effective in preventing head trauma (*perceived benefit*) and that the costs (*perceived barriers*) are minimal compared to the benefits of wearing a helmet—they are free from the County Health Department and the tight chin strap is a small price to pay for her safety. So Ginny decides to wear a helmet when biking. To remind herself to do so (*cues to action*) she places a Post-it on her handlebars stating "WEAR MY HELMET." She feels confident she can wear her helmet (*self-efficacy*) because she observes other bikers wearing theirs. In addition, when she received a helmet from the County Health Department, she received instructions on how to wear the helmet correctly so as to protect her head in case of an accident.

Self-Efficacy Theory

Self-efficacy is the amount of confidence an individual has about performing a particular task or activity. The greater your confidence that you can carry out an activity, including overcoming any barriers, the greater is the likelihood that you will actually perform that activity. According to Albert Bandura,[22] the more confident an individual is in his or her ability to stop smoking, the greater is the probability that that person will actually quit. Self-efficacy is important because it influences how much effort you will put into performing a task and the level of your performance. According to self-efficacy theory, people's beliefs about their capabilities are a better predictor of their accomplishments than are their actual knowledge, skills, or past accomplishments.

Because self-efficacy is so important, the question arises as to how one can increase one's confidence or self-efficacy in performing healthy behaviors. Bandura describes four ways to increase self-efficacy:

1. *Performance attainment.* Nothing succeeds like success. The most effective method of improving self-efficacy is successfully carrying out an activity. If you were able to exercise, even for a short time yesterday, then you will have more confidence that you can exercise today. If you do well on your first exam, then you will have greater confidence (self-efficacy) that you will do well on your next one. Recall from our description of shaping that breaking a complex behavior into small steps makes change possible.

2. *Vicarious experience.* All of us are influenced by observing other people. If we see someone similar to ourselves overcome an alcohol problem, we are more likely to believe (i.e., have greater confidence) that we too can overcome a similar problem. Being exposed to successful models who are similar to us and accomplish goals or overcome obstacles similar to ours is a very powerful tool for increasing self-efficacy.

3. *Verbal persuasion.* This approach is commonly used to encourage individuals to make changes in their health practices. People are assured that they have the ability to make changes in their own lives. "You can do it!" Though limited in its ability to produce long-lasting changes, verbal persuasion can bolster a person's confidence.

4. *Physiological state.* We receive information from our physiological state when determining our level of stress. If you feel very anxious (e.g., you have sweaty

palms) about a situation, you are not likely to feel confident about doing well in that situation. If you are perspiring heavily and shaking before an audition, you are not likely to feel confident about doing well at the audition. By learning to relax, you can reduce stress and increase your self-efficacy.

Goal-Setting Theory

Goal-Setting Theory

A conceptualization of how one successfully achieves goals. Among considerations are the difficulty of the goal, proximal and distal goals, and self-efficacy.

Self-efficacy is also an important construct in **Goal-Setting theory.** Goal-Setting theory identifies several variables that are associated with successfully achieving goals. These include[23]

- The highest level of effort occurs when the goal is moderately difficult, rather than when it is very easy or very hard. If it is too hard, you might become discouraged and lose confidence in your ability to meet the goal. If it is too easy, you might lose interest in pursuing the goal.

- Proximal and distal goals should be established. Proximal goals are steps to be achieved along the way to the long-range, or distal, goal. If you identify smaller goals to be achieved, you will be likely to achieve them, thereby reinforcing your efforts toward reaching the long-range goal.

- People with high self-efficacy set higher goals than people with lower self-efficacy. They are also more committed to achieving the goal, use more effective strategies, and respond to negative feedback better than do those with lower self-efficacy.

- The belief that one can attain the goal (self-efficacy), and the importance ascribed to attaining that goal, are related to successfully achieving the goal. Consequently, enhancing self-efficacy is one of the keys in Goal-Setting theory.[24]

- Core properties of effective goal setting include how specific and how difficult the goal is, the anticipated effects of achieving the goal, and feedback along the way.

How can you set and achieve goals that are important to you? How can you become more confident that you can attain these goals—self-efficacious? What strategies have you learned in this chapter, and elsewhere in this book, that can help you do this?

Theories of behavior change can help you take charge of your stress-related behaviors. Now it is up to you to do so. The information in this chapter can help you be less distressed over behaviors you wish to change but have not been able to eliminate. Try these methods. Modify them to fit your circumstances, and continue your search for better health and a satisfying lifestyle.

Coping in Today's World

Weight Watchers is one of the most successful weight loss programs. One of the primary reasons that people who join Weight Watchers are able to manage their weight is that the program is based on the tenets and principles of Goal-Setting theory. Among these are

- *Proximal* and *distal* goals are set. Proximal goals include the number of pounds to be lost in one week and one month. Distal goals specify the total weight loss desired over time.

- *Self-monitoring* is encouraged. This occurs through keeping a record of one's weight over a period of time and noticing changes. Foods eaten are also listed daily since they must

follow a regimen outlined in written materials distributed to those who sign up for the program.

- *Social support* is employed through attendance at meetings with others also trying to manage their weight. Strategies are suggested to help attendees meet their weight goals, and encouragement is offered.

- *Self-efficacy* is enhanced when others who have met their weight goals serve as role models, and when program participants, through self-monitoring strategies, record their weight loss, thereby reinforcing the belief that their weight goal can be met.

summary

- By decreasing stressful behaviors and increasing healthy behaviors, you can better manage the stress in your life.

- To decrease stressful behaviors, it is useful to identify the barriers that prevent changing these behaviors. Once the barriers are identified, strategies can be developed to eliminate or reduce them.

- Perceptions of control over your health influence whether you engage in healthy behaviors. If you perceive you have control over your health, you are more apt to engage in healthy behaviors than if you believe your health is a function of luck, chance, fate, or powerful others.

- Self-monitoring is observing and recording your behavior. Self-monitoring health and lifestyle behaviors can increase your awareness of your behavior, which is the first step in decreasing stressful behaviors.

- Tailoring a health-behavior program offers a way to maximize your success by allowing you to fit the program into your particular circumstances.

- The use of material and social reinforcement, or rewards, increases the likelihood that healthy behaviors will be repeated.

- Self-contracting and contracting with a significant other formalizes a commitment to engage in a particular behavior. Contracts have proved to be an effective means of decreasing stressful behaviors.

- Shaping a behavior is the gradual introduction of various components of a program. This technique is particularly helpful when a person has difficulty carrying out a total program—for example, a weight control or exercise program. A reminder system can also be helpful.

- Self-help groups have been formed to offer emotional support and information to individuals with similar health and lifestyle problems. Professional help has also been found valuable in assisting people to decrease their stressful behavior.

- There are several behavior change theories that can be used to explain and change health behavior. Among these are stages of change theory, self-efficacy theory, and the Health Belief model.

- The Stages of Change theory postulates people are at different points in motivation to change. These points—stages of readiness to change—are precontemplation, contemplation, decision/determination, action, and maintenance.

- Self-efficacy theory states that the more confident people are that they can perform a behavior, termed their *self-efficacy,* the more likely they are to perform that behavior.

- The Health Belief model states that health behavior is a function of one's perception of (1) the susceptibility of developing a severe condition, (2) whether there are behaviors that are effective in preventing that condition from developing, (3) whether barriers to engaging in these behaviors can be overcome, (4) whether there are cues to spur one to engage in those behaviors, and (5) if one feels confident in the ability to effectively perform the recommended behaviors.

- Goal-Setting theory explains how goals can be attained by recognizing variables affecting goal achievement. These variables include the amount of effort required to achieve the goal, the establishment of proximal (short-range) and distal (long-term) goals, self-efficacy, and the perceived importance of achieving the goal.

internet resources

Top Five Stress Triggers **http://healthnews.ediets.com/ health-topics/stress-emotions/top-5-stress-triggers.html** *Discusses stress triggers of finances, health, family, weather, and loneliness and how they lead to a stress reaction. Strategies for responding to these stress triggers are offered.*

Stresscure.org **www.stresscure.org** *Presents information regarding stress, stress relief, stress symptoms, stress*

anxiety, stress causes, stress effects, relaxation, and stress tests.

Stress Cure **www.stresscure.com** *Contains a Health Resource Network for general stress information as well as strategies for coping with stress.*

references

1. Karen Glanz, Barbara K. Rimer, and Frances Marcus Lewis, eds., *Health Behavior and Health Education: Theory, Research, and Practice* (San Francisco: Jossey-Bass, 2008).

2. Jodi S. Holtrop and Amy Slonim, "Sticking to It: A Multifactor Cancer Risk-Reduction Program for Low-Income Clients," *Journal of Health Education* 31(2000): 122–27.

3. Jerrold S. Greenberg, George B. Dintiman, and Barbee Myers Oakes, *Physical Fitness and Wellness,* 3rd ed. (Champaign, IL: Human Kinetics, 2004).

4. S. M. Noar, C. N. Benac, and M. S. Harris, "Does Tailoring Matter? Meta-Analytic Review of Tailored Print Health Behavior Change Interventions," *Psychological Bulletin* 133(2007): 673–93.

5. Natasha Singer, "Better Health, with a Little Help from Our Friends," *The New York Times: Research*. September 19, 2010, p. BU3.

6. Teresa E. Seeman, Tina M. Lusignolo, Marilyn Albert, and Lisa Beckman, "Social Relationships, Social Support, and Patterns of Cognitive Aging in Healthy, High-Functioning Older Adults: MacArthur Studies of Successful Aging," *Health Psychology* 20(2001): 243–55.

7. J. Salmon, M. Jorna, C. Hume, L. Arundell, N. Chahine, M. Tienstra, and D. A. Crawford, "Translational Research Intervention to Reduce Screen Behaviours and Promote Physical Activity Among Children: Switch-2-Activity," *Health Promotion International* 26(2011): 311–21.

8. Vicki S. Coon, Jeffrey C. Valentine, and Harris M. Cooper, "Interventions to Increase Physical Activity Among Aging Adults," *Annals of Behavioral Medicine* 24(2002): 190–200.

9. Emily B. Kahn, Leigh T. Ramsey, Ross C. Brownson, Gregory W. Heath, Elizabeth H. Howze, Kenneth E. Powell, Elaine J. Stone, Mummy W. Rajab, Phaedra Corso, and the Task Force on Community Preventive Services, "The Effectiveness of Interventions to Increase Physical Activity: A Systematic Review," *American Journal of Preventive Medicine* 22(2002): 73–107.

10. National Heart, Lung and Blood Institute. *Behavior Changes Helpful for Weight Loss: Guide to Behavior Change.* 2005. Available at: www.weight-loss-i.com/weight-loss-behavior-change.htm.

11. James Prochaska, C. C. DiClemente, and J. D. Norcross, "In Search of How People Change, Applications to Addictive Behaviors," *American Psychologist* 47(1992): 1102–14.

12. M. D. Anatchkova, C. A. Redding, and J. S. Rossi, "Development and Validation of Transtheoretical Model Measures for Bulgarian Adolescent Smokers," *Substance Use and Misuse* 42(2007): 23–41.

13. Y. H. Kim, "Adolescents' Smoking Behavior and Its Relationships with Psychological Constructs Based on Transtheoretical Model: A Cross-Sectional Survey," *International Journal of Nursing Studies* 43(2006): 439–46.

14. A. Schumann, T. Kohlmann, H. J. Rumph, U. Hapke, U. John, and C. Meyer, "Longitudinal Relationships Among Transtheoretical Model Constructs for Smokers in the Precontemplation and Contemplation Stages of Change," *Annals of Behavioral Medicine* 30(2005): 12–20.

15. C. L. Macnee and S. McCabe, "The Transtheoretical Model of Behavior Change and Smokers in Southern Appalachia," *Nursing Research* 53(2004): 243–50.

16. C. L. Kohler, L. Fish, and S. L. Davies, "Transtheoretical Model of Change Among Hospitalized African American Smokers," *American Journal of Health Behavior* 28(2004): 145–50.

17. J. R. Thompson, C. Horton, and C. Flores, "Advancing Diabetes Self-Management in the Mexican American Population: A Community Health Worker Model in a Primary Care Setting," *Diabetes Education* 33, Supplement 6(2007): 1595–1655.

18. A. K. Jenum, et al., "Promoting Physical Activity in a Low-Income Multiethnic District: Effects of a Community Intervention Study to Reduce Risk Factors for Type 2 Diabetes and Cardiovascular Disease: A Community Intervention Reducing Inactivity," *Diabetes Care* 29(2006): 1605–12.

19. M. S. Aloia, J. T. Arendt, C. Stepnowsky, J. Hecht, and B. Borrelli, "Predicting Treatment Adherence in Obstructive Sleep Apnea Using Principles of Behavior Change," *Journal of Clinical Sleep Medicine* 1(2005): 346–53.

20. K. Rooney, C. Hunt, L. Humphreys, D. Harding, M. Mullen, and J. Kearney, "Prediction of Outcome for Veterans with Post-Traumatic Disorder Using Constructs from the Transtheoretical Model of Behaviour Change," *Australian and New Zealand Journal of Psychiatry* 41(2007): 590–97.

21. S. B. Kennedy, S. Nolen, J. Applewhite, E. Waiters, and J. Vanderhoff, "Condom Use Behaviors Among 18–24 Year Old Urban African American Males: A Qualitative Study," *AIDS Care* 19(2007): 1032–38.

22. Albert Bandura, *Self-Efficacy: The Exercise of Control* (New York: W. H. Freeman, 1997).

23. E. A. Locke and G. P. Latham, "Building a Practically Useful Theory of Goal Setting and Task Motivation: A 35 Year Odyssey," *American Psychologist* 57(2002): 705–17.

24. A. Bandura and E. A. Locke, "Negative Self-Efficacy and Goal Effects Revisited," *Journal of Applied Psychology* 88(2003): 87–99.

LAB ASSESSMENT 14.1

Are Your Behaviors Healthy?

This is not a pass-fail test. The purpose of the questionnaire is simply to tell you how well you are doing at staying healthy. Some of the behaviors covered in the test may not apply to persons with certain chronic diseases or disabilities. Such persons may require special instructions from their physician or other health professional.

Directions: The questionnaire has six sections: safety; alcohol, tobacco, and other drugs; sexual behavior; eating habits; exercise/fitness; and stress control. Complete one section at a time by circling the number corresponding to the answer that best describes your behavior. Then add the numbers you have circled to determine your score for that section. Write the score on the line provided at the end of each section. The highest score you can get for each section is 100.

Safety

Within the **last school year**, how often did you:

(Please mark the appropriate column for each row.)

Columns: N/A didn't do this within the last 12 months — Never — Rarely — Sometimes — Most of the time — Always (5 1 2 3 4 5)

Wear a seatbelt when you rode in a car?						
Wear a helmet when you rode a bicycle?						
Wear a helmet when you rode a motorcycle?						
Wear a helmet when you were inline skating?						

total _____

Multiply total by 5: Safety score _____

Alcohol, Tobacco, and Other Drugs

Within the **last 30 days,** on how many days did you use:

(Please mark the appropriate column for each row.)

Columns: Never used — Have used, but not in last 30 days — 1–2 days — 3–5 days — 6–9 days — 10–19 days — 20–29 days — All 30 days (11 10 9 8 7 6 5 4)

Cigarettes								
Cigars								
Smokeless tobacco								
Alcohol (beer, wine, liquor)								
Marijuana (pot, hash, hash oil)								
Cocaine (crack, rock, freebase)								
Amphetamines (diet pills, speed, meth, crank)								
Rohypnol (roofies), GHB, or Liquid X (intentional use)								
Other drugs								

Alcohol, Tobacco, and Drugs score _____

Sexual Behavior

Within the **last 30 days,** if you are sexually active and unmarried, how often did you or your partner(s) use a condom during:

(Please mark the appropriate column for each row.)

Columns: Never did this sexual activity — Have not done this during last 30 days — Never — Rarely — Sometimes — Mostly — Always (10 10 2 4 6 8 10)

Oral sex?						
Vaginal intercourse?						
Anal intercourse?						

total _____

Multiply total by 3: Sexual Behavior score _____

Eating Habits

How many servings of fruits and vegetables do you usually have **per day** (1 serving = 1 medium piece of fruit, 1/2 cup chopped, cooked, or canned fruits/vegetables, 3/4 cup fruit/vegetable juice, small bowl of salad greens, or 1/2 cup dried fruit)?

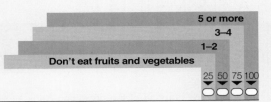

	5 or more
	3–4
	1–2
Don't eat fruits and vegetables	

25 50 75 100

Eating Habits score _____

Exercise/Fitness

On how many of the **past 7 days** did you:

(Please mark the appropriate column for each row.)

	3 days	4 days
	2 days	5 days
	1 day	6 days
	0 days	7 days

3 4 5 6 7 8 9 10

	3	4	5	6	7	8	9	10
Participate in vigorous exercise for at least 20 minutes or moderate exercise for at least 30 minutes?	○	○	○	○	○	○	○	○
Do exercises to strengthen or tone your muscles, such as push-ups, sit-ups, or weightlifting?	○	○	○	○	○	○	○	○
Get enough sleep so that you felt rested when you woke up in the morning?	○	○	○	○	○	○	○	○

total _____

Multiply total by 3: Exercise/Fitness score _____

Stress Control

(Please mark the appropriate column for each row.)

	Always
	Often
	Sometimes
Rarely/Never	

1 2 3 4

	1	2	3	4
I have a job or do other work that I enjoy.	○	○	○	○
I find it easy to relax and express my feelings freely.	○	○	○	○
I recognize early, and prepare for, events or situations likely to be stressful for me.	○	○	○	○
I have close friends, relatives, or others whom I can talk to about personal matters and call on for help when needed.	○	○	○	○
I participate in group activities (such as community organizations) or hobbies that I enjoy.	○	○	○	○

Multiply total by 5: Stress Control score _____

Scoring: There is no total score for this questionnaire. Consider each section separately. You are trying to identify aspects of your health behavior that you can improve in order to be healthier and to reduce the risk of illness. Let's see what your scores reveal.

Scores of 80–100

Excellent! Your answers show that you are aware of the importance of this area to your health. More important, you are putting your knowledge to work by practicing good health habits. As long as you continue to do so, this area should not pose a serious health risk. It's likely that you are setting an example for your family and friends to follow. Since you got a very high score on this part of the questionnaire, you may want to consider other areas where your scores indicate room for improvement.

Scores of 60–79

Your health practices in this area are good, but there is room for improvement. Look again at the items you answered with "sometimes" or "almost never." What changes can you make to improve your score? Even a small change can often help you achieve better health.

Scores of 40–59

Your health may be at risk. Would you like more information about the risks you are facing and the reasons why it is important for you to change these behaviors? Perhaps you need help in deciding how to make the changes you desire. In either case, help is available.

Scores of 0–39

You may be taking serious and unnecessary risks with your health. Perhaps you are not aware of the risks and what to do about them. You can easily get the information and help you need to improve.

LAB ASSESSMENT 14.2

Are Your Lifestyle Behaviors Healthy?

Directions: Use the scale below to describe how often you engage in the behaviors listed.

2 = almost always

1 = sometimes

0 = almost never

_____ 1. I go out and meet new people.

_____ 2. I am able to ask for help from others.

_____ 3. I listen intently to other people.

_____ 4. I am able to communicate with others.

_____ 5. I avoid needless arguments.

_____ 6. I am able to say I am sorry.

_____ 7. I spend time with friends.

_____ 8. I am punctual in writing friends.

_____ 9. I play a musical instrument.

_____ 10. I participate in artistic activities.

_____ 11. I participate in sports.

_____ 12. I travel to different places.

_____ 13. I am involved with hobbies.

_____ 14. I do volunteer work for worthwhile causes.

_____ 15. I am not afraid to try something new.

_____ 16. I enjoy talking in front of groups of people.

_____ 17. I am on time for meetings and appointments.

_____ 18. I do my work/studying on time.

_____ 19. I punctually do my day-to-day chores.

_____ 20. I am able to save money.

Once you have completed this questionnaire, examine the items for which you chose 0. From those items, choose two lifestyle behaviors that may cause you stress and that you would like to change. Use the strategies presented in this chapter to help you make that change.

Directions: Below are listed a number of possible factors—barriers—that may have kept *you* from engaging in certain health and lifestyle behaviors. Choose one health or lifestyle behavior you would like to change. For example, you may want to exercise more or drink less alcohol. For each of the barriers to performing that behavior listed below, circle a number from 1 to 7 that represents the degree to which that barrier affects your adopting this behavior.

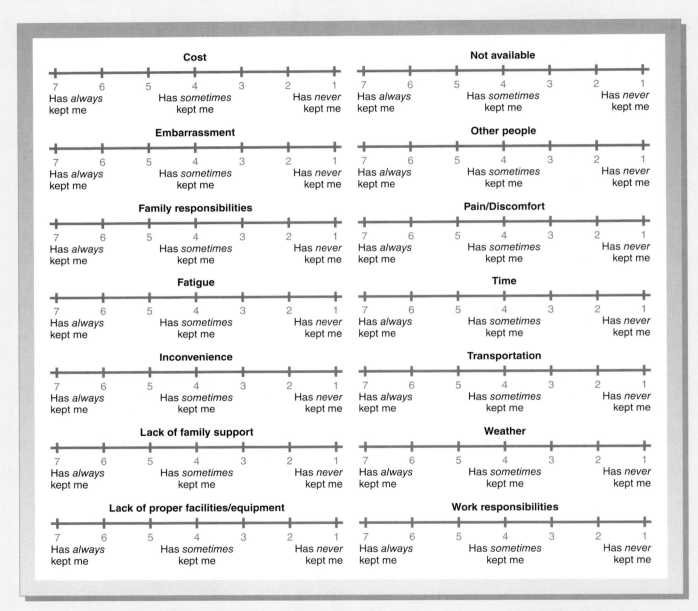

You now have information concerning some barriers and obstacles that have impeded your adopting certain health and lifestyle behaviors. The items for which you circled 7, 6, or 5 are major obstacles to performing the particular behavior that you are interested in changing. Use this information when employing the behavior change strategies described in this chapter. Responding to barriers to behavior change will result in your being more likely to successfully make changes.

Source: From "An Empirical Investigation of Exercise Behavior in Adult Women" by M. P. Noland and R. H. L. Feldman in *Health Education* 16(1985): 29–33. Reproduced with permission of AMERICAN ASSOCIATION FOR HEALTH EDUCATION via Copyright Clearance Center.

LAB ASSESSMENT 14.4

Decreasing Stressful Behaviors: A Guide

To assist you in making changes in your behaviors, use this guide, which is based on the material in this chapter.

1. Behavior I would like to change: _____

   _____

2. What barriers are preventing me from making these changes? _____

   _____

   _____

3. Techniques to decrease stressful behaviors:

   a. Self-monitoring: How often do I do this behavior? _____

   b. Contract: If I do this behavior _____

      then I will receive this reward _____

   c. Significant other: Who will be witness to this contract? _____

      _____

   d. Tailoring: When is the best time to do this behavior? _____

      _____

      Where is the best place to do this behavior?

   e. Social reinforcement: Who will reward me? _____

      How will that person socially reward me? _____

   f. Material reinforcement: What type of material rewards? _____

   g. Shaping: I will change my behavior in steps. List the steps:

      (1) _____

      (2) _____

      (3) _____

      (4) _____

   h. Reminders: What aids can I use to remind me to do this behavior (e.g., calendar)?

      _____

   i. Self-help groups: What self-help groups are available for my particular concern?

      _____

   j. Professional help: Do I need professional help with my problem? If so, where is it available?

      _____

LAB ASSESSMENT 14.5

Can You Use Behavior Change Theory to Change Your Behavior?

Two behavior change theories were presented in this chapter: Stages of Change theory and the Health Belief model. To determine if you are able to use these theories to manage your health and stress-related behaviors, complete the information requested below.

Identify a health- or stress-related behavior you would like to change. This could be either something you do currently that you would prefer not to do (e.g., overdo partying), or something you do not do now that you would prefer to do (e.g., exercise regularly).

Health Behavior: _____

Stages of Change Theory

1. Regarding to the health behavior you want to change, at which stage of change do you think you find yourself?

   _____

2. What strategies will you employ to encourage you to move to the next stage of change?

   a. _____

   b. _____

   c. _____

   d. _____

   e. _____

Health Belief Model

For each construct of the Health Belief model, devise a strategy to help facilitate the behavior change you desire.

Constructs	Behavior Change Strategy
Perceived susceptibility	1. 2. 3.
Perceived severity	1. 2. 3.
Perceived benefits	1. 2. 3.
Perceived barriers	1. 2. 3.

Cues to action	1.
	2.
	3.
Self-efficacy	1.
	2.
	3.

Now the question is, will you actually employ these strategies and take control of your health and stress-related behaviors? You now have the tools to do so. Whether you receive the benefits of healthier behaviors or the consequences of maintaining unhealthy behaviors is up to you.

Diversity and Stress

W hat do you know, Jew boy?" That's what my son heard from a classmate on the school bus in junior high school. After we notified the school—hate crimes and discriminatory acts were especially targeted that school year—and had a discussion with that student's parents, we were assured that comment would not be made again. Still, there was no way to assure my son that he would not be the object of other acts of prejudice—for example, when he wanted to rush a fraternity or when he went after a job he desired.

My son cannot be visually identified as Jewish (although his last name does the job pretty well—Greenberg has never been mistaken as Irish), so he might escape prejudice he would otherwise experience. Imagine the potential for prejudice and discrimination when someone is physically, and therefore visually, identifiable as a minority—African American, Native American, Asian American, or Hispanic, for example. I recently returned from a trip to Japan, where I was easily recognized as "different" from the typical Japanese. I experienced, for the first time, what many minorities experience every day.

This chapter considers the relationship between diversity and stress. We consider such factors as health, poverty, education, and family structure as they relate to race and ethnicity, cultural background, gender, age, sexual orientation, and physical and mental challenges. We begin with the realization that membership in a minority group often comes with a cost. It is frequently associated with poorer health, lower education, lower socioeconomic status, higher unemployment, and an atypical family structure. Of course, many people of color, the elderly, and people with physical and mental challenges excel—but often against tremendous odds. Certainly, they are the exceptions, but they are also sources of hope, especially to young people who come from similar backgrounds and circumstances and are motivated to make themselves successful. There is no denying the burden associated with being considered a minority in the United States, but those of you who are minorities are not inevitably heading toward a disadvantaged future. Although you may unjustly be swimming upstream, there are role models who have swum ahead of you and who are now on the banks of the river, enjoying the rewards of their effort.

Diverse Populations

Among the diverse populations this chapter considers are racial and ethnic minorities. When these populations are grouped together, they constitute a significant segment of our society today and the Census Bureau expects it will constitute an even greater percentage of the population in years to come (see Figure 15.1). You can see how the population is projected to change. In fact, in the year 2010, Hispanics outdistanced African Americans as the largest minority group in the United States. Other changes will occur as well. The population will increase by 42 percent from 2010 to 2050 to a whopping 439 million. Eighty-nine million of these U.S. citizens will be older than 65. That is approximately 20 percent of the population (as compared with 12.9 percent in 2010). And there will be an additional 26 million children under 18 years of age by the year 2050, comprising 23 percent of the population.

Figure 15.1

United States Population, 2010 and 2050

Source: U.S. Census Bureau, 2008. *Percent of Projected Population by Race and Hispanic Origin for the United States: 2010–2050.* Available at: www.census.gov/population/www/projections/summarytables.html

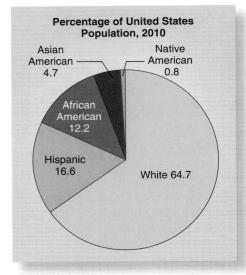

Percentage of United States Population, 2010

Asian American 4.7
Native American 0.8
African American 12.2
Hispanic 16.6
White 64.7

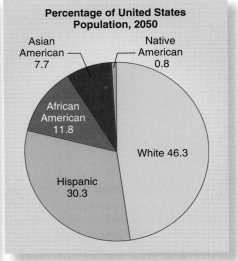

Percentage of United States Population, 2050

Asian American 7.7
Native American 0.8
African American 11.8
Hispanic 30.3
White 46.3

race

A group of people with similar physical traits, blood types, genetic patterns, and inherited characteristics.

ethnicity

A group of people having a common heritage such as common customs, characteristics, language, and history.

The complexity of discussing diverse populations can be best understood by starting with a definition of race and ethnicity. **Race** distinguishes people by a variety of variables such as physical traits (e.g., hair, eyes, skin color), blood types, genetic patterns, and inherited characteristics unique to a population. **Ethnicity** refers to a group having a common heritage as distinguished by customs, characteristics, language, and a common history. Hispanic is an example of an ethnic group.

Now that seems to be fairly straightforward; however, it is anything but. For example, Hispanic is a term of convenience used by the government to classify people. The reason for this classification is to be able to serve specific needs of specific populations. So, for example, if data indicate a specific health problem among that ethnic group, early intervention is possible. The problem is that these ethnic terms are often too encompassing. Relative to the Hispanic population in the United States, there is quite a difference in culture, education, health status, and so on, between those originally from Peru, for example, and those from Mexico, or those from El Salvador and those from Bolivia. The same can be said of the Asian American population. Asian Americans from Japan differ from Asian Americans from China, or Korea, or Vietnam. Cambodian, Laotian, and Hmong Asian immigrants have little in common with Chinese and Japanese Americans who have been in this country for generations.

That said, the problem I faced in writing this chapter can be better understood, and the limitations better appreciated. The data presented in this chapter comply with governmental categories for the sake of convenience; they are the only kinds of data available. When the data can be made more specific, they are presented that way.

For the purposes of this chapter, diverse populations include African Americans, Hispanics, Asian Americans, Native Americans, the elderly, gays and lesbians, and people with disabilities. You might argue that a particular population has been omitted or that one included should be deleted, but someone had to make a judgment as to what was feasible for this chapter, given its space limitations and focus. In this case, that someone was me. Still, if you are interested in learning more about these minority populations or others, you can consult the works cited in the "References" section at the end of this chapter.

Positive Aspects of Minority Status

In this section, a discussion of the health status of minorities is presented. As you will learn, in general, minorities experience poorer health, greater poverty, poorer education, and a range of unique problems. That can be depressing and, if you are a member of a minority group, disturbing. But not to be lost in this chapter on diversity are the major contributions of minority groups to the health and well-being of all of us.

If we were to look at the Asian American community, for example, we could point to acupuncture's adoption by the medical establishment as a mainstream practice and the contribution that has made to the health of Americans of many different ethnic, racial, cultural, and religious backgrounds. Or we could point to the introduction of herbal medicines, or the use of such relaxation techniques as meditation, or many other contributions that have enhanced American life. The respect for authority, the value of education, self-discipline, modesty, and the sense of responsibility toward the elderly are examples of other contributions made by Asian Americans to their own community and models of behavior for other Americans.

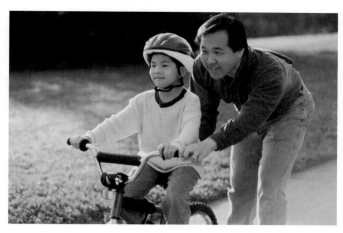

Culture can have significant effects on families. Asian American families, for example, are noted for close family ties and value of educational achievement.

Native Americans have helped us understand the concept of *holism* that has sprung into the holistic movement. Harmony and health have long been concepts embraced by Native Americans.[1] They helped the rest of us recognize that all things are physical, spiritual, emotional, and social, and that to remain healthy, there needs to be harmony (balance) among them. Furthermore, this sense of harmony translates into a belief in the oneness with all things—that is, harmony with others and with the universe. The concern for the environment, a traditional focus of Native Americans, can be seen as stemming from this worldview.

Latinos have demonstrated to the rest of us the value of social and family support. Although this sometimes turns into a deficit (e.g., when medical care is not sought early enough and, instead, family members' advice is relied on), Latino families often feel responsible for one another, make themselves available to one another, and protect one another from potentially harmful elements (such as homelessness). And the family to which they feel connected is an extended one (aunts, uncles, cousins, etc.). It would not be unusual, for example, to find a Hispanic family, without much room in their home for their own family, housing immigrant family members new to the United States. In addition, the spiritual aspects of health, the importance of which recent empirical studies support, has always been at the forefront in the Latino community. The church is a central part of daily life and a resource during stressful times.

Similar to Latinos, for African Americans, the church plays a major function in the community. African Americans often participate in the activities of the church by serving on various committees and contributing to community service efforts. These kinds of institutions and the activities they organize and the support they provide contribute a great deal toward managing stress. Churches provide emotional support and often provide resources as well (e.g., financial assistance). These institutions, their congregants, and their activities provide a model that the rest of the population would be wise to emulate. The value placed on enjoying one's life through activities such as sports, the arts, and social interactions is another contribution that African Americans make to our society. It has been stated repeatedly in this book that stress management requires a comprehensive approach. That point is so important that the word *comprehensive* appears in the title. Certainly, African Americans appreciate this point and model its value for the rest of us.

An Introduction to Problems Faced by Minorities

One of the reviewers of this chapter suggested it is too negative—that is, too many disturbing statistics are presented and problems are emphasized. If that is the case, I offer no apology. It angers me that minorities in the greatest country in the world suffer disproportionately from poor health, poverty, low educational levels, infant mortality, crime and violence, and so forth. I present the data that follow without sugarcoating the reality of what they mean. And that meaning is that minorities in the United States of America, and probably elsewhere in the world, are disadvantaged in significant ways that result in a great deal of stress.

Stressors Challenging Minorities

Minorities experience stressors that create unique challenges for them and that affect their health. In fact, minorities report higher levels of stress than white adults. In one study, the Commonwealth Fund conducted a survey and found 36 percent of minorities reported high levels of stress, whereas only 26 percent of white adults reported such high levels of stress.[2] The stressors found particularly higher for minorities than for white adults concerned money (25 percent versus 17 percent), fear of crime or violence (18 percent versus 8 percent), their spouse or partner (11 percent versus 6 percent), and mistreatment of a family member for race or cultural reasons (5 percent versus less than 0.5 percent). Furthermore, minorities were more likely to have been physically assaulted than Caucasians sometime within the past five years (12 percent versus 9 percent).

Racism

Among the most significant of these stressors is racism. Racial prejudice rests on the belief that one's own race is superior to another's race. Among the myriad effects of racism are anger, stroke, heart attack, and a number of other diseases associated with high blood pressure, as well as cancer.[3-5] In fact, discrimination in general has been found related to low birthweight in babies,[6] respiratory problems,[7] somatic complaints,[8] self-rated health,[9,10] mental health,[11,12] and chronic health conditions.[13,14]

Culture Conflicts

When someone leaves one culture and enters another, there is a need to "fit in." The immigrant seeks to learn the new cultural standards of behavior and the new reward system in order to be successful in the new environment. Complicating this difficult transition is the realization that some of the new culture's standards are at odds with the norms and values of the native culture. When that is the case, what should be the adaptation strategy? Ignore the new culture's standards and norms, and remain faithful to the familiar traditional standards and norms? By way of example, some Asian cultures value obedience and respect and teach these traits to their children. However, when Asians emigrate to the United States—a culture that values independence, assertiveness, and competitiveness—the traits they were taught to value are not necessarily those that will facilitate their becoming fully acculturated and successful. They are caught in a clash of cultures.

Culture clashes can occur in a number of different ways. Irujo presented some examples of common culture clashes that occur in the United States:[15]

> Not looking another person in the eye is a recognition of that person's authority for African-Americans, while whites interpret this as shiftiness and unreliability.
>
> Differences in gaze behavior may cause some misunderstandings. Latinos interpret a direct gaze as having sexual connotations, and a steady stare with raised eyebrows as anger.
>
> Africans, Arabs, and Hispanic Americans touch a great deal in interpersonal relationships, whereas in Britain, Japan, and the United States there is very little touching. Touching in certain circumstances causes embarrassment and discomfort.

Culture clash was evident in a poll of Latinos conducted by the *The Washington Post* in collaboration with the Henry J. Kaiser Foundation and Harvard University.[16] More than 2,000 Latinos, and a comparable number of non-Hispanic whites and African Americans who were used for comparison purposes, were interviewed regarding their views and lifestyles. Nearly 90 percent stated they believed it was important to maintain their native culture, and almost 60 percent said they had little or nothing in common with Anglos or African Americans. Most also believed that discrimination directed toward Latinos was a significant problem. Imagine trying to succeed in a culture you perceive in this way.

Acculturation Stressors

As has been shown, entering a new culture often requires a great deal of adaptation, which often results in stress and ill health. That may explain the higher blood pressure, mental illness, and higher rates of attempted suicide among immigrants when compared with the population in their country of origin.[17,18] One of these adaptations relates to language. Language barriers can interfere with obtaining employment, or result in menial jobs with low salaries. This is in spite of many immigrants having been highly educated and respected professionals in their original countries. The resulting low self-esteem is only one of the effects of this situation. Another is the need to work long hours to support a family, necessitating being away from the family and the supervision and upbringing of children. For example, although Asian Americans are thought to be one of the most economically successful minority groups in America, they receive less income per education level than white workers, requiring them to work longer hours for the same rewards.[19] Like a chain reaction, when the parents are away from home working long hours, the children may suffer the consequences.

Children usually acculturate faster than their parents. Their original culture is not as ingrained, and children tend to be more malleable in general. When children become "Americanized" and their parents adjust more slowly, clashes often occur within families. For example, children may want to be more independent than their original culture allowed, or they may want to wear clothing that reveals more of the body than their country of origin found acceptable, or they may not want to speak their native language at home, preferring to speak English. However, their parents may feel quite differently and remain steadfast in requiring their children to behave in a manner consistent with their traditional cultural standards and values. Both children and parents may feel the effects of this stress.

Other Acculturation Stressors

In addition to language, employment, and family cultural clashes, minorities often live in inner cities, where they may experience a particular type of prejudice, racial profiling. For example, in 2009, an African American Harvard professor, Henry Gates, came home late at night, couldn't find his keys, and eventually entered his house in the dark. A neighbor, seeing Professor Gates and another man enter his house in the dark, called the police. From there, the parties involved offer different accounts of what happened. The police officer said he was doing his job by questioning Professor Gates and asking for identification to make sure the person he was speaking with was not a burglar. However, Professor Gates accused the police officer of racial profiling—assuming an African American man could not own such an expensive home in an upscale neighborhood. President Obama, seemingly wanting to engage the country in a discussion of racial profiling, brought the professor and the police officer to the White House for a meeting in an attempt at conciliation.

In addition, crime and violence are more prevalent in the inner cities and are therefore encountered disproportionately by minorities. A subset of crime is crimes against people on the basis of their race, ethnicity, sexual orientation, or religion. These are called **hate crimes.** Unfortunately, hate crimes are additional stressors with which minorities must cope. In 2009, 8,336 people were the victims of hate crimes in the United States. Of these hate crimes that were racially motivated, violence was directed at: 72 percent against African Americans, 17 percent against whites, 4 percent against Asian Americans, and 2 percent against American Indians.[20]

hate crimes
Crimes against people based on their race, ethnicity, sexual orientation, or religion.

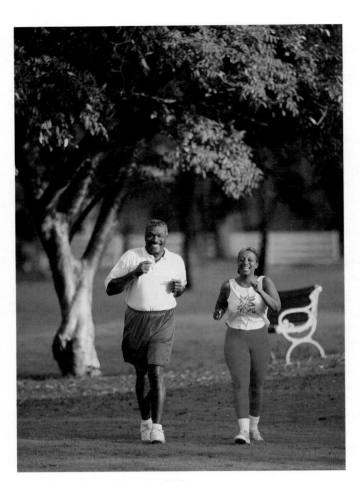

Exercise is an effective strategy to maintain health and decrease health disparities.

These stressors that challenge minorities have the potential to have an effect physiologically and psychologically, as do all stressors. We next explore the health-related implications of stress for minority individuals and minority communities.

Health Status

One of the most dramatic differences between minority populations and European Americans (whites) is health. Imagine how stressful it is to realize that a tremendous disparity exists in health status between minorities and the general population, especially if you are a member of a minority group. This was recognized by the government in the early 1990s: The economically disadvantaged—low income, poorly educated, nonprofessional—and women seem to be at higher risk for both psychosocial and psychophysiologic stress reactions, with the unemployed and the part-time employed minorities at higher risk for psychophysiologic distress.[21] In fact, when the national health objectives were developed for the year 2010, one of the two overarching goals was to "eliminate health disparities."[22]

Health disparities are defined as

a particular type of health difference that is closely linked with social, economic, and/or environmental disadvantage. Health disparities adversely affect groups of people who have systematically experienced greater obstacles to health based on their racial or ethnic group; religion; socioeconomic status; gender; age; mental health; cognitive, sensory, or physical disability; sexual orientation or gender identity; geographic location; or other characteristics historically linked to discrimination or exclusion.[23]

It is clear that racism can have negative health effects, and to surmise that so do sexism, ageism, and prejudice and discrimination by socioeconomic status and physical abilities is not unreasonable. In this chapter, we look at several indices of health as they are related to minorities.

National Health Objectives and Diversity

Whereas health objectives for the nation have been developed each decade since 1990, the year 2010 objectives took a different path than in the past. For the first time, the nation committed itself to the elimination of health disparities. Recognizing the gap in health status between those who are advantaged and those who are not is nothing new. The federal government has had a goal of closing that gap in previous editions of the nation's health objectives. However, the government committed to eliminating that gap altogether by 2010.

The 2020 national health objectives continue to include achieving health equity, eliminating disparities, and improving the health of all groups as overarching goals.[24] In particular, the 2020 national health objectives seek health equality for Americans of different races and ethnicities, genders, sexual identity and orientation, disability status or special health care needs, and geographic location (rural and urban).

Gender[25,26]

- Men have a life expectancy that is almost five years less than women.
- Men have a higher death rate for each of the leading causes of death.
- Women are at a greater risk of Alzheimer's disease than men, and are 1.5 times as likely to be affected by depression.

Race and Ethnicity[27]

- African American men were 1.3 times as likely to have new cases of lung and prostate cancer, and over two times more likely to die from it, compared to non-Hispanic white men.
- African American women were 10 percent less likely to have been diagnosed with breast cancer; however, they were 34 percent more likely to die from breast cancer, compared to non-Hispanic white women.
- African American adults are twice as likely as non-Hispanic white adults to have been diagnosed with diabetes by a physician.
- African American men were 30 percent more likely to die from heart disease, as compared to non-Hispanic white men, and African Americans are 1.5 times as likely as non-Hispanic whites to have high blood pressure.
- African American women are 1.7 times as likely as non-Hispanic white women to be obese.
- African Americans had 2.3 times the infant mortality rate of non-Hispanic whites.
- Hispanic men and women have higher incidence and mortality rates for stomach and liver cancer.
- Hispanic women were twice as likely as non-Hispanic white women to be diagnosed with cervical cancer.
- Hispanics were 1.6 times as likely as non-Hispanic whites to die from diabetes.
- Hispanic males have almost three times the AIDS rate as non-Hispanic white males, and Hispanic females have almost five times the AIDS rate as non-Hispanic white females.
- Asian/Pacific Islander men are twice as likely to die from stomach cancer as compared to the non-Hispanic white population, and Asian/Pacific Islander women are 2.6 times as likely to die from the same disease.
- Asian women had a higher case rate for AIDS than white women.
- The total number of reported AIDS cases has declined for the white population; however, it has continued to increase for Asian Americans.
- American Indian/Alaska Native adults were 2.3 times as likely as white adults to be diagnosed with diabetes and twice as likely as non-Hispanic whites to die from diabetes.
- American Indian/Alaska Native adults are 60 percent more likely to have a stroke than their white adult counterparts.

Disability[28,29]

- Adults with a disability were less likely to report excellent or very good health and more likely to report fair or poor health (40.3 percent versus 9.9 percent), compared with adults without disability.

Although infant mortality rates have declined in recent years in the United States, proportionately more African American infants than white infants die.

- People with disabilities have fewer days of vitality.
- People with disabilities have lower rates of physical activity and higher rates of obesity.

Sexual Orientation[30–34]

- Approximately 54 percent of cumulative AIDS cases are men who have sex with men.
- Research indicates that illicit drugs are used more often among lesbians than heterosexual women.
- Tobacco and smoking products are used more often by lesbians than by heterosexual women.
- Depression and anxiety affect gay men at a higher rate than the general population.

Infant Mortality

The disparity in health status is no more evident than in the rates of infant mortality. In 2009, the **infant mortality** rate in the United States was 6.4 deaths per 1,000 live births. When broken down, the rate for whites was 4.0, whereas for African Americans it was 12.7.[35] The reasons for this difference are varied. For example, African American pregnant women on average obtain prenatal care later, are more likely to live in poverty, and are generally less educated than their white counterparts. The rate for Hispanics is 5.4.

In addition to the reasons stated above, cost and access to health care are significant contributors to late prenatal care and, as a result, to a high infant mortality rate. Minorities are disproportionately represented among those lacking health insurance. Because most private health insurance is obtained through one's employer, and minorities have a higher unemployment rate than does the general population, it is not surprising that minorities have low health insurance rates. Individuals without health insurance—pregnant women as well as others—tend to postpone health care until a problem presents itself.

Also, there is often a lack of health care facilities within easy access of minority populations. I established a community-campus health partnership with a city near my university and serve as chair of that partnership. Ninety-seven percent of that city's population of 5,000 is African American. The city has only one health care provider, a dentist. To obtain health care, residents must travel out of the city. This is just one example of the barriers that minority groups in communities across the United States encounter in their attempt to obtain health care.

Life Expectancy

Life expectancy is the number of years a person is expected to live. Life expectancy at birth in the United States in 2010 was 78.3 years. However, for white males, life expectancy in 2010 was 5.1 years longer than for African American males (78.9 compared with 73.8). And life expectancy for white females was 4.1 years longer than for African American females (81.3 compared with 77.2). However, the gap is getting narrower. Whereas overall life expectancy increased by 2.9 years between 1990 and 2010, the increase for white males was 3.8 years, compared with African American males' increase of 5.7 years. The increase for white females was 1.9 years; for African American females it was 3.6 years.[36]

Years of Potential Life Lost

Years of potential life lost is a measure of premature death. When we look at the causes of premature death among various minority populations, differences emerge. For the general population, heart disease, cancer, and stroke are the leading causes

---

infant mortality
Death of infants before one year of age.

life expectancy
At his or her birth, years a person is expected to live.

years of potential life lost
The number of years between when a person is expected to live and the age of death; a measure of premature death.

Table 15.1 Leading Causes of Death

Cause of Death	White	African American	Native American	Asian/Pacific Islander	Hispanic
			Rank		
Diseases of the heart	1	1	1	2	1
Stroke	3	3	6	3	4
Cancers	2	2	2	1	2
Lung disease	4	8	7	6	8
Pneumonia and influenza	8	—	10	7	9
Liver disease	—	9	5	—	6
Diabetes mellitus	7	5	4	5	5
Kidney disease	9	7	9	8	—
HIV infection (AIDS)	—	9	—	—	—
Unintentional injuries	5	4	3	4	3
Suicide	10	—	8	9	—
Homicide	—	6	—	—	7
Perinatal diseases	—	—	—	—	10
Alzheimer's disease	6	—	—	10	—
Septicemia (blood poisoning)	—	10	—	—	—

Source: National Center for Health Statistics. *Health, United States*, 2009 (Hyattsville, MD: National Center for Health Statistics, 2010), 198–99.

of death, and lung disease and unintentional injuries rank fourth and fifth. This varies, though, for different minorities (see Table 15.1). For example, AIDS is the ninth leading cause of death among African American males, but it does not rank in the top ten among Native American males. And there are significant differences between males and females.

High Blood Pressure

Essential hypertension is characterized by high blood pressure of unknown origin. It is estimated that 90 percent of high blood pressure can be classified as essential, yet high blood pressure does not affect all people to the same degree or in the same manner. Essential hypertension occurs in 18 percent of white males, but it is found in 27 percent of African American males. It occurs in 16 percent of white females, but it occurs in 24 percent of African American females.[37] As a result, proportionately more African Americans die of heart disease (199 per 100,000 population) than do white Americans (133 per 100,000 population). When broken down by gender and ethnicity, diseases of the heart result in almost twice as many years of potential life lost for African American men than for white men, and almost three times as many years of potential life lost for African American women than for white women. Consequently, one of the national health objectives established by the U.S. Department of Health and Human Services is to encourage at least 95 percent of African American hypertensive men aged 18 through 34 to take action to control their blood pressure.

It is interesting to note that Hispanics have a lower rate of coronary heart disease than do whites, both men and women. Furthermore, although heart disease is the leading cause of death for Asian/Pacific Islander Americans, Asian Americans are at a lower risk of dying from coronary heart disease than are other minority groups or whites.

The mechanism for African Americans' being at increased risk of developing hypertension has been studied, and some interesting findings have emerged. Several researchers have found that when African Americans are exposed to stress in the laboratory—for example, by experiencing extreme cold, playing an electronic video game, riding an exercise bicycle, or performing mathematical functions—they react with greater increases in blood pressure than do whites.[38–40] Other research indicates that African Americans may produce fewer endorphins than whites when stressed.[41] This combination may explain the disparity in prevalence of high blood pressure.

On the other hand, studies to identify the reason African Americans have higher blood pressure than whites have found confounding results. Some researchers argue that high blood pressure is a result of urbanization. For example, researchers found that when people move from a traditional tribal society to an urban, westernized lifestyle, their blood pressure rises. An example of this finding is a study that found that when Kenyans moved to Nairobi they had higher blood pressures than people living in the villages, even if they had been in the city for only one month.[42] A related factor might be the neighborhood in which African Americans often live. For example, a study conducted in four U.S. communities found people living in the neighborhoods with the lowest median house prices tended to have the highest blood pressure.[43] Still another study[44] found depression associated with high blood pressure in African Americans but experiencing discrimination was not. Although 80 percent of the African American subjects reported having experienced some discrimination, blood pressure was actually higher in subjects who reported no discrimination. Confused by this finding, the researchers suggested that the people who reported no discrimination were actually in a state of denial and found the topic too painful to acknowledge. Investigations continue to answer the question as to why African Americans experience hypertension to a greater extent than do other Americans.

Acquired Immune Deficiency Syndrome (AIDS)

AIDS
Acquired immune deficiency syndrome.

human immunodeficiency virus
The virus that causes acquired immune deficiency syndrome (AIDS).

As of 2007, there were 1,051,875 persons with **AIDS** reported to the Federal Centers for Disease Control and Prevention.[45] Of these, 810,676 were adult or adolescent males, 198,544 were adult or adolescent females, and 9,209 were children. However, as with other indices of health, rates of HIV (**human immunodeficiency virus**) infection vary greatly in subgroups of the population. For example, whereas African Americans make up approximately 12 percent of the population, they comprised 40 percent of the reported AIDS cases in 2007. Among children reported with HIV infection in 2007, 62 percent were African American. In the United States in 2005, 8,562 African Americans died of AIDS.[46] The AIDS death rate for African American males ages 24 to 44 is approximately six times that for white males, and almost nine times that of white males ages 45 to 64. Even more alarming, the AIDS death rate for African American females ages 24 to 44 is approximately fifteen times that for white females, and eighteen times that of white females ages 45 to 64.[47] Among women with AIDS, 64 percent are African American.[48]

There is also variation in the HIV death rate by gender. For example, the death rate from AIDS in 2006 for American males aged 25 to 44 was almost double that for females. The death rate from HIV infection was 7.6 for Hispanic males and 2.5 for Hispanic females aged 25–44. And the HIV death rate was 32.9 for African American males and 19.9 for African American females aged 25–44.

Cancer

Several cancers are more prevalent among particular groups of Americans than others. For example, African Americans are more likely to develop and die from cancer than any other racial or ethnic population.[49] Whereas the death rate from cancer for African Americans is 170.4 per 1,000 population, it is 101.7 for whites, and 51 for Hispanics. In particular, lung, colorectal, prostate, and breast cancer death rates are significantly higher among African Americans. Hispanics have significantly lower cancer death rates for these cancers than whites or African Americans.

Although Hispanics have low cancer rates overall, they have higher rates of cancer of the uterus, cervix, liver, and stomach.[50] Similarly, Asian Americans and Pacific Islanders have low overall cancer rates. Yet, they have the highest incidence of and death rates from liver and stomach cancers of all racial and ethnic groups. Lastly, American Indians and Alaska Natives have higher incidence rates of lung and colorectal cancer, both men and women, than whites. American Indians and Alaska Natives also have greater rates of new diagnoses for cancers of the kidney, stomach, liver, cervix, and gallbladder than whites.[51]

Mental Health

One mental health issue that varies by subpopulation is suicide. The suicide rate differs dramatically by ethnicity, race, and culture. For example, in 2006, the suicide rate for males aged 15 to 24 was 35.7 for Native Americans, 11.6 for Hispanics, 17.1 for Caucasians, 10.6 for African Americans, and 12.0 for Asian Americans.[52]

Homicide also varies by ethnicity, gender, and cultural background. The death rate from homicide in 2005 for African American men and women was significantly higher than for other groups; the death rate was higher for men than for women; and it decreased as people reached their thirties.[53]

Part of the problem with homicides and unintentional injuries is the number of firearms in American homes. It is estimated by the U.S. Bureau of Alcohol, Tobacco, and Firearms that 200 million firearms exist in the United States and that approximately 50 percent of all households contain a firearm. In 2007, almost 721 deaths occurred by firearm accidents, in addition to firearm deaths by homicide and suicide.[54] Making matters even worse, in any one month approximately 5.2 percent of high school students carry a gun to school; 7.8 percent of white male students, 11.2 percent of African American male students, and 10.4 percent of Hispanic male students reported they had taken a gun to school within the past month.[55] Imagine how stressful it can be to attend a school in which a gun might go off at any time!

When other weapons are considered, the picture is even more alarming. The national Youth Risk Behavior Study[56] found that 18 percent of high school students carried a weapon (for example, a gun, knife, or club) to school in the previous month. That included 28.5 percent of all male students; highest among white males (30.3 percent), Hispanic males (28.2 percent), and African American males (24.6 percent).

Poverty and Educational Level

Because poverty and low educational level are related, we discuss these stressful conditions together. Both are associated with poorer health. Across all ethnic and cultural groups, the higher the educational level, the better the health status is. Because higher educational level is associated with higher income, poverty is also a cause of poor health: the lower the socioeconomic level, the poorer the health status. Table 15.2 shows the number and percentage of people and families in the United States below the poverty level as of 2008. Notice the disparity in the poverty level among whites and minority groups.

Surely, poverty is caused by many factors. Still, racism, ageism, and other "isms" can be included in that mix. For example, women working full time earn 80 percent of what men earn.[57] That figure becomes even worse when ageism is included: Older women workers (35 years of age and older) earn only 75 percent of what older male workers earn. Just 9 percent of women earned $1,500 or more per week, compared to 18 percent of men. Furthermore, poverty in old age is more prevalent among women than among men.

The stressful effects of being African American described by Dowd and Bengston remain true to this day: "Being old in an industrialized society is burden enough; being old *and* a member of a minority group is seen by many as constituting double jeopardy."[58]

Table 15.2
Persons and Families Below the Poverty Level, 2006

	Percentage Below Poverty Level (%)	Number Below Poverty Level
All Persons		
All races	13.2%	39,829,000
White	11.2	26,990,000
African American	24.7	9,379,000
Hispanic	23.2	10,981,000
Asian	11.8	1,578,000
Children Under 18		
All races	18.5	13,507,000
White	15.3	8,441,000
African American	34.4	3,781,000
Hispanic	30.3	4,888,000
Asian or Pacific Islander	14.2	430,000

Source: U.S. Census Bureau, *Statistical Abstracts of the United States:* 2011 (Washington, D.C.: U.S. Census Bureau, 2011), p. 464–65.

Imagine the stress felt by a person with a physical disability seeking employment only to discover that he or she is unable to find work because of the disabling condition, or a 60-year-old worker laid off due to a downturn in the economy who finds other companies unwilling to hire and train a person whom they perceive to be near retirement, or a young woman who cannot find a job because of employers' notions that she might soon become pregnant, thereby requiring time away from the job. Even though all of these actions are discriminatory, abhorrent, and illegal, many employers ignore the law and express their prejudices through their hiring practices. This behavior has implication for stress, health, and quality of life.

Family Life

In this section we consider two important factors related to stress: homelessness and family structure, as well as the needs of mixed race and international college students.

Homelessness

I will never forget the time I was asked to organize a presentation on homelessness at a national conference in Chicago. The presentation was in the Gold Room of a fancy downtown hotel. It was called the Gold Room because of the gold trim on the walls and moldings and the gold chandeliers hanging from the ceiling. To describe this room as opulent is an understatement. The irony of discussing homelessness in the Gold Room was, to say the least, an embarrassment.

Getting exact figures on homelessness is difficult. However, according to some estimates, on any given night between 444,000 and 842,000 people in the United States are homeless, and up to 3.5 million experience homelessness sometime during the year.[59] What is even more disturbing is that rather than decreasing, homelessness is actually increasing.[60] A U.S. Conference of Mayors survey[61] of homelessness in 30 cities found that families with children under 18 years of age accounted for 33 percent of the urban homeless, and 1 percent of the urban homeless are unaccompanied minors. Single men comprised 68 percent of the urban homeless and single women 33 percent. The number of homeless families increased dramatically throughout the 1990s. Families with children are the fastest-growing segment of the homeless population.[62] Families with children constitute 23 percent of the homeless.[63] Families, single mothers, and children make up the largest group of homeless people in rural areas.[64]

Every night, large numbers of Americans experience the stress of homelessness, and many of the homeless are families that include children.

The homeless population in urban areas is comprised of 42 percent African Americans, 38 percent Caucasians, 20 percent Hispanics, 4 percent Native Americans, and 2 percent Asian Americans.[65] In rural areas, the homeless consist of Caucasians more than other racial or ethnic groups.[66]

Homelessness results from many factors. Predominant among them are domestic violence and lack of employment or minimum-wage jobs. Fifty percent of cities surveyed identified domestic violence as a primary cause of homelessness.[67] Furthermore, when people are employed in minimum-wage jobs, they cannot afford housing. In fact, a minimum-wage worker would have to work 87 hours a week to afford a two-bedroom apartment at 30 percent of his or her income. Interestingly, approximately 15 percent of the homeless are employed. Obviously, these workers are not earning enough to avoid homelessness.[68]

Family Structure

For many reasons, there are differences in the stress experienced by minority families. For example, higher socioeconomic status affords some families the option of day care, time away from parental responsibilities, a lack of stress about money for food and shelter, and less concern about the ability to afford adequate health care. Consequently, they report fewer divorces and a higher percentage of two-parent families. In contrast, people living at poverty levels—we have already shown that minorities are disproportionately represented in this population—experience the stress of trying to afford the very basics, much less anything beyond that. These families, perhaps as a result of the increased stress they encounter, are statistically different. For example, in 2009, 60 percent of African American children were living with either one parent or no parent, 32 percent of Hispanic children were living with either one or no parent, and 35 percent of white children came from one- or no-parent families. Furthermore, in 2009, African American adults were found more likely to be single (43 percent of African American men and 41 percent of African American women were never married). For Hispanic adults the percentages of the never married were 38 percent for males and 26 percent for females. The comparable figures for whites were 27 percent for men and 29 percent for women.[69]

This discussion should not be interpreted to mean that minorities are the only families headed by one parent. In 2009, only 71 percent of households with children under the age of 18 consisted of a married couple and their children.

How Colleges Can Help Mixed Race Students with Identity Stress

In 1990, there were 964,000 interracial marriages in the United States, 1.8 percent of all marriages. By 2009, there were 2,437,000 interracial marriages, 4 percent of all marriages.[a] A study by the Pew Research Foundation reported that in 2008 one in seven new marriages was between spouses of different races or ethnicities. The result of the increase in interracial marriages is an influx of mixed race college students. Researchers have found that those of mixed race often feel racially stigmatized which affects their well-being.[b] One of the stressors experienced by interracial students is to develop a sense of identity. Too often society demands conformity to a preconceived racial category. Who am I? Where do I belong?

A model of how mixed race students develop a sense of identity proposes several different positions, called *border crossings*. These border crossing are:[c]

- Having *both feet in both groups* or being able to merge multiple perspectives simultaneously.

- *Situational ethnicity* or consciously switching between racial groups depending on the situation.

- *Sitting on the border* or adopting a multiracial perspective.

- Creating a *home base in one identity* but periodically becoming involved in others.

Colleges and universities can help students with identity stress in a number of ways. For example, providing opportunities to explore race and ethnicity in courses and through assigned projects encourages students—those of mixed race and others—to think about the complexity of these issues and explore their place in this constellation. In reviewing studies on colleges' attempts to respond to the issue of mixed race, one researcher concludes that courses, texts, workshops, lectures, and informal learning experiences that deal directly with the mixed race experience provide students—of any racial heritage—opportunities to expose the myth of racial purity.[d]

Does your campus offer these experiences? If not, how can you encourage your campus's decision makers to better respond to the needs of the rising number of mixed-race college students?

[a]U.S. Census Bureau. *Statistical Abstracts of the United States:* 2011 (Washington, DC: U.S. Census Bureau, 2010), 54.
[b]Diane T. Sanchez and Julie A. Garcia, "When Race Matters: Racially Stigmatized Others and Perceiving Race as a Biological Construct Affect Biracial People's Daily Well-Being," *Personal Social Psychological Bulletin* 35(2009): 1154–64.
[c]M. P. P. Root, "The Multiracial Experience: Racial Borders as a Significant Frontier in Race Relations." In P. P. Root, *The Multiracial Experience: Racial Borders as the New Frontier* (Thousand Oaks, CA: Sage, 1996), xiii–xxviii.
[d]Kristen A. Renn, "Understanding the Identities of Mixed-Race College Students through a Developmental Ecology Lens," *Journal of College Student Development* 44(2003): 383–403.

The importance of family structure becomes evident when we consider child health. Research over the past decade clearly shows that marital dissolution and childbearing outside of marriage often have long-term negative effects on children. Children who grow up with two parents do better in many ways than children who grow up with only one. For example, children from one-parent homes have lower intellectual test scores and are more likely to drop out of school. Girls from such families are more prone to become single mothers in their teens, and boys from such families are more prone to engage in antisocial behavior. These differences are seen in children from many social classes and ethnic groups.[70]

The *National Study of the Changing Workforce*[71] found that one-third of the workforce reported one or two symptoms of depression, therefore being at risk for clinical depression. In addition, 41 percent of employees reported experiencing three or more indicators of stress *sometimes, often,* or *very often.* The Families and Work Institute suggests these data provide an early warning sign that there could be an increase in stress-related illnesses among the American workforce. In fact, they continue, data from the *National Study of the Changing Workforce* also indicate that the frequency of minor health problems, such as headaches, upset stomachs, or trouble sleeping, has increased—conditions that can be caused or aggravated by stress. Another study found that 20 percent of those early in their careers, 33 percent of those in mid-career, and 38 percent in late-career reported feeling burned out.[72] If these families reported such a high level of stress feelings, imagine the stress experienced by minority families: families with only one parent present, families living in poverty, families with lower levels of education and job training, and families who are discriminated against only too regularly.

Age and Physical Challenges

Elders and individuals with physical challenges fare no better when it comes to stereotyping and stress.

Elders

In many other countries—Japan is a good example—elderly citizens are revered for their experience and knowledge. Unfortunately, in the United States, when people become old, they are expected to retire, to step aside and let younger people contribute to society's evolution. However, retirees need not be inactive. Many take part-time jobs and have sufficient time to do the things they were not able to do when working full-time. Still, ageism can make a person feel useless or worse—a burden. That must be a very stressful feeling!

The federal government has established health objectives specifically for older adults. One of the goals of these objectives is to increase the productive years of

Stress and the International Student

It is reported that in the 2003–2004 school year international students made up 4.3 percent of U.S. higher education enrollment. That is a total of 572,509 international students enrolled in colleges or universities across the United States.[a] When coming to the United States to study, many international students are faced with an unfamiliar culture to which they need to adapt. In one study,[b] the most significant adjustment these students faced was related to cultural differences, language challenges, and the U.S. educational system; whereas finances, homesickness, and health issues seemed insignificant. However, other researchers found that the more homesickness, the poorer adjustment.[c] Furthermore, many international students may perceive that significant academic demands are being placed upon them, and this can be a huge source of stress.[d] The perceived need for academic superiority is often the result of a desire to please the family or because financial assistance they receive may require academically high standards. Other potential sources of stress and anxiety for these students, especially those lacking language proficiency skills, are the expectation of class participation, group work, and oral presentations.[b]

Potential stressors for international students include language barriers and lack of knowledge of the host culture. However, language skills may be the most stressful because of the effect they can have on the social and academic performance of a student. Lack of English language proficiency may affect multicultural students' desire to interact socially, creating doubt about their ability to be successful in their new environment. In addition, since language proficiency is such an important factor, difficulty with it can negatively affect the self-concept and self-efficacy of students, which, in turn, negatively affects their academic performance.

Researchers have found that the quality of relationships international students have with faculty and with other students affects the mental well-being of students undergoing stress. Furthermore, in one study, asking for help was cited by international students as one of the strategies for positive adjustment.[e] However, international students experience difficulty seeking assistance from others. Rather, they prefer to seek help from family and friends, not wanting to divulge personal information to strangers, that is, people not from their culture.[b] Recognizing this reluctance to ask for help, although colleges and universities often have an office on campus devoted to providing support for international students, it is recommended that faculty purposely seek out international students in their courses and offer assistance. Another recommended strategy is to establish mentoring programs whereby international students are paired with native students. Not only does it appear that international students benefit from mentoring programs but so may the U.S. students. This reciprocal relationship contributes to cultural awareness and sensitivity by both international and U.S. students.[b]

[a]International student and total U.S. enrollment. Institute of International Education. 2004. Available at: http://opendoors .iienetwork.org/?p=49931.

[b]L. Zhai, "Studying International Students: Adjustment Issues and Social Support." 2002. ERIC Document 474481.

[c]Y. W. Ying, and L. H. Liese, "Initial Adjustment of Taiwanese Students to the United States," *Journal of Cross Cultural Psychology,* 25(1994): 466–77.

[d]Monique Olivas and Chi-Sing Li, "Understanding Stressors of International Students in Higher Education: What College Counselors and Personnel Need to Know," *Journal of Instructional Psychology* 33(2006): 217–22.

[e]W. C. Tseng and F. B. Newton, "International Students' Strategies for Well-being." *College Student Journal* 36(2002): 591–97.

elders and their years of quality life. One objective is to reduce the proportion of older adults who have moderate to severe functional limitations. When the objectives were developed, 28.3 percent of older Americans had moderate or severe functional limitations. The national objectives seek to reduce that to 25.5 percent.

People with Physical and Mental Challenges

Too often we do not appreciate something until we have lost it. Recently, while playing basketball, a friend struck me in my eye with his thumb. I had never experienced such pain in my life! It turned out that the scratch on the cornea and the cut on the white of my eye were the least of my worries. The blow had so traumatized the eye muscles that I had double vision. The ophthalmologist guessed that time would heal the muscles and restore my vision to normal. I only half believed him. Luckily, he was right and I was wrong. Four months later, I was able to reach for something, confident I would grab it rather than its phantom image. During those four months, though, the double vision led to headaches, dizziness, and nausea. Now I *really* appreciate my eyesight and the complexity of lining up two eyes to see one image.

People with physically challenging conditions experience the hardship I experienced (usually to a much greater degree), but their condition is not temporary. How cruel it is to add to their burden by subjecting them to discriminatory attitudes and practices that create even greater stress than they would normally experience, yet that is what too often occurs. Again, although it is against the law to discriminate because of physical challenges, too many employers still do. Although access to buildings and accommodations to allow for greater mobility have been created, too many barriers still exist. And in spite of such heroic accomplishments as completing a marathon in a wheelchair or running across the country on an artificial leg, too much disrespect for persons with physical challenges still exists. Recognizing the necessity of responding to the needs of people with various challenges, the federal government established health objectives specifically for this population. Among these national health objectives are to increase the proportion of adults with disabilities who report sufficient social and emotional support, and reduce the proportion of people with disabilities who report serious psychological distress.[73]

The effects of gender bias, age discrimination, and prejudice against people with various physical and mental challenges can be devastating for people who wish only to be treated equally and fairly—that is, to be given an equal opportunity to experience the American dream. However, more women live in poverty than do men, as do more of the female elderly and more of the female physically challenged. We have already explored the relationship between poverty and poor health. One might argue that treating our compatriots in this biased manner not only has negative consequences for them but also diminishes us. Anyone who has ever helped people in need knows the feeling experienced by doing the helping. When we behave in a discriminatory fashion, we deprive ourselves of the opportunity to have this feeling and are thereby less happy, proud, and self-respectful than we might be.

Sexual Orientation

Still another group experiencing discrimination and, as a result, stressful consequences are gays, lesbians, and transgenders. The Federal Bureau of Investigation reports 1,482 hate crimes stemming from sexual orientation bias.[74] Ten percent of these hate crimes occurred in schools or colleges. In fact, gay and lesbian verbal, physical, and sexual harassment was described by one expert as widespread in U.S. schools.[75]

Sexual orientation discrimination has significant stress and health-related consequences. For example, when gay men's incidences of harassment, discrimination, and violence were studied over a six-month period, 11 percent reported experiencing discrimination, and 5 percent reported physical violence.[76] These experiences were associated with lower self-esteem and increased suicide ideation. In another study, it was found that gays had a high prevalence of psychological symptoms of distress, including suicide ideation (17 percent), anxiety (44 percent), and depression (80 percent).[77] These researchers concluded that sexual orientation bias leads to social alienation, low self-esteem, and symptoms of psychological distress.

More and more colleges and universities are recognizing the need to respond to sexual orientation bias. One manifestation of this concern is the establishment of fraternities and sororities for gay and lesbian students. As of 2003, for instance, there were approximately two dozen gay fraternities in the United States, about half of which developed since 1998.[78] Some states have even passed legislation allowing for same-sex marriages, although the great majority have not, and same-sex marriage is still not federally sanctioned.

Coping in Today's World

As we discussed in this chapter, there is wide variation in the health of subgroups of Americans. We call these variations *health disparities*. Here is some additional information on that topic:

- In 2006, African Americans had the highest age-adjusted all-causes death rate of all races or ethnicities. In addition, African Americans had the highest age-adjusted death rate for heart disease, cancer, diabetes, and HIV/AIDS (see table below).

2006 age-adjusted death rates for selected causes of death, per 100,000 population

	All populations	African Americans	Asian Americans & Pacific Islanders
All causes	776.5	982.0	428.6
Heart disease	200.2	257.7	108.5
Cancer	180.7	217.4	106.5
Diabetes	23.3	45.1	15.8
Unintentional injury	39.8	38.3	16.9
HIV disease	4.0	18.6	0.6

Source: Health, United States, 2008 Table 28, updated November 2009.

- In 2007, non-Hispanic black persons 18 years of age and over were less likely than non-Hispanic white persons to have received a flu shot during the past 12 months (non-Hispanic black: 38.1 percent; non-Hispanic white: 49.9 percent), and were also less likely to have ever received a pneumococcal vaccination (non-Hispanic black: 43.7 percent; non-Hispanic white: 60.1 percent).

- In 2008, African American adults were almost four times as likely to be obese as Asian adults (African American:

36.1 percent, white: 26.5 percent, Asian American: 9.4 percent). African American women were particularly impacted, with 42.1 percent of African American women 18 years of age and over obese in 2008.

- According to the U.S. Census, blacks make up approximately 13.5 percent of the U.S. population. However, in 2007, blacks accounted for 21,754 (51 percent) of the estimated 42,655 new HIV/AIDS diagnoses in the United States.

- Systemic Lupus Erythematosus is three times more common in black women than in white women. Black and Hispanic/Latina women tend to develop symptoms at an earlier age than other women. African Americans have more severe organ problems, especially with their kidneys.

- Cancer death rates are highest among black women, followed by white, American Indian/Alaska Native, Hispanic, and Asian/Pacific Islander women.

- The rate of new cancer cases is highest among black men, followed by white, Hispanic, Asian/Pacific Islander, and American Indian/Alaska Native men. Death rates are highest among black men, followed by white, Hispanic, American Indian/Alaska Native, and Asian/Pacific Islander men.

Several reasons are proposed to explain why health disparities exist. Among these are racism and discrimination, disproportionate poverty and low education levels among certain minorities, inadequate health insurance, lack of minority medical care providers (in particular, physicians), communication barriers, and bias among physicians and nurses.

summary

- Cultural diversity is related to stress and, in turn, to health and well-being.

- Although in 2000 approximately three-quarters of the U.S. population was white, it is projected that by the year 2050 just over 52 percent will be white. Estimates are that, by 2050, 23 percent of Americans will be Hispanic, 14 percent will be African American, and 10 percent will be Asian American.

- Diversity is related to such health indices as infant mortality, life expectancy, years of potential life lost, hypertension, AIDS, cancer, and mental health.

- The infant mortality rate for the general population is 6.7 deaths per 1,000 live births. However, it is 13.3 for African Americans. For whites, the infant mortality rate is 5.7, for Hispanics it is 5.6, for Native Americans it is 8.7, and for Asian Americans it is 4.9.

- Life expectancy at birth for the general population is 77.8 years. However, for white males, life expectancy is 6 years longer than for African American males (75.7 compared with 69.5). And life expectancy for white females is 4.3 years longer than for African American females (80.8 compared with 76.5).

- The major causes of death vary somewhat by ethnicity and race, cultural background, and gender. For example, AIDS is the ninth leading cause of death among African Americans, but it is not included in the top ten causes of death for whites, Native Americans, Asian Americans, or Hispanics.

- High blood pressure and AIDS affect African Americans to a greater extent than they affect other subgroups of the population. African Americans have a disproportionate incidence of high blood pressure and comprise 40 percent of the AIDS cases.

- The suicide rate for Native American male youths aged 15 to 24 (32.7 deaths per 100,000) was significantly higher than for white, African Americans, Hispanic, and Asian American males.

- Poverty is also associated with poor health. Although 12 percent of the general population lives in poverty, 24 percent of African Americans, 21 percent of Hispanics, and 10 percent of Asian/Pacific Islanders live in poverty. By contrast, 10 percent of white Americans live in poverty.

- Rather than decreasing, homelessness is actually increasing. On any given night, some estimates are that between 444,000 and 842,000 people in the United States are homeless and up to 3.5 million experience homelessness sometime during the year. The number of homeless families has increased dramatically. Families with children are the fastest-growing segment of the homeless population. Families with children under eighteen years of age account for 33 percent of the urban homeless, and 1 percent of the urban homeless are unaccompanied children.

- Nearly 61 percent of African American children live with one parent only, 30 percent of Hispanic children live with only one parent, and 23 percent of white children come from one-parent families. Furthermore, African American adults are more likely to be single (42 percent of African American men and 39 percent of African American women are unmarried). The comparable figures for whites are 27 percent for men and 19 percent for women.

- Sexual orientation bias is prevalent and has significant stress and health-related consequences. The Federal Bureau of Investigation reports 1,265 hate crimes stemming from sexual orientation bias. This form of discrimination is associated with lower self-esteem, increased suicide ideation, increased anxiety and depression, and social isolation.

internet resources

NASP Resources: Recommended Diversity Websites **www .nasponline.org/resources/culturalcompetence/ diversitywebsites.aspx** *A listing of numerous websites related to different cultures. Included are programs to enhance cultural diversity.*

DiversityInc **http://diversityinc.com/** *An online magazine that provides news, resources, and commentary on the role of diversity. Focus is on diversity in the workplace but also includes articles on diversity in general.*

Psychological Stress and Cancer **www.oncolink.upenn.edu/ coping/index.cfm** *Includes Web links and resources to contact for additional information when coping with cancer.*

The Wellness Community **www.thewellnesscommunity.org** *Description of the services provided by The Wellness Community, a nonprofit organization whose mission is to help reduce stress for people with cancer and their families through free programs that offer* emotional support and education. Includes a list of facilities by state.

HIV and Depression **www.psycom.net/depression.central .hiv.html** *A central clearinghouse for information on all types of depressive disorders and on the most*

effective treatments for individuals suffering from depression related to HIV status.

Office of Minority Health Resource Center **www.omhrc.gov** *Provides statistics and resources regarding minorities.*

references

1. Raymond Nakamura, *Health in America: A Multicultural Perspective* (Dubuque, IA: Kendall Hunt, 2003).

2. The Commonwealth Fund, *A Comparative Survey of Minority Health* (New York: The Commonwealth Fund). www.cmwf .org:80/minhlth.html

3. C. Lee, S. L. Ayers, and J. J. Kronenfeld, "The Association between Perceived Provider Discrimination, Healthcare Utilization and Health Status in Racial and Ethnic Minorities," *Ethnicity and Disease* 19(2009): 330–37.

4. R. Benkert, R. Peters, N. Tate, and E. Dinardo, "Trust of Nurse Practitioners And Physicians Among African Americans With Hypertension," *Journal of the American Academy of Nurse Practitioners* 20(2008): 273–80.

5. M. K. Canales, D. Weiner, M. Samos, N. S. Wampler, A. Cunha, and B. Geer, "Multi-Generational Perspectives on Health, Cancer, and Biomedicine: Northeastern Native American Perspectives Shaped by Mistrust," *Journal of Health Care for the Poor and Underserved* 22(2011): 894–911.

6. C. Giurgescu, B. L. McFarlin, J. Lomax, C. Craddock, and A. Albrecht, "Racial Discrimination and the Black-White Gap in Adverse Birth Outcomes: A Review." *Journal of Midwifery and Women's Health* 56(2011): 362–70.

7. S. Karlsen and J. Y. Nazroo, "Relation Between Racial Discrimination, Social Class, and Health Among Ethnic Minority Groups," *American Journal of Public Health* 92(2002): 624–31.

8. T. L. Bowen-Reid and J. P. Harrell, "Racist Experiences and Health Outcomes: An Examination of Spirituality as a Buffer," *Journal of Black Psychology* 28(2002): 18–36.

9. J. Schultz, B. Israel, D. Williams, E. Parker, A. Becker, and S. James, "Social Inequalities, Stressors and Self-Reported Health Status Among African American and White Women in the Detroit Metropolitan Area," *Social Science and Medicine* 51(2000): 1639–53.

10. J. Stuber, S. D. Galea, J. Ahern, S. Blaney, and C. Fuller, "The Association Between Multiple Domains of Discrimination and Self-Assessed Health: A Multilevel Analysis of Latinos and Blacks in Four Low-Income New York City Neighborhoods," *Health Services Research* 38(2003): 1735–60.

11. H. Landrine, E. A. Klonoff, I. Corrall, S. Fernandez, and S. Roesch, "Conceptualizing and Measuring Ethnic Discrimination in Health Research," *Journal of Behavioral Medicine* 29(2006): 79–94.

12. S. Noh and V. Kaspar, "Perceived Discrimination and Depression: Moderating Effects of Coping, Acculturation, and Ethnic Support," *American Journal of Public Health* 93(2003): 232–38.

13. G. C. Gee, J. Chen, M. Spencer, et al. "Social Support as a Buffer for Perceived Unfair Treatment Among Filipino Americans: Differences Between San Francisco and Honolulu," *American Journal of Public Health* 93(2003): 677–84.

14. C. G. Gilbert, M. S. Spencer, J. Chen, and David Takeuchi, "A Nationwide Study of Discrimination and Chronic Health Conditions Among Asian Americans," *American Journal of Public Health* 97(2007): 1275–82.

15. Suzzane Irujo, "An Introduction to Intercultural Differences and Similarities in Nonverbal Communication." In *Toward Multiculturalism,* ed. J. Wurzel (Yarmouth, ME: Intercultural Press, 1988), 142–50.

16. Amy Goldstein and Roberto Suro, "A Journey of Stages: Assimilation's Pull Is Still Strong, but Its Pace Varies," *The Washington Post,* January 16, 2000, A1.

17. Guillermina Jasso, Douglas S. Massey, Mark R. Rosenzweig, and James P. Smith, "Immigrant Health—Selectivity and Acculturation," Paper prepared for *National Academy of Science Conference on Racial and Ethnic Disparities in Health,* 2004. Available at http://129.3.20.41/eps/lab/papers/0412/0412002.pdf

18. Annette E. Maxwell, "Acculturation," *Encyclopedia of Public Health,* 2009. Available at www.enotes.com/public-health-encyclopedia/acculturation

19. Jef Akst, "Life Sciences Salary Survey 2009," *The Scientist* 23(2009): 43.

20. Federal Bureau of Investigation, *Hate Crime Statistics, 2009* (Washington, D.C.: U.S. Department of Justice, 2009).

21. U.S. Public Health Service, *Healthy People 2000: National Health Promotion and Disease Objectives* (Washington, D.C.: U.S. Department of Health and Human Services, September 1992), 215.

22. U.S. Public Health Service, *Healthy People: The Surgeon General's Report on Health Promotion and Disease Prevention* (Washington, D.C.: U.S. Government Printing Office, 1999).

23. U.S. Department of Health and Human Services, The Secretary's Advisory Committee on National Health Promotion and Disease Prevention Objectives for 2020. Phase I report: Recommendations for the framework and format of Healthy People 2020. Section IV. Advisory Committee Findings and Recommendations. Available at: www.healthypeople.gov/ hp2020/advisory/PhaseI/sec4.htm#_Toc211942917

24. U.S. Department of Health and Human Services, *Healthy People 2020* (Washington, DC: U.S Department of Health and Human Services, 2011). Available at: www.healthypeople .gov/2020/default.aspx

25. U.S. Census Bureau, *Statistical Abstracts of the United States: 2011* (Washington, DC: U.S. Census Bureau, 2010).

26. National Center for Health Statistics, *Health, United States, 2009* (Hyattsville, MD: National Center for Health Statistics, 2010).

27. Office of Minority Health, *Data Statistics*. 2011. Available at: http://minorityhealth.hhs.gov/templates/browse .aspx?lvl=1&lvlID=5

28. Racial/Ethnic Disparities in Self-Rated Health Status Among Adults with and Without Disabilities—United States, 2004–2006. *MMWR* 57(2008): 1069–73.

29. Office of Disease Prevention and Health Promotion, *Healthy People 2010* (Washington, DC: U.S Department of Health and Human Services, 2000).

30. Statistics, *Youth Pride Inc.* 2010. Available at: www .youthprideri.org/Resources/Statistics/tabid/227/Default.aspx

31. Centers for Disease Control and Prevention, *Gay and Bisexual Men's Health*. 2010. Available at: www.cdc.gov/msmhealth/ substance-abuse.htm

32. Centers for Disease Control and Prevention, *Lesbian, Gay, Bisexual and Transgender Health*. 2009. Available at: www.cdc .gov/Features/LGBT/

33. Ten Things Lesbians Should Discuss with Their Health Care Providers, *Center for Research on Health and Sexual Orientation*. 2002. Available at: www.publichealth.pitt.edu/ docs/10things_lesbi.pdf

34. Ten Things Gay Men Should Discuss with Their Health Care Providers, *Center for Research on Health and Sexual Orientation*. 2002. Available at: www.publichealth.pitt.edu/ docs/10things_gay.pdf

35. Kenneth D. Kochanek, Jiaquan Xu, Sherry L. Murphy, Arialdi M. Miniño, and Hsiang-Ching Kung, Deaths: Preliminary Data for 2009. *National Vital Statistics Report* 59(2011): 6.

36. National Center for Health Statistics, Health, United States (2010), 176.

37. National Center for Health Statistics (2010), 293.

38. N. B. Anderson, "Racial Differences in Stress-Induced Cardiovascular Reactivity and Hypertension: Current Status and Substantive Issues," *Psychological Bulletin* 105(1989): 89–105.

39. K. C. Light and A. Sherman, "Race, Borderline Hypertension, and Hemodynamic Responses to Behavioral Stress Before and After Beta-Andrenergic Blockade," *Health Psychology* 8(1989): 577–95.

40. N. B. Anderson, et al., "Race, Parental History of Hypertension, and Patterns of Cardiovascular Reactivity in Women," *Psychophysiology* 26(1989): 39–47.

41. M. McNeilly and A. Zeichner, "Neuropeptide and Cardiovascular Response to Intravenous Catheterization in Normotensive and Hypertensive Blacks and Whites," *Health Psychology* 8(1989): 487–501.

42. N. R. Poulter, K. T. Khaw, B. E. Hopwood, et al. The Kenyan Luo Migration Study: Observations on the Initiation of a Rise in Blood Pressure, *British Medical Journal* 300(1990): 967–72.

43. A. V. Diez-Roux, F. J. Nieto, C. Muntaner, et al. Neighborhood Environments and Coronary Heart Disease: A Multilevel Analysis. *American Journal of Epidemiology* 146(1997): 48–63.

44. N. Krieger and S. Sidney, Racial Discrimination and Blood Pressure: The CARDIA Study of Young Black and White Adults, *American Journal of Public Health* 86(1996): 1370–78.

45. Centers for Disease Control and Prevention, *HIV/AIDS Surveillance Report, 2007*, vol. 19 (Atlanta, GA: U.S. Dept. of Health and Human Services, Centers for Disease Control and Prevention, 2009).

46. Ibid.

47. National Center for Health Statistics, *Health, United States, 2009* (Hyattsville, MD: National Center for Health Statistics, 2010), 230.

48. Centers for Disease Control and Prevention, "Cases of HIV Infection and AIDS in the United States and Dependent Areas, by Race/Ethnicity, 2003–2007," *HIV/AIDS Surveillance Supplemental Report* 14(2009): 5.

49. American Cancer Society, *Facts and Figures, 2011* (Atlanta, GA: American Cancer Society, 2011).

50. American Cancer Society, *Cancer Facts and Figures for Hispanics/Latinos 2009–2011* (Atlanta, GA: American Cancer Society, 2011).

51. American Cancer Society, *Cancer Disparities: Key Statistics*. 2008. Available at: www.cancer.org/Cancer/news/Features/ cancer-disparities-key-statistics

52. National Center for Health Statistics, *Health, United States, 2009*, 240–241

53. U.S. Census Bureau, *Statistical Abstract of the United States, 2011* (Washington, D.C.: U.S. Government Printing Office, 2010).

54. Jiaquan Xu, Kenneth D. Kochanek, and Betzaida Tejada-Vera, "Deaths: Preliminary Data for 2007," *National Vital Statistics Reports* 58(April 19, 2009): 20.

55. "Youth Risk Behavior Surveillance—United States, 2007," *Morbidity and Mortality Weekly Report* 57(2008): 8.

56. Ibid.

57. United States Department of Labor, *Highlights of Women's Earnings in 2009*, (2010). Available at www.bls.gov/cps/ cpswom2009.pdf

58. J. J. Dowd and V. L. Bengston, "Aging in Minority Populations: An Examination of the Double Jeopardy Hypothesis." In *Aging, the Individual, and Society: Readings in Social Gerontology*, ed. J. S. Quadango (New York: St. Martin's Press, 1984).

59. National Coalition for the Homeless, "How Many People Experience Homelessness?" *NCH Fact Sheet* (2009): 2.

60. Ibid.

61. National Law Center for Homelessness and Poverty, "Homelessness and Poverty in America: Overview," 2010. www.nlchp.org/hapia.cfm

62. National Coalition for the Homeless, "Who Is Homeless?" *NCH Fact Sheet* (2009).

63. U.S. Conference of Mayors, *A Status Report on Hunger and Homelessness in America's Cities: A 23-City Survey,* December 2007, 18. Available at http://usmayors.org/HHSurvey2007/hhsurvey07.pdf

64. Marjorie Robertson, Natalie Harris, Nancy Fritz, Rebecca Noftsinger, and Pamela Fischer, "Rural Homelessness," *2007 National Symposium on Homelessness Research,* 2007, 10. Available at www.huduser.org/publications/pdf/p8.pdf

65. National Coalition for the Homeless, "Who Is Homeless?" *NCH Fact Sheet* (2009).

66. National Coalition for the Homeless. "Who Is Homeless?"

67. National Coalition for the Homeless, "Who Is Homeless?" 3.

68. National Law Center for Homelessness and Poverty, "Homelessness and Poverty in America."

69. U.S. Census Bureau, *Statistical Abstract of the United States, 2011* (Washington, D.C.: U.S. Government Printing Office, 2010), 52, 56.

70. National Institute of Mental Health, "Family Process and Social Networks." In *Basic Behavioral Science Research for Mental Health* (Washington, D.C.: National Institute of Mental Health, updated June 1, 1999). www.nimh.nih.gov/publicat/baschap6.cfm

71. Kersten Aumann and Ellen Galinsky, *National Study of the Changing Workforce, 2008: The State of Health in the American Workforce: Does Having an Effective Workplace Matter?* (Families and Work Institute, 2009). Available at: www.familiesandwork.org/site/research/reports/HealthReport.pdf

72. Marcie Pitt-Catsouphes, Michael A. Smyer, Christina Matz-Costa, and Katherine Kane, *The National Study Report: Phase II of The National Study of Business Strategy and Workforce,* 2007. Available at http://agingandwork.bc.edu/documents/RH04_NationalStudy_03-07_000.pdf

73. Office of Disease Prevention and Health Promotion, *Healthy People 2020.*

74. Federal Bureau of Investigation, *Hate Crime Statistics.* 2009. Available at: www2.fbi.gov/ucr/hc2009/victims.html.

75. M. Sadowski, "Sexual Minority Student Benefit from School-Based Support—Where It Exists," *Harvard Education Letter, Research Online* (September/October 2001). Available at: www.edletter.org/current/

76. D. M. Huebner, G. M. Rebchook, and S. M. Kegeles, "Experiences of Harassment, Discrimination, and Physical Violence Among Young Gay and Bisexual Men," *American Journal of Public Health* 94(2004): 1200–03.

77. R. M. Díaz, G. Ayala, E. Bein, J. Henne, and B. V. Marin, "The Impact of Homophobia, Poverty, and Racism on the Mental Health of Gay and Bisexual Latino Men: Findings from 3 US Cities," *American Journal of Public Health* 91(2001): 927–32.

78. J. S. Greenberg, C. E. Bruess, and S. W. C. Conklin, *Exploring the Dimensions of Human Sexuality,* 3rd ed. (Sudbury, MA: Jones and Bartlett, 2007), 452.

LAB ASSESSMENT 15.1

How Has Prejudice Affected Your Level of Stress?

Almost everyone has experienced prejudice. Some of us have been the victims of bias because of our skin color, others because of our sex, some because of our religion, and others because of our physical appearance. Maybe we have a disability that has resulted in us being the brunt of prejudice, or perhaps we have been disadvantaged because of our athletic ability or intellectual capacity. When we experience prejudiced behavior, our stress levels rise. Recalling the stress model presented in Chapter 5, the biased actions become the life situation that is perceived as distressing. In turn, we experience emotional arousal (e.g., anger), which leads to physiological arousal (e.g., increased muscle tension). The consequences could be the development of a psychosomatic illness or any of the other potential consequences described in Chapter 3.

Describe an instance when you experienced prejudice against you.

_____

_____

_____

_____

How did you react? What did you do?

_____

_____

_____

_____

What were the consequences you experienced? Think of physical, psychological, and social consequences.

_____

_____

_____

_____

Describe how you could have reacted in a more appropriate or healthier way.

_____

_____

_____

_____

The next time you experience prejudicial behavior, think of this exercise and try to react in a way that is healthier for you. You cannot control the other person, but you can always control your reaction to the behavior of that other person. As you have learned throughout this book, no one forces you to perceive life situations as distressing. Instead, you could laugh at the stupidity of the biased person, or pray for him or her. Even if that does not change that person, it will prevent you from getting ill over it.

LAB ASSESSMENT 15.2

What Biases Do You Possess?

Although we may profess we are unbiased, and we would prefer to be so, all of us have our prejudices. Some of us feel uncomfortable with people who are different from us. As a result, we hang around those who are more like we are. If you doubt the truth of this statement, think of who eats lunch together in a school cafeteria. Do the popular kids sit together? Do different ethnic groups congregate together? Which socioeconomic groups socialize with one another, or join the same organizations? It is when this discomfort hurtfully excludes others that it becomes especially problematic.

When have you acted in a prejudicial way?

_____

_____

_____

_____

How do you feel now about having acted that way?

_____

_____

_____

_____

How would you prefer to act if a similar situation presents itself in the future?

_____

_____

_____

_____

If you see someone else behaving in a biased fashion, would you do something about that? If not, why not? If you would do something, what would that be?

_____

_____

_____

_____

If we admit to our own biases, we will be more likely to recognize them when they crop up and prevent them from resulting in a prejudiced behavior toward someone else. In that case, we will have prevented both the other person and ourselves from experiencing a stressful response.

LAB ASSESSMENT 15.3

How Well Do You Know Diverse Groups and Individuals?

Studies show that college students tend to hang out with other students who are similar to themselves. With most campuses having such a diverse group of students, it would be unfortunate to miss out on the opportunity to know, understand, and be comfortable with people who are different from yourself. To assist with that task, identify below a group on campus with which you have little contact and whom you would like to know better. This may be a gay fraternity or organization, or a racial group, an ethnic group, or a religious organization.

Group: _____

Next, identify what you would like to know about this group and its members by listing questions you want to ask:

1. _____

2. _____

3. _____

4. _____

5. _____

Then arrange to meet with an officer of this group to whom you can explain your intent. Ask if you can attend a meeting of the group and/or interview group members. Find out if the group keeps minutes of their meetings and, if so, whether you can read the minutes from the past year. Make sure that these and other activities answer the questions you listed above.

Analysis

What did you learn about this group that you did not know beforehand?

_____

_____

_____

_____

_____

Which stereotypes about this group were verified and which were not?

_____

_____

_____

_____

_____

How have your thoughts, beliefs, and feelings about this group been reinforced or changed?

_____

_____

_____

_____

You might consider sharing the answers to the questions above with the group. In that way, this Lab Assessment will serve not only as an educational tool for you but also for the group.

Specific Applications

16 Occupational Stress

It was over dinner in a seafood restaurant with fishnets and lobster cages on the walls that my father-in-law was bemoaning his choice of professions. Witnessed by a stuffed marlin looking at us from across the room, he was expressing his envy of his physician friends who "made $300,000 a year, worked three days a week, and played golf the rest of the time." I was surprised to hear him speak this way because he always seemed to me to be excited about his law practice and proud that he was a second-generation attorney in business with his son. "If I had to do it all over again, I'd be a physician," he said as his eyes wandered upward and his mind visualized how delightful that kind of life would have been. When he lowered his eyes, they fell upon me and the inevitable question fell from his lips. "What would you be if you had to do it all over again?" Well, that was some time ago. Even after Ralph retired, he still looked back, wondering how life might have been. In spite of the years that have passed, my answer to his question remains the same. "I'd do just what I am doing now." Upon some study I learned that my answer is not uncommon among my fellow college professors. It seems that "professoring" is consistently reported to be a satisfying profession by its practitioners. Being a professor is accompanied by certain traits associated with low-stress occupations. This chapter will discuss these characteristics in particular and occupational stress in general.

By the way, what would you do if you could start all over?

What Is Occupational Stress?

occupational stress
The combination of sources of stress at work, individual characteristics, and extraorganizational stressors.

Occupational stress is an extremely difficult construct to define. Obviously, it is stress on the job, but stress on the job occurs in a person. Here is where we run into problems because any worker brings to the job a level of predisposition to be stressed. One way to depict the complexity of occupational stress is shown in Figure 16.1.

We shall soon consider some of the sources of work stress in detail. For now, note that several sources of occupational stress exist. Some of these stressors are intrinsic to the job. Some are related to the employee's role within the organization, some to career development, some to relationships at work, and some to the structure and climate of the organization.

Interacting with these work stressors are the individual's characteristics. These are brought to the workplace rather than being a function of it, but they are important ingredients in occupational stress, nevertheless. These characteristics include the worker's levels of anxiety and neuroticism, tolerance of ambiguity, and Type A behavior pattern.

Added to this brew are the sources of stress that come from outside the workplace and outside the worker. These extraorganizational sources of stress stem from family problems, life crises, financial matters, and environmental factors. Mix it all up and out come symptoms of occupational health problems that may develop into full-blown disease.

This model of occupational stress, as complex as it appears, is simplified by limiting the examples of stress at work, individual characteristics, and extraorganizational

Time pressure at work can make us so tense we can become ill.

Figure 16.1 Occupational stress model.

Source: Cary L. Cooper and Judi Marshall, "Occupational Sources of Stress: A Review of the Literature Relating to Coronary Heart Disease and Mental Ill Health," in *Journal of Occupational Psychology* 49(1976) 11–28. Reproduced with permission of Blackwell Publishing Ltd.

sources of stress. Many others could be included. Further, the interaction of these three factors is depicted as evenly weighted. In actuality, different workplaces have different levels of intrinsic job stressors and career development stressors. Different workers have different levels of anxiety and tolerances of ambiguity, and different workers experience different amounts of family and financial problems. To assume that all of these ingredients can be quantified is naive.

Another way of looking at occupational stress utilizes the Occupational Stress Evaluation Grid.[1] Although developed in 1977, the grid is still a good way to understand occupational stress and stressors. This grid, presented in Table 16.1, recognizes that occupational stressors occur in different contexts—sociocultural, organizational, work setting, interpersonal, psychological, biological, and physical/ environmental. The grid identifies formal and informal means of intervening for each of these levels of stressors. Like the model of occupational stress presented in Figure 16.1, the Occupational Stress Evaluation Grid recognizes occupational stress to be a more complex construct than merely inclusive of some sources of stress at work.

Occupational Stress Cycle

Before proceeding, answer the questions in Lab 16.1 (at the end of this chapter) to get a better handle on occupational stress. If you are presently employed, answer these questions as they relate to your job. If you are not now working but have worked, answer these questions as they relate to your last job. If you have never worked, write me immediately to let me know your secret. In the meantime, answer these questions as you think they relate to a loved one who is presently working.

Table 16.1 Occupational Stress Evaluation Grid

Context	Stressors	Interventions Formal	Informal
Sociocultural	Racism, sexism Ecological shifts Economic downturns Political changes Military crises	Elections Lobbying/political action Political changes Trade associations	Grass roots organizing Petitions Demonstrations Migration Spouse employment
Organizational	Hiring policies Plant closings Layoffs, relocation Automation, market shifts, retraining Organizational priorities	Corporate decision Reorganization New management model Management consultant (in-service/retraining)	Social activities Contests, incentives Manager involvement and ties with workers Continuing education Moonlighting
Work setting	Task (time, speed, autonomy, creativity) Supervision Coworkers Ergonomics Participation in decision making	Supervisor meetings Health/safety meetings Union grievance Employee involvement Quality circles Job redesign In-service training	Slow down/speed up Redefine tasks Support of other workers Sabotage, theft Quit, change jobs
Interpersonal	Divorce, separation, marital discord Conflict, family/friend Death, illness in family Intergenerational conflict Legal/financial difficulties Early parenthood	Legal/financial services Leave of absence Counseling, psychotherapy Insurance plans Family therapy Loans/credit unions Day care	Seek social support/advice Seek legal/financial assistance Self-help groups Vacation/sick days Child care
Psychological	Neurosis, mental illness Disturbance of affect, cognition, or behavior Ineffective coping skills Poor self-image Poor communication Addictive behavior	Employee assistance (referral/in house) Counseling, psychotherapy Medication Supervisory training Stress management workshop	Seek support from friends, family, church Self-help groups/books Self-medication Recreation, leisure Sexual activity "Mental health" days
Biological	Disease, disability Sleep, appetite disturbance Chemical dependency Biochemical imbalance Pregnancy	Preplacement screening Counseling Medical treatment Health education Employee assistance Maternity leave	Change sleep/wake habits Bag lunch Self-medication Cosmetics Diets, exercise Consult physician
Physical/environmental	Poor air, climate Noise exposure Toxic substance exposure Poor lighting Radiation exposure Poor equipment design Bad architecture	Protective clothing/equipment Climate control Health/safety committee Interior decoration Muzak Union grievance	Own equipment, decoration Walkman, radio Consult personal physician Letters of complaint

Source: M. J. Smith et al., "A Review of NIOSH Psychological Stress Research—1977," *NIOSH Proceedings of Occupational Stress Conference* (Cincinnati, OH: National Institute of Occupational Health and Safety, March 1978), 27–28.

Now, before you get to Lab 16.1, I need to make one point. When I talk with groups of people about occupational stress, inevitably a woman raises her hand to say she's never worked and therefore can't answer these questions. Upon further investigation, we find she worked very hard but never received an outright salary. She was a mother, laundered, cleaned, arranged car pools, and counseled. If you are a woman or a man and work at home, answer these questions for that occupation.

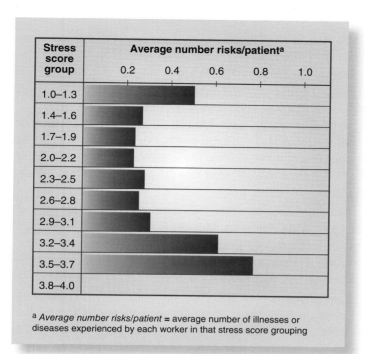

Figure 16.2

Percentage distribution of stress scores.

Stress score group	Average number risks/patient[a]				
	0.2	0.4	0.6	0.8	1.0
1.0–1.3					
1.4–1.6					
1.7–1.9					
2.0–2.2					
2.3–2.5					
2.6–2.8					
2.9–3.1					
3.2–3.4					
3.5–3.7					
3.8–4.0					

[a] *Average number risks/patient* = average number of illnesses or diseases experienced by each worker in that stress score grouping

Figure 16.2 depicts the relationship between the scores on Lab 16.1 and the incidence of disease when 1,540 workers were studied.[2] The expectation that a large amount of stress would be associated with a greater incidence of disease was supported. However, a small amount of stress was also associated with a greater incidence of disease. In other words, there was an optimal amount of stress (not too little and not too much) that was found to be healthiest. Several hypotheses can be offered to explain this finding. However, the one I think most plausible is that low scores on this instrument mean these respondents felt underutilized and unneeded. They felt little responsibility and believed their jobs were not very important. They could easily be replaced. Believing this created a great deal of stress rather than a little, but this type of stress was not measured by the scale. Further support for this interpretation can be found later in this chapter.

Why Is Occupational Stress of Concern?

One reason occupational stress receives so much attention is that businesses are genuinely beginning to care about employee welfare. You don't buy that? Well, how about this? Work stress is costing businesses billions of dollars. Sounds more plausible, doesn't it?

The costs of occupational stress to the organizations are primarily related to sickness and absenteeism, reduced productivity, worker replacement costs and training, and additional retirement costs. There may be further costs due to damage in production or equipment, costs in connection with grievance and litigation, and a potential public loss of goodwill toward the organization.

The costs of occupational stress to society are related to medical costs and possible hospitalization, benefits and Social Security costs in connection with premature retirement, as well as potential loss of productive workers. Job stress is estimated to cost American companies more than $300 billion a year in health costs, absenteeism, and poor performance.[3]

Employees trained over a long period of time, at great cost, may break down when stressed on the job. They may make poor decisions, miss days of work, begin abusing alcohol and other drugs, or die and have to be replaced by other workers who need training. All of this is costly.

In the 2007 Unscheduled Absence Survey, absences attributed to stress tripled between 1995 (6 percent) and 2007(13 percent).[4] In addition, absenteeism attributed to "entitlement mentality" (workers call in sick but are not). In 2007, more than 66 percent of the time when workers called in "sick," they were not sick.

Stress is being encountered at ever-increasing rates. Of the stress Americans experience, one study found 82 percent complained that work was their biggest source of stress.[5] Thirty-five percent of American workers also reported their jobs negatively affected their physical or emotional well-being.[6] In 2007, human resources managers were asked, "Do you believe your workforce is stressed?" They responded that 45 percent of their employees had high levels of stress, 42 percent had constant but manageable stress levels, and 13 percent had some stress. When workers were asked the same question, 60 percent stated they had high levels of stress, with extreme fatigue and a sense that they were out of control. Another third responded that they had constant but manageable stress levels. Only 7 percent reported they had low stress levels.[7] Recognizing occupational stress to be more than just an American phenomenon, the World Health Organization considered it to be "the twentieth century disease" indicating it was prevalent in almost every occupation around the world and had become a "global epidemic."

To make matters worse, American workers take fewer vacation days than do workers in other developed countries. As shown in Table 16.2, American workers receive an average of 13 vacation days a year. That is significantly less than in other developed countries. To make matters worse, each year 34 percent of Americans do not take all of the vacation days they earn. On average, they give back three vacation days. Since 40 percent of American workers regularly work more than

	United States	Great Britain	France	Germany	Spain
Number of Vacation Days Received	13	26	38	27	30
Average Number of Vacation Days Each Employed Person Gives Back	3	2	2	2	3
Percentage of Workers Who Do Not Take All of Their Vacation Days	34%	21%	22%	24%	23%
Total Estimated Vacation Days Given Back Each Year	436 Million				
Total Estimated Value of Vacation Days Given Back	$63.33 Billion				

Table 16.2
Vacation Days Earned and Used

Source: Expedia, 2009 *International Vacation Deprivation Survey Results* (2009). Available at http://media.expedia.com/media/content/expus/graphics/promos/vacations/Expedia_International_Vacation_Deprivation_Survey_2009.pdf

40 hours a week, they really need these vacation days. Then, when they do take vacation, 24 percent check their work voice and e-mail, and one-fourth have trouble coping with stress from work at some point during their vacations.[8] Furthermore, while vacationing, 43 percent of American workers do at least some work, using their laptops (41 percent), cellular phones (30 percent), personal computers (10 percent), or PDAs (7 percent).[9] Researchers argue that the high value placed on hard work and productivity in the United States and a strong work ethic have led to this unfortunate vacation-time disparity.[10]

Not the least of the factors giving rise to the tremendous increase in occupational stress is the development of technological advances. Although many Americans enjoy the fact that they are never out of reach—given their cell phones, smartphones, fax machines, laptop and iPad, e-mail addresses, and beepers and pagers—being "always on call" can be quite stressful in itself. The extent of this problem is evident in the results of a Gallup poll that found that, on average, workers receive 190 messages a day, by telephone, e-mail, voicemail, interoffice mail, regular mail, fax, Post-it notes, phone message slips, pager, overnight courier, and cell phone[11]—and this was in 1998! Just imagine what the sitvation is like today.

High-Stress Jobs

Researcher Robert Karasek and colleagues studied job stress and found the most stressful jobs are those that allow for very little decision making yet place a high psychological demand on the worker. Examples of psychological demands are having to work quickly and having a huge workload. Is the occupation you're training for one that expects a lot of you but does not allow you to make enough decisions about how you'll function on the job? If so, perhaps you want to reconsider whether you want to experience the stress and strain that job might entail.

Source: Robert A. Karasek, et al., "Job Characteristics in Relation to the Prevalence of Myocardial Infarction in the U.S. Health Examination Survey (HES) and the Health and Nutrition Examination Survey (HANES)," *American Journal of Public Health* 78(1988): 910–18.

Stress is a prevalent concern for American workers. The National Institute for Occupational Safety and Health (NIOSH) reports that 40 percent of employees believe their jobs are *very* or *extremely* stressful and at least 26 percent of employees feel burned out. Furthermore, the American Psychological Association reports that job stress costs U.S. companies $300 billion a year in absenteeism, productivity loss, turnover, and health care costs. (See Figure 16.3.)

Stress is also of concern in other parts of the world. A study in Europe found that work stress was so prevalent as to be a major problem. When the European Foundation for the Improvement of Living and Working Conditions conducted its Second European Survey they found that one in four workers felt stressed by work, one in five felt fatigue, and one in eight suffered from headaches.

The survey also found that work stress is experienced somewhat differently in different countries. For example, about 50 percent of Dutch workers reported a high work pace. In England, about 67 percent of workers reported that stress was the most serious problem in their working lives. Furthermore, British doctors and nurses believed stress was increasing and 20 percent had considered suicide. English teachers also experience a great deal of stress. More than half of them have considered leaving the teaching profession. Swedish teachers feel similarly. In fact, 75 percent of Swedish teachers considered the psychological demands of their jobs extremely high.

The lesson to be learned by the Second European Survey is that work stress is a problem throughout the world, one that needs immediate attention and alleviation if the health and well-being of our workforce is to be protected.

Sources: National Institute for Occupational Safety and Health, *Stressed at Work* (Washington, D.C.: National Institute for Occupational Safety and Health, 2006).
American Psychological Association, *Why Focus on Employee Health and Well-being?* 2006. Available at www.phwa.org/background
"More Than One Worker in Four Feels Stressed by Work," *Euro Review on Research in Health and Safety at Work,* 1997.

Figure 16.3

Increased risk as a result of stressful workplaces.[a]

[a]"Stressful workplaces" are defined as those with *high demand and low control* or *high effort and low reward.*

Source: Adapted from *The Business Case for a Healthy Workplace,* 2011 with permission of Workplace Safety & Prevention Services, Mississauga, Canada.

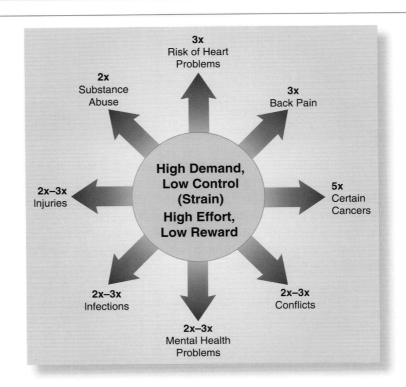

Gender and Occupational Stress

Researchers have begun to identify sources of stress particularly experienced by women: career blocks, sexual harassment, male-dominated organizational structures and climates, performance pressure, gender stereotyping, isolation, and lack of role models. One researcher found women reported job stress related to opportunities for personal development, rates of pay, keeping up with new ideas, business travel, and the accumulative effect of minor tasks.[12] One study of managers found that females tended to experience stressors emotionally.[13] Their stress was due to pressure to meet expectations to be responsible for people both inside and outside the home. By contrast, males tended to focus on themselves and regard other things as beyond their control.

Female workers take on more of the household work, and the accompanying stress, than do male workers. However, between 1992 and 2008, some of these practices have changed. Whereas in 1992, only 40 percent of married men stated they shared housecleaning chores equally with their spouses, by 2008, 53 percent stated they did. And yet, as shown in Table 16.3, women did not perceive a significant change between 1992 and 2008 in who did the housecleaning. In terms of cooking, in 1992, 34 percent of married men stated they shared equally in the responsibility for cooking, whereas in 2008, 55 percent stated they did. As with housecleaning, there is a discrepancy between women's and men's perceptions. Table 16.3 shows that although women do agree that men have taken on more responsibility for cooking, men's and women's perceptions differ on how much additional responsibility. Likewise for responsibility for child care. As noted in a study by the Family and Work Institute,

> . . . despite changes in the behavior of married men, employed married women still spend significantly more time than their husbands doing chores and caring for children, which is to say they are much more likely than their husbands to work "two shifts"—one at their paid job and one at home.[14]

Table 16.3 Division of Family Household Work: Housecleaning, Cooking, and Child Care

Gender	Who Takes Responsibility for Cleaning?	1992	2008
Men	I do or share equally	40%	53%
	My spouse/partner does	51	36
	Others do	9	10
Women	I do	73	71
	My spouse/partner does or shares equally	18	21
	Others do	9	8
Gender	**Who Takes Responsibility for Cooking?**	**1992**	**2008**
Men	I do or share equally	34%	55%
	My spouse/partner does	56	35
	Others do	9	7
Women	I do	75	67
	My spouse/partner does or shares equally	15	26
	Others do	9	6
Gender	**Who Takes Responsibility for Child Care?**	**1992**	**2008**
Men	I do or share equally	41%	49%
	My spouse/partner does	58	46
	Others do	1	4
Women	I do	73	66
	My spouse/partner does or shares equally	21	30
	Others do	6	4

Source: Families and Work Institute, *National Study of the Changing Workforce, 1992, 2008.*

And single moms experience even more distress without a spouse to help with household chores and childrearing. Furthermore, single mothers are working five more hours a week—a total of forty-four hours a week—than were single mothers in 1977.[15]

Women also tend to cope with occupational stressors differently than do men. Women request[16] and receive more social support[17,18] than men. They also use social support to cope with occupational stressors more than do men.[19] Some researchers believe that women have been socialized to be more nurturing and emotionally involved than men, and that encourages them to care about people, express their emotions, and seek more social support,[20] whereas men have been socialized to develop action skills such as risk-taking, assertiveness, and calmness in the face of danger.[21]

Many married and employed women with substantial household responsibilities intentionally limit their career aspirations and purposefully reduce their involvement in work, in comparison with their male counterparts.[22] The occupational stress that male workers experience has been found to be related to their concerns about the power structure within the organization that employs them. Female workers, in contrast, experience occupational stress when there is a conflict between job requirements and family responsibilities.[23]

Stress management experts recommend that work organizations develop a culture that employees perceive to be supportive of their efforts to balance their career and family lives.[24] Many companies are trying to do so. Those that are recognized for these efforts—an article listed the top ten healthiest companies for women[25]—are well positioned to recruit and retain top-notch workers of both genders.

Disease and Occupational Stress

The link between occupational stress and disease is a difficult one to prove since this relationship is complicated by the workers' characteristics and stressors outside of the workplace. There is, however, evidence that supports the conclusion that occupational stress is related to illness and disease. This evidence falls into two categories: evidence of the physiological effects of occupational stress and evidence of disease states associated with occupational stress.

Physiological Effects

Several studies have shown that physiological arousal accompanies occupational stress. For example, several investigators have found the work environment associated with hypertension,[26,27] serum cholesterol,[28] cardiovascular disease,[29,30] musculoskeletal disorders,[31] development of the common cold,[32] injury and illness,[33] decreased effectiveness of the immunological system,[34,35] and ingestion of alcohol.[36]

An interesting finding is that the amount of work does not seem as critical to health as the control the worker has over the work rate or related work processes. For example, in a classical study, Karasak and colleagues found that workers in jobs with higher workload and pacing demands, and very little control of these demands, have increased rates of coronary heart disease and higher blood pressure than workers in jobs not so characterized.[37,38]

Disease States

Many studies have implicated occupational stress in the development of illness and disease. Given the increase in blood pressure, serum cholesterol, catecholamines,

When a job demands too much work in too little time, stress can develop.

and plasma fibrinogen, it should be no surprise to learn that occupational stress is related to coronary heart disease.[39, 40] And it is related to death from heart disease.[41] It is also associated with obesity,[42] probably because people eat as a way of relieving stress at work. Those workers experiencing occupational stress report low levels of job satisfaction and more psychosomatic symptoms,[43, 44] as well as feelings of anger and alienation.[45, 46]

The impact of work stress can be so devastating that researchers find higher rates of heart attacks on Mondays than on any other day of the week, and the fewest heart attacks on Fridays (TGIF).[47] Why ruin the weekend? Other researchers found that heart attacks occur most often during holidays, such as New Year's, and attribute a good portion of that to stress surrounding those occasions.[48]

Psychological Effects

Occupational stress also has consequences for psychological health. Some occupational stressors can result in low self-confidence, increased job tension, and lower job satisfaction.[49] A summary of 96 studies of the psychological effects of occupational stress found that absenteeism and poor job performance are related to stress on the job.[50] In addition, job stress has been found to lead to depression and anxiety.[51]

Occupational Stressors

Workers report more occupational stress when work objectives are unclear, when they have conflicting demands placed upon them, when they have too little or too much to do, when they have little input into decisions that affect them, and when they are responsible for other workers' professional development.

Two Alternative Occupational Stress Models

One way of conceptualizing work stress is the *demand-control* model described in this chapter. The demand-control model conceives of stress as the result of high job demands and low job control. You can imagine how frustrating, and stressful, it would be to be expected to be highly productive while at the same time not being able to decide how to do that. In a sense, the manner in which you are evaluated (meeting the high job demands) depends on factors beyond your control. How unfair that must feel!

Another way of conceptualizing work stress is the *effort-reward imbalance* model. The effort-reward imbalance model conceives of work stress as a function of too great a work effort required to do the job accompanied by low reward for a job well done. This model considers such effort as high workload on one end of the equation and such rewards as salary, esteem, and occupational status on the other. According to the effort-reward imbalance model, "demanding tasks under insecure conditions, lack of promotion, and low wages compared to qualifications may in the long run threaten workers' health and well-being."[a]

Perhaps occupational stress is a combination of the factors included in each of these models. High work demand, low job control, and lack of accompanying reward are all probably factors that contribute to work stress.

[a]"Chronic Load Is Dangerous for Health and Well-Being," *Euro Review on Research in Health and Safety at Work,* 1997, 13.

Figure 16.4

The effect of participation on work-related criteria measures.

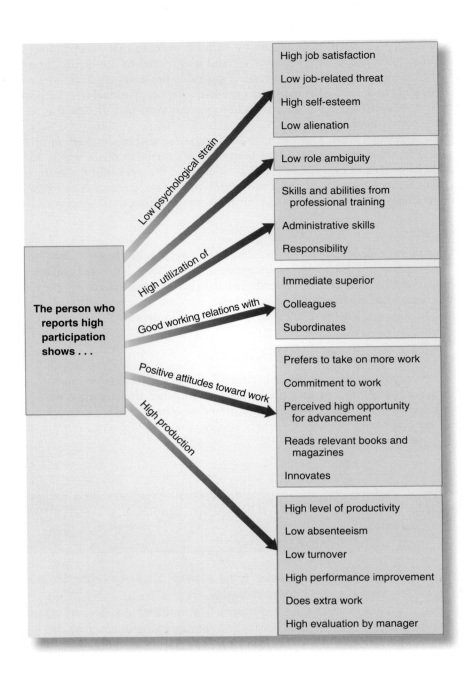

Lack of Participation

One of the factors of the workplace and of the organization's modus operandi that is related to stress is the degree of participation. Workers' perceptions of the degree of their participation in the decision-making process, the degree to which they are consulted on issues affecting the organization, and their involvement in establishing rules of behavior at work have proved to be related to job satisfaction, job-related feelings of threat, and feelings of self-esteem.[52,53] And these variables can affect workers' health. Figure 16.4 depicts the effects of high participation on the job. Low participation can be expected to have the opposite effect.

Role Problems

A clear sense of your role in an organization and a sense that you can "play the part" are important in keeping stress at a minimum. A variety of role-related problems may arise for workers who lack these feelings.[54]

Figure 16.5

Role conflict: which demands to meet?

Role Overload

When job demands are so great that the worker feels an inability to cope, stress will develop. You can imagine the feeling of having too much to do in too little time.

Role Insufficiency

When workers lack the training, education, skills, or experience to accomplish the job, they feel stressed. A poor fit between workers' talents and the organization's expectations creates disharmony and dissatisfaction.

Role Ambiguity

When aspects of the job and workplace are unclear, frustration and stress are likely to develop. Workers should know the criteria for career advancement, the priorities of the organization, and generally what is expected of them.

Role Conflict

Sometimes workers get caught in a bind. Two supervisors each expect something different. The worker may be faced with conflicting demands (see Figure 16.5). This is the "damned if you do, damned if you don't" dilemma. Such a situation is a factor in occupational stress.

Job Dissatisfaction

The factors that are typically thought related to dissatisfaction on the job are salary and conditions of the workplace (e.g., noise, poor lighting, poor ventilation, crowding, etc.). However, even if workers were paid well and worked in hygienic conditions, they might still be dissatisfied. A class of work-related factors, called **motivational factors,** can affect job satisfaction. These factors include the degree of stimulating tasks involved, the amount of recognition for jobs done well, relationships with fellow workers, and the amount of encouragement to take on responsibility (see Figure 16.6, which is based on Maslow's Hierarchy of Needs). Unfortunately, many unions ignore these factors when negotiating a contract. Obviously, some of these motivational factors would be difficult to ensure in writing. They're important enough, however, to try for.

motivational factors
Variables associated with job satisfaction; includes working on stimulating tasks, being recognized for work well done, and positive relationships with work colleagues.

Figure 16.6

Human needs and their job-related satisfiers.

Self-realization needs	Job-related satisfiers
Reaching your potential Independence Creativity Self-expression	Involvement in planning your work Freedom to make decisions affecting work Creative work to perform Opportunities for growth and development
Esteem needs	**Job-related satisfiers**
Responsibility Self-respect Recognition Sense of accomplishment	Status symbols Merit awards Challenging work Sharing in decisions Opportunity for advancement
Social needs	**Job-related satisfiers**
Companionship Acceptance Love and affection Group membership	Opportunities for interaction with others Team spirit Friendly coworkers
Safety needs	**Job-related satisfiers**
Security for self and possessions Avoidance of risks Avoidance of harm Avoidance of pain	Safe working conditions Seniority Fringe benefits Proper supervision Sound company policies, programs, and practices
Physical needs	**Job-related satisfiers**
Food Clothing Shelter Comfort Self-preservation	Pleasant working conditions Adequate wage or salary Rest periods Labor-saving devices Efficient work methods

Job satisfaction is important if for no other reason than that it is associated with higher levels of job performance, lower levels of absenteeism, less tardiness, less turnover, and increased life satisfaction.[55] And yet, job satisfaction has declined significantly in recent years. In 2007, the Conference Board[56] reported that fewer than half of Americans are satisfied with their jobs, down from 61 percent 20 years ago. Fewer than 30 percent expressed contentment with their workload and with their work/life balance. Research studies have found that low levels of job demands (for example, work load) and high levels of job control (for example, autonomy) are associated with job satisfaction.[57,58] Likewise, high job demand and low control are associated with low job satisfaction. Given the amount of time people spend at work and on work-related activities, it is unfortunate so many are not satisfied with their jobs. This spills over into their home lives and leads to increased stress.

The Work Environment

In some places of work, hazards create stress. Dangerous tasks or work settings, toxic chemicals, high noise levels, dust, overcooling, unpleasant odors, and other stressful factors can lead to illness or disease. An interesting source you might want to consult if you are interested in this aspect of occupational stress is a book entitled *Monitoring for Health Hazards at Work*.[59]

The Workaholic

Too much work, even if you enjoy it, can itself be an occupational stressor. Some people either enjoy their work so much or find so little pleasure in their nonworking lives that they immerse themselves in their jobs. Their jobs consume them. If you've ever wondered whether you're a **workaholic**—or if you think you might be working or living with one—complete Lab 16.2 at the end of this chapter and see.

One cause of workaholism is a matter of *identity*. Too many people identify more with their roles as workers than with their roles as individual persons. Are you a person who happens to be a student, or are you a student who happens to be a person? The answer to this question determines your priorities and how you allocate your time. The self-worth of some workers is a function of what they produce. Some professors may judge their self-worth by how many articles they publish or by how many awards they receive. Do you judge yourself by your grades or by the number of credits you have accumulated? Or do you consider what kind of a friend you are or how much you contribute to your family and community? A strong personal identity offers the best way to prevent workaholism and other occupational stressors from negatively impacting on your life.

Workaholism has serious health consequences. A variety of health problems including exhaustion, anxiety, and high blood pressure are attributed to workaholism. Longer work hours also increase chances of weight gain, smoking, alcohol consumption, high blood pressure, and cardiovascular disease. Furthermore, workaholics are less likely to rate themselves as very satisfied with their health.[60] Another study found workaholism has a major effect on marital cohesion.[61]

To combat workaholism, try these tips:

1. Focus on the work you most love doing, and try to find ways to stop doing, delegate, or minimize the parts of your work you dislike.

2. Ask yourself, "What work would I do for free?" Then try to evolve your work in that direction.

3. Use your time; don't let it use you. Decide how much time you want to spend working; then limit your work time accordingly. For example, you might arrange to stop working at 5:30 p.m. by making a commitment to go running with a friend every workday at 5:45. Arrangements like these help workaholics return to feeling more refreshed—and more productive.

4. Build friendships at work. Arrange to spend quality time with coworkers.

5. Schedule open time into your work life. If, for instance, you now schedule work-related appointments every 30 minutes, try to evolve toward scheduling them every 45 minutes instead.

6. Learn to say no to new demands on your time. If this is difficult, say that you'd like some time to think about it; then say no later.

7. Decorate your workplace to create an environment that pleases you. You deserve it.

workaholic
Immersing oneself excessively in work at the expense of nonwork activities.

We each need time alone. A chance to get away and relax can be rejuvenating. When did you last sit and do nothing?

8. Try to stay in touch with the positive aspects of your work: the pleasure of doing work that fulfills you, the freedom, the opportunity to be of service to others, or other aspects of your work you find rewarding.

9. Heavy involvement in work usually entitles you to have a good deal to say about the way you work. How might you change or restructure your work to make it feel more fulfilling?

In addition to these suggestions, remember that the workaholic enjoys work and therefore might not notice the harm it is doing. Family members often suffer more than the workaholic. Time is taken away from them and family responsibilities accrue to them because of the workaholic's work style. To intervene between workaholism and poor family health, time should be scheduled for family activities that will get the workaholic away from the telephone, the computer, and job commitments. Hiking and backpacking are useful for this purpose.

Burnout

burnout
An adverse stress reaction to work with psychological, psychophysiological, and behavioral components.

Too much work or frequent frustration at work can lead to a syndrome of physical and emotional exhaustion. This syndrome is called **burnout.** Burnout is a prolonged response to chronic emotional and interpersonal stressors on the job and includes three dimensions: emotional exhaustion, depersonalization, and lack of personal accomplishment.[62] *Emotional exhaustion* refers to feeling emotionally depleted and tired. *Depersonalization* refers to feeling detached from the work and worksite. And *lack of personal accomplishment* refers to feeling incompetent and lacking achievement at work. One of the culprits in the development of burnout is workaholism. In fact, some experts believe workaholics are addicted to work, as are drug addicts to drugs and cigarette smokers to tobacco.[63] This addiction results in their working excessively, ignoring other aspects of their lives, and eventually burnout. There is also evidence that high job demands (for example, work overload and time pressures) and lack of resources to meet those demands are antecedents to burnout.[64] Other factors related to burnout are lack of control at work, insufficient reward, breakdown of the work community, and absence of fairness (that is, a lack of trust, openness, and respect at work). The symptoms of burnout include:

1. *Diminished sense of humor:* inability to laugh at daily, on-the-job situations.

2. *Skipping rest and food breaks:* continually having no time for coffee or lunch breaks to restore stamina.

3. *Increased overtime and no vacation:* indispensable to the organization; reluctant to say *no* to working on scheduled off-days.

4. *Increased physical complaints:* fatigue, irritability, muscle tension, stomach upset, and susceptibility to illness.

5. *Social withdrawal:* pulling away from coworkers, peers, family members.

6. *Changed job performance:* increased absenteeism, tardiness, use of sick leave, and decreased efficiency or productivity.

7. *Self-medication:* increased use of alcohol, tranquilizers, and other mood-altering drugs.

8. *Internal changes:* emotional exhaustion, loss of self-esteem, depression, frustration, and a "trapped" feeling.

Complete Lab 16.3 at the end of this chapter to determine if you are experiencing burnout.

A different way of looking at how burnout develops involves a progressive five-stage approach:

Stage one (the honeymoon). At this stage, the worker is usually satisfied with the job and the tasks involved and remains enthusiastic toward the work. However, as this stage continues, the tasks become unenjoyable and the worker loses energy.

Stage two (fuel shortage). At this stage, fatigue sets in, and the worker may respond by abusing drugs. Difficulty sleeping is another symptom of this stage.

Stage three (chronic symptoms). At this stage, overwork leads to physical effects that include constant exhaustion and susceptibility to disease and psychological effects that include acute anger and feelings of depression.

Stage four (crisis). At this stage, actual illness can develop that results in the worker not being able to attend to the job. Relationships at home may also be affected due to a sense of pessimism, self-doubt, or obsession with problems.

Stage five (hitting the wall). At this stage, the physical and psychological problems can become severe enough to cause illness that is life threatening. The worker now has so many problems at work that his or her career is actually threatened.

What can one do about burnout? One expert suggests the following:

1. *"What do I work for?"* List all things—material and abstract—that you get out of your job. Identify your motivations, the value and meaning of your job.

2. *"I really want to do that."* List all activities you like and rank them in order of importance. Then note the last time you engaged in each.

3. *Create a support group.* Friends or coworkers meet on a regular basis.

4. *Start a physical self-care program.* Include exercise, nutrition, and elimination of destructive habits such as smoking.

5. *Start a psychological self-care program.* Include training in relaxation, negotiation, time management, and assertiveness.

6. *Do something silly every day.* Roller skate, play tiddlywinks, blow bubbles, or make a funny face. Relax, smile, and avoid taking yourself too seriously.[65]

Have you had it with school? With work? Are you near burnout? If so, will you do something about it? You're in control of yourself and your feelings. You can exercise this control. You don't have to suffer from burnout if you choose not to.

Women and Work Outside the Home

Women in the workplace experience some unique stressors. For example, they do not make as much money as men do, and they are more likely to be subjected to sexual harassment.

Although the work women do inside the home may be as important as (or more important than) the work they do outside, this section focuses on outside work.

Before proceeding, it may be interesting to see how much you know about women's economic roles. Decide which of the following statements are true and which are false:

1. Women get paid the same amount of money as men when they do the same job.
2. Women get paid the same amount of money as men when they have a comparable educational level.
3. Men are sexually harassed on the job about as often as are women.
4. Traditionally female occupations have become inundated with many males.
5. Women in racial, ethnic, and other minority groups have salaries comparable to those of minority men.

If you answered that all five statements are false, you get an honorary membership in the Burbank Friends of Truth Museum. If you answered that all are true, you get a stuffed male chauvinist pig for Christmas or Chanukah.

Statistics clearly demonstrate women are disadvantaged in the world of work, minority women particularly so. They make less money than their male counterparts, even when they perform similar jobs and have similar educational backgrounds. As though that weren't enough of an insult, women are subjected to sexual harassment and sexual discrimination at work to a much greater extent than are men.

Types of Jobs and Wages

Although a large number of women are working outside the home (72 percent),[66] they are still predominantly employed in traditional women's roles. Preschool and kindergarten teachers, teacher assistants, registered and LPN nurses, dental hygienists, dental assistants, medical assistants, maids and housekeeping cleaners, hairdressers, child care workers, bookkeepers, receptionists, secretaries, and typists or word processors are occupations still made up of more than 90 percent women.[67]

Just as stressful is the fact that women earn less than men in almost all job categories and at all ages. This discrepancy holds up even in comparisons of men and women with the same levels of education. In 2009, the weekly median earnings of females was $657 compared to $819 for males. The annual median earnings of female workers in management, business, and financial occupations was $46,039, whereas it was $65,278 for men in these occupations. For professionals, the annual median earnings of females was $38,649 and of male professionals, $60,123. Even in the traditional female service occupations, females earned less than males ($13,229 compared with $20,344).[68] In the year 2008, the U.S. Bureau of Labor reported women earned 80 cents on the dollar compared with men.[69]

Also alarming, though unfortunately not surprising, is the penalty minority workers pay. Minority men earn less money than do white men, and minority women earn less than do white women. These differences involve significant amounts of money.

Last, women who work outside the home must also work inside the home. When children are involved, the stress associated with working can be magnified, yet more and more women with young children are entering the labor force. In 2008, 67 percent of married women with children younger than 18 were in the labor force, as were approximately 74 percent of married women with children between the ages of 6 and 17. Sixty percent of married women with children under 6 years of age were employed outside the home in 2008.[70]

Coping with Work Stress

My wife complains that when she shares a problem with me, I immediately suggest several ways to solve that problem. When she shares that problem with a female friend, her friend empathizes with her, acknowledges her feelings, and listens. This is not surprising in view of what we know about how women cope with stress—in particular, work stress—and how they cope differently than men. Women tend to use emotion-focused coping more than men.[71] They also request and receive more social support than do men as a means of coping with work stress.[72] Studies indicate that when social support is high, women report greater job satisfaction, greater family satisfaction, and less family interference with their work than do men.[73] Furthermore, women's coping involves interpersonal relationships more than does men's coping.[74,75]

Women and Retirement

The experiences of women in retirement also differ from those of men. For example, whereas over 65 percent of men receive pensions, only 33 percent of women do, and women's pension benefits average approximately 60 percent those of men.[76] With more and more women entering the workforce, it is expected this situation will change for the next generation of Americans. Still, that leaves a lot of women currently wrestling with their financial health. To exacerbate women's financial situation in retirement, almost one-third of men do not select joint-survivor life insurance options that would provide income for their spouses when their husbands are deceased, that in spite of women living an average of five years longer than men. Divorce also has significant implication for women in retirement.

Some Facts About Women and Retirement

- Women are more likely to work in part-time jobs that don't qualify for a retirement plan.

- Working women are more likely than men to interrupt their careers to take care of family members. Therefore, they work fewer years and contribute less toward their retirement, resulting in lower lifetime savings.

- Of the 62 million wage and salaried women (ages 21 to 64) working in the United States, just 45 percent participated in a retirement plan. Even small amounts can earn interest and add up over time.

- On average, a female retiring at age 65 can expect to live another 19 years, 3 years longer than a man retiring at the same age. Savings can increase a woman's chances of having enough money to last during her retirement.

- Women invest more conservatively than men, therefore accumulating less retirement assets.

- Women earn less than men. Because retirement benefits are based on accumulated earnings during a working career, this *gender wage gap* quickly turns into a *retirement wage gap*. Women with pensions receive about half the amount men do each year.

Source: Employee Benefits Security Administration, U.S. Department of Labor. *Women and Retirement Savings.* 2011. Available at: www.dol.gov/ebsa/publications/women.html; Stephanie Loiacono, "Overcome the Retirement 'Gender Gap,'". *Investipedia.* 2009. Available at: www.investopedia.com/articles/retirement/08/women-savings.asp#axzz1Y7PplUEq.

Divorced women earn less money than women in intact households and receive less social security income in their later years.

Not surprisingly, older women are disproportionately represented in poverty status. Whereas 6.7 percent of men 65 years of age and older were classified as living in poverty in 2008, 11.9 percent of women in that age group were so classified.[77] One expert concludes that older women are poor because the retirement system is based on earnings and women have low earnings, husbands' benefits cease or are significantly lower when he dies, and the shift to 401(k) plans rather than defined pensions disadvantages lower-wage earners.[78] Several solutions have been proposed. Among these are for women to save more and/or to retire at later ages so they accumulate more in their retirement accounts. One problem with women saving more is that they tend to be more conservative than men in their investments. The result is they can expect to accumulate less retirement savings than men.[79] Still, for women to have to strategize differently from men to assure their financial wherewithal when they are older seems unfair.

Family-Friendly Work-Related Policies

Soon you will be graduating and looking for a job. How would you react if, during an interview, you were told you can write out your grocery list, bring it to work in the morning, and someone will shop and deliver your groceries to you before you leave work that day? Sound absurd? Well, there actually are companies that provide

Benefits of Job Stress Management Programs

Summarizing research findings pertaining to the benefits to business of conducting occupational stress management programs, the Canadian Institute of Stress reports the following:[a]

- 18 percent reduction in absences.
- 32 percent reduction in grievances.
- 52 percent reduction in disability time.
- 7 percent improvement in productivity.
- 13 percent improvement in service quality.

Based on these and other findings, businesses can annually save the following:[b]

- $700 million in stress-related absences.
- $2.22 billion in lost productivity due to mental illness.
- $6.6 billion in lost productivity due to all forms of clinical and subclinical mental illness.
- $1.1 billion in absenteeism due to work–family conflict.

[a]Canadian Institute of Stress, Bell Canada Operations Services Research. *Our Reputation for Worldclass Results*. 2007. Available at: www.stresscanada.org/reputation.html.
[b]Joan Burton, "The Business Case for a Healthy Workplace," *Industrial Accident Prevention Association*, 2007. Available at: www.uml.edu/centers/cph-new/job-stress/Documents/fd_business_case_healthy_workplace%5B1%5D.pdf

that service to their employees. These and other family-friendly policies are designed to respond to some of the conflicts between employees' work and home lives that cause occupational stress. They also respond to companies' needs to recruit and retain the best workers, and allow them to focus on their work so they can be more productive. Several family-friendly policies are described below.

Job Sharing

Some businesses allow workers to share the responsibility of one full-time position, with the salary, vacation and leave, pension rights, and fringe benefits divided between them.[80] Job sharing, though, is not synonymous with part-time work. With job sharing, employees communicate with each other, coordinate their work tasks and responsibilities, and agree on their work schedules. Workers might split weeks working half a week each, or split days in which one employee works in the morning and the other in the afternoon. Job sharing has advantages for parents who want to spend more time with their children than a full-time position allows. It also affords students the opportunity to work while pursuing their studies. Advantages to businesses include being able to recruit talented employees who are not ready to work full-time, and to retain employees whose situations change and prevent them from working full-time—for example, needing to take care of an elderly relative. Furthermore, job sharing helps employers get the best of two people's skills and experience for the price of one, curbs absenteeism, and diminishes stress-related disorders.

The Family and Medical Leave Act

To help employees cope with the stress resulting from major family crises, in 1993 the U.S. Congress passed the Family and Medical Leave Act, and it was signed into law by President Clinton. The Family and Medical Leave Act requires companies to

1. Allow employees as much as twelve weeks of unpaid leave during any 12-month period for the birth of a child, to care for a spouse or parent who becomes seriously ill, or to care for themselves if their own health condition prevents them from performing job responsibilities.

2. Allow employees who choose to take a leave to return to their former jobs or to an equivalent position upon their return to work.

3. Keep providing workers with health care benefits although workers on leave do not have to be paid. However, if workers do not return when their leave expires, the business can recapture from the former worker the health care premiums they paid during the leave.

To be eligible,

1. Employees must work for a business that has 50 or more workers.

2. Employees must have worked for the business for at least one year and for at least 1,250 hours (25 hours a week).

3. Employees can be required to provide documentation of the reason for their leave. Up to three medical opinions on the need for the leave can be requested by the employer.

Working from home can help alleviate some work-related stress.

Flexible Work Schedules

In 2004, the most current data available shows 27 million full-time workers, almost 15 percent of the workforce, had flexible work schedules that allowed them to vary the time they began or ended work.[81] Of these workers, 16 percent chose this arrangement to facilitate family responsibilities and 11 percent to allow for child care. Some companies also allow workers to work a longer work day, but work only four days a week. Flexible scheduling allows workers to avoid rush hour traffic, to take care of family responsibilities such as taking children to school, and to work when the worksite is less hectic. In a national study,[82] it was found that many different types of flexible work options are provided by companies. For example,

- 68 percent allow workers to alter starting and quitting times.
- 78 percent give workers control of when they take breaks.
- 77 percent give employees time off for important personal and family needs without loss of pay.
- 39 percent allow employees to work a compressed work week for at least part of the year.
- 39 percent allow workers to decide which shifts they work.

Home-Based Work

Thirty-four percent of employers allow their full-time employees to work from their homes occasionally and 31 percent allow this arrangement on a regular basis.[83] Approximately 24 percent of workers did some or all of their work at home.[84] As they work at home, 80 percent use a computer, slightly fewer use a telephone, and 70 percent use the Internet or e-mail. Working at home responds to the needs of employees who have family commitments such as child or elder care, eliminates the time and inconvenience of a commute to work, and allows employees to arrange a flexible work schedule when needed.[85]

Health Promotion Programs

Employers are concerned with the health of their workforce for several reasons, one of which is the recognition that "organizations are composed of employees and, without these employees, there would be no organization."[86] Another reason is the high cost of health insurance. If workers remain healthy, they access the health care system less frequently and, as a result, the company's health insurance premiums do not increase as much. This is why many businesses offer health promotion programs. In fact, 93 percent of businesses with 200 or more employees provide some type of program designed to promote health.[87] In a review of health-promotion programs, it was concluded that for every dollar spent on these programs, $3.48 was saved. Furthermore, it was found that increases in health insurance rates and absenteeism were related to high levels of stress, excessive body weight, and the presence of multiple risk factors (for example, smoking).[88]

These programs also increase *presenteeism,* that is, focus and function while at work. Workers who are more *present* are more productive. In terms of stress management programs in particular, researchers have concluded that they improve employee well-being, improve productivity, increase presenteeism, and decrease absenteeism.[89]

Examples of worksite health-promotion programs abound. For instance, King County, Washington provides each county worksite $25 per employee, and sites have decided to use those funds to purchase gym equipment, pay for a yoga instructor, purchase walking maps and pedometers, or arrange for weekly delivery of organic produce.[90] A Weight Watchers program offered by King County resulted in employees losing a collective 5,700 pounds. Agora, Inc., of Baltimore, Maryland, conducted weight loss competitions resulting in employees losing a collective 1,000 pounds. Argon also offers an on-site gym and free classes with a personal trainer.

Child and Elder Care

More and more companies offer child care programs to alleviate stress associated with leaving children during work. Chase Manhattan Bank was one of these. In the 1990s, workers for the bank received up to 20 days of free care per child each year. A cost analysis found this program saved Chase Manhattan $825,000 in 1996.[91] Parents did not miss work because of the need to care for a child, did not worry about the child's welfare during the workday, could therefore concentrate on work-related tasks, and did not become ill because of stress about the welfare of the child. AOL also operated several child care centers for their employees with approximately 310 children enrolled. Even so, there was a wait list of over 400.

Some companies even opened their own elementary schools for workers' children. Hewlett-Packard in Santa Rosa, California, and Target in Minneapolis are examples of such enterprises. Most of these schools were a collaboration between the local school system—which supplied teachers, curricula, and instructional materials—and the company, which usually owned the land, built the school, maintained the school, and paid the utilities. American Bankers Insurance Group opened a company school in Miami in 1987. It costs the company $140,000 annually to operate it, yet it saved the company $475,000 per year because it decreased employee absenteeism and turnover. Job turnover among parents whose children attended the school was 6 percent, versus a 13.3 percent rate for the company as a whole.[92]

Like child care, some organizations offer elder care. For example, Freddie Mac and Verizon provided advisors and consultation for employees experiencing elder care needs. They discussed available facilities, financial issues, and legal considerations. Twenty-two of the largest corporations in America—including IBM, Lucent Technologies, Xerox, AT&T, Hewlett Packard, Deloitte, Price Waterhouse, and Exxon Mobil—formed an alliance to offer quality child and elder care for their employees.[93] These organizations recognized that more and more workers are caring for elderly relatives.[94] Being distracted with thoughts of how the elder is doing while the worker is at work decreases presenteeism and diminishes productivity. And having to manage the needs of elderly relatives increases absenteeism.

Other Policies

Still other perks are being offered to help workers alleviate stress. For example, some companies offer free chair massages at workers' desks. A unique approach has been adopted by Texas Instruments (TI) in Dallas. TI offers concierge service for its workers. An employee can call the concierge to set up a birthday party for a child, for example. The employee pays the cost of the party, but Texas Instruments pays for the concierge service. Approximately 1,500 employees used the service during the first two months it was made available.[95]

At J.C. Penney's of Plano, Texas, employees can pick up a chef-prepared take-home meal as they leave work. This increases morale, decreases absenteeism, and helps with recruitment and retention of employees. And at AOL, special parking is set aside at the front of all buildings for pregnant women employees, nurse-coaches are available to advise new parents via e-mail or telephone, lactation counseling is offered, and parenting workshops are provided.

Work-Family Balance

The reason these family-friendly policies are necessary is due to the effects of work on employees' family lives, and the effects of employees' family lives on their work. In the winter, workers come to work and hang up their coats on coat racks. They can then proceed with their work tasks unencumbered. They also come to work with stress from outside of work. Yet, *there ain't no stress rack!* Workers *wear* their stress all day at work and, not surprisingly, this affects their productivity, decision making, and relationships at work. Conversely, employees who have a stressful day at work bring that home with them, the consequences being increased arguing, physical and emotional unavailability, and marital dissatisfaction. This can be especially problematic for dual career couples. The number of dual career couples has increased over the years, primarily as a result of the increase in employment of women. In 1970, 40.8 percent of women worked outside the home, whereas in 2009, 54.4 percent of women worked outside the home.[96] In 2009, 66 percent of both parents in married couples with children under 18 years of age worked outside the home. In spite of this workload, the time parents spend with their children has actually increased. Something has to give. What is it? Time for themselves. Fathers spend 1.3 hours on themselves during a typical work day. Mothers spend a measly 0.9 hours on themselves during a typical work day. This does not make for marital and family harmony. Throw in the need for many families to care for elderly family members and the situation becomes critical.

These issues are classified as work-family balance issues. Work-family balance is satisfaction and good functioning at work and at home with a minimum of role conflict.[97] Several theories explain the effects of a work-family imbalance.[98] The *spillover* theory states that a change in one domain results in a comparable change in the other domain. For example, having poor relationships at work will lead to poor relationships at home. In an example of the spillover theory, researchers have found that both job distress and work overload were related to the intention to leave one's marriage.[99] The *compensation* theory states that when one domain is not working out well, time and other resources are spent on the other domain. For example, being dissatisfied at work leads to more time spent at home, or being unhappy at home leads to more time spent at work. Lastly, the *resource drain* theory states that the use of resources (time, energy) in one domain limits the availability of resources for the other domain. For example, time and energy spent at work are time and energy not available to spend with the family.

Working in the Home

The bank was a typical one: leather upholstered chairs, wooden gates with swinging doors, red carpet, caged-in tellers, and cheap replicas of attractive paintings on the walls. It didn't look like a studio setting, yet a TV camera hanging conspicuously in the corner of the room recorded all the exciting goings-on. I was there with my wife, seeking approval of a mortgage well beyond our means but just this side of our aspirations. The bank manager, who to her credit sized up the situation quickly, was asking all the usual embarrassing questions—"How much did you make last year? Can you prove it? To whom do you owe money? Is your car paid for?"

Well, the trouble was just beginning. It soon came time for my wife to answer the same questions. The first one did it—"Do you work?" How innocent those three little words sounded. Nevertheless, I knew what to expect as I leaned back in my chair in an unconscious nonverbal expression that said "I don't want any part of this one!"

"I most certainly do," was my wife's answer.

"How much do you earn?"

"I don't earn anything. I work at home."

"Oh, you're just a housewife."

"No, I'm not *just* a housewife."

"Sorry, I didn't mean any offense."

Sorry or not, the damage was done. Had I bothered to, I'm sure I could have objectively verified what I knew to be my wife's biomedical condition—elevated

When men and women work full time outside of the home, women still do more than an equal share of work inside the home.

blood pressure, increased heart rate, rapid and shallow breathing, and tense muscles. By now you recognize the stress response.

One of the stressors women experience is the denigration of their homemaking role. My wife's term—domestic engineer—is an accurate one. Full-time homemaking is difficult, is tiring, and requires a great deal of skill, time, effort, creativity, and commitment. Although there is nothing that makes women more suited than men for this role, tradition has made full-time homemaking a job done predominantly by women. In recent years, more attention has been paid to men who occupy this role, and their designation—househusband—is as demeaning as the female version—housewife. Men and women who work as full-time homemakers are certainly not married to the house, and their priorities aren't there, either. Rather, their homemaking role is designed to make themselves and those with whom they live feel comfortable. They organize car pools, umpire baseball games, place Band-Aids on wounds that heal better for their loving care, and do other varied and meaningful tasks such as watching over the family's health and nutrition.

That some people, men and women, downplay the significance and value of homemaking is unfortunate. Certainly this role is not one that everyone would choose, but it is a role that many women and some men occupy by choice and perform exceptionally well. It is an extremely important role that can be divided by members of the family or performed by one person.

The stressors associated with domestic engineering are similar to other occupational stressors: too much to do in too little time (role overload), not being specifically trained for many of the tasks (role insufficiency), having to answer to too many different family members' demands (role conflict), and not being clear about all that is expected (role ambiguity). When the denigration of the role is added to these stressors, the load may become too much to bear, and illness and disease may occur.

Women with children face another stressor. One day, after years of mothering, the last child moves out. For women who see the empty nest as offering an opportunity to do things that they didn't have time to do before, obstacles may present themselves. Some employers may view empty-nester applicants as lacking in experience. Career counselors, however, have been helping women market themselves as well-trained and abundantly experienced in organizational skills, time management, interpersonal relationships, problem solving, and purchasing. How many employers would not want to hire an applicant who has demonstrated an ability to handle challenging, difficult chores requiring a great deal of skill, time, effort, creativity, and commitment? These are the traits that I used several paragraphs earlier to describe homemaking.

Interventions

More and more businesses are offering health promotion programs with stress management as a primary component. One of the national health objectives for the year 2020 is to increase the proportion of employees who have access to workplace programs that prevent or reduce employee stress. In 1992, 37 percent provided employee stress programs.[100]

Using our stress model, we know we can intervene between occupational stress and its negative consequences by changing life situations, our perceptions or cognitive appraisal of those situations, or our emotional reactions, or by doing something physical to use up the stress by-products. This section will describe how to specifically apply these interventions.

Life-Situation Interventions

If you dislike your job and it is causing you either to feel ill or to behave in ways that are detrimental to your career or your home life, you can always quit that job. Short of that, you can ask for a change in job responsibilities, or you can request a less stressful job within the same organization. If you are experiencing burnout, learn to organize your time better and to say no when asked to take on additional responsibilities. In addition, some stress-reducing rules might help:

1. Don't take work home.
2. Establish a techno-free time during which your cell phone is off and you do not check for e-mail messages or instant messages.
3. Take a full hour for lunch.
4. Do not discuss business over lunch.
5. Discuss your feelings about occupational stress with whomever is close by whenever those feelings develop.

Perception Interventions

Recognizing that your perceptions of your occupational stress are as important as the actual events precipitating that stress, you will need to intervene in these perceptions. These suggestions should help:

1. *Look for the humor in your stressors at work.* A resourceful teacher, frustrated by inane memos from the principal with which she was repeatedly

and unmercifully bombarded, kept a file of these memos and eventually wrote a very humorous and successful book based upon them. The principal may not have found humor in this teacher's survival technique, but the teacher sure did; besides, she had tenure.

2. *Try to see things for what they really are.* Here's an example, but keep this between us. Publishers are notorious for requesting manuscripts from authors by certain *firm* deadline dates. Unfortunately, too often these manuscripts sit on an editor's desk before being processed. Through some bitter experiences, I have learned that publishers' *deadlines* are really not deadlines. Rather, they are dates *close* to when they would like to receive a manuscript and, knowing that many authors will be late with their sub-missions, these editors have selected dates with a margin for delay. I have learned to allow myself more time to get a job done when I have been able to perceive that I really have more time to complete that work than I first thought. You can use that strategy as well. Perhaps you, too, have "deadlines" that really aren't deadlines.

3. *Distinguish between need and desire.* For example, "I *must* get this task com-pleted" might be more truthfully stated as "I *wish* I could get this task completed."

4. *Separate your self-worth from the task.* If you fail at a task, it does not mean you are a failure.

5. *Identify situations and employ the appropriate style of coping.* Lazarus and Folkman differentiated between **problem-focused coping** and **emotion-focused coping**.[101] Problem-focused coping is the use of activities specific to getting the task accomplished, whereas emotion-focused coping is the use of activities to feel better about the task. If you employed problem-focused coping for a task that was beyond your accomplishment (e.g., turning in a 200-page treatise on the migratory habits of aardvarks for tomorrow's class), you would only frustrate yourself and become distressed. Given such an impossible task, you would do better to joke about it, discuss your feelings with a friend, or leave a real aardvark in your professor's mailbox with a note instructing him or her to observe this creature's migratory habits and get back to you. Conversely, if a task can be accomplished but you dillydally by joking and partying with friends, you are employing emotion-focused coping when you should have engaged in activities to get the task done (problem-focused coping). Perceiving what is called for in a particular situation will allow you to better determine which method of coping is most appropriate.

problem-focused coping
The use of activities specific to getting a task done.

emotion-focused coping
The use of activities to feel better about the task.

Emotional Arousal Interventions

Relaxation techniques, if done regularly, can help prevent occupational stress from making you ill, creating disharmony in your relationships at work or at home, or leading to your abuse of alcohol or other drugs, as well as prevent the other harmful consequences of occupational stress. I have had participants in my classes and workshops tell me they have found out-of-the-way places at work where they meditate during part of their lunch hour or during breaks in the workday. Others have had to leave the worksite but have found nearby parks or golf courses, where they, too, practice a relaxation technique. Still others have been able to get their companies to establish one area as the relaxation area—usually an infrequently used lounge or work area. You can use a relaxation tech-nique to intervene at this level if you choose to. Be ingenious, be assertive, be committed to caring for you.

I conducted lunchtime seminars for various businesses as a representative of the Ronald McDonald House. The intent was to offer a free, yet valued, service for which the participants were so grateful that they contributed to the Ronald McDonald House during charity fund-raising campaigns and at other times during the year. Well, sometimes I was unavailable at the time when the business requested a seminar. On those occasions, I asked a student to conduct the seminar for me. I am delighted to report that these students have done an excellent job. After all, they did not want to embarrass themselves, so they learned the material extremely well and prepared an educational and interesting presentation. What a wonderful opportunity they had. Not only did they provide a service to a community organization, but at the same time they learned more about stress, and they added a line on their résumés that made them more marketable when they graduated. If there ever was a win-win situation, this was it.

As long as students have enough time to prepare for the presentation, and work in groups so they can learn from one another, they can do an excellent job. After all, they are enrolled in a stress management course and the presentations they prepare, being limited to one hour, are relatively basic.

You do not have to wait to be invited to conduct a stress management seminar for a community business establishment. You can initiate such requests by letting businesses know of your availability and willingness to run a stress management seminar for them. You can do this by sending out letters to various businesses, by arranging for meetings with directors of health promotion or human resources staff, or by developing a one-page flyer announcing the availability of stress management lunchtime seminars. In this way, you will be contributing to your community's health while deriving many benefits for yourself.

Physiological Arousal Interventions

Exercise is an excellent way to use up the stress products created by occupational stress. Recognizing this, many businesses have built gymnasiums or outside exercise areas (for example, running tracks or par courses). If you have these facilities at work, use them. If not, you can join an exercise club (if you need the company of others) or exercise on your own.

Managing Occupational Stress

In conclusion, occupational stress may be difficult to define and measure because of the personal stressors people bring to their jobs and their varying personality characteristics, but we all know when we are experiencing it. Fortunately, we can manage occupational stress by using the stress model to set up roadblocks between occupational stress and illness and disease. We can change jobs (life-situation intervention), perceive the stressors associated with our jobs as challenges rather than burdens to bear (perception intervention), practice relaxation techniques regularly (emotional arousal intervention), and exercise regularly to use up the accumulated products of stress (physiological arousal intervention). But whether we do anything is our own choice. "Grinning and bearing it" won't help; neither will always complaining about jobs or bosses. Help is available, and reading this book is a good start.

Coping in Today's World

What Americans value most is inherently stressful. That is the argument made by two experts on stress.[a] Americans value the *work ethic* and believe that hard work leads to success, prosperity, well-being, and the good life. Material acquisitions (a large house, fancy car, etc.) are proof of our ability, achievements, accomplishments, and righteousness.[b] This value leads to constant change—moving from one house to another, from one job to another, from one profession to another. Change is also reflected in the organization as it, too, seeks to accomplish more and more. As a result, there is rightsizing, downsizing, merging, reinventing, and the use of the latest technological tools. And this constant change is stressful.

Striving to *get ahead,* the American societal norm of competitiveness comes into play. We try to distinguish ourselves from other workers by working harder and longer, and the result is often social isolation in the workplace. Such a work environment can result in feelings of distress and loneliness that affect our health and that of the organization.[c]

Another American value is individualism, which is based on freedom and liberty. If we are competing against other workers as individuals, we need control and autonomy. When we don't obtain this control, we are likely to experience stress-related illness and disease. In fact, numerous studies have found a relationship not only between job stress—defined by the demand-control model—and cardiovascular disease, but also with obesity.[d]

One way to counteract these forces is to create a different type of workplace. As stated by Peterson and Wilson,[e] ". . . when managers lead by persuasion rather than command-control tactics, they facilitate both organizational and employee health outcomes. When workers are communicated to about the meaning and purpose of their work, they are better able to perform and less likely to be vulnerable to the hassles and changes within the workplace." When looking for a job, you might want to interview prospective employees to determine if these conditions exist at that workplace.

[a]M. Peterson and J. F. Wilson, "Work Stress in America," *International Journal of Stress Management* 11(2004): 911–13.
[b]M. A. Ledeen, *Tocqueville on American Character* (New York: St. Martin's Press, 2000).
[c]M. Peterson and J. Wilson, "The Culture–Work–Health Model: A Theoretical Conceptualization," *American Journal of Health Behavior* 26(2002): 16–24.
[d]P. A. Schulte, G. R. Wagner, A. Ostry, et al., "Work, Obesity, and Occupational Safety and Health," *American Journal of Public Health* 97(2007): 428–36.
[e]Peterson and Wilson, "The Culture–Work–Health Model," 109–10.

summary

- Too little occupational stress is almost as unhealthy as too much. There is an optimal level of occupational stress that is desirable.

- Occupational stress consists of a mix of worksite stressors, the individual's characteristics, and extraorganizational stressors. These stressors can lead to symptoms of occupational ill health or to actual disease.

- Businesses have become interested in occupational stress because it costs them money to ignore it due to employees' ill health, poor decision making, and absenteeism. In addition, stress management programs are used to attract prospective employees whom the company is recruiting.

- Workers report more occupational stress when work objectives are unclear, when conflicting demands are placed upon them, when they have too little or too much to do, when they have little input in decisions that affect them, and when they are responsible for other workers' development.

- Role problems that can result in occupational stress include role overload, role insufficiency, role ambiguity, and role conflict.

- Workaholics spend much of their time working, often eat while working, prefer work to play, and can and do work anytime and anywhere. They are intense and energetic and have difficulty sleeping and taking vacations.

- Burnout is a syndrome of physical and emotional exhaustion; it is an adverse work stress reaction with psychological, psychophysiological, and behavioral components. Symptoms include diminished sense of humor, skipping rest and food breaks, increased overtime and no vacations, increased physical complaints, social withdrawal, diminishing job performance, self-medication, and psychological changes such as depression or a "trapped" feeling.

- More and more women are working outside the home. Given that many of these women have more than their share of responsibilities in the home, and that many have young children, that they experience the effects of occupational stress should be no surprise.

- Part of the stress experienced by women who work outside the home relates to the fact that, at each educational level and for comparable jobs, women earn less than men. In addition, women are still predominantly employed in traditional women's roles (nurse, dental hygienist, cashier, secretary, waitress, and child care worker).

- The stress associated with domestic engineering (home-making) can be similar to the stress resulting from other jobs. Such components of occupational stress as role overload, role conflict, role insufficiency, and role ambiguity may be present in the homemaking situation, just as they can be associated with many jobs outside the home.

- Life situation, perception, and emotional and physiological arousal interventions can be effective in managing sex-role stress.

internet resources

Job Stress Network **www.workhealth.org** *Information about and related to job strain and work stress, by the Center for Social Epidemiology, a private nonprofit foundation whose purpose is to promote public awareness of the role of environmental and occupational stress in the etiology of cardiovascular disease.*

18 Ways to Survive Your Company's Reorganization, Takeover, Downsizing, or Other Major Change **www .stresscure.com/jobstress/reorg.html** *An article that offers practical suggestions for coping with the stresses related to major changes in the workplace.*

NIOSH/Stress at Work **www.cdc.gov/niosh/docs/99–101** */Developed by the National Institute for Occupational Safety and Health, this site provides information about current NIOSH activities in the area of work, stress, and health and provides access to resources to help prevent stressful working conditions.*

American Institute of Stress **www.stressorg/job.htm** *Facts and figures about job stress and reference to current information about occupational stress.*

references

1. Jefferson A. Singer, Michael S. Neale, and Gary E. Schwartz, "The Nuts and Bolts of Assessing Occupational Stress: A Collaborative Effort with Labor." In *Stress Management in Work Settings*, ed. Lawrence R. Murphy and Theodore F. Schoenborn (Washington, D.C.: National Institute for Occupational Safety and Health, 1987), 3–29.

2. Clinton G. Weiman, "A Study of the Occupational Stressor and the Incidence of Disease/Risk," *NIOSH Proceeding: Reducing Occupational Stress* (Cincinnati: National Institute for Occupational Safety and Health, April 1978), 55.

3. P. J. Rosch (Ed.), "The Quandary of Job Stress Compensation," *Health and Stress* 3(2001): 1–4.

4. CCH Inc., *2007 CCH Unscheduled Absence Survey* (Riverside, CA: CCH Inc., 2007).

5. Marlin Company, *Attitudes in the American Workplace VII* (North Haven, CT: Marlin Company, 2001).

6. Ibid.

7. J. Hudson, *Stress Disconnect: 60 Percent of Employees Report High Levels of Stress; Managers Beg to Differ*. ComPsych, 2007. Available at http://compsych.com/jsp/en_US/content/press Release/2007/stressDisconnect.jsp

8. Expedia, Expedia.com. *2009 International Vacation Deprivation Survey Results*, 2009. Available at http://media.expedia.com/ media/content/expus/graphics/promos/vacations/Expedia_ International_Vacation_Deprivation_Survey_2009.pdf

9. Steelcase, *Steelcase Workplace Index Survey Reveals Growing Trend of Working on Vacation*, 2006. Available at www.steelcase .com/na/workplace_index_survey_reveals_News.aspx?f=25748

10. Michael Peterson and John F. Wilson, "Work Stress in America," *International Journal of Stress Management* 11(2004): 911–13.

11. Kirstin Downey Grimsley, "Message Overload Taking Toll on Workers," *The Washington Post*, May 5, 1998, C13.

12. Martin Loosemore and Tom Waters, "Gender Differences in Occupational Stress Among Professionals in the Construction Industry," *Journal of Management in Engineering* 20(2004): 126–32.

13. Yoshi Iwasaki, Kelly J. MacKay, and Janice Ristock, "Gender-Based Analysis of Stress Among Professional Managers: An Exploratory Qualitative Study," *International Journal of Stress Management* 11(2004): 56–79.

14. Family and Work Institute, *Generation & Gender in the Workplace* (New York: Family Work Institute, 2002), 12. www .familiesandwork.org/site/research/reports/genandgender.pdf

15. Ibid., 4.

16. A. L. Day and H. A. Livingstone, "Gender Differences in Perceptions of Stressors and Utilization of Social Support Among University Students," *Canadian Journal of Behavioural Science* 35(2003): 73–83.

17. H. T. Krajewski and R. D. Goffin, "Predicting Occupational Coping Responses: The Interactive Effect of Gender and Work Stressors Context," *Journal of Occupational Health Psychology* 10(2005): 44–53.

18. E. Torkelson and T. Muhonen, "Coping Strategies and Health Symptoms Among Women and Men in a Downsizing Organization," *Psychology Reports* 92(2003): 899–907.

19. M. G. Gonzalez-Morales, J. M. Rodriguez, and E. R. Greenglass, "Coping and Distress in Organizations: The Role of Gender in Work and Stress," *International Journal of Stress Management* 13(2006): 228–48.

20. D. Nelson and R. J. Burke, "A Framework for Examining Gender, Work Stress, and Health." In *Gender, Work Stress and Health,* ed. D. Nelson and R. J. Burke (Washington, D.C.: American Psychological Association, 2002), 2–14.

21. R. J. Burke, "Men, Masculinity and Health." In *Gender, Work Stress and Health,* ed. D. Nelson and R. J. Burke (Washington, D.C.: American Psychological Association, 2002), 35–54.

22. S. D. Friedman and J. H. Greenhaus, *Allies or Enemies? How Choices About Work and Family Affect the Quality of Men's and Women's Lives* (New York: Oxford University Press, 2000).

23. Peter R. Vagg, Charles D. Spielberger, and Carol F. Wasala, "Effects of Organizational Level and Gender on Stress in the Workplace," *International Journal of Stress Management* 9(2002): 243–61.

24. Michael P. O'Driscoll, Steven Poelmans, Paul E. Spector, Thomas Kalliath, Tammy D. Allen, Cary L. Cooper, and Juan I. Sanchez, "Family-Responsive Interventions Perceived Organizational and Supervisor Support, Work-Family Conflict, and Psychological Strain," *International Journal of Stress Management* 10(2003): 326–44.

25. Lambeth Hochwald, "The Top 10 Healthiest Companies for Women," *Health,* July/August 2003, 148–55, 202.

26. A. Steptoe, "Impact of Job and Marital Strain on Ambulatory Blood Pressure," *American Journal of Hypertension* 18(2005): 1138.

27. H. Riese, L. J. Van Doornen, I. L. Houtman, and E. J. De Geus, "Job Strain in Relation to Ambulatory Blood Pressure, Heart Rate, and Heart Rate Variability Among Female Nurses," *Scandinavian Journal of Work, Environment & Health* 30(2004): 477–85.

28. Y. Kobayashi, T. Hirose, Y. Tada, A. Tsutsumi, and N. Kawakami, "Relationship Between Two Job Stress Models and Coronary Risk Factors Among Japanese Part-Time Female Employees of a Retail Company," *Journal of Occupational Health* 47(2005): 201–10.

29. J. Siegrist. "Perceived Rewards at Work and Cardiovascular Health," *Psychosomatic Medicine* 73(2011): 434–435.

30. K. Fujishiro, A. V. Diez Roux, P. Landsbergis, S. Baron, R. G. Barr, J. D. Kaufman, J. F. Polak, and K. Hinckley Stukovsky, "Associations of Occupation, Job Control and Job Demands with Intima-Media Thickness: The Multi-Ethnic Study of Atherosclerosis (MESA)," *Occupational and Environmental Medicine* 68(2011): 319–26.

31. T. R. Waters, R. B. Dick, and E. F. Krieg, Jr. "Trends in Work-Related Musculoskeletal Disorders: A Comparison of Risk Factors for Symptoms Using Quality of Work Life Data from the 2002 and 2006 General Social Survey," *Journal of Occupational and Environmental Medicine* 53(2011): 1013–24.

32. A. Nakata, M. Takahashi, M. Irie, T. Ray, N. G. Swanson, "Job Satisfaction, Common Cold, And Sickness Absence Among White-Collar Employees: A Cross-Sectional Survey," *Industrial Health* 49(2011): 116–21.

33. L. P. Brown, K. M. Rospenda, R. K. Sokas, L. Conroy, S. Freels, and N. G. Swanson, "Evaluating the Association of Workplace Psychosocial Stressors with Occupational Injury, Illness, and Assault," *Journal of Occupational and Environmental Hygiene* 8(2011): 31–37.

34. A. Nakata, M. Takahashi, M. Irie, and N. G. Swanson, "Job Satisfaction Is Associated with Elevated Natural Killer Cell Immunity Among Healthy White-Collar Employees," *Brain Behavior and Immunity;* 24(November 2010): 1268–75.

35. K. M. Lee, D. Kang, K. Yoon, S. Y. Kim, H. Kim, H. S. Yoon, D. B. Trout, and J. J. Hurrell, Jr. "A Pilot Study on the Association Between Job Stress and Repeated Measures of Immunological Biomarkers in Female Nurses," *International Archives of Occupational and Environmental Health* 83(2010): 779–89.

36. Jenny Head, Stephen A. Stansfeld, and Johannes Siegrist. "The Psychosocial Work Environment and Alcohol Dependence: A Prospective Study," *Occupational and Environmental Medicine* 61(2004): 219–24.

37. R. A. Karasek, J. Schwartz, and T. Theorell, *Job Characteristics, Occupation, and Coronary Heart Disease,* Final report on contract no. R-01-0H00906 (Cincinnati, OH: National Institute for Occupational Safety and Health, 1982).

38. Robert A. Karasek, et al., "Job Characteristics in Relation to the Prevalence of Myocardial Infarction in the U.S. Health Examination Survey (HES) and the Health and Nutrition Examination Survey (HANES)," *American Journal of Public Health* 78(1988): 910–18.

39. H. X. Wang, C. Leineweber, R. Kirkeeide, B. Svane, K. Schenck-Gustafsson, T. Theorell, and K. Orth-Gomér, "Psychosocial Stress and Atherosclerosis: Family and Work Stress Accelerate Progression of Coronary Disease in Women. The Stockholm Female Coronary Angiography Study," *Journal of Internal Medicine* 261(2007): 245–54.

40. M. Kivimäki, M. Virtanen, M. Elovainio, A. Kouvonen, A. Väänänen, and J. Vahtera, "Work Stress in the Etiology of Coronary Heart Disease—A Meta-Analysis," *Scandinavian Journal of Work, Environment and Health* 32(2006): 431–42.

41. Heart Disease and Stress, *MedicineNet.com.* 2011. Available at: www.medicinenet.com/stress_and_heart_disease/article.htm.

42. P. A. Schulte, G. R. Wagner, A. Ostry, L. A. Blanciforti, R. G. Cutlip, K. M. Krajnak, M. Luster, A. E. Munson, J. P. O'Callaghan, C. G. Parks, P. P. Simeonova, and D. B. Miller, "Work, Obesity, and Occupational Safety and Health," *American Journal of Public Health* 97(2007): 428–36.

43. J. C. Cohrs, A. E. Abele, and D. E. Dette, "Integrating Situational and Dispositional Determinants of Job Satisfaction: Findings from Three Samples of Professionals," *Journal of Psychology* 140(2006): 363–95.

44. B. Gearhart, "The (Affective) Dispositional Approach to Job Satisfaction: Sorting Out the Policy Implications," *Journal of Organizational Behavior* 26(2005): 79–97.

45. Byoung-Suk Kweon, Roger S. Ulrich, Verrick D. Walker, and Louis G. Tassinary, "Anger and Stress: The Role of Landscape Posters in an Office Setting," *Environment and Behavior* 40(2008): 355–81.

46. R. J. Burke and M. P. Leiter, "Contemporary Organizational Realities and Professional Efficacy: Downsizing, Reorganization, and Transition." In *Coping, Health and Organizations,* ed. P. Deue, M. P. Leiter, and T. Cox (London: Taylor & Francis, 2000), 237–56.

47. HealthCore Physicians Group, *Heart Attacks*, 2006. Available at www.healthcoreweb.com/b_hrtattack.html

48. D. P. Phillips, J. R. Jarvinen, I. S. Abramson, and R. R. Phillips, "Cardiac Mortality Is Higher Around Christmas and New Year's Than at Any Other Time: The Holidays as a Risk Factor for Death," *Circulation* 110(2004): 3781–88.

49. F. G. Benavidesa, J. Benacha, A. V. Diez-Rouxb, and C. Romana, "How Do Types of Employment Relate to Health Indicators? Findings from the Second European Survey on Working Conditions," *Journal of Epidemiology and Community Health* 54(2000): 494–501.

50. D. C. Mohren, G. M. Swaen, I. Kant, C. P. van Schayck, and J. M. Galama, "Fatigue and Job Stress as Predictors for Sickness Absence During Common Infections," *International Journal of Behavioral Medicine* 12(2005): 11–20.

51. R. J. Driscoll and R. L. Tubbs, "Evaluation of Work Stress," *International Journal of Occupational and Environmental Health* 15(2009): 229.

52. Cohrs, Abele, and Dettie, 2006, op. cit.

53. L. Riolli and V. Savicki, "Impact of Fairness, Leadership, and Coping on Stress, Burnout, and Turnover in Organizational Change," *International Journal of Stress Management* 13(2006): 351–77.

54. D. Ortqvist and J. Wincent, "Prominent Consequences of Role Stress: A Meta-Analytic Review," *International Journal of Stress Management* 13(2006): 399–42.

55. C. L. Hulin and T. A. Judge, "Job Attitudes." In *Handbook of Psychology*, Vol. 12: *Industrial and Organizational Psychology*, ed. W. C. Borman, D. R. Ilgen, and R. J. Klimoski (Hoboken, NJ: Wiley, 2003), 255–76.

56. The Conference Board, *U.S. Job Satisfaction Declines, The Conference Board Reports*, Press Release, February 23, 2007. Available at www.conference-board.org/utilities/pressPrinterFriendly.cfm?press_ID=3075

57. P. P. M. Janssen, M. C. W. Peeters, J. de Jonge, I. Houkes, and G. E. R. Tummers, "Specific Relationships Between Job Demands, Job Resources and Psychological Outcomes and the Mediating Role of Negative Work-Home Interference," *Journal of Vocational Behavior* 65(2004): 411–29.

58. G. Pomaki, S. Maes, and L. ter Doest, "Work Conditions and Employees' Self-test Goals: Goal Processes Enhance Prediction of Psychological Distress and Well-being," *Personality and Social Psychology Bulletin* 30(2004): 685–94.

59. Indira Ashton and Frank Gill, *Monitoring for Health Hazards at Work* (New York: Wiley-Blackwell, 2000).

60. Anna Kemeny, "Driven to Excel: A Portrait of Canada's Workaholics," *Canadian Social Trends.* Ottawa, Ontario: Catalogue No. 11-008, 2002.

61. Bryan F. Robinson, Claudia Flowers, and Jane Carroll, "Work Stress and Marriage: Examining the Relationship Between Workaholism and Marital Cohesion," *International Journal of Stress Management* 8(2001): 165–75.

62. C. Maslach, W. B. Schaufeli, and M. P. Lester, "Job Burnout," *Annual Review of Psychology* 52(2001): 397–422.

63. D. S. Hamermesh and J. Stemrod, "The Economics of Workaholism: We Should Not Have Worked on This Paper," IZA Discussion Paper No. 1680, July 2005.

64. A. Rasku and U. Kinnunen, "Job Conditions and Wellness Among Finnish Upper Secondary School Teachers," *Psychology and Health* 8(2003): 414–46.

65. Pamela K. S. Patrick, *Health Care Worker Burnout: What It Is, What to Do About It* (Chicago: Blue Cross Association, Inquiry Books, 1981), 87–111.

66. U.S. Census Bureau, *Statistical Abstract of the United States, 2011* (Washington, D.C.: U.S. Government Printing Office, 2010), 377.

67. Ibid., 393–396.

68. Ibid., 422.

69. U.S. Department of Labor, *Women in the Labor Force: A Databook (2009 Edition).* 2009. Available at www.bls.gov/cps/wlf-intro-2009.pdf

70. U.S. Department of Labor, Bureau of Labor Statistics, *Families with Own Children: Employment Status of Parents by Age of Youngest Child and Family Type, 2007–08 Annual Averages.* May 27, 2009. Available at www.bls.gov/news.release/famee.t04.htm

71. P. Matud, "Gender Differences in Stress and Coping Style," *Personality and Individual Differences* 37(2004): 1401–05.

72. A. L. Day and H. A. Livingstone, "Gender Differences in Perceptions of Stressors and Utilization of Social Support Among University Students," *Canadian Journal of Behavioural Science* 35(2003): 73–83.

73. P. L. Perrewe and D. S. Carlson, "Do Men and Women Benefit from Social Support Equally? Results from a Field Examination Within the Work and Family Context." In *Gender, Work Stress and Health*, ed. D. L. Nelson and R. J. Burke (Washington, D.C.: American Psychological Association, 2002), 101–14.

74. H. T. Krajewski and R. D. Goffin, "Predicting Occupational Coping Responses: The Interactive Effect of Gender and Work Stressors Context," *Journal of Occupational Health Psychology* 10(2005): 44–53.

75. E. Torkelson and T. Muhonen, "Coping Strategies and Health Symptoms Among Women and Men in a Downsizing Organisation," *Psychology Reports* 92(2003): 899–907.

76. *Patterns Retirement—Gender and Retirement*, 2007. Available at www.medicine.jrank.org/pages/1493/Retirement-Patterns-Gender-retirement.html

77. U.S. Census Bureau, "2009 Annual Social and Economic Supplement," *Current Population Survey* (2009). Available at www.census.gov/hhes/www/cpstables/032009/pov/new01_100_01.htm

78. A. H. Munnell, "Why Are so Many Older Women Poor?" *Just the Facts on Retirement Issues* (April 2004). Available at www.bc.edu/crr/facts/jtf_10.pdf

79. John and Mark McNaughton, "Gender Differences in Risk Aversion and Expected Retirement Benefits," *Financial Analysis Journal* 63(2007): 52–62.

80. U. S. Department of Labor, *Work Hours: Job Sharing,* 2007. Available at www.dol.gov/dol/topic/workhours/jobsharing.htm

81. Bureau of Labor Statistics, *Workers on Flexible and Shift Schedules in 2004: Summary,* 2005. Available at www.bls.gov/cps/

82. J. T. Bond, C. Thompson, E. Galinsky, and D. Prottas, *Highlights of the National Study of the Changing Workforce* (New York: Family Work Institute, 2002). Available at www.familiesandwork.org/summary/nscw2002.pdf

83. Ibid.

84. Bureau of Labor Statistics, *Economic News Release: American Time Use Survey Summary.* 2011. Available at: www.bls.gov/news.release/atus.nr0.htm

85. Bureau of Labor Statistics, *Work at Home in 2004,* 2005. Available at www.bls.gov/cps/

86. M. J. Grawitch, M. Gottschalk, and D. C. Munz, "The Path to a Healthy Workplace: A Critical Review Linking Healthy Workplace Practices, Employee Well-being, and Organizational Improvements," *Consulting Psychology Journal: Practice and Research* 58(2006): 129–47.

87. Health Promotion Programs, *Inc.* 2011. Available at: www.inc.com/encyclopedia/health-promotion-programs.html.

88. S. G. Aldana, "Financial Impact of Health Promotion Programs: A Comprehensive Review of the Literature," *American Journal of Health Promotion* 15(2001): 296–320.

89. D. C. Munz, J. M. Kohler, and C. I. Greenberg, "Effectiveness of a Comprehensive Worksite Stress Management Program: Combining Organizational and Individual Interventions," *International Journal of Stress Management* 8(2001): 49–62.

90. "Incentives, Support Yield Health Results: Employers Making Room for Health Promotion in the Workplace," *The Nation's Health* (September, 2007): 1, 12–13.

91. K. D. Grimsley, "A Little Baby Powder on the Bottom Line," *The Washington Post,* July 17, 1998, F1, F5.

92. Kirstin Downey Grimsley, "At Work-Site Schools, Kids Learn While Parents Earn," *The Washington Post,* September 8, 1998, A1, A8.

93. K. D. Grimsley, "Companies See Results After 6 Years of Unusual Alliance on Work-Life Issues," *The Washington Post,* November 23, 1997, H1.

94. J. Bond and E. Galinsky, *How Can Employers Increase the Productivity and Retention of Entry-Level, Hourly Employees?* (New York: Family Work Institute, 2006). Available at www.familiesandwork.org/ site/research/reports/brief2.pdf

95. "Incentives, Support Yield Health Results," *The Nation's Health.*

96. U.S. Census Bureau, *Statistical Abstracts of the United States, 2011* (Washington, D.C.: U.S. Census Bureau, 2010), 378.

97. S. C. Clark, "Work Cultures and Work/Family Balance," *Journal of Vocational Behavior* 58(2001): 348–65.

98. M. R. Frone, "Work-Family Balance." In *Handbook of Occupational Health Psychology,* ed. J. C. Quick and L. E. Tetrick (Washington, D.C.: American Psychological Association, 2003).

99. C. M. Brotheridge and R. T. Lee, "Impact of Work-Family Interaction on General Well-Being: A Replication and Extension," *International Journal of Stress Management* 12(2005): 203–21.

100. Office of Disease Prevention and Health Promotion, *Healthy People 2010* (Washington, D.C.: Department of Health and Human Services, 2000).

101. Richard S. Lazarus and Susan Folkman, *Stress, Appraisal, and Coping* (New York: Springer, 1984).

LAB ASSESSMENT 16.1

Do You Have Occupational Stress?

Directions: For each question below, place the number that represents your answer in the space provided.

1 = never
2 = seldom
3 = sometimes
4 = frequently
5 = nearly all the time

_____ 1. How often do you feel that you have too little authority to carry out your responsibilities?

_____ 2. How often do you feel unclear about just what the scope and responsibilities of your job are?

_____ 3. How often do you not know what opportunities for advancement or promotion exist for you?

_____ 4. How often do you feel that you have too heavy a workload, one that you could not possibly finish during an ordinary workday?

_____ 5. How often do you think that you will not be able to satisfy the conflicting demands of various people around you?

_____ 6. How often do you feel that you are not fully qualified to handle your job?

_____ 7. How often do you not know what your superior thinks of you, how he or she evaluates your performance?

_____ 8. How often do you find yourself unable to get information needed to carry out your job?

_____ 9. How often do you worry about decisions that affect the lives of people you know?

_____ 10. How often do you feel that you may not be liked and accepted by people at work?

_____ 11. How often do you feel unable to influence your immediate supervisor's decisions and actions that affect you?

_____ 12. How often do you not know just what the people you work with expect of you?

_____ 13. How often do you think that the amount of work you have to do may interfere with how well it is done?

_____ 14. How often do you feel that you have to do things on the job that are against your better judgment?

_____ 15. How often do you feel that your job interferes with your family life?

Scoring: To score this occupational stress scale, add up your answers. The higher your score is, the greater is your occupational stress.

Interpretation of Scores

15–30 = low occupational stress
31–45 = somewhat low occupational stress
46–60 = somewhat high occupational stress
61–75 = high occupational stress

- If you scored above 60, you have a good chance of occupational stress resulting in illness or disease.

- If you scored between 46 and 60, you have a moderate chance of occupational stress resulting in illness or disease.

- If you scored between 31 and 45, you have a moderate chance to avoid occupational stress resulting in illness or disease.

- If you scored between 15 and 30, you have a good chance of occupational stress not resulting in illness or disease.

LAB ASSESSMENT 16.2

Are You a Workaholic?

Directions: Check "Yes" or "No" for each question as it applies to you.

Yes   No

____ ____ 1. *Do you get up early, no matter how late you go to bed?*

As one management consultant confessed, "I'd get home and work until [about] 2 a.m., and then get up at 5 a.m. and think, 'Gee, aren't I terrific!'"

____ ____ 2. *If you are eating lunch alone, do you read or work while you eat?*

Robert Moses, New York's long-time Parks Commissioner, reportedly considered lunches a bore and a bother because he couldn't bear to interrupt work. He used a large table as a desk so lunch could be served right there.

____ ____ 3. *Do you make daily lists of things to do?*

Ever-present appointment books and cluttered calendars are a hallmark of workaholics. Indeed, their main way of wasting time, admits Dr. Elizabeth Whelan, a Harvard University epidemiologist, may be looking for lost lists!

____ ____ 4. *Do you find it difficult to "do nothing"?*

It was claimed that David Mahoney, the hardworking chairman of Norton Simon Inc., abandoned transcendental meditation because he found it impossible to sit still for 20 minutes.

____ ____ 5. *Are you energetic and competitive?*

President Johnson once asked Doris Kearns, then a White House Fellow, if she were energetic. Kearns replied, "I hear you need only five hours of sleep, but I need only four, so it stands to reason that I've got even more energy than you."

____ ____ 6. *Do you work on weekends and holidays?*

In *Working*, author Studs Terkel related that the president of a Chicago radio station confessed that he regularly works in his home on weekends. But, he added, "When I do this on holidays, like Christmas, New Year's, and Thanksgiving, I have to sneak a bit so the family doesn't know what I'm doing."

____ ____ 7. *Can you work anytime and anywhere?*

Two associates at Cravath, Swaine and Moore, one of Manhattan's most prestigious law firms, were said to have bet about who could bill the most hours in a day. One worked around the clock, billed 24, and felt assured of victory. His competitor, however, having flown to California in the course of the day and worked on the plane, was able to bill 27.

____ ____ 8. *Do you find vacations "hard to take"?*

George Lois, the art director who heads Lois Pitts Gershon, an advertising agency, had to think awhile when I asked him when he had taken his last vacation. Finally, he recalled when it was: 1964—almost 14 years before!

____ ____ 9. *Do you dread retirement?*

After retiring from the ad agency where she had created such classic slogans as Clairol's "Does she . . . or doesn't she?" Shirley Polykoff started her own advertising agency. As president of Shirley Polykoff Advertising in New York she still—some six years later—has no plans to slow up or step down. She says, "I'm doing more now than I've ever done. I don't know how you retire if you're still healthy and exuberant about living. They'll have to carry me out in a box!"

____ ____ 10. *Do you really enjoy your work?*

As Joyce Carol Oates, the novelist, once told the *New York Times*, "I am not conscious of working especially hard, or of 'working' at all. . . . Writing and teaching have always been, for me, so richly rewarding that I do not think of them as work in the usual sense of the word."

If you answered "Yes" to fewer than five questions, you probably are not a workaholic.
If you answered "Yes" to six to nine questions, you may be a mild workaholic.
If you answered "Yes" to more than nine questions, you may be a full-fledged workaholic.
Refer back to the section "The Workaholic" for tips to combat workaholism.

Source: Machlowitz, Marilyn, Workaholics, 1st edition, © 1980, pp. 17–20. Reprinted by permission of Pearson Education, Inc., Upper Saddle River, NJ.

LAB ASSESSMENT 16.3

Do You Have Burnout or Brownout?

Directions: Determine whether you are suffering from burnout, or if you are only partway there (brownout). Complete the brownout inventory below and find out. For each statement, write a T if that statement is true for you or an F if it isn't.

_____ 1. Is your efficiency at work declining?

_____ 2. Have you lost some of your initiative at work?

_____ 3. Have you lost interest in your work?

_____ 4. Does work stress get to you more than it used to?

_____ 5. Do you feel fatigued or run down?

_____ 6. Do you get headaches?

_____ 7. Do you get stomachaches?

_____ 8. Have you lost weight recently?

_____ 9. Do you have trouble sleeping?

_____ 10. Do you experience shortness of breath?

_____ 11. Do you have frequently changing or depressive moods?

_____ 12. Are you easy to anger?

_____ 13. Do you get frustrated easily?

_____ 14. Are you more suspicious than you used to be?

_____ 15. Do you feel more helpless than you used to?

_____ 16. Are you using too many mood-altering drugs (e.g., tranquilizers or alcohol)?

_____ 17. Are you becoming more inflexible?

_____ 18. Are you becoming more critical of your own and others' competencies?

_____ 19. Are you working more but feeling that you're getting less done?

_____ 20. Have you lost some of your sense of humor?

If you answered *true* for more than half the statements, you may be experiencing brownout. If you answered *true* for 15 or more of these statements, you may be burning out (or already burned out). Recognize, however, that you can remedy this situation by employing the stress management suggestions described in this chapter.

Family Stress

17

I'll never forget the voice breaking with emotion, the tears being held back, as he eulogized his 42-year-old brother after his brother's premature death:

> My brother need not be idealized or enlarged in death beyond what he was in life. To be remembered simply as a good and decent man who saw wrong and tried to right it, who saw suffering and tried to heal it, who saw war and tried to stop it. Those of us who loved him and who take him to his rest today, pray that what he was to us, what he wished for others, may come to pass for all the world. As he said many times in many parts of this nation, to those he touched and who sought to touch him: Some men see things as they are. I dream things that never were and say, why not?

These words were spoken in New York City's St. Patrick's Cathedral in early June of 1968 as the nation stopped to mourn with Edward Kennedy the death of his brother Robert. As I listened to the eulogy and participated in the funeral, albeit from afar, I could not help thinking of *my* two brothers, Stephen and Mark. Stephen, the businessman bent on making a million dollars, and Mark, the musician and artist, are as different from me as they are from each other. And yet, we are family. We grew up sharing one bedroom, fought with each other regularly, and shared the sorrows and joys accompanying twenty-some years of life under one roof.

This chapter is about such bonds—family bonds—and how the changes in family life can be stressful. It describes ways to intervene between family stress and illness and disease.

The Family

A family is a set of intimate and personal relationships. These relationships may be legal (as in marriage) or extralegal (as in communal family groups). We speak of *a family of friends,* fraternity *brothers,* sorority *sisters,* and kissing *cousins,* using family-related terms to communicate the intimacy of these relationships. Our discussion, however, will be limited in this section to the **nuclear family**—a married couple and their children—and the **extended family**—relatives other than spouses and children.

Needs Satisfied by the Family

One of the functions of a family is to govern societal control of reproduction and child rearing. Although there are some marriage partners who do not have children—by choice or anatomical condition—for those who do have them, the societal expectation is that these children will be raised within a family structure. This family may take many forms, and, although some single women and lesbians choose to conceive children, the social expectation is still that a child will be born to a married couple.

The family may also provide economic support. Food, clothing, and shelter are provided by family members who assist one another in their various tasks and functions. For example, one family member might cook the food that another

nuclear family
A married couple and their children.

extended family
Relatives other than spouses and children.

419

In addition to dealing with important things, the effective family has fun together.

family member earns money to buy, or both marriage partners may take jobs outside the home to earn money to eat out. While children are growing up, they are supported by the more self-sufficient family members (parents, older siblings, or other relatives), and their physiological, safety, and security needs are provided for.

Lastly, the family may provide for many emotional needs. It can provide love, eliminate feelings of isolation, foster a sense of belonging, and teach you that others are concerned about and care for you. In a family you can really be yourself—even your worst self—and usually still feel you belong to the group. Your family may not like your behavior or your decisions, but you'll still be welcome for Thanksgiving dinner, so to speak. Families can also serve you well in times of crisis. As we noted earlier in this book, having people with whom you can discuss your problems (social support) can help prevent you from becoming ill from those problems.

These words describing the needs families can meet convey the role of the family only in an academic, intellectual sense. For many people, family life serves a real emotional need as well. They have been made to feel secure and loved and have developed a sense of belonging from their families. I'm reminded of a story I recently read in the newspaper of an automobile accident in which a family of five was involved. The car crash killed the father, mother, and two young children, but the two-year-old daughter, who wore a seat belt, survived. As I read the story, my heart went out to this child, and I felt her loss. By that, I do not mean I was concerned about who would care for her, feed her, or shelter her. Rather, I was feeling her *irreplaceable* loss—the loss of her blood relatives, whose connection with her could never be totally compensated. There's something about the family bond that makes it unique.

Now, having said all of that, we need to recognize that not all families function as described. Some parents are abusive, some family members are separated from each other, and some people are so impoverished (financially, emotionally, or morally) that the last thing on their minds is helping to satisfy family needs. There are single-parent families, blended families, and dysfunctional families. And there are families whose members just don't know any better or who are so busy providing some of the needs (e.g., economic support) that other needs go unmet (e.g., love). However, when the family is effective, it can be such a major influence that nothing can compare with its effect on your total existence and future.

The Changing Family

The predominant family style in America is the breadwinning father, homemaking mother, and resident children. Right? Wrong! Check out these surprising statistics about family life in 2009 America:[1]

- Just over 130 million U.S. adults (57 percent of the adult population) were married and living with a spouse.

- Among 25- to 29-year-olds, 61 percent of men (over 6.6 million) had never been married, as were 46 percent of women (4.8 million) never married.

- Only 21 percent of households met the stereotypical standard of a husband, wife, living with their own children.

- Just over 13 percent of adults (23 million) were currently divorced.

- 26 percent of all children under 18 lived with a single parent.

- Of children living with a single parent, 85 percent lived with their mothers, 44 percent of whom had never married and 30 percent who were divorced.

Covenant Marriages

In 1997, Louisiana passed a law requiring couples applying for marriage licenses to choose one of two types of marital contracts. The Standard Marital Contract allows married partners to divorce after living separately for six months, or immediately if one spouse is guilty of adultery, has been sentenced to prison, or dies. The Covenant Marital Contract allows the couple to divorce only after they have lived apart for two years or after one spouse commits adultery, is sentenced to prison for a felony, abandons the home for at least a year, or physically or sexually abuses the spouse or child, and the couple must participate in premarital counseling from either a member of the clergy or a counselor. In other words, with a Covenant Marital Contract, the couple waive their right to a no-fault (easily obtained) divorce. The intent is to require couples deciding to marry to consider their commitment and to make sure they are making the right decision, then, when problems in the marriage surface, as they do in most marriages, to encourage couples to work through these problems rather than take the easy route to divorce. However, opponents argue that marriages that are in trouble only create distress for the couple and negatively influence children.

If you were about to become married, which contract would you choose?

Fewer than half (43 percent) of married-couple households have children under 18 years of age living at home.[2] However, children older than 18 years of age also move back in with their parent(s) or never move out. Those who move out and return—because of divorce, economic hardship, or myriad other reasons—are sometimes referred to as **boomerang children.** Fifteen percent of family households had these children 18 or older living at home. Of family households with children under 18, 30 percent were maintained by single parents; there were almost 10 million mother-child family groups and 1.7 million father-child family groups. Furthermore, in the mother-child single-parent family groups, 43 percent of the mothers had never been married.[3] The types of households are depicted in Figure 17.1.

boomerang children

Children who leave home to live elsewhere but subsequently return to live with the parents.

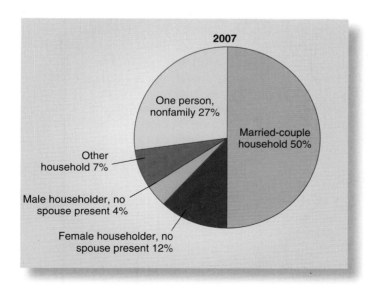

Figure 17.1

Households by Type, 2009

Source: U.S. Census Bureau. *Statistical Abstracts of the United States,* 2011 (Washington, D.C.: U.S. Census Bureau, 2010), 54.

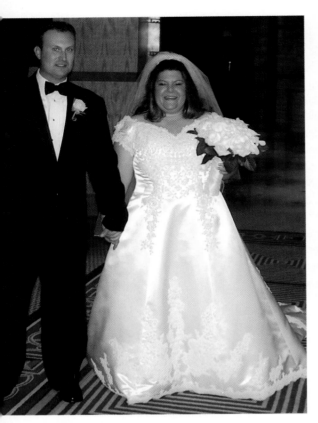

Marriage can be quite joyful, with couples sharing happy occasions. At the same time, marriage can be stressful as two people who lived apart now must accommodate each other.

cohabitation
Romantically involved couples living together although not married.

Marriage

Many aspects of marriage have remained unchanged for centuries, and many others have changed radically. June marriages are still the most popular, more adults still get married rather than remain single, marriage is still a legal entity requiring a marriage license and a marriage ceremony (either civil or religious), and more women still take their husband's last name than do not.

On the other hand, marriage has changed considerably over the years. People of the same sex may be legally married in some states. In 2009, 57 percent of the adult population were married and living with their spouses. Yet, a large number of adults have never married. Among people twenty to twenty-four years old, 87 percent of males have never married and 77 percent of females have never married.

Marriage can be quite joyful, but even in the best of marriages it can also be quite stressful. Are *you* ready for marriage? Complete Lab 17.1 at the end of this chapter to help you decide. What kind of person would you prefer to marry? Completing Lab 17.2 will help you answer that question.

Cohabitation

More and more people choose to live with someone with whom they are romantically involved but to whom they are not married. Between 1970 and 1976, the number of people living together with someone of the opposite sex without marrying doubled to 1.3 million people. Until around 1970, **cohabitation** was illegal in all 50 states. By 2008 it was reported that there were 5.6 million Americans cohabiting with someone of the opposite sex and another 565,000 same-sex cohabiting partners.[4] People between the ages of 20 and 24 are most likely to be currently cohabiting, with ages 25 to 29 next most likely.

About a third of all adults, and 4 in 10 under the age of 50, have been in a cohabiting relationship with someone with whom they were not married.[5] It is estimated that approximately 25 percent of unmarried women age 25 to 39 are currently living with a partner, and another 25 percent have lived with a partner sometime in the past.[6] Almost half of all first marriages are preceded by cohabitating, as compared to virtually none 50 years ago.[7] When asked why they decided to live together rather than marry, 21 percent of cohabiting couples stated they wanted to be sure this was the person for them, 15 percent responded the timing for marriage was not right, 12 percent reported it was convenient or easier than marriage, and 10 percent cohabited rather than marry for financial reasons.[8]

Cohabitation is prevalent on college campuses but is not exclusive to young adults. Many elderly people who are widowed are living together because of the financial benefits—their two separate Social Security checks may be larger than one check when remarried—or because they feel no need to formalize their union. The separated and divorced are also choosing to cohabit more than in the past.

Divorce

Table 17.1 shows the divorce rate from 1960 through 2008. As can be seen, the divorce rate rose consistently from 1960 to about 1981; it has been dropping ever since. As of 2008, 10 percent of Americans were divorced. That amounted to almost 23 million divorced men and women. When broken down by gender, 9 percent of men (almost 10 million) and 11 percent of women (over 13 million) were divorced.[9]

Year	Rate per 1,000 Population
2008	3.4
2007	3.6
2006	3.6
2005	3.6
2004	3.7
2003	3.8
2002	4.0
2001	4.0
2000	4.1
1995	4.4
1991	4.7
1985	5.0
1981	5.3
1975	4.8
1970	3.5
1965	2.5
1960	2.2

Table 17.1
Divorce Rates: United States, 1960 to 2008

Sources: National Center for Health Statistics, "Annual Summary of Births, Marriages, Divorces, and Deaths: United States, 1992," *Monthly Vital Statistics Report* 41(28 September 1993), 4–5; "National Center for Health Statistics, Births, Marriages, Divorces, and Deaths for 1995," Monthly Vital Statistics Report 44(24 July 1996) 1; National Center for Health Statistics, "Births, Marriages, Divorces, and Deaths for 1996," *Monthly Vital Statistics Report* 45(17 July 1997), 1; U.S. Census Bureau, Statistical Abstract of the United States, 1999; National Center for Health Statistics, "Births, Marriages, Divorces, and Deaths: Provisional Data for 2003," *National Vital Statistics Report* 52(10 June 2004), 1; National Center for Health Statistics, "Births, Marriages, Divorces, and Deaths: Provisional Data for 2006," *National Vital Statistics Reports* 55(August 28, 2007), 1. National Center for Health Statistics, "National Marriage and Divorce Rate Trends," *National Vital Statistics System*, 2009. Available at: www.cdc.gov/nchs/nvss/mardiv_tables.htm. B.Tejada-Vera and P. D. Sutton, "Births, Marriages, Divorces, and Deaths: Provisional Data for 2009." *National Vital Statistics Reports*, vol. 58, no. 25 (Hyattsville, MD: National Center for Health Statistics. 2010).

As you might guess, large numbers of children are affected by their parents' divorce. In 1970, merely 12 percent of children lived with one parent. By 2008, that number had increased to 31 percent.[10]

Single-Parent Families

The U.S. Census Bureau reports that the number of families maintained by one parent increased by 80 percent from 1970 to 1980. By 2010, approximately 31 percent of all families with children still at home were maintained by one parent.[11] Eighty-four percent of the one-parent families were headed by women in 2010. That amounts to over 12 million families. In addition, 2 million one-parent families were headed by men. This number of **single-parent families** is a result of increased marital separation, divorce, and out-of-wedlock pregnancies rather than widowhood. Further, in 2009, 61 percent of African American families with children at home, 33 percent of Hispanic families with children at home, and 23 percent of white families with children at home were maintained by one parent.[12]

single-parent families
Families in which the father or the mother is absent because of divorce, marital separation, out-of-wedlock pregnancy, or death.

Gay and Lesbian Families

Should gay and lesbian couples be allowed to adopt children? Some people argue that children raised in a gay or lesbian household are especially likely to adopt a homosexual lifestyle. They strongly lament the lack of male and female gender role models during children's developmental years. They warn that homosexuality is sinful, and they believe that children should not be allowed to be brought up in sinful homes.

Other people argue that there is no reason to believe, or evidence to indicate, that children raised by gays and lesbians are more likely than other children to become

Although most single-parent families are headed by women, men also can be, and often are, effective single parents.

Family Insight

To learn things about your family about which even you are unaware, try this activity: draw a picture of your family participating in some activity. Do this now on a separate piece of paper.

The next time you are with a group of people—perhaps in class—ask several people to look at your drawing and, on its back, write one sentence describing their perceptions of either the family in general or any member in particular. You will be surprised how people who may not know you or any other members of your family very well can be so accurate in their perceptions of your family. I'll give you some examples now of how this works, but, since these examples may influence what you draw, don't read on until your drawing is complete.

In one group that I asked to do this activity, a woman drew a picture of herself at the ironing board, with her husband on his back on the rug with their baby held up in his extended arms. Several written comments noted that it seemed she did the housework while her husband relaxed and had fun. She said, "Yes, you know, that's true. I'm going to speak to him about helping out."

Another group included a man who drew himself, his wife, and his son in some activity, with his daughter doing something else at some distance from the other three. Several comments suggested that the daughter seemed left out of family activities. The man thought about this for a while and agreed. He said he was going to make a conscious effort to include his daughter in family activities from then on.

When you have other people comment on your drawing, do not reject any comments without giving them thought. Perhaps you were not consciously aware of some aspects of your family dynamics but subconsciously attuned to them so that they were included in your drawing. Of course, those commenting on your drawings will probably not be psychoanalysts, but my experience is that their comments will be insightful. What's more, their comments will help you to begin improving your family's effectiveness and making your family life less stressful.

homosexuals themselves. Furthermore, they continue, gay and lesbian households can be as ethical, spiritual, or religious as any other household, for sexual orientation does not preclude a moral setting in which children can be raised.

One way in which gays and lesbians are reacting to this societal debate is by conceiving children through artificial insemination or other means. In that way, they need not seek the approval of adoption agencies to establish a family with children. Both gay couples and lesbian couples are parenting such children.

The right to raise children is not the only family-related stressor with which gays and lesbians must cope. Gay and lesbian marriage is another one. Several states have sanctioned marriage between homosexual couples. The first state supreme courts to rule bans on gay and lesbian marriages unconstitutional were those of Hawaii (1993) and Alaska (1998). However, the legislatures of both states later amended their state constitutions to outlaw gay marriage. Elsewhere, alarmed by the thought of state-sanctioned gay marriages, opponents were successful in convincing 37 states to adopt laws prohibiting legalized same-sex marriages.[13] Then in 2003 the Massachusetts Supreme Judicial Court ruled that "the right to marry means little if it does not include the right to marry the person of one's choice."[14] By a 4-to-3 vote, that court approved gay marriage. Since then, many gay couples have been married.

When the public was polled about gay marriage, most respondents were opposed to it.[15] Sixty-one percent stated that they were opposed to their state passing a law permitting same-sex marriage. Yet 50 percent opposed amending the United States Constitution to prohibit states from allowing these marriages, and 51 percent favored civil unions among same-sex couples. Civil unions would not be sanctioned marriages but would provide gay couples inheritance, insurance, pension, and other rights enjoyed by heterosexual couples.

It can be quite stressful for gays and lesbians, and their children, to be perceived as living an immoral, sinful life. Like other forms of bias, being singled out in this way can lead to stress reactivity, which in turn can result in negative consequences such as illness and disease.

Family Stressors

Although the family may not be dying—as some sociologists argue—it certainly is in transition. All the changes in family life previously cited need to be adapted to and are therefore stressful. Some of these stressors are discussed in this section.

The Dual-Career Family

More women who are married and have young children work outside the home than in previous generations. Whereas in 1980, 54 percent of married mothers with children worked outside the home, 70 percent did in 2009.[16] In 2009, 62 percent of married mothers with children under 6 years of age worked outside the home, and 76 percent with children between the ages of 6 and 13 worked outside the home.[17]

There are many reasons for the increase in dual-career families. Among these are that children are expensive to raise (see the next section). Day care, clothing, medical care, schooling, and other costs result in many families deciding that both spouses need to earn money. In addition, aspirations have increased from past generations. Many families want to have two cars, a big house, nice clothing, and all the latest in

Issue: Is Family Life Worse Than It Used to Be?

A Gallup poll prepared for the White House Conference on Families found 45 percent of Americans think family life has gotten worse. Of the 1,592 adults polled, 18 percent said they personally knew of a child-abuse situation, and 18 percent also knew of husband or wife abuse cases. Lastly, 25 percent reported that alcohol-related problems had adversely affected their family lives.

Others believed that, although it has certainly changed, family life has not worsened. Citing more equal sex roles and chores of family members, the greater opportunity for women to work outside the home, the increased availability of quality child-care services, and the positive effect of divorce upon children when the historical alternative has been to grow up with two parents constantly bickering, some people actually perceive the family to have evolved into a more effective unit.

Do you believe the family unit has worsened, or do you believe it has become more responsive to its members' needs? Why did you answer as you did?

technology (for example, iPods and iPhones, iPads, computers, Internet connection, large-screen high-definition televisions). One result is that, in spite of the increase in dual-career families, family debt keeps increasing, especially with the global recession of 2008–2009. In fact, it increased 5 percent from 2000 to 2009.[18]

Not only does a woman who works outside the home experience stress about juggling all of her responsibilities, but she is also bothered over what she is missing. As one mother who worked out of economic necessity put it a while ago: "Having to deal with a babysitter is very painful. All I can see is another woman holding, loving, and caring for my new baby. I am actually paying her to do all the things I wish I could be doing."[19] In one study,[20] women were asked, "Considering everything, what would be the ideal situation for you—working full-time, part-time, or not at all outside the home?" Whereas in 1997, 32 percent of working mothers responded that they would prefer to work full-time, in 2007 only 21 percent responded that way. Interestingly, when fathers were asked the same question, 72 percent answered they would prefer to work full-time. Clearly, many men who work outside the home and therefore have less contact with their children than they would wish may also have feelings similar to those expressed by the woman quoted above.

Both working parents must also adapt to a lifestyle in which they share housework and child-rearing responsibilities. Certainly, working women still assume more than their fair share of these responsibilities, and that imbalance can be stressful. Still, spouses of working women take on more of these chores, and working women take on fewer of these chores, than in households in which only men work outside the home.

Finally, in this equation, the child also must adapt to parents not being around as much. The child must cope with a babysitter or day care staff and learn to be more self-sufficient at an earlier age.

All of this is not to say that women or men should not or need not work outside the home. People who are trained for a career and not pursuing it may experience more stress than that associated with combining parenting, homemaking, and a career. If they feel more stress, the chances are that so will their spouses and children. However, that **dual-career families** are potentially stressful should not be denied.

dual-career family
A family in which both spouses work outside the home with careers of their own.

Children

A friend once warned me that children are geometric, rather than arithmetic, stressors. What he meant was that a couple who has a child has added stressors equivalent to two extra adults; a couple with one child who has another multiplies their stress by some number other than 1 or 2; and a couple with two children . . . Children are wonderful, but they certainly are stressful. This is understandable, since stress involves adjusting to change. Although all of us are changing, children are changing more rapidly, repeatedly, and dramatically than mature adults. Children's bodies are changing, their minds developing, and their social skills and life-space expanding. To expect such change not to be stressful is unrealistic.

Further, when children change, so does the family. Oftentimes, children are able to assume more responsibilities, take on more jobs, become more self-sufficient, and hold more firm opinions than when they were younger. These changes affect other members of the family. For example, when children become old enough to drive the family car, the parents no longer need to make themselves available for car pools. However, they must take on other stressors: "Will Johnny and the car both get home in one piece tonight?" This leads us to those notorious teenage years.

Parents who see their children approaching "teenagehood" sometimes find their knees knocking together, their hearts racing, and their headaches visiting more frequently. Teenagers may get involved with drugs, sex, vandalism, shoplifting, automobile accidents, or truancy; they may be impossible to discipline, talk with, or get to see very often; or they may have problems with their teachers, their friends, or their bosses. Or they may be companions, helpers, and interesting to talk with; they may be brilliant, committed to causes, and willing to persevere to

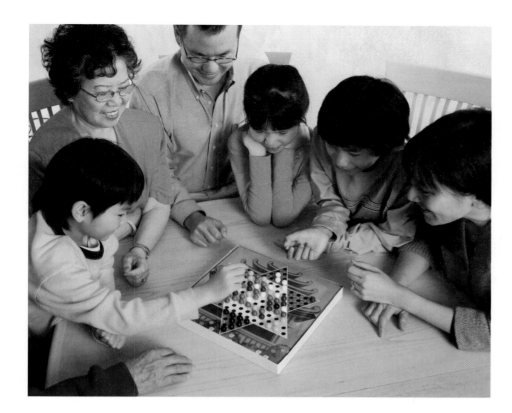

achieve goals; and they may be individuals of whom we are very, very proud. Lest we forget, these years are stressful for teenagers as well. A sobering piece of evidence of this is the number of attempted suicides by teenagers.

Other years of growing up may be stressful for parents and children, too. A while ago, the parent-child relationship was described as three-phased: bonding, detachment, and reunion.[21] During the *bonding* years, the child learns love, approval, and acceptance from the family. During the *detachment* years, the child learns independence and relies less on the family. The *reunion* years occur after the child is independent and is secure enough to rebond with the family. Bonding is a preteen phase, detachment a teen phase, and reunion a postteen phase. Each phase has its own stressors and its own joys.

Family Planning

A discussion of stress and children must include a discussion of planning for how many children to have. Two topics pertaining to this consideration are discussed in this section: contraception and abortion and their relationship to family stress.

When couples decide to control conception to limit the number of children they have, they must decide upon a method. There is no perfect method of birth control. Each has its advantages and disadvantages, and all should be studied before one is chosen. This choice, however, may generate disagreement between the sexual partners and cause distress. Who should be responsible for birth control, the man or the woman? How much inconvenience or interruption are they willing to tolerate in sexual activity? What religious proscriptions should they adhere to? How much risk—both in terms of their health and in terms of the chances of a pregnancy—are they willing to accept?

Once the decision about birth control is made, there is still the possibility of pregnancy. No method except abstinence is 100 percent effective. If unwanted pregnancy does occur, what then? Another child? An **abortion?** Give the baby up for adoption? These decisions, too, can be very stressful and more complicated than at first thought.

abortion
The termination of a pregnancy.

Helping Children Cope with Stress

The following is a list of online resources for families to help children manage the stress in today's world.

Afterschool Alliance

www.afterschoolalliance.org

This site provides links to many resources for helping youth deal with tragedy and terrorism, increase their cultural tolerance, and interpret media messages.

American Academy of Pediatrics

www.aap.org/advocacy/releases/disastercomm.htm

This site offers advice on communicating with children and adolescents about stressful events.

KidsHealth

http://kidshealth.org/parent/emotions/feelings/stress.html

Provides an online resource entitled *Childhood Stress* that discusses sources of stress, signs and symptoms of stress, and strategies to reduce stress experienced by children.

National Education Association

www.nea.org/tools/EW-Saving%20Kids%20from%20Stress.htm

NEA's web page includes *Helping Families and Children Cope with This National Tragedy.*

National Parent Teacher Association

www.pta.org/2563.htm

The National PTA offers a resource online entitled *Hints to Help Reduce Homework Stress.*

For more websites, visit the Online Learning Center at www.mhhe.com/greenberg13e.

Adoption

Some families experience the stress associated with the inability to conceive their own children. For these families, adoption is an alternative, although the adoption process itself can be a stressor.

There are two basic types of adoption. **Closed adoptions** are confidential; there is no contact between the birth parents and the adoptive parents. The identities of the birth parents and adoptive parents are kept secret from one another. In **open adoptions** there is contact between the birth and adoptive parents. In fact, the birth parents may even select the adoptive parents. This contact can occur regularly or intermittently throughout the child's upbringing.

Although there have been some highly publicized cases of birth parents seeking to reverse them, adoptions are legally binding and irreversible after a short, limited period of time. Birth parents sign "relinquishment papers" after the baby is born and, unless both birth parents did not sign these papers, the courts refuse to reverse adoptions.

Adoption agencies can be located through most religious organizations or by writing the National Council for Adoption at 225 N. Washington Street, Alexandria, VA 22314 or by telephoning them at (703) 299–6633. They will even accept collect calls from pregnant women. Their web address is www.adoptioncouncil.org.

Someone contemplating placing a child for adoption may want to discuss that decision with someone trusted to be helpful. Adopting a child can be stressful as well, as evidenced in the accompanying box.

closed adoption

Adoptions in which there is no contact between the birth parents and the adoptive parents.

open adoption

Adoptions where there is contact between the birth parents and the adoptive parents.

Some Things to Ask Yourself If You Are Thinking About Adopting a Child

Questions Regarding Personal Changes:
- Am I ready to be a parent? Do I feel as though I can deal with the additional responsibilities of caring for a child?
- What kind of lifestyle do I have? What kinds of changes will I need to make, such as adjustments to the amount of time I spend with friends and the hours that I keep? Do I feel good about making lifestyle changes to care for a baby?
- What are my personal goals and priorities concerning having a family, going to school, and/or having a career?

Questions Regarding Relationship Changes for the Couple:
- What are your expectations about dividing work around the house and caring for the baby?
- What are your plans for taking time off from work or school? How do you each feel about these plans?
- How do you feel about the way decisions are made in your relationship? Do you feel as though you need more input into the decision of whether or not to have a baby and when?
- How do you feel about the ways you and your partner share intimacy? Do you have any nonsexual (but perhaps still physical) ways to be intimate? Would you like to add some things that you can do for each other to show you care?
- How do you spend your time now as a couple? If you have a child, how will you continue to find time for yourselves individually and as a couple?

Questions Regarding Changes in Relationships with Parents:
- How do my partner and I get along with our parent(s)?
- Am I viewed as an adult by my parent(s)?
- In what ways do I want my child's life to be similar to or different from my childhood?
- If a parent is deceased or not in our lives, how does that affect us?

Questions Regarding Changes in Relationships with Those Outside of the Family:
- Am I prepared for changes in my friendships?
- Who could I go to for emotional support and knowledge if I had a baby?
- How would having a baby change things for me at work? If I do decide to have a baby, what would I need to do to prepare for this in the workplace (for instance, giving notice or asking for time off, or making changes to insurance)?

Questions Regarding New Demands Associated with Being a Parent:
- How do each of you react when you don't get enough sleep?
- What are the expectations that each of you have about being up during the night with a baby?
- Are there family members or friends who could help out, or would it be possible to hire someone to come and stay in the home and help with child care in the initial months?
- How do you respond to stress, and what helps you deal with stress?

Source: Amanda N. Holzworth and Heidi Liss Radunovich. *Questions to Ask as You Consider Parenthood: A Couples' Guide.* Gainesville, Florida: Department of Family, Youth and Community Science, Florida Cooperative Extension Service, IFAS, University of Florida, 2007. Available at http://edis.ifas.ufl.edu/fy928

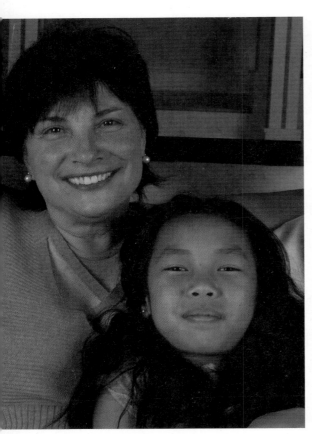

Adoption of children from other countries is a possibility for those wanting children and also wanting to respond to global needs.

Finding the Birth Parent

As adults, many adopted children seek to identify their birth parents. This search is fraught with stress related to the search itself and to the reactions of both the adoptive parents and the birth parents. There is a good deal of disagreement as to whether and how this process should be facilitated. Some experts believe that contacting the birth parents might make them feel guilty about the adoption years earlier, or that they might reject the adopted child—now an adult—and the child might develop unhealthy reactions to that rejection.

Before World War II, it was common practice for adoption records to be open. However, after the war, the combination of an increase in out-of-wedlock pregnancies and a conservative mood in the country resulted in adoption going "into the closet." Adoption records became sealed so secrecy could be maintained. Since then, a couple of states have opened adoption records to adoptees, although almost all states do not.[22] Yet, court orders can be obtained in many states to gain access to adoption records and, if both adoptee parents and birth parents agree, records may be unsealed in many other states.

Mobility

There was a time when the members of an extended family all lived in the same town and visited frequently. When I was growing up, a "family circle" met one Sunday a month. All the aunts, uncles, cousins, and Grandma Mary and Grandpa Barney gathered to talk, play cards, play ball, argue, and eat. We would sometimes pile into the back of my grandfather's pickup truck, sit on empty wooden milk crates, and be off for a day at the beach. We all felt close to one another and were caught up in one another's lives. I knew whom my cousin Marcia was dating, and she knew what sports I liked.

How times have changed! My children were born in Buffalo and now one lives in Seattle and the other in the Washington, D.C., area. We have no relatives living in either of these places. We make a point of renewing extended family ties once a year at a Passover seder rather than once a month, as when I was young. My children rarely played with their cousins and didn't know much about their relatives' lives. Their grandmother didn't come over every Friday night for dinner, as mine did. She lived 300 miles away. When they had a babysitter, it wasn't their cousin Larry from next door, as it was for me. Their babysitter was a nonrelative from a list of sitters we maintained ("supported" might be a more accurate term).

What's more, families pick up and move so often nowadays that even close friends who might serve as surrogate extended family are left elsewhere. New friendships need to be developed, and it takes time for these new relationships to become meaningful.

In addition to the lack of involvement with extended family, mobility has led to other stressors. When you move, you need to find new physicians, dentists, gas stations, shopping malls, libraries, and so forth. Many of your surroundings and habits change—and we know by now that change can be stressful.

Violence: A Family Matter

It is unfortunate that families, or for that matter anyone, cannot feel safe, yet that is the situation in many communities around the country. Street crime is on everyone's mind as our prisons expand in population and number, without any noticeable effect in limiting the crime and violence to which we are all subjected. This situation has resulted in additional stress in our already stressful lives and particularly in additional stress for families. Even our children are not immune to the devastating effects of violence.

Child Abuse

As if that weren't enough, domestic violence—violence among family members and violence occurring in the home—has also exploded. As early as 1994, the U.S. secretary of health and human services described domestic violence as a crisis, a plague, a sickness, an epidemic, and terrorism in the home.[23] According to the Centers for Disease Control and Prevention,[24] approximately 772,000 children were found to be victims of child abuse or neglect in calendar year 2008. Of this number, 71 percent suffered neglect, 16 percent were physically abused, 9 percent were sexually abused, 7 percent were emotionally or psychologically maltreated, and less than 1 percent were medically neglected. In 2008, 1,740 deaths occurred as a result of child abuse and neglect.[25] Child abuse and neglect are a result of drug abuse by family members, poverty and economic stress, and a lack of parenting skills.[26]

One reason children are the victims of violence may be the number of guns and firearms in U.S. homes and the improper care of those guns. There are approximately 192 million privately owned firearms in the United States, 65 million of which are handguns. In the United States in 2006, 29,674 people . . . were intentionally killed by firearms, either by others (43 percent were homicides) or by their own hands (57 percent were suicides).[27] And for every firearm fatality, there are estimated to be more than two nonfatal firearm injuries. Other countries' firearm deaths and injuries pale by comparison. For example, in 2006, firearms were used to murder 27 people in Australia, 190 people in Canada, 59 people in England and Wales, 194 people in Germany, and 60 people in Spain.[28] During that same year, 11,344 people in the United States were murdered by firearms.

Every Day in America: The Violent Lives of America's Children

5 children are killed by abuse or neglect.

5 children and youths under 20 commit suicide.

8 children and youths under 20 die from firearms.

186 children are arrested for violent crimes.

368 children are arrested for drug abuse.

1,240 public school children are corporally punished.

4,133 children are arrested.

Source: Children's Defense Fund, *Each Day in America. 2011.* Available at: www.childrensdefense.org/child-research-data-publications/each-day-in-america.html.

Waiting in traffic after a stressful day at work could add to violence at home. Although this is certainly no excuse for violence, stress can be defused in healthier ways.

Intimate Partner Violence

The Centers for Disease Control and Prevention's *National Center for Injury Prevention and Control* reports on statistics on violence by intimates.[29] Intimates are defined as spouses, ex-spouses, boyfriends, and girlfriends. Nearly 4.8 million incidents of intimate partner violence are experienced by women each year, and 2.9 million by men. However, since most incidents of intimate partner violence are not reported—only 20 percent of rapes and sexual assaults, 25 percent of physical assaults, and 50 percent of stalkings are reported—these data greatly underestimate the true magnitude of the problem. Over a lifetime, 11 percent of women and 2 percent of men report experiencing forced sex at some time in their lives. And 3 percent of women and 1 percent of men report experiencing unwanted sexual activity in the previous 12 months. Furthermore, 20 to 25 percent of women report experiencing an attempted or a completed rape while attending college.[30] And leaving one's abusive partner is often not a surefire way to prevent intimate partner violence. Women who are separated from their abusive partners are particularly at risk of violence. In these instances, restraining orders can be obtained through the courts mandating that the abuser have no contact with and remain a certain distance from the victimized partner. The costs of intimate partner violence are staggering, exceeding \$8.3 billion.[31]

As you might suspect, the perpetrators of intimate violence are not the most valued members of society. In fact, of those in jail, 78 percent of abusers have a prior criminal record, although not necessarily for intimate violence. Forty percent of jail inmates convicted of a violent crime against an intimate had a criminal justice status at the time of the crime; about 20 percent were on probation, 9 percent were under a restraining order, and just under 10 percent were on parole, pretrial release, or other status. They also have a history of drug and alcohol abuse. More than half the inmates serving time for violence against an intimate were using drugs or alcohol or both at the time of the incident. Battering men typically have low self-esteem, traditional sex role expectations, jealousy, a need to control, abusive family backgrounds, and a need to blame others.[32]

In addition to physical abuse, domestic violence can take other forms. The National Resource Center on Domestic Violence includes sexual abuse (forcing a partner to engage in unwanted sexual behaviors), emotional abuse (name calling, put downs, threatening, and stalking), and property/economic abuse (stealing or destroying property).[33]

There are things we can all do to help prevent family violence. Here are a few suggestions.

- Ask your local schools or school board to include dating violence in the curriculum.
- Call your local media and remind them to acknowledge Domestic Violence Awareness Month (October).
- Ask local businesses to display the telephone number of the National Domestic Violence Hotline (1-800-799-SAFE).
- Ask local clergy to offer sermons on domestic violence.

Financial Stressors

Another category of stressors experienced by many families relates to finances. Some families live in poverty and, as we have seen, that often results in poor physical and psychological health, low education, poor housing arrangements, being susceptible to acts of violence, and a range of other negative consequences. Even attempts to encourage people out of poverty by requiring them to work have not been as successful as hoped. For example, in the mid-1990s, the welfare laws were changed to set a limit on the amount of years someone could receive benefits without being employed. Touting the value of these new regulations, the government cited the number of former welfare recipients who became employed. What was left unsaid, however, was the number of Americans employed in minimum-wage or close to minimum-wage jobs who could not afford health insurance or health care for themselves or their children, did not have enough money from their salaries for decent housing accommodations, and generally could not support their families as they would like. Imagine how stressful being in this situation can be!

Even middle-class Americans encounter significant financial stressors. Too often people overspend and wind up with debt from which they have a hard time escaping. This is not unusual for college students who may be using a credit card independently for the first time. Given the high interest rates charged by many credit card companies, getting out from under credit card debt can be very difficult. But it is not only college students who overspend. Some middle-class Americans want to drive a nice, new car, or live in the best of neighborhoods, or wear the flashiest of clothes. Wanting these things creates no problem. It is purchasing them that does. Living within one's means is a developmental task that people need to learn, but too often it is learned at great financial and emotional cost. As is discussed in the "Interventions" section later in this chapter, budgeting goes a long way to help prevent or resolve financial problems.

Almost all families, but especially those that did not plan well, have financial concerns regarding the raising of children. The cost of raising a child through age 17 is $226,920 for a middle-income family.[34] These costs include housing, child care, health care, clothing, transportation, food, and miscellaneous expenses. And that is for *one* child! Add other children and the costs obviously increase. Furthermore, these costs do not include expenses for children beyond the age of 17, when they may be attending college or graduate or professional school (see Chapter 4), getting married with costs associated with a wedding, or needing financial assistance as they begin their careers at relatively low-paying jobs.

Prosperous families also experience financial stress. Although not as stressful in the same way as having to deal with poverty, *any* change in financial condition may be accompanied by stress. Maybe Aunt Abigail died and left a large

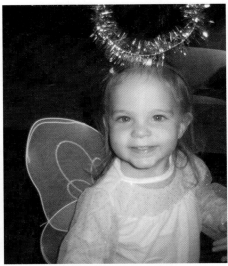

Whether they are angels or devils, and at some point all children are both, they cost a great deal to raise, and that can be quite stressful.

sum of cash to Mom or Dad. Maybe a killing was made in the stock market or some other investment. You now need to protect that money to minimize tax payments. This means tax shelters, real estate deals, money market funds, or other financial wizardry. The fear of losing the new wealth raises its head, and you must direct attention, time, and energy at preventing such a loss. In addition, you may go out and buy a new car, move into a bigger house in a better neighborhood, buy more fashionable clothing, or arrange for vacations to faraway places instead of visiting relatives nearby. While these may be lifestyle adaptations you feel good and are excited about, they are adjustments and changes, nevertheless. That means they are stressors with the potential to result in illness or disease.

Other Stressors

There are many other stressors for which space dictates only a mention. Over 50 percent of families in the United States are remarried or re-coupled families. On average, 1,300 new stepfamilies are formed each day.[35] In these and other families, disagreements between parents regarding how to discipline children can be stressful. How best to assist elderly parents—arrange nursing home care or have them live with you—creates stress for many families. Other families find their sexual lives stressful—for example, how often they should have sexual intercourse, who should initiate it, or which sexual activities they should engage in. Some parents are raising children alone or are in the midst of a divorce. Some parents, usually fathers, may be living apart from their children. I'm sure you can add to this list. Since family life is dynamic, it is always changing—and therefore stressful.

A Model of Family Stress

To intervene in family stress, it is necessary to have a clear understanding of the situation. I have developed a model of family stress (see Figure 17.2) to help with this task. People who have applied the model have found it useful to help appreciate the components and manifestations of stress in families they know.

This model demonstrates that stressors are occurring within the family but are screened through individuals who differ on a number of important variables. It also demonstrates how these individual family members are affected by stressors

Figure 17.2 Family Stress Model

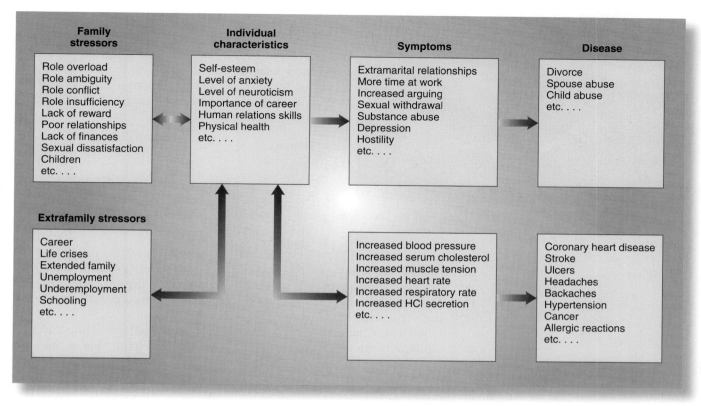

that occur outside the context of the family but that, nonetheless, affect how family stressors are perceived and reacted to. The result of the interaction of family stressors and extrafamily stressors upon differing family members may be signs and symptoms of family stress or full-blown family disease. Once this complex of family stress is understood, the interventions described in this chapter can be better tailored to meet each family's needs.

Interventions

Family stress can be prevented from resulting in illness and disease through employing life-situation interventions, perception interventions, emotional arousal interventions, and physiological arousal interventions.

Life-Situation Interventions

Lack of time is a major stressor in dual-career families. It prevents some chores from being done, takes time away from other family members, and creates stress when you hurry to complete as much as possible in the little time available. To manage this stress, you can seek the help of other family members or friends. For example, they can do some shopping for you or pick up the kids from soccer practice. You might also hire someone to do some of the less important chores, such as cleaning the house or doing the laundry, to free you to do the more important ones. Your first priority after work hours, whether you are male or female, should be your family. To maximize your time with the family, you can plan vacations for work holidays and weekends—vacations that will get you all away from friends and chores so you can focus more upon each other. Fishing trips and hiking excursions provide a relaxing setting and an opportunity for conversing with each other. Trips to fancy hotels, where the kids attend a day camp

Families both create stress and serve as social support networks to help us manage stress better.

and the parents golf all day, are not conducive to sharing meaningful family time together.

Marriage is said to be hard work. Maintaining all family relationships can be substituted for the word "marriage" in the previous sentence. Successful marriage partners share a commitment to their mates as demonstrated by the following traits from a study of married couples that asked about the qualities that made their marriages successful:[36]

1. Honesty
2. Love
3. Trust
4. Communication
5. Respect
6. Commitment

Perhaps all of us need to spend time and energy developing similar feelings for our families. To do so, though, requires a commitment to organize our lives so as to be together, sharing meaningful activities and developing a positive family history. The suggestions in this chapter should help.

For most of the family stressors described in this chapter, improving the communication between members of the family would be helpful. One of the most important prerequisites of communication, and one that is so obvious it is almost forgotten, is that you need to set aside time to communicate. Family members are usually involved in so many activities that they almost never have time to sit and talk and get to know one another. The kids are out playing, have practice for some team they are on, or are doing schoolwork. The parents are busy with their careers, sports, or friends. To make sure that time will be available for other family members, some families actually schedule it in. Other families set up weekly gripe sessions for any member to complain about anything bothering him or her. A while ago, I realized that I wasn't spending enough time with my son and, in particular, understanding what he was doing in school. I rearranged my time so we could spend 15 minutes together after dinner on Tuesdays and Thursdays (a time convenient to both of us). During that time, he showed me all of his schoolwork and pointed out how far he had gone in his textbooks. At other times, either my son or my daughter would sit on my lap and we would have a "conversation"—our key word for a discussion of our feelings. We would discuss what makes us happy, sad, frightened, angry, or any other emotion one of us suggested. Far from being the perfect parent, I cite these examples of our family life because they worked for us. Maybe they will work for you and your family.

Regarding stress associated with divorce, the best advice is to get involved with people. Also, work at maintaining your sense of self-worth. One author presents some advice to divorced parents:[37]

1. *Don't make your child the messenger:* Do not communicate through your child—speak directly to your ex-spouse.
2. *Don't make your child your therapist:* Do not share details about your divorce or your angry feelings about your ex-spouse with your child.

Parenting requires scheduling time to spend with the children.

3. *Listen to your child*: Try to understand his or her feelings. Do not tell your child what to think, or criticize your ex-spouse in front of your child.

4. *Avoid the third degree*: Do not grill your child or put him or her in the middle between you and your ex-spouse.

5. *Repair the damage you've already done*: Apologize and explain in detail what you've done wrong, and say you're sorry.

This advice will help the formation of a more positive relationship with the children and the ex-spouse and thereby decrease the stress experienced as a result of the divorce.

Regarding stress about family planning, you might want to talk with a counselor—for example, one at Planned Parenthood—to better understand your options. One of the best sources of information about family planning, which identifies the methods available, their effectiveness, and their advantages and disadvantages, is a book entitled *Contraceptive Technology,* written by Robert Hatcher and published by Ardent Media (P. O. Box 286, Cooper Station P. O., New York, NY 10276-0286). You might want to write for that book. If you have moral, ethical, or religious concerns about birth control, consult with your clergy. In addition to all of these steps, remember to involve your partner. To be less distressed over these decisions, you need to work together, relying on each other to help sort out all the issues involved.

Regarding the stress of living long distances from members of your extended family, you can plan vacations to visit them rather than going other places. You can also telephone them regularly. Regular phone calls will allow some time for small talk—important in getting to know each other—since less time between calls will mean there are fewer major issues to discuss. Another means of maintaining your connection with your extended family—less expensive than visiting—is exchanging letters with them. Notice I said *letters,* not cards. Birthday or anniversary cards won't serve the same purpose, nor will e-mail messages. Your relatives should know that you are making a special effort to communicate with them; then they will understand how important keeping in touch is to you and will be more apt to write back. Letters will better convey this need than will cards or e-mail.

Financial Stress Interventions

Financial stress can be devastating. It can undermine relationships between family members as they act out their frustrations on each other. Serious health consequences may result if medical care is postponed until it is absolutely necessary. Financial stress also may have negative psychological and emotional effects on family members' self-esteem and sense of control over their lives, and it may foster the development of anger and alienation. For these reasons financial stress interventions are highlighted in this chapter.

Perhaps the most valuable intervention is the formulation of a budget that guides financial decisions. Budgets can help prevent debt that, if unpaid, can result in bad credit and, sometimes, legal action. The budget can let you control your finances rather than let your finances control you. The correct way to establish a budget is to review how you spent money last year. For example, you could review canceled checks, bank records, and credit card records. Also, review income for the year. If you are not able to obtain records for the past year, or are not motivated to go back that far, do so for the previous two months. Then,

- Identify income you expect to acquire for each month in the present year.
- Identify anticipated expenses for each month.

- Try to set aside some money each month for savings, depending on the amount of income above expenses and your goals (savings are important to meet unforeseen emergencies or expenses).

- If you owe money, try to pay off some of your debt each month.

The percentage of your income that you spend in each category is an individual decision. The less you make, the greater is the percentage of income that you will have to spend on basic needs (e.g., shelter and food). However, as a general rule, you should spend between 20 to 35 percent on housing, 15 to 30 percent on food, 3 to 10 percent on clothing, 6 to 20 percent on transportation, 2 to 6 percent on entertainment, and 5 to 9 percent for savings.[38] If you find it difficult to stick to your budget, you can set up a system by which you place the money budgeted for each category in separate envelopes as you receive income. Of course, you can borrow from one envelope (category) for another, but if that happens too often, the budget will be destroyed.

Several other strategies should help:

- Control spending. Leave your checkbook and credits cards at home when not needed.

- Pay bills on time thereby avoiding interest charges (credit card interest rates are quite high).

- Review the budget periodically to make sure it is still appropriate.

- If eligible, enroll your children in state health insurance programs (states offer a Children's Health Insurance Program for low-income families).

- If you have too much debt, contact the Consumer Credit Counseling Service for help (1-800-251-2227).

- When making purchases, avoid the extended warranties. Appliances usually don't break during their three years' warranty period, and if breakdowns happen, the average cost of repairing the appliance is not much more than the average price paid for the warranty.[39]

- Compare gasoline prices at different gas stations rather than purchasing gas at the most convenient station.

- Shop around for the least expensive automobile and homeowner's or rental insurance.

- Consult organizational evaluations of products before purchasing them (e.g., Consumers Union).

- Only purchase telephone services that are necessary, and shop around for the best cell phone plans.

- Use generic drugs rather than brand-name drugs when generics are available.

Perception Interventions

Many perception interventions are applicable to family stress. For example, you can use selective awareness to perceive the changes in your family life as exciting, interesting, and challenging, and remind yourself that in the long run you will all be closer for having experienced these changes together. Viewed in this way, family transitions will be less stressful.

You can also "smell the roses"—that is, enjoy your family life as fully as possible. Sometimes, while I was reading, my daughter would climb onto my lap. My first inclination was to figure out a way to get her off without having her feel rejected so I could continue reading undisturbed, and she would grow up with one less psychological scar. Most of the time, however, I put down what I was reading and tried to appreciate Keri on my lap. I stopped to recognize that, in all too few more years, lap-sitting with her dad would be a thing of the past—my loss more than hers, I'm sure. With that realization, I wanted to soak up as much lap-sitting and appreciation from lap-sitting as I could get. The interesting thing, though, is that, with this attitude of "smelling the roses," *each* new phase of our relationship will be experienced fully. It may be lap-sitting today and boyfriend problems tomorrow. Because one phase is over, I need not be distressed over its loss if I experienced it to its fullest, since the next phase offers new wonders. Children will cause less stress if we wonder at them—if we watch them grow and marvel at their uniqueness.

Understanding of the Type A behavior pattern can be used to manage family stress. One characteristic of Type A people is that they are concerned with quantity more than with quality. They try to do many things, allowing the quality of each to suffer, rather than doing fewer things well. Generalizing this characteristic and relating it to stress caused by too little time to spend with family members, spend the limited time you have qualitatively. Talk with each other rather than watch television together. Go out for dinner rather than to a movie, where you can't converse. With elderly family members, try to get them to talk about the past and perhaps video-record or tape-record those discussions so they won't be lost to future generations. The elderly, you will find, have so many interesting stories and have experienced a world so different from ours that honoring their past in this manner will not only alleviate some of their stress— they will feel as though they have something worthwhile to offer—but will help us connect to the past from which we sprang. It will give us roots and help us to see that our lives are not just fleeting moments but, rather, a link in the chain of humankind.

As we discussed earlier in this chapter, wives do more housework per week than their husbands. One might argue that a fifty-fifty split of the housework between husbands and wives who work outside the home full-time would be the only fair arrangement. However, some women may have difficulty sharing home and parenting duties because of the fear of losing their identities as women and mothers. If you or someone you know is experiencing these concerns, discuss the quality-of-time versus quantity-of-time issue with them to better help them perceive the need to be willing to share routine household and parenting responsibilities. Only if they realize they are not superwomen and cannot do everything themselves will women who work outside the home free up time to improve their family relationships and decrease the potential for family stress. Men, too, need to perceive their limitations and delegate responsibilities to other family members when they are overburdened. However, as the data indicate, this need, at least at home, is not as much of a concern for men as it is for women.

Lastly, your perceptions of the control you can exercise over events that affect your life—your locus of control—influence how you respond to family stressors. If you work to develop internality, you will believe you can do something to experience less stress from your family life. You will, therefore, try some of the suggestions appearing in this chapter and even seek others. One of the best ways to develop internality is to try controlling some events and analyzing how that attempt fared. Was it successful? If so, why? If not, why not? Experience in actually exercising control over aspects of your life will reinforce your notion that such control is possible. Try some of the suggestions given in this section. Choose one that you think has the best chance of being successful and then move on to some others. You will find that you really can do something to manage family stress better.

Emotional Arousal Interventions

Family stress can be less unhealthy if you regularly practice some relaxation techniques. Any of the techniques described in this book will do. With family stress as your particular concern here, you might want to engage in relaxation as a family. Perhaps you can schedule a "relaxation time" when everyone in the family meditates. Maybe you can all take a yoga class together. Regular practice of relaxation will help you cope better with normal family transitions as well as with unusual and unanticipated family stressors.

Physiological Arousal Interventions

Like other stressors, family stressors increase serum cholesterol, heart rate, and blood pressure and change other body processes. Exercise can use these stress products in a healthy manner and prevent them from making you ill. Why not exercise as a family? You could bike, swim, play tennis, or even jog as a family.

Coping in Today's World

Want to maintain a healthy life? Get married! At least that is what data from the Centers for Disease Control and Prevention indicate. CDC researchers studied more than 127,000 Americans ages 18 and older and found that, regardless of the sub-group (age, sex, race, culture, education, or income), married adults were healthier than other adults.[a] Married adults were also less likely to experience health-related limitations in their activities than any other marital status group (never married, widowed, divorced or separated, or cohabiting).

Two theories suggest reasons for these data: The *marriage protection theory* states that married people have more advantages in terms of economic resources, social and psychological support, and support for healthy lifestyles. The *marital selection theory* states that healthier people get married and stay married. Another explanation may be that it is not marriage per se that provides this health benefit. Perhaps being in a long-term committed relationship is the key. We know, for example, that the importance of family to health is undisputed. We also know that *family* can take many forms. Maybe these marriage data are a reflection of family—not necessarily marriage. Can you think of other variables that might explain these data?

[a]C.A. Schoenborn, "Marital Status and Health: United States, 1999–2002." *Advance Data from the Vital and Health Statistics* 351(2004): 1.

summary

- A family is a unique set of intimate relationships.
- The nuclear family is a married couple and their children. The extended family includes relatives other than spouses and their children.
- The family satisfies several needs. These include the social control of reproduction and child rearing, economic support, security and safety needs, and the emotional needs of love and a sense of belonging.
- The family has changed in recent years. People are marrying later and more people are choosing to remain single. More people are cohabiting rather than marrying, and a large number of divorces are occurring, with more than 1 million children involved each year.
- Family stressors include financial concerns, dual-career marriages, increased mobility, child rearing, contraception decisions, separation from extended families, and violence.

- Family stress is a complex of family stressors, individual family members' characteristics, and extrafamily stressors. These can lead to symptoms of family stress or to stress-related illness.
- Effective communication and conflict resolution skills can help manage family stress.
- Adoption occurs in several formats. There are closed adoptions that are confidential, and open adoptions in which there is contact between the birth parents and the adoptive parents.
- Budgeting is an important strategy for managing family financial stress. As a general rule, 20 to 35 percent of income should be spent on housing, 15 to 30 percent on food, 3 to 10 percent on clothing, 6 to 20 percent on transportation, 2 to 6 percent on entertainment, and 5 to 9 percent set aside for savings.

internet resources

Stress Management Tip.com: Family Stress Management **www.stressmanagementtips.com/family.htm** *Discusses how to prevent family stress and tips to manage family stress when it occurs. Links to other stress management tips are also included.*

Stress and Infertility **www.asrm.org/uploadedFiles/ASRM_Content/Resources/Patient_Resources/Fact_**

Sheets_and_Info_Booklets/Stress-Fact.pdf *A fact sheet from the American Society of Reproductive Medicine describing the relationship between infertility and stress and what can be done to reduce stress, thereby enhancing reproductive health.*

references

1. U.S. Census Bureau, *Statistical Abstracts of the United States: 2011.* Washington, D.C.: U.S. Government Printing Office, 2010, 53.

2. Ibid., 56.

3. Ibid., 58.

4. Ibid., 55.

5. Pew Research Center, *As Marriage and Parenthood Drift Apart, Public is Concerned about Social Impact,* 2007. Available at http://pewresearch.org/pubs/526/marriage-parenthood

6. D. Popenoe and B.D. Whitehead, (2006), "The State of our Unions, 2006." *The National Marriage Project, Rutgers, The State University of New Jersey, 2006.* Available at http://marriage.rutgers.edu

7. J. Teachman, (2003). "Premarital sex, premarital cohabitation, and the risk of subsequent marital disruption among women." *Journal of Marriage and the Family,* 65: 444–55.

8. Pew Research Center, 2007.

9. U.S. Census Bureau, "America's Families and Living Arrangements, 2008." *Current Population Reports,* 2008, table A1. Available at www.census.gov/population/www/socdemo/hh-fam/cps2008 .html

10. U.S. Census Bureau, "America's Families and Living Arrangements, 2010," 2010, table C2.

11. U.S. Census Bureau, "America's Families and Living Arrangements, 2010," 2010, table C3.

12. U.S. Census Bureau, *Statistical Abstracts of the United States, 2011* (Washington, D.C.: U.S. Census Bureau, 2010), 58.

13. Charles Lane, "States' Recognition of Same-Sex Unions May Be Tested," *The Washington Post,* November 19, 2003, A8.

14. David Von Drehl, "Gay Marriage Is a Right, Massachusetts Court Rules," *The Washington Post,* November 19, 2003, Al.

15. Annenberg Public Policy Center, "American Public Remains Opposed to Same-Sex Marriages as They Begin in Massachusetts, Annenberg Data Show," *National Annenberg Election Survey.* www.annnenbergpublicpolicycenter.org

16. U.S. Census Bureau, *Statistical Abstracts of the United States, 2011* (Washington, D.C.: U.S. Census Bureau, 2010), 385.

17. Ibid.

18. Board of Governors of the Federal Reserve, "Statistics & Historical Data: Household Debt Service and Financial Obligations Ratios," *Federal Reserve Bulletin* 95(2009). Available at: www.federalreserve.gov/releases/housedebt/default.htm

19. Janet DiVittorio Morgan, "I Work Because I Have to." In *The Mothers' Book: Shared Experiences,* ed. Ronnie Friedland and Carol Kort (Boston: Houghton Mifflin, 1981), 96.

20. Pew Research Center, *Fewer Mothers Prefer Full-time Work,* 2007. Available at http://pewresearch.org/pubs/536/working-women

21. Jean Rosenbaum and Veryl Rosenbaum, *Living with Teenagers* (New York: Stein & Day, 1980).

22. Child Welfare Information Gateway, *Obtaining Birth and/or Adoption Records, 2009.* Available at www.childwelfare .gov/adoption/search/records.cfm

23. Don Colburn, "When Violence Begins at Home," *Washington Post Health,* March 15, 1994, 7.

24. Centers for Disease Control and Prevention, *Child Maltreatment.* 2010. Available at: www.cdc.gov/ violenceprevention/pdf/CM-DataSheet-a.pdf

25. Ibid.

26. V. Iannelli, "Preventing Child Abuse," About.com: Pediatrics, 2007. Available at http://pediatrics.about.com/od/ childabuse/a/05_prevnt_abuse.htm

27. Centers for Disease Control and Prevention, "WISQARS," *Injury Mortality Reports* (Washington, D.C.: National Center for Injury Prevention and Control, 2009).

28. Brady Campaign, *Firearm Facts,* 2009. Available at www .bradycampaign.org/facts/

29. Centers for Disease Control and Prevention, *Understanding Intimate Partner Violence, Fact Sheet, 2009.* 2009. Available at www.cdc.gov/violenceprevention/pdf/IPV_factsheet-a.pdf

30. Centers for Disease Control and Prevention, *Sexual Violence, Fact Sheet, 2009.* 2009. Available at www.cdc.gov/ violenceprevention/pdf/SV-DataSheet-a.pdf

31. W. Max, D. P. Rice, E. Finkelstein, R. A. Bardwell, and S. Leadbetter, "The Economic Toll of Intimate Partner Violence Against Women in the United States," *Violence and Victims* 19(2004): 259–72.

32. Jerold S. Greenberg, Clint E. Bruess, and Sarah T. Conklin, *Exploring the Dimensions of Human Sexuality* (Sudbury, MA: Jones & Bartlett, 2011), 540–544.

33. *Help End Domestic Violence,* National Resource Center on Domestic Violence, n.d.

34. U.S. Department of Agriculture, *Expenditures on Children by Families, 2010* (Washington, D.C.: U.S. Department of Agriculture, 2011).

35. Stepfamily Foundation, *Statistics,* 2009. Available at www .stepfamily.org/statistics.html

36. Sheri Stritof and Bob Stritof, "Marriage Qualities Survey Results," *Your Guide to Marriage,* June 2005. http://marriage .about.com/od/keysforsuccess/a/qualresults.htm

37. "The Top 5 Mistakes Divorced Parents Make," *WebMD the Magazine,* February, 2009. Available at www.webmd.com/parenting/ features/top-5-mistakes-divorced-parents-make?page=2

38. Consumer Action, *Budgeting and Planning: Building a Better Future.* 1993. Available at: www.consumer-action.org/english/articles/ budgeting_and_planning_building_a_better_future_english

39. Consumers Union, "Just Say No to Extended Warranties," *ConsumerReports.org.* 2009. Available at: www .consumerreports.org/cro/appliances/resource-center/ appliance-stores/extended-warranties/0708_store_war_1.htm

LAB ASSESSMENT 17.1

Are You Ready for Marriage?

Directions: The following questions are designed to assist you in clarifying your readiness for marriage. Although there are no absolutely "right" or "wrong" answers, these questions can help identify some issues for you to focus on as you think about marriage. Check the appropriate blank for each of the following questions.

Yes   No

_____ _____ 1. Even though you may accept advice from other people (parents, instructors, friends), do you make important decisions on your own?

_____ _____ 2. Do you have a good working knowledge of the physiology of human sexuality, and do you understand the emotional and interpersonal factors that are involved in sexual adjustment?

_____ _____ 3. Have you had the experience of contributing to or sharing in the financial support of yourself and at least one other person?

_____ _____ 4. Have you and someone with whom you have had an intimate relationship ever worked through disagreements to a definite conclusion that was acceptable to both of you?

_____ _____ 5. Are you usually free of jealousy?

_____ _____ 6. Have you thought carefully about the goals you will strive for in marriage?

_____ _____ 7. Do you find yourself able to give up gracefully something you wanted very much?

_____ _____ 8. Can you postpone something you want for the sake of later enjoyment?

_____ _____ 9. Do you generally feel embarrassed or uneasy about giving or receiving affection?

_____ _____ 10. Are your feelings easily hurt by criticism?

_____ _____ 11. In an argument, do you lose your temper easily?

_____ _____ 12. Do you frequently feel like rebelling against responsibilities (work, family, school, and so on)?

_____ _____ 13. Are you often sarcastic toward others?

_____ _____ 14. Do you find yourself strongly emphasizing the more glamorous aspects of marriage, such as its social components?

_____ _____ 15. Are you often homesick when you are away from your family?

Scoring and interpretation: In questions 1–8, the more yes responses you have, the readier you are for marriage. In questions 9–15, the more no responses you have, the readier you are for marriage. Each question can help you identify areas that need some attention before you enter into marriage.

- Questions 1, 3, 4, 6, 7, and 8 explore behaviors that will affect the success of your marriage.

- Question 2 concerns knowledge that will affect the success of your marriage. Knowledge about human sexuality is an important prerequisite to sexual adjustment in marriage.

- Questions 5, 9, 10, 11, 12, 13, 14, and 15 enable you to estimate your emotional readiness for marriage. Question 5, for example, explores jealousy, an emotion that has been shown to be destructive to marital stability. If you are a jealous person in general, it may be important for you to seek professional guidance in dealing with issues such as trust and self-esteem before you contemplate marriage.

If you scored low on some parts of this scale and wish to be married in the future, you might consider enrolling in a course on marriage and the family. You may be able to find such a course in the sociology or health sciences departments. Alternatively, churches, synagogues, and mosques often conduct workshops to prepare congregants for marriage.

Source: Questions adapted from L. A. Kirkendall and W. J. Adams, *The Students' Guide to Marriage and Family Life Literature*, 8th ed. (Dubuque, IA: Wm. C. Brown Communications, 1980), 157.

LAB ASSESSMENT 17.2

Who Is Your Ideal Mate?

Imagine you sign up at a dating service. When completing the required form, you are asked to describe your ideal mate. How would you respond to the following questions:

1. What does your partner do for leisure?

   _____

2. What does your partner look like?

   _____

3. What does your partner worry about?

   _____

4. On what does your partner enjoy spending money?

   _____

5. Describe your partner's personality?

   _____

6. About what is your partner passionate?

   _____

7. What angers your partner?

   _____

8. What are your partner's life goals?

   _____

9. What talents does your partner possess?

   _____

10. Why does your partner love you?

    _____

Once you understand what you want in a romantic partner, decisions regarding who you date and who you marry can be made more systematically. The result will be you getting involved in fewer dysfunctional, dissatisfying relationships. Recognizing that no one will possess all of the characteristics of your *ideal* partner, if you rank order the questions above so the one most important is ranked number 1, the second most important ranked number 2, and so on, you can further refine your relationship decisions. Taking control of your life—your stressors and even your relationships—is an important benefit of stress management.

Epilogue

Someone told me of a person who came home one evening holding the steering wheel of the family car, hair and clothes disheveled and speckled with glass from the windshield and smelling of engine oil, and who with a faint, halfhearted smile said to the waiting spouse, "Well, at least you won't have to waste your Fridays at the car wash any longer."

If only we could adopt that attitude toward the future and the stressors it will bring. Alvin Toffler wrote of the nature of the future in his classic book *Future Shock*.[1] Toffler described the rapid and pervasive changes that we will, and do, experience. As we have learned, such changes have the potential to elicit a stress response—that is, they're stressors.

The knowledge of today often becomes the misinformation of tomorrow. For example, most of us were taught and believed that parallel lines never meet, yet today physicists say that they do meet somewhere in infinity. We learned that eggs and liver were good for us and that we should eat them frequently, yet some cardiologists now believe that they contain so much cholesterol that we should limit how much of them we eat. Knowledge is expanding exponentially; new knowledge often replaces old "knowledge." This situation creates confusion—what do we believe? It creates frustration, one example of which is the oft-heard lament "Everything seems to cause cancer." It creates stress—how do we manage in a world that has so much scientific knowledge and technology that a few individuals could destroy it by pushing several buttons? Well, at least we wouldn't have to waste Fridays at the car wash.

In *The Third Wave*, Toffler continued describing a changing society, focusing upon the influence of science and technology on our daily lives.[2] I recalled Toffler's description of the effects that new forms of communication and computers would have upon us (e.g., we can now shop, bank, and work from computers in our homes or on the wireless network at the local coffee shop, and watch television programs on our smartphones) when I read of an experiment that took place during a football game. The Racine Gladiators were playing the Columbus Metros in a semipro football game way back in July of 1980. The cable TV system televising the game allowed subscribers to communicate through it instantaneously by punching buttons on a handheld control unit in their homes, and that is exactly what more than 5,000 viewers did. Prior to each play, the viewers voted on the next play they wanted their hometown Metros to run, out of a choice of five different plays. In 10 seconds the responses were tallied and flashed on a screen at the stadium—unseen by the players—and the vote was relayed to the quarterback. The Metros lost the game 10–7 but their coach said he probably couldn't have called the plays any better. "The times they are a-changing."

If we are going to survive and flourish in a rapidly changing society, we had better learn how to manage the inevitable stress. We must adjust our life situations to eliminate unnecessary stressors and to find comfort in rewarding routine and stable relationships and activities. We need to strengthen our families, do meaningful and enjoyable work, and organize our leisure time to be fun and recreating (which is where the word *recreation* comes from). Furthermore, we need to perceive those distressing life situations that we cannot change as less threatening and disturbing. This includes viewing ourselves as worthwhile beings, believing we can control many events and consequences in our lives, and considering life's tests as challenges and growth experiences rather than as plagues to be shunned, avoided, and forgotten.

Added to these recommendations must be the regular practice of relaxation and exercise. Relaxation skills provide a "reservoir of relaxation" from which we can draw when our lives become particularly stressful. These skills also serve to intervene between life situations that we perceive to be distressing and subsequent illnesses and diseases by diminishing the physiological arousal caused by stressors.

In the hope that this book enhances your ability to manage the stress in your life, I leave you with the following thought. This Persian proverb has meant much to me, and my hope is that it will also have significance for you. It is short, so you can easily commit it to memory:

I murmured because I had no shoes,
Until I met a man who had no feet.

notes

1. Alvin Toffler, *Future Shock* (New York: Random House, 1970).

2. Alvin Toffler, *The Third Wave* (New York: William Morrow & Co., 1980).

Glossary

A

A,B,C Lists: a time management technique in which tasks are prioritized. (p. 162)

ABCDE Technique: a method of coping with anxiety that consists of examining irrational beliefs. (p. 149)

Abortion: the termination of a pregnancy. (p. 427)

Acquaintance Rape: forcible sexual intercourse between people who know each other. (p. 89)

Acquired Immune Deficiency Syndrome (AIDS): a condition transmitted through sexual contact and the sharing of intravenous needles that leads to the mixing of blood or semen, in which the immune system becomes progressively ineffective. (p. 87)

Active Listening: paraphrasing the speaker's words and feelings; also called reflective listening. (p. 154)

Adrenal Cortex: the part of the adrenal gland that secretes corticoids. (p. 50)

Adrenal Medulla: the inner portion of the adrenal gland that secretes catecholamines. (p. 31)

Adrenocorticotropic Hormone (ACTH): activates the adrenal cortex to secrete corticoid hormones. (p. 28)

Aerobic Exercise: exercise of relatively long duration, using large muscle groups, that does not require more oxygen than can be inhaled. (p. 309)

Aggressive: acting in a way to get what one is entitled to, one's rights, but at the expense of someone else's rights. (p. 149)

AIDS: acquired immune deficiency syndrome. (p. 364)

Aldosterone: the primary mineralocorticoid secreted from the adrenal cortex that is responsible for an increase in blood pressure. (p. 30)

Allostatic Load: the cumulative biological wear and tear that results from responses to stress that seek to maintain body equilibrium. (p. 8)

Anaerobic Exercise: exercise of short duration that requires more oxygen than can be inhaled. (p. 309)

Anal Opening: the exit point for unusable food substances. (p. 36)

Anapanasati: a Zen practice that involves counting breaths as the object of focus during meditation. (p. 241)

Anorexia Nervosa: an eating disorder in which a person takes in so few calories as to potentially starve him- or herself to death. (pp. 92, 127)

Antibodies: substances produced by the body to fight antigens. (p. 56)

Antigen: a foreign substance irritating to the body. (p. 56)

Anxiety: an unrealistic fear that manifests itself in physiological arousal and behaviors to avoid or escape the anxiety-provoking stimulus. (p. 192)

Apoplexy: a lack of oxygen to the brain resulting from a blockage or rupture of a blood vessel; also called stroke. (p. 50)

Aqua Dynamics: a program consisting of structured exercises conducted in limited water areas. (p. 320)

Armchair Desensitization: a form of systematic desensitization in which the stimulus is imagined. (p. 196)

Aromatherapy: the use of plant material added to massage oil thought to have pharmacological qualities that improve health. (p. 288)

Arteriosclerosis: loss of elasticity of the coronary arteries. (p. 52)

Asanas: body positions used during the practice of yoga. (p. 289)

Assertive: acting in a way to get what one is entitled to, one's rights, but not at the expense of someone else's rights. (p. 150)

Atherosclerosis: clogging of the coronary arteries. (p. 52)

Attitude of Gratitude: focusing on things about which to be grateful. (p. 183)

Autogenic Meditation: visualization of relaxing images used during autogenic training. (p. 259)

Autogenic Training: a relaxation technique that involves imagining one's limbs to be heavy, warm, and tingling. (p. 253)

Autohypnosis: being able to place oneself in a hypnotic state. (p. 253)

Autoimmune Response: a physiological response in which the body turns on itself. (p. 58)

Autonomic Nervous System: controls such body processes as hormone balance, temperature, and width of blood vessels. (p. 27)

B

B Cells: a type of lymphocyte that produces antibodies. (p. 45)

Barriers: reasons given or situations that interfere with someone engaging in behaviors that he or she wishes to engage in. (p. 334)

Biofeedback: the use of electronic instruments or other techniques to monitor and change physiological parameters, many of which are regulated by the autonomic nervous system. (p. 281)

Body Scanning: a relaxation technique that searches for relaxed body parts and transports that sensation to less relaxed areas. (p. 286)

Boomerang Children: children who leave home to live elsewhere but subsequently return to live with the parents. (p. 421)

Bracing: the contraction of muscles for no obvious purpose. (pp. 6, 37)

Bulimia: an eating disorder characterized by binge eating followed by purging of food, such as by inducing vomiting or ingesting a laxative. (pp. 83, 127)

Burnout: an adverse stress reaction to work with psychological, psychophysiological, and behavioral components. (p. 396)

C

Carcinogens: cancer-causing agents. (p. 56)

Cerebellum: part of the subcortex responsible for coordination. (p. 26)

Cerebral Cortex: the upper part of the brain responsible for thinking functions. (p. 26)

Cerebral Hemorrhage: a rupture of a blood vessel in the brain. (p. 50)

Closed Adoption: adoptions in which there is no contact between the birth parents and the adoptive parents. (p. 428)

Cocreator Perception Deficiency (CCPD): the belief that one is either the victim of circumstances or the master of circumstances, each of which is erroneous. (p. 191)

Cognitive Appraisal: interpretation of a stressor. (p. 112)

Cognitive Restructuring: a method of coping with anxiety that involves thinking about an anxiety-provoking event as less threatening. (p. 196)

Cohabitation: romantically involved couples living together although not married. (p. 422)

Cold Turkey: stopping a behavior all at once. (p. 337)

Coping: engaging in a behavior or thought to respond to a demand. (p. 111)

Corticotropin Releasing Factor (CRF): released by hypothalamus and results in the release of adrenocorticotropic hormone. (p. 28)

Cortisol: the primary glucocorticoid secreted from the adrenal cortex that is responsible for an increase in blood glucose. (p. 30)

Course Overload: having too many courses or courses too difficult to complete well during one semester. (p. 79)

D

DESC Form: a formula for verbally expressing assertiveness consisting of a description of the situation, expression of feelings, specification of preferred change, and consequences of whether or not a change is made. (p. 151)

Diaphragmatic Breathing: deep breathing that expands the belly rather than just the chest. (p. 285)

Diastolic Blood Pressure: the pressure of the blood against the arterial walls when the heart is relaxed. (p. 49)

Diencephalon: part of the subcortex responsible for regulation of the emotions. (p. 26)

Distress: stress that results in negative consequences such as decreased performance growth. (pp. 5, 116)

Double-Blind Studies: research investigations in which neither the research subjects nor the data collectors are aware of who is in the control group and who is in the experimental group. (p. 224)

Dual-Career Family: a family in which both spouses work outside the home with careers of their own. (p. 426)

E

Electromyographic (EMG) Biofeedback: biofeedback that measures muscle contraction. (p. 282)

Emotion-Focused Coping: the use of activities to feel better about the task. (p. 407)

Emotional Intelligence: the ability to accurately identify and understand one's own emotional reactions and those of others, and to regulate one's emotions and to use them to make good decisions and act effectively. (p. 158)

Endocrine System: comprised of hormones that regulate physiological functions. (p. 28)

Endorphins: brain neurotransmitters that decrease pain and produce feelings of well-being. (p. 313)

Epinephrine: a catecholamine secreted by the adrenal medulla. (p. 31)

Erotic Love (Eros): a passionate, all-enveloping type of love recognized by the heart racing and other signs of excitement. (p. 83)

Esophagus: the food pipe. (p. 36)

Essential Hypertension: hypertension with no known cause. (p. 49)

Ethnicity: a group of people having a common heritage such as common customs, characteristics, language, and history. (p. 356)

Eustress: stress that results in positive consequences such as enhanced performance or personal growth. (pp. 5, 117)

Extended Family: relatives other than spouses and children. (p. 419)

External Locus of Control: the perception that one has little control over events that affect one's life. (p. 190)

F

Fear Hierarchy: a list of small steps to move through an anxiety-provoking stimulus. (p. 196)

Fight-or-Flight Response: the body's stress reaction that includes an increase in heart rate, respiration, blood pressure, and serum cholesterol. (p. 3)

Forgiveness: a sincere intention not to seek revenge or avoid the transgressor (*decisional forgiveness*) and replacing negative emotions such as resentment, hate, and anger with positive emotions such as compassion, empathy, and sympathy (*emotional forgiveness*). (p. 225)

G

Galvanic Skin Response (GSR): the electrodermal response or the electrical conductance of the skin. (p. 38)

Gastrointestinal (GI) System: the body system responsible for digestion. (p. 36)

General Adaptation Syndrome: the three stages of stress reaction described by Hans Selye. (p. 4)

Glucocorticoids: regulate metabolism of glucose. (p. 30)

Gluconeogenesis: the production of glucose from amino acids by the liver. (p. 30)

Goal-Setting Theory: a conceptualization of how one successfully achieves goals. Among considerations are the difficulty of the goal, proximal and distal goals, and self-efficacy. (p. 344)

Gray Matter: the cerebral cortex. (p. 27)

H

Hardy: a state of mind and body that includes three factors: commitment, control, and challenge. (p. 200)

Hassles: daily interactions with the environment that are essentially negative. (p. 140)

Hate Crimes: crimes against people based on their race, ethnicity, sexual orientation, or religion. (p. 359)

Health Behavior: activities that are taken by people who believe themselves to be healthy and that are designed to maintain health, a subclass of lifestyle behaviors. (p. 333)

Health Belief Model: a way of conceptualizing how people make decisions regarding their health behavior. Constructs include perceptions of *susceptibility* to and *severity* of illness or disease, *benefits* of the behavior and *barriers* to performing it, *cues* to encourage, and *confidence* in being able to perform the behavior. (p. 342)

High-Density Lipoprotein (HDL): sometimes termed *good cholesterol*, HDL helps to remove cholesterol from the body thereby lowering the chances of developing coronary heart disease. (p. 47)

Hippocampus: part of the brain that "sounds the alarm" that stress is present. (p. 29)

Hot Reactors: people who react to stress with an all-out physiological reaction. (p. 43)

Human Immunodeficiency Virus (HIV): the virus that causes acquired immune deficiency syndrome (AIDS). (pp. 87, 364)

Hydrochloric Acid: a substance found in the digestive system that helps break down food for digestion. (p. 36)

Hypercholesterolemia: high levels of cholesterol in the blood. (p. 47)

Hypoglycemia: a condition of low blood sugar. (p. 136)

Hypothalamus: part of the diencephalon that activates the autonomic nervous system. (p. 27)

I

Infant Mortality: death of infants before one year of age. (p. 362)

Instant Calming Sequence (ICS): a relaxation technique that elicits relaxation quickly in a five-step approach. (p. 292)

Intercessory Prayer: prayers that seek divine intervention either to prevent an occurrence or to help overcome it. (p. 223)

Internal Locus of Control: the perception that one has control over events that affect one's life. (p. 190)

Interventions: activities to prevent a stressor from resulting in negative consequences. (p. 111)

In Vivo **Desensitization** a form of systematic desensitization in which the stimulus is actually encountered. (p. 196)

J

Jacobsonian Relaxation: a relaxation technique involving contracting and relaxing muscle groups throughout the body; also called progressive relaxation or neuromuscular relaxation. (p. 262)

Jealousy: fear of losing one's property, such as a lover, friend, status, or power. (p. 91)

K

Koans: Unanswerable, illogical riddles used as the object of focus during meditation. (p. 241)

L

Large Intestine: part of the digestive system that receives unusable food substances from the small intestine. (p. 36)

Life Expectancy: at his or her birth, years a person is expected to live. (p. 362)

Lifestyle Behaviors: all of the activities in which people engage. (p. 333)

Limbic System: produces emotions, the "seat of emotions." (p. 27)

Locus of Control: the perception of the amount of control one has over events that affect one's life. (p. 334)

Low-Density Lipoprotein (LDL): sometimes termed *bad cholesterol*, too much LDL leads to a clogging of the arteries and, therefore, is related to the development of coronary heart disease. (p. 47)

Ludic Love (Ludus): a playful, flirtatious type of love involving no long commitment. (p. 83)

M

Mandala: a geometric figure used as the object of focus during meditation. (p. 240)

Manic Love (Mania): a combination of passionate love (eros) and flirtatious, playing love characterized by jealousy and irrational joy that usually does not result in a long commitment. (p. 83)

Mantra: a word that is the focus of meditation. (p. 241)

Massage: a relaxation technique that involves manipulating points in the body that are muscularly tense. (p. 288)

Material Reinforcement: rewarding a behavior with a tangible object. (p. 336)

Medulla Oblongata: part of the subcortex responsible for the regulation of the heartbeat and breathing. (p. 26)

Memory T and B Cells: cells left in the bloodstream and the lymphatic system to recognize and respond to future attacks to the body by the same invader. (p. 45)

Mindfulness: focusing attention on the present moment to relax. (p. 292)

Mineralocorticoids: regulate the balance between sodium and potassium. (p. 30)

Motivational Factors: variables associated with job satisfaction; includes working on stimulating tasks, being recognized for work well done, and positive relationships with work colleagues. (p. 393)

Myocardial Infarction: when a part of the heart dies because of a lack of oxygen. (p. 50)

N

Nadam: imagined sounds used as the object of focus during meditation. (p. 241)

Neuromuscular Relaxation: a relaxation technique involving contracting and relaxing muscle groups throughout the body; also called progressive relaxation or Jacobsonian relaxation. (pp. 6, 262)

Nonassertive: giving up what one is entitled to, one's rights, in order not to upset another person. (p. 149)

Norepinephrine: a catecholamine secreted by the adrenal medulla. (p. 31)

Nuclear Family: a married couple and their children. (p. 419)

O

Occupational Stress: the combination of sources of stress at work, individual characteristics, and extraorganizational stressors. (p. 382)

Open Adoption: adoptions where there is contact between the birth parents and the adoptive parents. (p. 428)

Oxytocin: a hormone secreted by the pituitary gland. (p. 29)

P

Panic Disorder: a condition in which feelings of terror arise from unrealistic fear, resulting in symptoms such as feeling numb, sweaty, weak, and faint. (p. 192)

Parasympathetic Nervous System: part of the autonomic nervous system responsible for conserving energy. (p. 33)

Perceptions: a person's cognitive interpretation of events. (p. 179)

Phagocytes: a type of white blood cell whose purpose is to destroy substances foreign to the body. (p. 45)

Physical Fitness: ability to do one's work and have energy remaining for recreational activities. Consists of muscular strength, muscular endurance, cardiorespiratory endurance, flexibility, body composition, and agility. (p. 310)

Plaque: debris that clogs coronary arteries. (p. 50)

Pons: part of the subcortex responsible for regulating sleep. (p. 26)

Pranayama: a Hindu practice that involves breathing as the object of focus during meditation. (pp. 241, 289)

Preattack: synonymous with prodrome. (p. 54)

Primary Appraisal: judging how much of a threat is involved, and how important is the outcome. (p. 111)

Primary Control: attempts to change a situation; similar to problem-focused coping. (p. 222)

Problem-focused Coping: the use of activities specific to getting a task done. (p. 407)

Prodrome: the constriction phase of a migraine headache; also called preattack. (p. 54)

Progressive Relaxation: a relaxation technique involving contracting and relaxing muscle groups throughout the body; also called neuromuscular relaxation or Jacobsonian relaxation. (pp. 6, 262)

Pseudostressors: food substances that produce a stresslike response; also called sympathomimetics. (p. 135)

Psychogenic: a physical disease caused by emotional stress without a microorganism involved. (p. 44)

Psychoneuroimmunology: the study of the illness-causing and healing effects of the mind on the body. (p. 44)

Psychophysiological: synonymous with psychosomatic. (p. 44)

Psychosomatic: conditions that have a mind and body component. (p. 44)

Q

Quieting Reflex (QR): a six-step relaxation technique that results in relaxation in seconds. (p. 291)

R

Race: a group of people with similar physical traits, blood types, genetic patterns, and inherited characteristics. (p. 356)

Reappraisal: evaluation of whether the response made to a demand/threat was effective. (p. 112)

Reflective Listening: paraphrasing the speaker's words and feelings; also called active listening. (p. 154)

Reflexology: a massage technique that massages a "reflex zone" in the foot in which damage to body parts is thought to be manifested. (p. 288)

Relaxation Response: the physiological state achieved when one is relaxed; the opposite of the stress reaction; also called the trophotropic response. (p. 243)

Religion: an organized entity in which people have common beliefs and engage in common practices relevant to spiritual matters. (p. 220)

Reminder System: a means of reminding oneself to perform a particular behavior. (p. 338)

Resiliency: the ability to identify and make use of strengths and assets to respond to challenges, thereby growing as an individual. (p. 199)

Reticular Activating System (RAS): a network of nerves that connects the mind and the body. (p. 27)

Rheumatoid Factor: a blood protein associated with rheumatoid arthritis. (p. 58)

S

Saliva: substance in the mouth that starts to break down food. (p. 36)

Secondary Appraisal: determining whether resources needed to meet the demand are available. (p. 112)

Secondary Control: attempts to control oneself or one's emotional reactions; similar to emotion-focused coping. (p. 222)

Self-Contracting: making a contract with oneself to change a behavior. (p. 337)

Self-Efficacy: confidence in the ability to manage a demand/threat. (p. 112)

Self-Esteem: how highly one regards oneself. (p. 188)

Self-Monitoring: the process of observing and recording behavior. (p. 335)

Sexually Transmitted Infections (STIs): diseases such as syphilis, gonorrhea, chlamydia, and genital warts that are transmitted through sexual activity. (p. 86)

Shaping: changing a behavior a little bit at a time. (p. 337)

Shiatsu: acupressure massage. (p. 288)

Shyness: to be afraid of people and being worried of what strangers and powerful others think of oneself. (p. 90)

Significant Other: another person who is important to an individual. (p. 337)

Single-Parent Families: families in which the father or the mother is absent because of divorce, marital separation, out-of-wedlock pregnancy, or death. (p. 423)

Skeletal Muscles: muscles attached to bones. (p. 37)

Small Intestine: part of the digestive system into which the esophagus empties. (p. 36)

Smooth Muscles: muscles that control the contraction of internal organs. (p. 37)

Social Phobia: overwhelming fear and excessive self-consciousness in everyday situations; a chronic fear of being watched by others and not performing well. Fear of public speaking is an example. (p. 193)

Social Reinforcement: rewarding a behavior with social approval by someone else. (p. 336)

Social Support: the presence of significant others with whom to discuss stressors. (p. 139)

Somatogenic: a psychosomatic disease that results from the mind increasing the body's susceptibility to disease-causing microbes or natural degenerative processes. (p. 44)

Specific Phobia: an intense fear of a specific situation that poses little or no actual danger. Fear of elevators is an example. (p. 194)

Sphygmomanometer: an instrument used to measure blood pressure. (p. 49)

Spiritual Disease: a condition in which people are not true to their spiritual selves and are living a "life story" that is inconsistent with their beliefs and values. (p. 229)

Spiritual Health: adherence to religious doctrine; the ability to discover and express one's purpose in life; to experience love, joy, peace, and fullfillment; or to achieve and help others to achieve full potential. (p. 219)

Spirituality: a person's view of life's meaning, direction, purpose, and connectedness to other things, other people, and the past and future. (p. 220)

State Anxiety: anxiety that is either temporary in nature or specific to a particular stimulus. (p. 192)

Storgic Love (Storge): a calm, companionate type of love conceiving of a long commitment. (p. 83)

Strain: the physical, psychological, and behavioral outcomes of stress reactivity. (p. 71)

Stress: the combination of a stressor, stress reactivity, and strain. (pp. 13, 111)

Stressor: something with the potential to cause a stress reaction. (p. 3)

Stroke: a lack of oxygen to the brain resulting from a blockage or rupture of a blood vessel; also called apoplexy. (p. 50)

Subcortex: the lower part of the brain responsible for various physiological processes necessary to stay alive. (p. 26)

Suppressor T Cells: cells whose purpose is to halt the immune response. (p. 45)

Sympathetic Nervous System: part of the autonomic nervous system responsible for expending energy. (p. 33)

Sympathomimetics: synonymous with pseudostressors. (p. 135)

Systematic Desensitization: either imagining or encountering an anxiety-provoking stimulus while practicing relaxation. (p. 195)

Systolic Blood Pressure: the pressure of the blood as it leaves the heart. (p. 49)

T

T Cells: a type of lymphocyte whose purpose is to destroy substances foreign to the body by puncturing invaded body cells and killing the cells and foreign substances. (p. 45)

T-Lymphocytes: a part of the immune system that destroys mutant cells. (p. 56)

Tai Chi: an exercise and relaxation technique developed in China that involves focused, slow, rhythmic movement. (p. 295)

Tailoring: making a behavior change program specific to the life of the individual. (p. 336)

Target Heart Rate Range: the low and the high heart rate during exercise to strive toward. (p. 316)

Temporomandibular (TMJ) Syndrome: the interference with the smooth functioning of the jaw. (p. 59)

Thalamus: part of the diencephalon that relays sensory impulses to the cerebral cortex. (p. 26)

Thermal Biofeedback: biofeedback that measures temperature. (p. 283)

Thyroid Gland: an endocrine gland that secretes the hormone thyroxin. (p. 31)

Thyrotropic Hormone (TTH): stimulates the thyroid gland to secrete thyroxin. (p. 28)

Thyrotropic Hormone Releasing Factor (TRF): released by hypothalamus and stimulates the pituitary gland to secrete thyrotropic hormone. (p. 28)

Trait Anxiety: a general sense of anxiety not specific to a particular stimulus. (p. 192)

Transcendental Meditation (TM): a relaxation technique involving the use of a sanskrit word as the object of focus. (p. 240)

Trophotropic Response: the physiological state achieved when one is relaxed; also called the relaxation response. (p. 243)

Type A Behavior Pattern: a cluster of behaviors associated with the development of coronary heart disease that includes excessive competitiveness, free-floating hostility, and a sense of time urgency and is associated with the development of coronary heart disease. (pp. 51, 185)

Type B Behavior Pattern: behavior pattern that is not excessively competitive, no free-floating hostility and no sense of time urgency. Also develops coronary heart disease. (p. 186)

Type C: a personality type proposed to be associated with the development of cancer. Characterized by denial and suppression of emotions, in particular anger, resentment, and hostility, and pathological niceness. (p. 189)

Type D: a personality type associated with the development of and death from coronary heart disease. Characterized by negative emotion and inhibited self-expression. (p. 189)

U

Uplifts: positive events that make us feel good. (p. 140)

V

Vasopressin (ADH): a hormone secreted by the pituitary gland. (p. 29)

W

Workaholic: immersing oneself excessively in work at the expense of nonwork activities. (p. 395)

Y

Years of Potential Life Lost: the number of years between when a person is expected to live and the age of death; a measure of premature death. (p. 362)

Yoga: a set of Hindu relaxation techniques. (p. 288)

Photo Credits

Index

For a comprehensive list of all the references used in this text, go to **www.mhhe.com/greenberg13e**.

biofeedback, 6, 271, 281–285
    defined, 281
    EMG, 282–283
    how to arrange training, 285
    phases, 282
    physiological effects, 282–283
    psychological effects, 283
    relaxing, 283–284
    thermal, 283
Biofeedback Webzine, 300
blood pressure, 30, 36, 49, 363
BMI (body mass index), 134
body brace, 283
body composition, 310
body language, 156
body mass index (BMI), 134
body scanning, 286–288
body's reaction to stress. *See* stress
    psychophysiology
bonding years, 427
bone marrow transplant, 293
boomerang kids, 299, 421
Booth-Kewley, Stephanie, 45
bracing
    back pain, 58
    defined, 6, 37
    health effects, 7
    muscle spasms, 58
    progressive relaxation, 261–262
    signs of, 262
brain, 25–29
    anatomy, 26, 27
    evolution of, 28
    exercise, and, 314
    meditation, and, 243, 247
    music, and, 294
    neuroplasticity, 247
    RAS, 27
    stress, and, 29
brainstem, 26
brainstorming, 155
breakups, 90–91
breathing exercises, 286. *See also* diaphragmatic
    breathing
Brosse, Therese, 6, 242
brownout, 417
bruxism, 59
Budzynski, Thomas, 6
bulimia nervosa, 92–93, 134
burnout, 369, 388, 396–397
Burt, John, 191
"but," 157

C

caffeine, 135
calcium, 53, 136
calcium channel blockers, 53
CAM (complementary and alternative
    medicine), 61, 271
campus health centers, 100
Camus, Albert, 292
cancer, 6, 56, 131, 132, 364–365
cancer-prone personality, 46
cancer survivors, 297
candidiasis, 87
Cannon, Walter, 3

carcinogen, 56
cardiac muscle, 53
cardiorespiratory endurance, 310, 317
cardiorespiratory exercise, 325
cardiorespiratory fitness, 317
cardiovascular disease, 132
cardiovascular system, 35–36
cat pose, 289
cavemen, 9
CCPD (cocreator perception deficiency), 191
Center for Spirituality at Work, 231
cerebellum, 26, 27
cerebral cortex, 26, 27
cerebral hemorrhage, 50
cerebral subcortex, 26, 27
challenge, 200
chanting, 138
Chaplin, Charlie, 184
child abuse, 431
chlamydia, 87
cholesterol, 36, 47
ChooseMyPlate.gov, 129
chronic dysregulation, 8
church nurse, 230
closed adoption, 428
clown care unit, 65
cobra pose, 290
cocreator perception deficiency (CCPD), 191
cognitive appraisal, 111, 113
cognitive behavioral therapy, 63, 92, 193, 271
cognitive restructuring, 133, 196–197
cohabitation, 422
cold feet, 35
cold turkey, 337
collaborative religious approach to increasing
    control, 223
college affinity card agreements, 82
college students, 76–99
    acquaintance rape, 87–89
    breakups, 90–91
    career and school, 93–94
    course overload, 78
    Credit CARD Act, 82
    credit cards, 80–81, 82
    eating disorders, 91–93
    emotional arousal interventions,
        100–101
    family and school, 94
    finances, 75, 76
    friendship, 82–83
    grades, 77
    hassles, 140
    HIV/AIDS, 86
    international students, 370
    jealousy, 90
    life-situation interventions, 97–99
    love, 83–84
    minorities, 95
    mixed race students, 368
    older students, 93–94
    perception interventions, 99–100
    physiological arousal interventions, 101
    safety, 96
    self-doubt, 94–95
    service-learning, 226–228
    sex, 84–85
    shyness, 89–90

sources of funding, 79
spirituality, 222
STIs, 86–87
stress-related illness, 45
student load debt, 79, 81
time management, 164
younger students, 76–93
color breathing, 286
Combs, Sean "P. Diddy," 19
comforting sounds, 137–138
commitment, 118–120, 200
common cold, 48
communication, 155–158
community centers, 166
community involvement. *See* "Getting involved in
    your community" boxes
community service, 17, 226, 227
compensation theory, 404
complementary and alternative medicine
    (CAM), 61, 271
*Complete Idiot's Guide to Mindfulness,
    The,* 293
compliments, 179–180
comprehensive stress management, 114–115
computer relaxation, 295
conflict resolution, 152–155
Conflict Resolution Information Source, 167
consciousness meditation, 246
Consortium for Research on Emotional
    Intelligence in Organizations, 158
Consumer Credit Counseling Service, 438
contemplation stage, 341
Contraceptive Technology (Hatcher), 437
contract of commitment, 119
contracting with a significant other, 337
control
    behavior change, 334
    biofeedback, 283
    CCPD, 191
    hardiness, 200
    responsibility, 191
    spirituality, 222–223
    stress management, 117–118
conversion opportunity score, 175
Cooper, Robert, 292
Copernicus, 33
coping, 110–111
Coping in Today's World
    airport noise/flight path, 38
    anger, 19
    brain neuroplasticity, 247
    CAM therapies, 271
    church nurse, 230
    clown care unit, 65
    exercise, 328
    health disparities, 372
    health ministries in African American
        churches, 230
    hostility, 201
    humor, 120
    marriage, 143, 441
    relaxation technique, 299
    satisfaction with life scale, 166
    unethical behavior, 101
    Weight Watchers, 344
    work-related values, 409
coronary bypass surgery, 53

coronary heart disease, 51–53, 131
coronary heart disease-prone personality, 46
corporate scandals, 101
corpse pose, 290
corpus callosum, 26
corticotropin releasing factor (CRF), 28
cortisol, 30, 31, 135
Cosby, Bill, 184
course overload, 78
Cousins, Norman, 184
covenant marriage, 421
crane prose, 290
Credit Card Accountability, Responsibility, and
        Disclosure (CARD) Act, 82
Credit CARD Act, 82
credit cards, 80–81, 82
CRF (corticotropin releasing factor), 28
cues to action, 342
culture clashes, 358–359
cyber-disinhibition, 158

D

daily hassles, 140
daily record of activity, 161
Darwin's theory of evolution, 33
Date.com, 84
date rape, 87–89
decibel ratings, 138
decision/determination stage, 341
decisional forgiveness, 225
decreasing stressful behavior, 333–354
        barriers to action, 334
        control, 334
        health-behavior assessment, 333
        methods. See behavior management
                techniques
        theory. See behavior change theories
deferring religious approach to increasing
        control, 223
definitions (glossary), G–1 to G–5
delegating, 162
demand-control model, 391
Denollet, Johan, 7, 189
dentists, 51
depersonalization, 396
DESC form, 151–152
desensitization procedure, 196–197
detachment years, 427
developmental assets, 199
diabetes, 132, 136
diaphragmatic breathing, 285–286
diary
        diet, 133
        stress, 125–126
        time, 161
diastolic blood pressure, 30, 36, 49
diencephalon, 26, 27
diet. See nutrition
diet diary, 133
diet-related chronic diseases, 132
direct effect theory, 164
disabilities, persons with, 361–362, 371
disease. See illness/disease
"'Disease-Prone Personality,' The" (Friedman/
        Booth-Kewley), 45
distress, 5, 115

diversity and stress, 355–380
        acculturation stressors, 359
        AIDS/HIV, 364
        cancer, 364–365
        culture clashes, 358–359
        disabilities, persons with, 361–362, 371
        diverse populations, 355–356
        elderly persons, 369–371
        family structure, 367–369
        hate crimes, 359, 371
        health, 360–362, 372
        high blood pressure, 363–364
        homelessness, 366–367
        homicide, 365
        infant mortality, 362
        inner cities, 359
        life expectancy, 362
        national health objectives, 360
        positive aspects of minority status, 356–357
        poverty, 365, 366
        racial profiling, 359
        racism, 358
        sexual orientation. See gays, lesbians and
                transgenders
        suicide, 365
        years of potential life lost, 362–363
        See also gender differences; race and ethnicity
DiversityInc, 373
divorce, 422–423, 436–437
dogs, 298
domestic engineer, 405
domestic violence, 432–433
Dopamine, 313
Dossey, Larry, 220
double-blind studies, 224
dual-career family, 425–426
Dunbar, Flanders, 50
duration, 11
Dworkin, Barry, 283
dynamic stretching, 323, 324
dyspnea, 254
dysregulation of systems, 8

E

easy pose, 290
eating disorders, 91–93, 127, 134
Edelman, Marion Wright, 17, 227
education loans, 79
educational level, 365
effleurage, 288
effort-reward imbalance model, 391
80/20 rule, 162
elderly persons
        cohabitation, 422
        earnings potential, 365
        elder care at work, 403
        exercise, 325–327
        functional limitations, 369–371
        poverty, 365, 400
electromyographic (EMG) biofeedback,
        282–283
Ellis, Albert, 197
Emerson, Ralph Waldo, 17, 225
EMG biofeedback, 282–283
emotion-focused coping, 110, 407
emotional arousal, 112, 113

emotional arousal interventions
        college students, 100–101
        family stress, 440
        occupational stress, 407
emotional exhaustion, 396
emotional forgiveness, 225
emotional health, 16
emotional intelligence, 158–159, 160
employment. See occupational stress
endocrine glands, 29
endocrine system, 28, 29–32
endorphins, 313
energy expenditure chart, 312
Engel, George, 6
Enron, 101
entitlement mentality, 386
environmental health, 16
environmental planning, 194–195, 197
environmental stressors, 10
epinephrine, 31, 32
Epstein, Robert, 115
Erikson, Erik, 228
erotic love (eros), 83
esophagus, 36
essential hypertension, 49, 363
esteem needs, 394
ethnic food pyramids, 131
ethnicity, 356. See also race and ethnicity
eustress, 5, 115–116
eustressors, 116
everyday hassles, 140
*Everything You Wanted to Know About Sex but
        Were Afraid to Ask*, 36
exercise and health, 308–332
        ACSM guidelines, 325
        aerobic/anaerobic exercise, 309
        bicycling, 321
        body's release of chemical substances, 313
        cardiorespiratory fitness, 317
        CDC guidelines, 326
        clothing, 318
        cognitive functioning, 314
        competition and enjoyment, 319–320
        cool-down, 318
        elderly persons, 325–327
        equipment, 319
        exercise myths and facts, 332
        fluids, 319
        jogging, 322, 323
        know your body, 319
        PAR-Q, 315
        physical activity pyramid, 328
        physical health, 309–311, 314
        principles of exercise, 316
        psychological health, 311–313
        rope jumping, 320–321
        starting an exercise program, 317–318
        stretching, 322–324
        swimming, 320
        train *vs.* strain, 318
        walking, 321–322
        warm-up, 318
        work-related benefits, 313
        See also physiological arousal interventions
exercise benefit zone (EBZ), 316
exercises/activities. See student exercises/activities
exhaustion phase, 5

homosexuality. *See* gays, lesbians, and transgenders
hostility, 52, 186, 201
hot reactors, 43
household work, 389
househusband, 405
How to Master Stress, 121
HPV, 87
human immunodeficiency virus (HIV), 86, 364
human papillomavirus (HPV), 87
humor, 120, 184–185, 208
humorous videotapes, 44
hurdlers knee raise, 324
hurricanes, 63
hydrochloric acid, 36, 37, 53
hypercholesterolemia, 47
hypertension, 30, 36, 49–50, 132, 363–364
hypoglycemia, 136
hypothalamus, 26–27, 29

I

"I" statements, 157–158
ICS (instant calming sequence), 292
illness/disease
    allergies, 56–57
    backache, 58–59
    cancer, 56
    college students, 45
    coronary heart disease, 51–53
    hot reactors, 43
    hypertension, 49–50
    immunological system, 44–46
    migraine headache, 54–55
    miscarriage, 64
    nutrition, 131, 132
    obesity, 60
    personality type, 185–188, 189
    psychosomatic disease, 43–44
    PTSD, 62–64
    rheumatoid arthritis, 58
    serum cholesterol, 47–48
    sports injuries, 64–65
    stroke, 50–51
    tension headache, 55
    TMJ syndrome, 59–60
    ulcers, 53–54
    U-shaped curve, 14
imagery, 259–261
immunological system, 7, 44–46
impatience/irritability (II), 186
in vivo desensitization, 196
Indian yogis, 6
individualism, 409
infant mortality, 362
inner cities, 359
Insight Meditation (Salzberg/Goldstein), 247
instant calming sequence (ICS), 292
insulin, 136
integrity *vs.* despair, 228–229
intercessory prayer, 221, 223
internal locus of control, 190
international food guide pyramids, 131
international students, 370
interpersonal hostility assessment technique, 200
interracial marriage, 368
interruptions, 163

interventions
    defined, 110
    emotional arousal. *See* emotional arousal interventions
    life events. *See* life-situation interventions
    perception. *See* perception interventions
    physiological arousal. *See* physiological arousal interventions
intimate partner violence, 432–433
iPod, 137
irrational beliefs, 197, 198
irritable bowel syndrome, 37
isometric squeeze exercises, 266

J

Jacobian relaxation, 262. *See also* progressive relaxation
Jacobson, Edmund, 6, 262
Jaffe, Hirschel, 328
jealousy, 90, 99
job satisfaction, 393–394
job sharing, 401
job stress. *See* occupational stress
job stress management programs, 400
Job Stress Network, 39, 410
jogging, 322, 323
jumping rope, 320–321
junk mail, 163

K

Kabat-Zinn, Jon, 220, 293
Karasek, Robert, 387
Kennedy, Edward, 419
Kiddie QR, 291
KidsHealth, 428
Kiecolt-Glaser, J. K., 7
killer T cells, 45, 46
kneading, 288
koans, 241

L

lab assessments
    active listening, 174–175
    assertiveness, 169–170
    autogenic training, 277
    behavior change, 347–351
    behavior change theory, 352–353
    bias, 378
    budgeting while in school, 105
    burnout/brownout, 417
    causing others stress, 305
    conflict resolution, 171
    diverse groups and individuals, 379–380
    emotional intelligence, 176–177
    eustress, 123
    exercise myths and facts, 332
    forgiveness, 237
    friendships, 106
    hassles, 148
    health indices, 73
    healthy behaviors, 347–348
    imagery, 278
    irrational beliefs, 217–218
    life-change-unit (LCU) score, 146, 147
    life events, 147

lifestyle behaviors, 349
locus of control, 212
lover, 107
marriage, 443
mate, 444
meditation, 251
occupational stress, 415
pet therapy, 306
physical self-esteem, 211
physiological reactions to stress, 42
prejudice, 377
progressive relaxation, 279
PTSD, 71
resting metabolic rate (RMR), 145
roadblocks to exercise, 331
roadblocks to healthy behaviors, 350
self-esteem, 210
sense of humor, 207–208
social physique anxiety, 216
social support, 172–173
spirituality, 235–236
stress and illness, 72
stress psychophysiology, 41
stressful events, 146
stressors, 23, 24
test anxiety, 214–215
trait anxiety, 213
Type A personality, 209
workaholic, 416
lack of personal accomplishment, 396
large intestine, 36
Latinos, 357. *See also* Race and ethnicity
laughter, 184, 185, 202
Lazarus, Richard, 110
Lazarus' model of appraisal, 111
LDL (low-density lipoprotein), 47
Learning Meditation (website), 248
leg reclining lunge, 290
leg swing, 324
lesbians. *See* gays, lesbians, and transgenders
LeShan, Lawrence, 6, 56
lie detector test, 38
life-change units (LCU), 138, 146, 147
life events, 138–140
life-events scale, 138, 146, 147
life-events theory, 8
life expectancy, 362
life-situation interventions, 125–178
    assertiveness, 149–152
    college students, 97–99
    communication, 155–158
    conflict resolution, 152–155
    eliminating unnecessary stressors, 125–127
    emotional intelligence, 158–159, 160
    family stress, 435–437
    hassles, 140
    interpersonal matters, 149–178
    intrapersonal matters, 125–148
    life events, 138–140
    noise, 137–138
    nutrition. *See* nutrition
    occupational stress, 406
    social support networking, 163–166
    success analysis, 140–142
    technostress, 159–160
    time management, 160–163
lifestyle behaviors, 333, 349

social support theory, 223–224
volunteerism, 225–226, 227
Spirituality in Higher Education (website), 231
sports injuries, 64–65
Stafford loans, 79
stage of exhaustion, 5
stage of resistance, 5
stages of change theory, 341–342
state anxiety, 192
static stretching, 323
stationary bicycle, 321
Steinmetz, Jenny, 266
STIs (sexually transmitted infections),
    85–87
stop to smell the roses, 181
storgic love (storge), 83
strain, 11
stress
    body's reaction. See stress psychophysiology
    brain damage, 29
    causes, 10
    defined, 5, 12–13
    demand, 110–111
    effects of, 10
    model of, 111–113
    performance, and, 115
Stress and Communication, 167
Stress and Infertility, 441
stress appraisal, 110, 111
stress buffering theory, 164
Stress Cure, 121, 345
stress diary, 125–126
Stress Education Center, 20, 271
Stress in College: Common Causes of Stress in
    College, 102
Stress Less, 143
stress management
    blood pressure, 50
    comprehensive, 114–115
    confidence, 190
    eliminate unnecessary stressors, 125–127
    goals, 14
    historical overview, 3–7
    interventions. See interventions
    pet therapy, 296–299
    wise vs. smart, 125
Stress Management and Relaxation Central
    (website), 300
Stress Management Associates, 271
Stress Management for Patient and Physician, 66
stress management goals, 14
Stress Management Information, 202
stress management seminar, 408
Stress Management Tip.com: Family Stress
    Management, 441
stress management workshops, 228
stress model, 112–113
Stress of Life, The (Selye), 4
stress phrases, 35
stress portfolio
    autogenic training, 277
    focusing on the positive, 180
    managing anxiety formula, 198–199
    meditation, 251
    progressive relaxation, 279
    satisfaction with life scale, 166
    setting goals, 161

sexual behavior, 84–87
    stress diary, 125–126
stress products, 10
stress profile vs. healthy profile, 13
stress psychophysiology, 25–42
    autonomic nervous system, 33–34
    brain, 25–29
    cardiovascular system, 35–36
    endocrine system, 29–32
    GI system, 36–37
    muscles, 37
    skin, 38
stress reactivity, 11, 12, 112, 120
stress reactivity pathways, 28
stress-related hormones, 32
stress-related illness. See illness/disease
stress-related national health objectives, 227–228
stress theory
    hardiness theory, 8
    life-events theory, 8
    social support theory, 8
Stresscure.org, 345
stressors
    defined, 3, 9
    domestic engineering, 405–406
    eliminate, 125–127
    family, 425–424, 435
    minorities, and, 358–360
    modern-day, 299
    occupational, 384, 391–395
    questions to ask, 126–127
    types, 10
stretching, 322–324
stretching neck muscles, 265
striving to get ahead, 409
Stroebel, Charles, 291
stroke, 50–51
student exercises/activities
    community involvement. See "Getting
        involved in your community" boxes
        control, 118
    daily record of activity, 161
    forgiveness, 226
    portfolio. See stress portfolio
    stress reactivity, 12
    success chart, 141
    target heart rate range, 316
    workbook. See your personal stress profile and
        activity workbook
    See also lab assessments
student load debt, 79, 81
students. See college students
Study Guides and Strategies: Time
    Management, 167
subcortex, 26, 27
subsidized Stafford loans, 79
Success: You Can Make It Happen (Swell), 140
success analysis, 140–142
success chart, 141
sugar, 136
suicide, 365
sulcus, 26
suppressor T cells, 45, 46
Swedish massage, 288
swimming, 320
symbolic stressors, 10
sympathetic nervous system, 33, 34

sympathomimetics, 135
synovial membrane, 58
syphilis, 87
systematic desensitization, 63, 195–196, 197
systolic blood pressure, 30, 36, 49

T

T cells, 45, 46
T-lymphocytes, 56
T tubules, 53
tai chi, 295–296
taiji, 295
taijiquan, 295
tailoring, 335–336
Take Five: Relaxation at Your Fingertips, 295
taking charge, 127
talk therapy, 63
target heart rate change, 316
task-oriented coping, 110
Taylor, Shelly, 7, 11
tea, 135
techno-cocoons, 158
technostress, 159–160
telephone operators, 299
temporal lobe, 27
temporomandibular joint, 59
temporomandibular (TMJ) syndrome, 59–60
tend-and-befriend, 11, 32
tension headache, 55
terminology (glossary), G–1 to G–5
test anxiety, 192
testis, 29
thalamus, 26, 27
The Wellness Community, 373
theobromine, 135
theophylline, 135
thermal biofeedback, 283
Third Wave, The (Toffler), E–1
thoracic breathing, 285
thought management, 115
thought stopping, 195, 197
three Cs, 200
thymus, 29
thyroid gland, 29, 31
thyrotropic hormone (TTH), 28
thyrotropic hormone releasing factor (TRF), 28
thyroxin, 28, 32
TIA. See transient ischemic attack (TIA)
Tibetan Buddhists, 240
tightening calf muscles, 265
tightening facial muscles, 265
time diary, 161
time management, 160–163
    assessing how you spend time, 161
    college students, 164
    delegating, 162
    evaluating tasks once, 163
    interruptions, 163
    investing time, 163
    junk mail, 163
    maximizing your rewards, 162
    meditation, 246–247
    prioritizing, 162
    saying "no," 162
    scheduling, 162
    setting goals, 161